voices of
THE WOMEN'S HEALTH MOVEMENT

VOLUME ONE

BARBARA SEAMAN

with LAURA ELDRIDGE

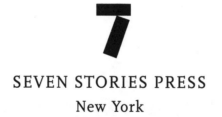

SEVEN STORIES PRESS
New York

Seven Stories Press
140 Watts Street
New York, NY 10013
www.sevenstories.com

College professors may order examination copies of Seven Stories Press titles for a free six-month trial period. To order, visit http://www.sevenstories.com/textbook or send a fax on school letterhead to (212) 226-1411.

Book design by Jon Gilbert

Library of Congress Cataloging-in-Publication Data

Voices of the women's health movement / edited by Barbara Seaman ; with Laura Eldridge.
    p. cm.
  Includes bibliographical references and index.
  ISBN 978-1-60980-444-2 (v. 1) -- ISBN 978-1-60980-446-6 (v. 2)
  1. Women--Health and hygiene. 2. Women--Health and hygiene--History. I. Seaman, Barbara. II. Eldridge, Laura.
  [DNLM: 1. Women's Health--United States--Collected Works. 2. Feminism--United States--Collected Works. 3. Feminism--history--United States--Collected Works. 4. History, 19th Century--United States--Collected Works. 5. History, 20th Century--United States--Collected Works. 6. Women's Health--history--United States--Collected Works. 7. Women's Rights--United States--Collected Works. 8. Women's Rights--history--United States--Collected Works. WA 309]
  RA564.85.V65 2012
  362.1082--dc22
                        2010016341

Printed in the United States of America

9 8 7 6 5 4 3 2 1

voices of

THE WOMEN'S
HEALTH
MOVEMENT

VOLUME ONE

Contents

CHAPTER 2: TAKING OUR BODIES BACK:
THE WOMEN'S HEALTH MOVEMENT

CHAPTER 3: BIRTH CONTROL

CHAPTER 4: MENSTRUATION

CHAPTER 5: PREGNANCY AND BIRTHING

CHAPTER 6: MOTHERHOOD

CHAPTER 7: MENOPAUSE AND AGING

CHAPTER 8: GYNECOLOGICAL SURGERY

CHAPTER 9: ABORTION

CHAPTER 10: LESBIAN, BISEXUAL, AND TRANSGENDER HEALTH

CHAPTER 11: GENDER AND MEDICINE

To My Daughter, Elana Felicia
—Barbara

To My Grandmothers, Grace, Ellen, and Ray
—Laura

Acknowledgments

FIRST AND FOREMOST, thanks to our agent, Valerie Borchardt, who is generous and patient with her time and good advice, and also to Anne and Georges Borchardt.

Many thanks to our editor, Theresa Noll, whose talent and calm never cease to amaze us—this book bears evidence of her vision and hard work in every section. Our gratitude goes also to Amy Scholder, who helped us to imagine what the book might look like and saw our plans realized. Our deepest admiration and thanks to Dan Simon, who we have been fortunate to know and work with for many years.

Barbara thanks her co-founders of the National Women's Health Network: Alice Wolfson, Belita Cowan, Phylis Chesler, PhD, and Mary Howell, MD. Also to Cindy Pearson, Olivia Cousins, PhD, and Amy Allina who carried on our goals. We are grateful to Phil Corfman, MD, and Richard Crout, MD (who stood up for informed consent in women's health care), Judy Norsigian (OBOS), Pat Cody and Sybil Shainwald (on behalf of DES families), Maryann Napoli (Center for Medical Consumers), Susan Wood, PhD (formerly of the FDA), and Nancy Krieger, PhD.

We are grateful also to Andrea Tone, Leonore Tiefer, Shere Hite, Gloria Steinem, Congresswoman Carolyn Maloney, Minna Elias, Sheryl Burt Ruzek, Barbara Brenner, Barbara Ehrenreich, Alice Yaker, Suzanne Parisian, MD, Byllye Avery, Susan Love, MD, David Michaels, PhD, Devra Lee Davis, PhD, Carolyn Westhoff, MD, Elizabeth Siegel Watkins, PhD, Pat Cody, Gordon Guyatt, MD, Bruce Stadel, Diane Meier, MD, Ben Loehnen, Jennifer Baumgardner, Nikki Scheuer, Sheila and Donald Bandman, Judge Emily Jane Goodman, Daniel Simon, Thomas Hartman, E. Neil Schachter, Debra Chase, Tara Parker Pope, Senator Ron Wyden, Nora Coffey, Warren Bell, MD, Alan Cassels, Wendy Armstrong, Colleen Fuller, Anne Rochon-Ford, Leora Tanenbaum, Abby Lippman, PhD, Harriet Rosenberg, PhD, Amy Richards, Pam Martens, Ariel Olive, Ann Fuller, Barbara Mintzes, Aubrey Blumsohn, MD, Frances C. Whittelsey, K-K Seaman, Ronnie Eldridge, Mavra Stark, Joan Michel, and Linda K. Nathan.

To our top-notch assistants: Sara Germain was relentless in helping us contact authors and choose selections. Megan Buckley, Helen Lowery, Reed Eldridge, and Seven Stories' Daniella Gitlin were all helpful at crucial moments. Thanks to Kim Chung, who against all odds kept our computers running, and Maria Tylutki, who made sure everything else around the office was organized and as efficient as possible. And as always we are grateful to Agata Rumprecht-Behrens, who knows where things are better than either of us and who helps with whatever project we are working on despite her own busy schedule.

ADDITIONAL ACKNOWLEDGMENTS FROM BARBARA:
My deepest gratitude to Dr. Susan Love, Dr. Neil Schachter, Deborah Chase, and Dr. Diane Meier.

I am grateful to Ruth Gruber, my stepmother; my sisters, Elaine Rosner Jeria and Jeri Drucker, and Jeri's husband Ernest Drucker, PhD; my children, Noah, Shira, and Elana; my sons-in-law, Urs Bamert and Timothy Walsh; my cousins, Amelia Rosner and Richard Hyfler; and Jesse Drucker, Nell Casey, and Henry Jeria.

All my love to my grandchildren, Sophia Bamert, Idalia Bamert, Liam Walsh, and Ezekiel Walsh.

ADDITIONAL ACKNOWLEDGMENTS FROM LAURA:
I would like to thank Irene Xanthoudakis, Rebecca Kraut, Lauren Porsch, Molly Barry, Rachel Fisher, Rumela Mitra, Helen Lowery, April Timko, Nicole Richman, Stephanie Kirk, Chi-Hyun Kim, Susan Masry, Rob Tennant, Rabbi Sari Laufer, Leonore Tiefer, Danie Greenwell, Alisa Kraut, Brian Cooke, Chris Rugen, Kim Jordan, Jenny Tomczak, Caroline Cruz, Amy Troy, Melissa Barrett, Jennifer Smith-Garvin, Karla Wiehagen, Anne Taylor, Kate Jefferson, Chad and Sonya Cooper, Miriam Silberstein, and Katie Walker.

Much, much love goes to my brothers, David, Reed, and Peter, my dearest friends, and to my grandfather Paul Eldridge, Sr.

My gratitude to the Seaman family, who have supported me through the years, and given me the chance to love and grieve my dear friend properly. They are like a second family and I am blessed to have them in my life.

Many thanks to Sheldon, Beth, Marnie, Zachary, and Josh Weinberg, and to the entire Weinberg/Josell/Alperin family.

My parents Paul and Susan Eldridge are my best examples of how to lead meaningful, ethical lives. They have given me big shoes to fill and helped me as best they could to be up to the task. My son, Levi Jacob, has blessed and challenged me in countless ways. Jeremy Weinberg has been an unending source of love, patience, and support. His kindness, intelligence, and humor are the great pleasures of my life, and I am truly fortunate to have him as my partner in everything I undertake.

Introduction

WHEN ELIZABETH CADY STANTON decided to re-set her son's collarbone in the mid-nineteenth century she wasn't trying to be radical, she was trying to be a good mother. She wasn't trying to empower female healing and reject the mostly male medical establishment. She was trying to respond to the unalleviated pain of a cherished love one.

In addition to her tireless writing and activism, Stanton was a mother of five children. Never daunted, Stanton moved her writing desk into the nursery and worked in between spending time with her brood. When her eldest son Daniel was born with a dislocated collarbone, the Stantons tried to get him the best medical care. Repeated doctors' visits resulted in bandaging and treatments that actually made the problem worse. When a nurse helping Daniel refused to respond to the fact that his hand was turning blue from the bandages, saying, "I shall never interfere with the doctor," Stanton sprang into action. She replaced the doctor only to be disappointed a second time. She wasn't about to be fooled a third time, and, to the nurse's shock, took off her son's bandages and with arnica (a homeopathic remedy) and gentle pressure re-dressed her son's bones. She concluded, "I learned another lesson in self-reliance. I trusted neither men nor books absolutely after this . . . but continued to use my 'mother's instinct,' if 'reason' is too dignified a term to apply to a woman's thoughts."

Her decisiveness goes to the heart of women's health activism. It is almost always born of personal experience, often a social injustice acted out on the body. It is inherently and un-self-consciously radical. Throughout human history—and more recently the nineteenth and twentieth centuries, we have witnessed brilliant and courageous examples of women taking control of their bodies and health choices. These experiences have often led to a greater sense of autonomy and equality. In many ways, it is an original rebellion.

In these days as we debate the basic right of human beings to have medical care, it is an often-made point that one of the simplest ways to control a citizenry is through access to health services. Women have known this for a long time, and the process of coming to understand and reject this system of control often helps them to see themselves as independent agents in a larger sense.

In the nineteenth century, medical services were consolidated by doctors taken with new and changing medical technologies. As physicians and scientists pioneered surgeries, pharmaceuticals, and new mental health practices, they pushed out traditional (often female) providers, including midwives and makers of alternative medicines. Because these doctors were almost entirely male, they treated distinctively female body parts and health issues as disease. Male bodies were healthy and female ones were pathological. Nineteenth- and early twentieth-century ideas of the hysterical woman appall our twenty-first century sensibilities, but they haven't entirely gone away. The way that menopause has been treated as a disease state is evidence that while there is now a different language used to misinterpret and medicate women's bodies, the tendency persists.

When Elizabeth Cady Stanton and the other first-wave feminists abandoned the recommendations of physicians, they were creating a model of resistance that lived on in small pockets of activism throughout the twentieth century and then was taken up again in major ways in the 1970s. I was lucky enough to be a part of that movement.

When we talk about the "women's health movement," we are, of course, talking about many movements. We can look to the work of women who writer Susan Brownmiller has termed our "heroic antecedents," daring women in past centuries who stood up against a culture that discouraged open speech about health problems, or who provided alternative care when none was available. We can speak specifically about the second-wave women's movement in the 1970s and look at the foundational writings that have changed the landscape of women's health. And we can listen to the voices of young activists who help us to understand the new issues we face today.

So many of my friends recall sitting in rooms where secrets were shared among women. Typically any shameful feelings we may have had lifted as we learned that our private experiences often turned out to be universal.

I remember the voices: "Yes, I had an illegal abortion." "Yes, I was raped." "Yes, my neighbor (brother, father, uncle, priest, doctor, therapist, teacher) hassled me sexually." "Yes, I faked orgasms." "Yes, every birth control method I've ever used was a disaster." "Yes, my gynecologist makes me feel uncomfortable, but I can't admit it, he's so esteemed. His pelvic exams are so rough it hurts." "Yes, I took a drug that made me very sick, but my doctor told me to keep taking it."

Women talked, listened, and spread the word. We went back to our communities, started our own women's groups, consciousness-raising groups, and know-your-body courses. By 1975, there were nearly 2,000 official women's self-help projects scattered around the United States and countless unofficial ones.

Do women talk less to each other now than they did then? The very possibility is troubling.

If I have a single hope for this book it is that the women who read it be inspired to talk among themselves about health, since women who talk to each other about health will go on to talk to each other about anything and everything.

At the turn of the millennium, a Barnard College senior asked Judy Norsigian of *Our Bodies, Ourselves* what she hopes to see when the continuously updated volume celebrates its fiftieth anniversary in the year 2020. Norsigian answered, "The creation of a health and a medical care system that is far more responsive to women's needs and accessible to all women regardless of age, income, sexual preference, race, etc. . . . And using technology in the most appropriate way—that is science-based, not profit-based . . ." People need to be in control of their own health. But in order for that to be possible, they must have information from a trustworthy source.

I asked Cindy Pearson, executive director of the National Women's Health Network, what she thinks about patients taking their health into their own hands. "Thirty years ago," Pearson said, "if anyone talked about a bad experience they had with the health care system . . . the response would usually be 'You need a better doctor. . . .'" Today, in part through the hard-won battles of consumer advocates, AIDS activists, and the feminist health movement, among others, that isn't the only answer. Pearson continues, "People talked about finding a good doctor but then realized good doctors aren't the answer, informed patients are the answer."

We believe that within the yin and yang of these two thoughtful responses there is to be found the right approach: good science combined with leadership from the patients' points of view. What makes a good doctor these days isn't always easy to say. But if there is one quality we should all be looking for in our doctors, it is the willingness to listen seriously to their patients.

In the Beginning

WHEN I WAS GROWING UP in New York City in the 1940s and '50s, there was no women's movement per se. There was, however, the memory of a women's movement. And all around me were women who had been a part of it—suffragettes who organized and protested for the vote. My future mother-in-law, Sylvia Seaman, was one who marched to win women's basic enfranchisement. My aunt, Gertrude Weil Klein, was a union rabble-rouser from way back who went to jail with Eugene V. Debs. When I was a child she would always marvel at how I thought women voting was normal. She chided that I couldn't possibly appreciate it, and warned me not to forget the past despite the beautiful future I was growing up in. I think we in the now-older generation of feminists tend to get frustrated with young women because they don't (and can't) understand what it "was like." It's important to remember that it is a mark of our success—and not their failure—that they sometimes take freedoms for which we had to fight for granted.

There were women in my aunt's generation who weren't suffragettes or part of an organized women's movement, but who have nonetheless been amazing examples of the scope and diversity possible in female lives. My stepmother Ruth Gruber was one of these women. At the age of twenty she became the youngest person in the world to hold a PhD, and only a few years later the first American reporter of any gender to be allowed to enter the Soviet Arctic. It was women like Ruth—educated and brave, with exciting careers—for whom Betty Friedan was scouring the pages of women's magazines when she got mad enough to write *The Feminine Mystique*. Betty had grown up reading stories about ambitious young women who did great things—often in the city, and often involving a career in journalism. This character disappeared after World War II to be replaced by domestic goddesses and suburban royalty. Images of independent women may have become few and far between, but they weren't gone. And neither was the energy and widespread desire to expand rights and options for women.

Both kinds of women are so important—the generations of movement women, who come together in waves to make change at pivotal moments, and the strong individuals who move against the daunting tide of social injustice and backlash. Although my women's movement wasn't the same as Elizabeth Cady Stanton's, they had things in common. There is continuity between generations of determined folks working for basic equality and dignity for all people. The memory of courageous individuals is part of this; it perpetuates possibility, and it opens up space for the new generation to find the issues that connect them with the past as well as the ones that are distinctly theirs. It also lets them know that achieving change is possible through example.

Witches, Midwives, and Nurses: A History of Women Healers

BARBARA EHRENREICH AND DEIRDRE ENGLISH

Barbara Ehrenreich and Deirdre English, *Witches, Midwives, and Nurses: A History of Women Healers*, New York: Feminist Press, 1973. Reprinted by permission.

Barbara Ehrenreich and Deirdre English's Witches, Midwives, and Nurses: A History of Women Healers, *a 45-page pamphlet published in 1973, revealed some of the thuggish tactics powerful males often used to oust women (and alternative providers) from medical and midwifery practice, as well as the extreme—even lunatic—treatments offered by these more formally trained physicians. Defenders of orthodox medicine dismissed and tried to discredit Barbara and Deirdre's influential work, but a decade later, confirmation emerged in the form of a book that won the 1984 Pulitzer Prize for General Nonfiction,* The Social Transformation of American Medicine: The Rise of a Sovereign Profession and the Making of a Vast Industry *by Princeton University sociologist Paul Starr. Starr confirmed that in the US colonies, "women were expected to deal with illness in the home and to keep a stock of remedies on hand; in the fall they put away medicinal herbs as they stored preserves.*

Care of the sick was part of the domestic economy for which the wife assumed responsibility . . . in worrisome cases perhaps bringing in an older woman who had a reputation for skill with the sick." Many guides to domestic medicine were available: "They argued that medicine was filled with unnecessary obscurity and complexity, and should be made intelligible and practicable."

In contrast to home remedies, Starr recapitulates the teachings of Dr. Benjamin Rush, the revolutionary leader, who "greatly influenced future generations of physicians at the University of Pennsylvania." Rush maintained that there was but one disease, "morbid excitement induced by capillary tension," and its one remedy was "to deplete the body by letting blood with the lancet and emptying out the stomach and bowels with the use of powerful emetics and cathartics. Patients could be bled until unconscious and given heavy doses of the cathartic calomel (mercurous chloride) until they salivated."

"Heroic" therapy of this type "dominated American medical practice in the first decades of the 19th century," Starr reminds us, which helps explain why, by the 1830s, many states revoked the rights to licensure they had first granted to orthodox doctors around the time of the revolution.

INTRODUCTION

Women have always been healers. They were the unlicensed doctors and anatomists of Western history. They were abortionists, nurses, and counselors. They were pharmacists, cultivating healing herbs and exchanging the secrets of their uses. They were midwives, traveling from home to home and village to village. For centuries women were doctors without degrees, barred from books and lectures, learning from each other, and passing on experience from neighbor to neighbor and mother to daughter. They were called "wise women" by the people, witches or charlatans by the authorities. Medicine is part of our heritage as women, our history, and our birthright.

Today, however, health care is the property of

male professionals. Ninety-three percent of the doctors in the United States are men; and almost all the top directors and administrators of health institutions. Women are still in the overall majority—70 percent of health workers are women—but we have been incorporated as *workers* into an industry where the bosses are men. We are no longer independent practitioners, known by our own names, for our own work. We are, for the most part, institutional fixtures, filling faceless job slots: clerk, dietary aide, technician, and maid.

When we are allowed to participate in the healing process, we can do so only as nurses. And nurses of every rank from aide up are just "ancillary workers" in relation to the doctors (from the Latin *ancilla,* maid servant). From the nurse's aide, whose menial tasks are spelled out with industrial precision, to the "professional" nurse, who translates the doctors' orders into the aide's tasks, nurses share the status of a uniformed maid service to the dominant male professionals.

Our subservience is reinforced by our ignorance, and our ignorance is *enforced.* Nurses are taught not to question, not to challenge. "The doctor knows best." He is the shaman, in touch with the forbidden, mystically complex world of Science, which we have been taught is beyond our grasp. Women health workers are alienated from the scientific substance of their work, restricted to the "womanly" business of nurturing and housekeeping—a passive, silent majority.

We are told that our subservience is biologically ordained: women are inherently nurse-like and not doctor-like. Sometimes we even try to console ourselves with the theory that we were defeated by anatomy before we were defeated by men, that women have been so trapped by the cycles of menstruation and reproduction that they have never been free and creative agents outside their homes. Another myth, fostered by conventional medical histories, is that male professionals won out on the strength of their superior technology.

According to these accounts, (male) science more or less automatically replaced (female) superstition—which from then on was called "old wives' tales."

But history belies these theories. Women have been autonomous healers, often the only healers for women and the poor. And we found, in the periods we have studied, that, if anything, it was the male professionals who clung to untested doctrines and ritualistic practices—and it was the woman healers who represented a more humane, empirical approach to healing.

Our position in the health system today is not "natural." It is a condition which has to be explained. In this pamphlet we have asked: How did we arrive at our present position of subservience from our former position of leadership?

We learned this much: that the suppression of women health workers and the rise to dominance of male professionals was not a "natural" process, resulting automatically from changes in medical science, nor was it the result women's failure to take on healing work. It was an active *takeover* by male professionals. And it was not science that enabled men to win out: The critical battles took place long before the development of modern scientific technology.

The stakes of the struggle were high: Political and economic monopolization of medicine meant control over its institutional organizations, its theory and practice, its profits and prestige. And the stakes are even higher today, when total control of medicine means potential power to determine who will live and will die, who is fertile and who is sterile, who is "mad" and who sane.

The suppression of female healers by the medical establishment was a political struggle, first, in that it is part of the history of sex struggle in general. The status of women healers has risen and fallen with the status of women. When women healers were attacked, they were attacked as *women;* when they fought back, they fought back in solidarity with all women.

It was a political struggle, second, in that it

was part of a *class* struggle. Women healers were people's doctors, and their medicine was part of a people's subculture. To this very day women's medical practice has thrived in the midst of rebellious lower-class movements which have struggled to be free from the established authorities. Male professionals, on the other hand, served the ruling class—both medically and politically. Their interests have been advanced by the universities, the philanthropic foundations, and the law. They owe their victory not so much to their own efforts, but to the intervention of the ruling class they served.

This pamphlet represents a beginning of the research which will have to be done to recapture our history as health workers. It is a fragmentary account, assembled from sources which were usually sketchy and often biased, by women who are in no sense "professional" historians. We confined ourselves to Western history, since the institutions we confront today are the products of Western civilization. We are far from being able to present a complete chronological history. Instead, we looked at two separate, important phases in the male takeover of health care: the suppression of witches in medieval Europe, and the rise of the male medical profession in nineteenth-century America.

To know our history is to begin to see how to take up the struggle again.

WITCHCRAFT AND MEDICINE IN THE MIDDLE AGES

Witches lived and were burned long before the development of modern medical technology. The great majority of them were healers serving the peasant population, and their suppression marks one of the opening struggles in the history of man's suppression of women as healers.

The other side of the suppression of witches as healers was the creation of a new male medical profession, under the protection and patronage of the ruling classes. This new European medical profession played an important role in the witch-hunts, supporting the witches' prosecutors with "medical" reasoning:

> Because the Medieval Church, with the support of kings, princes and secular authorities, controlled medical education and practice, the inquisition [witch-hunts] constitutes, among other things, an early instance of the "professional" repudiating the skills and interfering with the rights of the "nonprofessional" to minister to the poor.[1]

The witch-hunts left a lasting effect: An aspect of the female has ever since been associated with the witch, and an aura of contamination has remained—especially around the midwife and other women healers. This early and devastating exclusion of women from independent healing roles was a violent precedent and warning: It was to become a theme of our history. The women's health movement of today has ancient roots in the medieval covens, and its opponents have as their ancestors those who ruthlessly forced the elimination of witches.

THE WITCH CRAZE The age of witch-hunting spanned more than four centuries (from the fourteenth to the seventeenth century) in its sweep from Germany to England. It was born in feudalism and lasted—gaining in virulence—well into the "age of reason." The witch craze took different forms at different times and places, but never lost its essential character: that of a ruling-class campaign of terror directed against the female peasant population. Witches represented a political, religious, and sexual threat to the Protestant and Catholic churches alike, as well as to the state.

The extent of the witch craze is startling: In the late fifteenth and early sixteenth centuries there were thousands upon thousands of executions—usually live burnings at the stake—in Germany, Italy, and other countries. In the mid-sixteenth century the terror spread to France, and finally to England. One writer has estimated the number of executions at an average of 600 a year for certain German cities—or two a day, "leaving out Sundays."

Nine hundred witches were destroyed in a single year in the Wertzberg area, and 1,000 in and around Como. At Toulouse, 400 were put to death in a day. In the Bishopric of Trier, in 1585, two villages were left with only one female inhabitant each. Many writers have estimated the total number killed to have been in the millions. Women made up some 85 percent of those executed—old women, young women, and children.*

Their scope alone suggests that the witch-hunts represent a deep-seated social phenomenon which goes far beyond the history of medicine. In locale and timing, the most virulent witch-hunts were associated with periods of great social upheaval shaking feudalism at its roots—mass peasant up-risings and conspiracies, the beginnings of capitalism, the rise of Protestantism. There is fragmentary evidence—which feminists ought to follow up—suggesting that in some areas witchcraft represented a female-led peasant rebellion. Here we can't attempt to explore the historical context of the witch-hunts in any depth. But we do have to get beyond some common myths about the witch craze—myths which rob the "witch" of any dignity and put blame on her and the peasants she served.

Unfortunately, the witch herself—poor and illiterate—did not leave us her story. It was recorded, like all history, by the educated elite, so today we know the witch only through the eyes of her persecutors.

Two of the most common theories of the witch-hunts are basically *medical* interpretations, attributing the witch craze to unexplainable outbreaks of mass hysteria. One version has it that the peasantry went mad. According to this, the witch craze was an epidemic of mass hatred and panic cast in images of a blood-lusty peasant bearing flaming torches. Another psychiatric interpretation holds that the witches themselves were insane. . . .

But, in fact, the witch craze was neither a lynching party nor a mass suicide by hysterical women. Rather, it followed well-ordered, legalistic procedures. The witch-hunts were well-organized campaigns, initiated, financed, and executed by church and state. To Catholic and Protestant witch-hunters alike, the unquestioned authority on how to conduct a witch-hunt was the *Malleus Maleficarum* or *Hammer of Witches*, written in 1487 by the Reverends Kramer and Sprenger (the "beloved sons" of Pope Innocent VIII). For three centuries this sadistic book lay on the bench of every judge, every witch-hunter. In a long section on judicial proceedings, the instructions make it clear how the "hysteria" was set off:

> The job of initiating a witch trial was to be performed by either the vicar (priest) or judge of the county. . . . Anyone failing to report a witch faced both excommunication and a long list of temporal punishments. . . .

Kramer and Sprenger gave detailed instructions about the use of tortures to force confessions and further accusations. Commonly, the accused was stripped naked and shaved of all her body hair, then subjected to thumbscrews and the rack, spikes and bone-crushing "boots," starvation and beatings. The point is obvious: The witch craze did not arise spontaneously in the peasantry. It was a calculated ruling-class campaign of terrorization.

THE CRIMES OF THE WITCHES Who were the witches, then, and what were their "crimes" that could arouse such vicious upper-class suppression? . . . Three central accusations emerge repeatedly in the history of witchcraft throughout northern Europe: First, witches are accused of every conceivable sexual crime against men. Quite simply, they are "accused" of female sexuality. Second, they are

---

*We are omitting from this discussion any mention of the New England witch trials in the 1600s. These trials occurred on a relatively small scale, very late in the history of witch-hunts, and in an entirely different social context than the earlier European witch craze.

accused of being organized. Third, they are accused of having magical powers affecting health—of harming, but also of healing. They were often charged specifically with possessing medical and obstetrical skills.

First, consider the charge of sexual crimes. The medieval Catholic church elevated sexism to a point of principle: the *Malleus* declares, "When a woman thinks alone, she thinks evil." The misogyny of the church, if not proved by the witch craze itself, is demonstrated by its teaching that in intercourse the male deposits in the female a homunculus, or "little person," complete with soul, which is simply housed in the womb for nine months, without acquiring any attributes of the mother. The homunculus is not really safe, however, until it reaches male hands again, when a priest baptizes it, ensuring the salvation of its immortal soul. Another depressing fantasy of some medieval religious thinkers was that upon resurrection all human beings would be reborn as men!

The church associated women with sex, and all pleasure in sex was condemned, because it could only come from the devil. Witches were supposed to have gotten pleasure from copulation with the devil (despite the icy-cold organ he was reputed to possess) and they in turn infected men. Lust in either man or wife, then, was blamed on the female. On the other hand, witches were accused of making men impotent and of causing their penises to disappear. As for female sexuality, witches were accused, in effect, of giving contraceptive aid and of performing abortions:

> Now there are, as it is said in the Papal Bull, seven methods by which they infect with witchcraft the venereal act and the conception of the womb: First, by inclining the minds of men to inordinate passion; second, by obstructing their generative force; third, by removing the members accommodated to that act; fourth, by changing men into beasts by their magic act; fifth, by destroying the generative in women; sixth, by procuring abortion; seventh, by offering children to the devils, besides other animals and fruits of the earth with which they work much harm. . . .[2]

In the eyes of the church, all the witch's power was ultimately derived from her sexuality. Her career began with sexual intercourse with the devil. Each witch was confirmed at a general meeting (the witches' sabbath) at which the devil presided, often in the form of a goat, and had intercourse with the neophytes. In return for her powers, the witch promised to serve him faithfully. (In the imagination of the church even evil could only be thought of as ultimately male-directed!) As the *Malleus* makes clear, the devil almost always acts through the female, just as he did in Eden:

> All witchcraft comes from carnal lust, which in women is insatiable. . . . Wherefore for the sake of fulfilling their lusts they consort with devils . . . it is sufficiently clear that it is no matter for wonder that there are more women than men found infected with the heresy of witchcraft. . . . And blessed be the Highest Who has so far preserved the male sex from so great a crime. . . .

Not only were the witches women, they were women who seemed to be organized into an enormous secret society. A witch who was a proved member of the "devil's party" was more dreadful than one who had acted alone, and the witch-hunting literature is obsessed with the question of what went on at the witches' "sabbaths." (Eating of unbaptised babies? Bestialism and mass orgies? So went their lurid speculations. . . .)

In fact, there is evidence that women accused of being witches did meet locally in small groups and that these groups came together in crowds of hundreds or thousands on festival days. Some writers speculate that the meetings were occasions for trading herbal lore and passing on the news. We have little evidence about the political significance of the witches' organizations, but it's hard to imagine that they weren't connected to the peasant rebellions of the time. Any peasant organization, just being an organization, would attract dissidents, increase communication between villages, and build a spirit of collectivity and autonomy among the peasants.

WITCHES AS HEALERS We come now to the most fantastic accusation of all. The witch is accused not only of murdering and poisoning, sex crimes and conspiracy, but of *helping and healing. . . .*

Witch-healers were often the only general medical practitioners for a people who had no doctors and no hospitals and who were bitterly afflicted with poverty and disease. In particular, the association of the witch and the midwife was strong: "No one does more harm to the Catholic church than midwives," wrote witch-hunters Kramer and Sprenger. . . .

When faced with the misery of the poor, the church turned to the dogma that experience in this world is fleeting and unimportant. But there was a double standard at work, for the church was not against medical care for the upper class. Kings and nobles had their court physicians, who were men, sometimes even priests. The real issue was control: Male upper-class healing under the auspices of the church was acceptable; female healing as part of a peasant subculture was not.

The church saw its attack on peasant healers as an attack on *magic,* not medicine. The devil was believed to have real power on earth, and the use of that power by peasant women—whether for good or evil—was frightening to the church and state. The greater their satanic powers to help themselves, the less they were dependent on God and the church and the more they were potentially able to use their powers against God's order. Magic charms were thought to be at least as effective as prayer in healing the sick, but prayer was church-sanctioned and controlled while incantations and charms were not. Thus magic cures, even when successful, were an accused interference with the will of God, achieved

with the help of the devil, and the cure itself was evil. There was no problem in distinguishing God's cures from the devil's, for obviously the Lord would work through priests and doctors rather than through peasant women.

The wise woman, or witch, had a host of remedies which had been tested in years of use. Many of the herbal remedies developed by witches still have their place in modern pharmacology. They had painkillers, digestive aids, and anti-inflammatory agents. They used ergot for the pain of labor at a time when the church held that pain in labor was the Lord's just punishment for Eve's original sin. Ergot derivatives are the principal drugs used today to hasten labor and aid in the recovery from childbirth. Belladonna—still used today as an antispasmodic—was used by the witch-healers to inhibit uterine contractions when miscarriage threatened. Digitalis, still an important drug in treating heart ailments, is said to have been discovered by an English witch. . . .

The witch-healer's methods were as great a threat (to the Catholic Church, if not Protestant) as her results, for the witch was an empiricist: She relied on her senses rather than on faith or doctrine, she believed in trial and error, cause and effect. Her attitude was not religiously passive, but actively inquiring. She trusted her ability to find ways to deal with disease, pregnancy, and childbirth—whether through medications or charms. In short, her magic was the science of her time.

The church, by contrast was deeply anti-empirical. It discredited the value of the material world and had a profound distrust of the senses. There was no point in looking for natural laws that govern physical phenomena, for the world is created anew by God in every instant. Kramer and Sprenger, in the *Malleus,* quote St. Augustine on the deceptiveness of the senses:

> Now the motive of the will is something perceived through the senses or the intellect, both of which are subject to the power of the devil. . . .

The senses are the devil's playground, the arena into which he will try to lure men away from Faith and into the conceits of the intellect or the delusions of carnality.

In the persecution of the witch, the anti-empiricist and misogynist antisexual obsessions of the church coincide: Empiricism and sexuality both represent a surrender to the senses, a betrayal of faith. The witch was a triple threat to the church: She was a woman, and not ashamed of it. She appeared to be part of an organized underground of peasant women. And she was a healer whose practice was based in empirical study. In the face of the repressive fatalism of Christianity, she held out the hope of change in this world.

THE RISE OF THE EUROPEAN MEDICAL PROFESSION
While witches practiced among the people, the ruling classes were cultivating their own breed of secular healers: the university-trained physicians. In the century that preceded the beginning of the "witch craze"—the thirteenth century—European medicine became firmly established as a secular science and a *profession*. The medical profession was actively engaged in the elimination of female healers—their exclusion from the universities, for example—long before the witch-hunts began.

For eight long centuries, from the fifth to the thirteenth, the otherworldly, antimedical stance of the church had stood in the way of the development of medicine as a respectable profession. Then, in the thirteenth century, there was a revival of learning, touched off by contact with the Arab world. Medical schools appeared in the universities, and more and more young men of means sought medical training. The church imposed strict controls on the new profession, and allowed it to develop only within the terms set by Catholic doctrine. University-trained physicians were not permitted to practice without calling in a priest to aid and advise them, or to treat a patient who refused confession. By the fourteenth century their practice was in demand among the wealthy,

as long as they continued to take pains to show that their attentions to the body did not jeopardize the soul. In fact, accounts of their medical training make it seem more likely that they jeopardized the *body*.

There was nothing in late medieval medical training that conflicted with church doctrine, and little that we would recognize as "science." Medical students, like other scholarly gentlemen, spent years studying Plato, Aristotle, and Christian theology. Their medical theory was largely restricted to the works of Galen, the ancient Roman physician who stressed the theory of "complexions" or "temperaments" of men, "wherefore the choleric are wrathful, the sanguine are kindly, the melancholy are envious," and so on. While a student, a doctor rarely saw any patients at all, and no experimentation of any kind was taught. Medicine was sharply differentiated from surgery, which was almost everywhere considered a degrading, menial craft, and the dissection of bodies was almost unheard of.

Confronted with a sick person, the university-trained physician had little to go on but superstition. Bleeding was a common practice, especially in the case of wounds. Leeches were applied according to the time, the hour, the air, and other similar considerations. Medical theories were often grounded more in "logic" than in observation: "Some foods brought on good humors, and others, evil humors. For example, nasturtium, mustard, and garlic produced reddish bile; lentils, cabbage, and the meat of old goats and beeves begot black bile." Incantations, and quasi-religious rituals were thought to be effective: The physician to Edward II, who held a bachelor's degree in theology and a doctorate in medicine from Oxford, prescribed for toothache writing on the jaws of the patient, "In the name of the Father, the Son, and the Holy Ghost, Amen," or touching a needle to a caterpillar and then to the tooth. . . .

Such was the state of medical "science" at the time when witch-healers were persecuted for being practitioners of "magic." It was witches who developed an extensive understanding of bones and muscles, herbs and drugs, while physicians were still deriving their prognoses from astrology and alchemists were trying to turn lead into gold. So great was the witches' knowledge that in 1527, Paracelsus, considered the "father of modern medicine," burned his text on pharmaceuticals, confessing that he "had learned from the Sorceress all he knew."

THE SUPPRESSION OF WOMEN HEALERS The establishment of medicine as a profession requiring university training made it easy to bar women legally from practice. With few exceptions, the universities were closed to women (even to upper-class women who could afford them), and licensing laws were established to prohibit all but university-trained doctors from practice. It was impossible to enforce the licensing laws consistently since there was only a handful of university-trained doctors compared to the great mass of lay healers. But the laws *could* be used selectively. Their first target was not the peasant healer, but the better-off, literate woman healer who competed for the same urban clientele as that of the university-trained doctors.

Take, for example, the case of Jacoba Félicie, brought to trial in 1322 by the Faculty of Medicine at the University of Paris, on charges of illegal practice. Jacoba was literate and had received some unspecified "special training" in medicine. That her patients were well off is evident from the fact that (as they testified in court) they had consulted well-known university-trained physicians before turning to her. The primary accusations brought against her were that

> . . . she would cure her patient of internal illness and wounds or of external abscesses. She would visit the sick assiduously and continue to examine the urine in the manner on physicians, feel the pulse, and touch the body and limbs.

Six witnesses affirmed that Jacoba had cured them, even after numerous doctors had given up, and one patient declared that she was wiser in the art of surgery and medicine than any master physician or surgeon in Paris. But these testimonials were used against her, for the charge was not that she was incompetent, but that—as a woman—she dared to cure at all.

Along the same lines, English physicians sent a petition to Parliament bewailing the "worthless and presumptuous women who usurped the profession" and asking the imposition of fines and "long imprisonment" on any woman who attempted to "use the practyse of Fisyk." By the fourteenth century, the medical profession's campaign against urban, educated women healers was virtually complete throughout Europe. Male doctors had won a clear monopoly over the practice of medicine among the upper classes (except for obstetrics, which remained the province of female midwives even among the upper classes for another three centuries). They were ready to take a key role in the elimination of the great mass of female healers—the "witches."

The partnership between church, state, and medical profession reached full bloom in the witch trials. The doctor was held up as the medical "expert," giving an aura of science to the whole proceeding. He was asked to make judgments about whether certain women were witches and whether certain afflictions had been caused by witchcraft. The *Malleus* says: "And if it is asked how it is possible to distinguish whether an illness is caused by witchcraft or by some natural physical defect, we answer that the first [way] is by means of the *judgment of doctors*" [emphasis added]. In the witch-hunts, the church explicitly legitimized the doctors' professionalism, denouncing nonprofessional healing as equivalent to heresy: "If a woman dare to cure *without having studied*, she is a witch and must die." . . .

The distinction between "female" superstition and "male" medicine was made final by the very roles of the doctor and witch at the trial. The trial in one stroke established the male physician on a moral and intellectual plane vastly above the female healer he was called to judge. It placed him on the side of God and law, a professional on par with lawyers and theologians, while it placed her on the side of darkness, evil, and magic. He owed his new status not to medical school or scientific achievements of his own, but to the church and state he served so well.

THE AFTERMATH Witch-hunts did not eliminate the lower-class woman healer, but they branded her forever as superstitious and possibly malevolent. So thoroughly was she discredited among the emerging middle classes that in the seventeenth and eighteenth centuries it was possible for male practitioners to make serious inroads into that last preserve of female healing—midwifery. Nonprofessional male practitioners—"barber-surgeons"—led the assault in England, claiming technical superiority on the basis of their use of the obstetrical forceps. (The forceps were legally classified as a surgical instrument, and women were legally barred from surgical practice.) In the hands of the barber-surgeons, obstetrical practice among the middle class was quickly transformed from a neighborly service into a lucrative business, which real physicians entered in force in the late eighteenth century. Female midwives in England organized and charged the male intruders with commercialism and dangerous misuse of the forceps. But it was too late—the women were easily put down as ignorant "old wives" clinging to the superstitions of the past.

WOMEN AND THE RISE OF THE AMERICAN MEDICAL PROFESSION

In the United States, the male takeover of healing roles started later than in England or France, but ultimately went much further. . . . By the turn of the century, medicine here was closed to all but a tiny minority of necessarily tough and well-heeled women. What was left was nursing, and this was in no way a substitute for the autonomous roles women had enjoyed as midwives and general healers.

The question is not so much how women got "left out" of medicine and left with nursing, but how did these categories arise at all? To put it another way: How did one particular set of healers, who happened to be male, white, and middle-class, manage to oust all the competing folk healers, midwives, and other practitioners who had dominated the American medical scene in the early 1800s?

The conventional answer given by medical historians is, of course, that there always was one *true* American medical profession—a small band of men whose scientific and moral authority flowed in a unbroken stream from Hippocrates, Galen, and the great European medical scholars. In frontier America these doctors had to combat not only the routine problems of sickness and death but the abuses of a host of lay practitioners—usually depicted as women, ex-slaves, Indians, and drunken patent medicine salesmen. Fortunately for the medical profession, in the late nineteenth century the American public suddenly developed a healthy respect for the doctors' scientific knowledge, outgrew its earlier faith in quacks, and granted the true medical profession a lasting monopoly of the healing arts.

But the real answer is not in this made-up drama of science versus ignorance and superstition. It's part of the nineteenth century's long story of class and sex struggles for power in all areas of life. When women had a place in medicine, it was in a *people's* medicine. When that people's medicine was destroyed, there was no place for women—except in the subservient role of nurses. The set of healers who became *the* medical profession was distinguished not so much by its associations with modern science as by its associations with the emerging American business establishment. With all due respect to Pasteur, Koch, and the other great European medical researchers of the nineteenth century, it was the Carnegies and the Rockefellers who intervened to secure the final victory of the American medical profession. . . .

In western Europe, university-trained physicians already had a centuries-old monopoly over the right to heal. But in America, medical practice was traditionally open to anyone who could demonstrate healing skills—regardless of formal training, race, or sex. Ann Hutchinson, the dissenting religious leader of the 1600s, was a practitioner of "general physik," as were many other ministers and their wives. The medical historian Joseph Kett reports that "one of the most respected medical men in the late eighteenth century Windsor, Connecticut, for example, was a freed Negro called 'Dr. Primus.' In New Jersey, medical practice, except in extraordinary cases, was mainly in the hands women as late as 1818."

Women frequently went into joint practices with their husbands: the husband handling the surgery, the wife the midwifery and gynecology, and everything else shared. Or a woman might go into practice after developing skills through caring for family members or through an apprenticeship with a relative or other established healer. . . .

ENTER THE DOCTOR In the early 1800s there was also a growing number of formally trained doctors who took great pains to distinguish themselves from the host of lay practitioners. The most important real distinction was that the formally trained, or "regular" doctors, as they called themselves, were male, usually middle-class, and almost always more expensive than the lay competition. The regulars' practices were largely confined to middle- and upper-class people who could afford the prestige of being treated by a "gentlemen" of their own class. By 1800, fashion even dictated that upper- and middle-class women employ male regular doctors for obstetrical care—a custom which plainer people regarded as grossly indecent.

In terms of medical skills and theory, the so-called regulars had nothing to recommend them over the lay practitioners. Their "formal training" meant little even by European standards of the time: Medical programs varied in length from a few months to two years; many medical schools had no clinical facilities; high school diplomas were not required for admission to medical schools. Not that serious academic training would have helped much anyway—there was no body of medical science to be trained in. Instead, the regulars were taught to treat most ills by "heroic" measures: massive bleeding, huge doses of laxatives, calomel (a laxative containing mercury) and, later, opium. (The European medical profession had little better to offer at this time.) There is no doubt that these "cures" were often either fatal or more injurious than the original disease. . . .

The lay practitioners were undoubtedly safer and more effective than the regulars. They preferred mild herbal medications, dietary changes, and hand-holding to heroic interventions. Maybe they didn't know any more than the regulars, but at least they were less likely to do the patient harm. Left alone, they might well have displaced the regular doctors with even middle-class consumers in time. But they didn't know the right people. The regulars, with their close ties to the upper class, had legislative clout. By 1830, 13 states had passed medical licensing laws outlawing "irregular" practice and establishing the regulars as the only legal healers.

It was a premature move. There was not popular support for the idea of medical professionalism, much less for the particular set of healers who claimed it. And there was no way to enforce the new laws. The trusted healers of the common people could not just be legislated out of practice. Worse still for the regulars, this early grab for medical monopoly inspired mass indignation in the form of a radical, popular health movement which came close to smashing medical elitism in America once and for all.

THE POPULAR HEALTH MOVEMENT The popular health movement of the 1830s and 1840s is usually dismissed in conventional medical histories as the high tide of quackery and medical cultism. In reality it was the medical front of a general social upheaval stirred up by feminist and working-class movements. Women were the backbone of the popular health movement. "Ladies' Physiological Societies," the equivalent of our know-your-body courses, sprang up everywhere, bringing rapt audiences simple instructions in anatomy and personal hygiene. The emphasis was on preventive care, as opposed to the murderous "cures" practiced by the regular doctors. The movement ran up the banner for frequent bathing (regarded as a vice by many regular doctors of the time), loose-fitting female clothing, whole-grain cereals, temperance, and a host of other issues women could relate to. And, at about the time Margaret Sanger's mother was a little girl, some elements of the movement were already pushing birth control.

The movement was a radical assault on medical elitism and an affirmation of the traditional people's medicine. "Every man his own doctor," was the slogan of one wing of the movement, and they made it very clear that they meant every woman too. The regular, licensed, doctors were attacked as members of "parasitic, non-producing classes," who survived only because of the upper class's "lurid taste" for calomel and bleeding. Universities (where the elite of the regular doctors were trained) were denounced as places where students "learn to look upon labor as servile and demeaning" and to identify with the upper class. Working-class radicals rallied to the cause, linking "King-craft, Priest-craft, Lawyer-craft, and Doctor-craft" as the four great evils of the time. In New York State, the movement was represented in the legislature by a member of the Workingmen's Party, who took every opportunity to assail the "privileged doctors."

The regular doctors quickly found themselves outnumbered and cornered. From the left wing of the popular health movement came a total rejection of "doctoring" as a paid occupation—much less as an overpaid "profession." From the moderate wing came a host of new medical philosophies, or sects to compete with the regulars on their own terms: eclecticism, Grahamism, homeopathy, plus many minor ones. The new sects set up their own medical schools (emphasizing preventive care and mild herbal cures), and started graduating their own doctors. In this context of medical ferment, the old regulars began to look like just another sect, a sect whose particular philosophy happened to lean toward calomel, bleeding, and the other standbys of "heroic" medicine. It was impossible to tell who were the "real" doctors, and by the 1840s, medical licensing laws had been repealed in almost all of the states.

The peak of the popular health movement coincided with the beginnings of an organized feminist movement, and the two were so closely linked that it's hard to tell where one began and the other left off. "This crusade for women's health [the popular health movement] was related both in cause and effect to the demand for women's rights in general, and at the health and feminist movements become indistinguishable at this point," according to Richard Shryock, the well-known medical historian. The health movement was concerned with women's rights in general, and the women's movement was particularly concerned with health and with women's access to medical training.

In fact, leaders of both groups used the prevailing sex stereotypes to argue that women were even better equipped to be doctors than men. "We cannot deny that women possess superior capacities for the science of medicine," wrote Samuel Thomson, a health movement leader, in 1834. (However, he felt surgery and the care of males should be reserved for male practitioners.) Feminists, like Sarah Hale, went further, exclaiming in 1852: "Talk about this [medicine] being the appropriate sphere for man and his alone! With tenfold more plausibility and reason we say it is the appropriate sphere for woman, and hers alone."

The new medical sects' schools did, in fact, open their doors to women at a time when regular medical training was all but closed to them. For example, Harriet Hunt was denied admission to Harvard Medical College, and instead went to a sectarian school for her formal training. (Actually, the Harvard faculty had voted to admit her—along with some black male students—but the students threatened to riot if they came.) The regular physicians could take the credit for training Elizabeth Blackwell, America's first female "regular," but her alma mater (a small school in upstate New York) quickly passes a resolution barring further female students. The first generally co-ed medical schools was the "irregular" Eclectic Central Medical College of New York, in Syracuse. Finally, the first two all-female medical colleges, one in Boston and one in Philadelphia, were themselves "irregular."

Feminist researchers should really find out more about the popular health movement. From the perspective of our movement today, it's probably more relevant than the women's suffrage struggle. To us, the most tantalizing aspects of the movement are:

1. That it represented both class struggle and feminist struggle. Today it's stylish in some quarters to write off purely feminist issues as middle-class concerns. But in the popular health movement we see a coming together of feminist and working-class energies. Is this because the popular health movement naturally attracted dissidents of all kinds, or was there some deeper identity of purpose?

2. It was not just a movement for more and better medical care, but for a radically different kind of health care: It was a substantive challenge to the prevailing medical dogma, practice, and theory. Today we tend to confine our critiques to the organization of medical care and assume that the scientific substratum of medicine is unassailable. We too should be developing the capability for the critical study of medical "science"—at least as it relates to women.

DOCTORS ON THE OFFENSIVE At its height in the 1830s and 1840s, the popular health movement had the regular doctors—the professional ancestors of today's physicians—running scared. Later in the nineteenth century, as the grassroots energy

ebbed and the movement degenerated into a set of competing sects, the regulars went back on the offensive. In 1848, they pulled together their first national organization, pretentiously named the *American* Medical Association (AMA). County and state medical societies, many of which had practically disbanded during the height of medical anarchy in the 1830s and 1840s, began to re-form.

Throughout the latter part of the nineteenth century, the regulars relentlessly attacked lay practitioners, sectarian doctors, and women practitioners in general. The attacks were linked: Women practitioners could be attacked because of their sectarian leanings; sects could be attacked because of their openness to women. The arguments against women doctors ranged from the paternalistic (how could a respectable woman travel at night to a medical emergency?) to the hard-core sexist. . . .

The virulence of the American sexist opposition to women in medicine has no parallel in Europe. This is probably because, first, fewer European women were aspiring to medical careers at this time. Second, feminist movements were nowhere as strong as in the United States, and here the male doctors rightly associated the entrance of women into medicine with organized feminism. And, third, the European medical profession was already more firmly established and hence less afraid of competition.

The rare woman who did make it into a regular medical school faced one sexist hurdle after another. First, there was the continuous harassment—often lewd—by the male students. There were professors who wouldn't discuss anatomy with a lady present. . . .

Having completed her academic work, the would-be woman doctor usually found the next steps blocked. Hospitals were usually closed to women doctors, and even if they weren't, the internships were not open to women. If she finally did make it into practice, she found her brother "regulars" unwilling to refer patients to her and absolutely opposed to her membership in their medical societies.

And so it is all the stranger to us, and all the

sadder, that what we might call the "women's health movement" began, in the late nineteenth century, to dissociate itself from its popular health movement past and to strive for respectability. Members of irregular sects were purged from the faculties of the women's medical colleges. Female medical leaders such as Elizabeth Blackwell joined male "regulars" in demanding an end to lay midwifery and "a complete medical education" for all who practiced obstetrics. All this at a time when the regulars still had little or no "scientific" advantage over the sect doctors or lay healers.

The explanation, we suppose, was that the women who were likely to seek formal medical training at this time were middle-class. They must have found it easier to identify with the middle-class regular doctors than with lower-class women healers or with the sectarian medical groups (which had earlier been identified with radical movements). The shift in allegiance was probably made all the easier by the fact that, in the cities, female lay practitioners were increasingly likely to be immigrants. (At the same time, the possibilities for a cross-class women's movement on *any* issue were vanishing as working-class women went into the factories and middle-class women settled into Victorian ladyhood.) Whatever the exact explanation, the result was that middle-class women had given up the substantive attack on male medicine, and accepted the terms set by the emerging male medical profession.

PROFESSIONAL VICTORY The regulars were still in no condition to make another bid for medical monopoly. For one thing, they still couldn't claim to have any uniquely effective methods or special body of knowledge. Besides, an occupational group doesn't gain a professional monopoly on the basis of technical superiority alone. A recognized profession is not just a group of self-proclaimed experts; it is a group which has authority *in the law* to select its own members and regulate their practice, i.e., to monopolize a certain field without outside interference. How does a particular group gain full professional status? In the words of sociologist Elliot Freidson:

> A profession attains and maintains its position by virtue of the protection and patronage of some elite segment of society which has been persuaded that there is some special value in its work.

In other words, professions are the creation of a ruling class. To become *the* medical profession, the regular doctors needed above all, ruling-class patronage.

By a lucky coincidence for the regulars, both the science and the patronage became available around the same time, at the turn of the century. French and especially German scientists brought forth the germ theory of disease which provided, for the first time in human history, a rational basis for disease prevention and therapy. While the run-of-the-mill American doctor was still mumbling about "humors" and dosing people with calomel, a tiny medical elite was traveling to German universities to learn the new science. They returned to the United States filled with reformist zeal. In 1893 German-trained doctors (funded by local philanthropists) set up the first . . . German-style medical school, Johns Hopkins.

As far as curriculum was concerned, the big innovation at Hopkins was integrating lab work in basic science with expanded clinical training. Other reforms included hiring full-time faculty, emphasizing research, and closely associating the medical school with a full university. Johns Hopkins also introduced the modern pattern of medical education—four years of medical school following four years of college—which of course barred most working-class and poor people from the possibility of a medical education.

Meanwhile the United States was emerging as the industrial leader of the world. Fortunes built on oil, coal, and the ruthless exploitation of American workers were maturing into financial empires. For the first time in American history, there were sufficient concentrations of corporate wealth to allow for massive organized philanthropy, i.e., organized ruling-class intervention in the social, cultural, and political life of the nation. Foundations were created as the lasting instrument of this intervention—the Rockefeller and Carnegie foundations appeared in the first decade of the twentieth century. One of the earliest and highest items on their agenda was medical "reform," the creation of a respectable, scientific American medical profession.

The group of American medical practitioners that the foundations chose to put their money behind was, naturally enough, the scientific elite of the regular doctors. (Many of these men were themselves ruling-class, and all were urbane, university-trained gentlemen.) Starting in 1903, foundation money began to pour into medical schools by the millions. The conditions were clear: conform to the Johns Hopkins model or close. To get the message across, the Carnegie Corporation sent a staff man, Abraham Flexner, out on a national tour of medical schools—from Harvard right down to the last third-rate commercial schools.

Flexner almost singlehandedly decided which schools would get the money—and hence survive. For the bigger and better schools (i.e., those which already had enough money to begin to institute the prescribed reforms), there was the promise of fat foundation grants. Harvard was one of the lucky winners, and its president could say smugly in 1907, "Gentlemen, the way to get endowments for medicine is to improve medical education." As for the smaller, poorer schools, which included most of the sectarian schools and special schools for blacks and women—Flexner did not consider them worth saving. Their options were to close, or to remain open and face public denunciation in the report Flexner was preparing.

The Flexner report, published in 1910, was the foundations' ultimatum to American medicine. In its wake, medical schools closed by the score, including six of America's eight black medical schools and the majority of the "irregular" schools which had been a haven for female students. Medicine was established once and for all as a branch of "higher" learning, accessible only through lengthy and expensive university training. It's certainly true that as medical knowledge grew, lengthier training did become necessary. But Flexner and the foundations had no intention of making such training available to the great mass of lay healers and "irregular" doctors. Instead, doors were slammed shut to blacks, to the majority of women, and to poor white men. (Flexner in his report bewailed the fact that any "crude boy or jaded clerk" had been able to seek medical training.) Medicine had become a white, male, middle-class occupation.

But it was more than an occupation. It had become, at last, a profession. To be more precise, one particular group of healers, the regular doctors, was now *the* medical profession. Their victory was not based on any skills of their own: the run-of-the-mill regular doctor did not suddenly acquire a knowledge of medical science with the publication of the Flexner report. But he did acquire the *mystique* of science. So what if his own alma mater had been condemned in the Flexner report, wasn't he a member of the AMA, and wasn't it in the forefront of scientific reform? The doctor had become—thanks to some foreign scientists and eastern foundations—the "man of science": beyond criticism, beyond regulation, very nearly beyond competition.

OUTLAWING THE MIDWIVES In state after state, new, tough, licensing laws sealed the doctor's monopoly on medical practice. All that was left was to drive out the last holdouts of the old people's medicine—the midwives. In 1910, about 50 percent of all babies were delivered by midwives—most were blacks or working-class immigrants. It was an intolerable situation to the newly emerging obstetrical specialty. For one thing, every poor woman who went to a midwife was one more case lost to academic teaching and research. America's vast lower-class resource of obstetrical "teaching material" was being wasted on ignorant midwives. Besides which, poor women were spending an estimated $5 million a year on midwives—$5 million which could have been going to "professionals."

Publicly, however, the obstetricians launched their attacks on midwives in the name of science and reform. Midwives were ridiculed as "hopelessly dirty, ignorant and incompetent." Specifically, they were held responsible for the prevalence of puerperal sepsis (uterine infections) and neonatal ophthalmia (blindness due to parental infection with gonorrhea). Both conditions were easily preventable by techniques well within the grasp of the least literate midwife (hand-washing for puerperal sepsis, and eye drops for the ophthalmia). So the obvious solution for a truly public-spirited obstetrical profession would have been to make the appropriate preventive techniques known and available to the mass of midwives. This is in fact what happened in England, Germany, and most other European nations: Midwifery was upgraded through training to become an established, independent occupation.

But the American obstetricians had no real commitment to improved obstetrical care. In fact, a study by a Johns Hopkins professor in 1912 indicated that most American doctors were *less* competent than the midwives. Not only were the doctors themselves unreliable about preventing sepsis and ophthalmia but they also tended to be too ready to use surgical techniques that endangered mother or child. If anyone, then, deserved a legal monopoly on obstetrical care, it was the midwives, not the MDs. But the doctors had power, the midwives didn't. Under intense pressure from the medical profession, state after state passed laws outlawing midwifery and restricting the practice of obstetrics to doctors. For poor and working-class women, this actually meant worse—or no—obstetrical care. (For instance, a study of infant mortality rates in Washington showed an increase in infant mortality in the years immediately following the passage of the law forbidding midwifery.) For the new, male medical profession, the ban on midwives meant one less source of competition. Women had been routed from their last foothold as independent practitioners.

THE LADY WITH THE LAMP The only remaining occupation for women in health was nursing. Nursing had not always existed as a paid occupation—it had to be invented. In the early nineteenth century, a "nurse" was simply a woman who happened to be nursing someone—a sick child or an aging relative. There were hospitals, and they did employ nurses. But the hospitals of the time served largely as refuges for the dying poor, with only token care provided. Hospital nurses, history has it, were a disreputable lot, prone to drunkenness, prostitution, and thievery. And conditions in the hospitals were often scandalous. In the late 1870s a committee investigating New York's Bellevue Hospital could not find a bar of soap on the premises.

If nursing was not exactly an attractive field to women workers, it was a wide open arena for women *reformers.* To reform hospital care, you had to reform nursing, and to make nursing acceptable to doctors and to women "of good character," it had to be given a completely new image. Florence Nightingale got her chance in the battle-front hospitals of the Crimean War, where she replaced the old camp-follower "nurses" with a bevy of disciplined, sober, middle-aged ladies. Dorothea Dix, an American hospital reformer, introduced the new breed of nurses in the Union hospitals of the Civil War.

The new nurse—"the lady with the lamp," selflessly tending the wounded —caught the popular imagination. Real nursing schools began to appear in England right after the Crimean War, and in the United States right after the Civil War. At the same time, the number of hospitals began to increase to keep pace with the needs of medical education. Medical students needed hospitals to train in; good hospitals, as the doctors were learning, needed good nurses.

In fact, the first American nursing schools did their best to recruit actual upper-class women as students. Miss Euphemia Van Rensselear, of an old aristocratic New York family, graced Bellevue's first class. And at Johns Hopkins, where Isabel Hampton trained nurses in the University Hospital, a leading doctor could only complain that:

Miss Hampton has been most successful in getting probationers [students] of the upper class; but unfortunately, she selects them altogether for their good looks and the House staff is by this time in a sad state.

Let us look a little more closely at the women who invented nursing, because, in a very real sense, nursing as we know it today is the product of their oppression as upper-class Victorian women. Dorothea Dix was an heiress of substantial means. Florence Nightingale and Louisa Schuyler (the moving force behind the creation of America's first Nightingale-style nursing school) were genuine aristocrats. They were refugees from the enforced leisure of Victorian ladyhood. Dix and Nightingale did not begin to carve out their reform careers until they were in their thirties, and faced with the prospect of a long, useless spinsterhood. They focused their energies on the care of the sick because this was a "natural" and acceptable interest for ladies of their class.

Nightingale and her immediate disciples left nursing with the indelible stamp of their own class biases. Training emphasized character, not skills. The finished products, the Nightingale nurse, was simply the ideal lady, transplanted from home to the hospital and absolved of reproductive responsibilities. To the doctor, she brought the wifely virtue of absolute obedience. To the patient, she brought the selfless devotion of a mother. To the lower level hospital employees, she brought the firm but kindly discipline of a household manager accustomed to dealing with servants.

But, despite the glamorous "lady with the lamp" image, most of nursing work was just low-paid, heavy-duty housework. Before long, most nursing schools were attracting only women from working-class and lower-middle-class homes, whose only other options were factory or clerical work. But the philosophy of nursing education did not change—after all, the educators were still middle- and upper-class women. If anything, they toughened their insistence on ladylike character development, and the socialization of nurses became what it has been for most of the twentieth century: the imposition of upper-class cultural values on working-class women. (For example, until recently, most nursing students were taught such upper-class graces as tea pouring, art appreciation, etc. Practical nurses are still taught to wear girdles, use makeup, and in general mimic the behavior of a "better" class of women.)

But the Nightingale nurse was not just the projection of upper-class ladyhood onto the working world. She embodied the very spirit of femininity as defined by sexist Victorian society—she was Woman. The inventors of nursing saw it as a natural vocation for women, second only to motherhood. When a group of English nurses proposed that nursing model itself after the medical profession, with exams and licensing, Nightingale responded that "nurses cannot be registered and examined *any more than mothers*" [emphasis added]. Or, as one historian of nursing put it, nearly a century later, "Woman is an instinctive nurse, taught by Mother Nurse" (Victor Robinson, *White Caps: The Story of Nursing*). If women were instinctive nurses, they were not, in the Nightingale view, instinctive doctors. She wrote of the few female physicians of her time: "They have only tried to be men, and they have succeeded only in being third-rate men." Indeed, as the number of nursing students rose in the late nineteenth century, the number of female medical students began to decline. Woman had found her place in the health system.

Just as the feminist movement had not opposed the rise of medical professionalism, it did not challenge nursing as an oppressive female role. In fact, feminists of the late nineteenth century were themselves beginning to celebrate the nurse-mother image of femininity. The American women's movement had given up the struggle for full sexual equality to focus exclusively on the vote, and to get it, they were ready to adopt the most sexist tenets of Victorian ideology: women need the vote, they argued, not because they are human, but because they are mothers. "Woman is the mother of the race," gushed Boston feminist Julia Ward Howe, "the guardian of its helpless infancy, its earliest teacher, its most zealous champion. Woman is also the homemaker, upon her devolve the details which bless and beautify family life." And so on, in paeans too painful to quote.

The women's movement dropped its earlier emphasis on opening up the professions to women: Why forsake motherhood for the petty pursuits of males? And of course the impetus to attack professionalism itself as inherently sexist and elitist was long since dead. Instead, they turned to professionalizing women's natural functions. Housework was glamorized in the new discipline of "domestic science." Motherhood was held out as a vocation requiring much the same preparation and skill as nursing or teaching.

So while some women were professionalizing women's domestic roles, others were "domesticizing" professional roles, like nursing, teaching, and, later, social work. For the woman who chose to express her feminine drives outside of the home, these occupations were presented as simple extensions of women's "natural" domestic role. Conversely the woman who remained at home was encouraged to see herself as a kind of nurse, teacher, and counselor practicing within the limits of the family. And so the middle-class feminists of the late 1800s dissolved away some of the harsher contradictions of sexism.

THE DOCTOR NEEDS A NURSE Of course, the women's movement was not in a position to decide on the future of nursing anyway. Only the medical profession was. At first, male doctors were a little skeptical about the new Nightingale nurses—perhaps suspecting that this was just one more feminine attempt to infiltrate medicine. But they were soon won over by the nurses' unflagging obedience. (Nightingale was a little obsessive on this point. When she arrived in the Crimea with her newly trained nurses, the doctors at first ignored them all. Nightingale refused to let her

women lift a finger to help the thousands of sick and wounded soldiers until the doctors gave an order. Impressed, the doctors finally relented and set the nurses to cleaning up the hospital.) To the beleaguered doctors of the nineteenth century, nursing was a godsend. Here at last was a kind of health worker who did not want to compete with the "regulars," did not have a medical doctrine to push, and who seemed to have no other mission in life but to serve.

While the average regular doctor was making nurses welcome, the new scientific practitioners of the early twentieth century were making them *necessary*. The new, post-Flexner physician, was even less likely than his predecessors to stand around and watch the progress of his "cures." He diagnosed, he prescribed, he moved on. He could not waste his talents, or his expensive academic training in the tedious details of bedside care. For this he needed a patient, obedient helper, someone who was not above the most menial tasks—in short, a nurse.

Healing, in its fullest sense, consists of both curing and caring, doctoring *and* nursing. The old lay healers of an earlier time had combined both functions, and were valued for both. (For example, midwives not only presided at the delivery, but lived in until the new mother was ready to resume care of her children.) But with the development of scientific medicine, and the modern medical profession, the two functions were split irrevocably. Curing became the exclusive province of the doctor; caring was relegated to the nurse. All credit for the patient's recovery went to the doctor and his "quick fix," for only the doctor participated in the mystique of science. The nurse's activities, on the other hand, were barely distinguishable from those of a servant. She had no power, no magic, and no claim to the credit.

Doctoring and nursing arose as complementary functions, and the society which defined nursing as feminine could readily see doctoring as intrinsically "masculine." If the nurse was idealized woman, the doctor was idealized man—combining intellect and action, abstract theory and hard-headed pragmatism. The very qualities which fitted Woman for nursing barred her from doctoring, and vice versa. Her tenderness and innate spirituality were out of place in the harsh, linear world of science. His decisiveness and curiosity made him unfit for long hours of patient nurturing.

These stereotypes have proved to be almost unbreakable. Today's leaders of the American Nursing Association may insist that nursing is no longer a feminine vocation but a neuter "profession." They may call for more male nurses to change the "image," insist that nursing requires almost as much academic preparation as medicine, and so on. But the drive to "professionalize" nursing is, at best, a flight from the reality of sexism in the health system. At worst, it is sexist itself, deepening the division among women health workers and bolstering a hierarchy controlled by men.

CONCLUSION

We have our own moment of history to work out, our own struggles. What can we learn from the past that will help us—in a women's health movement—today? These are some of our conclusions:

➤ We have not been passive bystanders in the history of medicine. The present system was born in and shaped by the competition between male and female healers. The medical profession in particular is not just another institution which happens to discriminate against us: It is a fortress designed and erected to exclude us. This means to us that the sexism of the health system is not incidental, not just the reflection of the sexism of society in general or the sexism of individual doctors. It is historically older than medical science itself; it is deep-rooted, institutional sexism.

➤ Our enemy is not just "men" or their individual male chauvinism. It is the whole class system which enabled male, upper-class healers to win out and which forced us into subservience. Institutional sexism is sustained by a class system which supports male power.

➤ There is no historically consistent justification for the exclusion of women from healing roles. Witches were attacked for being pragmatic, empirical, and immoral. But in the nineteenth century the rhetoric reversed. Women became too unscientific, delicate, and sentimental. The *stereotypes* change to suit male convenience—*we* don't—and there is nothing in our "innate feminine nature" to justify our present subservience.

➤ Men maintain their power in the health system through their monopoly of scientific knowledge. We are mystified by science, taught to believe that it is hopelessly beyond our grasp. In our frustration, we are sometimes tempted to reject *science*, rather than to challenge the men who hoard it. But medical science could be a liberating force, giving us real control over own bodies and power in our lives as health workers. At this point in our history, every effort to take hold of and share medical knowledge is a critical part of our struggle—know-your-body courses and literature, self-help projects, counseling, women's free clinics.

➤ Professionalism in medicine is nothing more than the institutionalization of a male upper-class monopoly. We must never confuse professionalism with expertise. Expertise is something to work for and to share; professionalism is—by definition—elitist and exclusive, sexist, racist and classist. In the American past, women who sought formal medical training were too ready to accept the professionalism that went with it. They made *their* gains in status—but only on the backs of their less privileged sisters: midwives, nurses, and lay healers. Our goal today should never be to open up the exclusive medical profession to women, but to open up medicine to all women.

➤ This means that we must begin to break down the distinctions and barriers between women health workers and women consumers. We should build shared concerns: consumers aware of women's needs as workers, workers in touch with women's needs as consumers. Women workers can play a leadership role in collective self-help and self-teaching projects, and in attacks on health institutions. But they need support and solidarity from a strong women's consumer movement.

➤ Our oppression as women health workers today is inextricably linked to our oppression as women. Nursing, our predominate role in the health system, is simply a workplace extension of our roles as wife and mother. The nurse is socialized to believe that rebellion violates not only her "professionalism," but her very femininity. This means that the male medical elite has a very special stake in the maintenance of sexism in the society at large: doctors are the bosses in an industry where the workers are primarily women. Sexism in the society at large insures that the female majority of the health workforce are "good" workers—docile and passive. Take away sexism and you take away one of the mainstays of the health hierarchy.

What this means to us in practice is that in the health system there is no way to separate worker organizing from feminist organizing. To reach out to women health workers as *workers* is to reach out to them as *women*.

NOTES

1. Thomas Szasz, *The Manufacture of Madness* (Syracuse, NY: Syracuse University Press, 1997).

2. Heinrich Kramer and Jacob Sprenger, *Malleus Maleficarum* [*Hammer of Witches*] (n.p.: 1487).

Out of Conflict Comes Strength and Healing: Women's Health Movements

HELEN I. MARIESKIND

Adapted from Helen I. Marieskind, *Women in the Health System: Patients, Providers, and Programs*, St. Louis, Missouri: C. V. Mosby, 1980. Reprinted by permission.

Helen Marieskind, founding editor of the journal Women and Health, *chose her surname to honor her mother, Marie. (*Kind *is the German word for "child.") With similar devotion she honors the* names and the work of some superstar women healers in history. (Hey, girlfriend, how about that Hildegard of Bingen?!)

Conflict and activism in women's health care have a long history; ancient issues remain with us. In 3500 BCE, Egyptian midwives, *jatromaiai*, proudly protected their rights to practice surgery and internal medicine, distinguishing themselves from the strictly obstetrical practice of the *maiai*. Greece had many skilled women physicians, but by the third century BCE, their service as abortionists, the influence of Hippocrates, and the growth of the Pythagorean school combined to prohibit them from practice. Women "picketed the courthouse," winning the right to practice and acquittal of their favorite, Agnodice, arrested for practicing gynecology as a man.

The growth of Christianity led to a deepening conviction by men of the church that women should keep out of public and religious affairs, and major conflicts over women's role in health care delivery and in the nature of health care began in earnest. Saint Augustine had written, "educated women should take care of the sick," but by the Council of Nantes in 660 CE, women were termed "soulless brutes." Thus began centuries of denying education to women and male dominance in medicine.

Only a few women—usually the wealthy, nobility, or clerics—were educated. Many of these women turned to monastic life, becoming medical missionaries with their monasteries as centers of healing. For example, the English princess Walpurga (c. 710–77), always depicted with a flask of urine and bandages, treated the poor at the monastery she founded in Germany. Hildegard of Bingen (1098–1179), who is best known today for her enchanting music, entered monastic life at age eight. In 1147, at age fifty, Hildegard built a new convent near Bingen, on the Rhine. Hildegard wielded great power, corresponding with popes, emperors, and kings. Fiery and prophetic, she published her theories on the chemistry and circulation of blood, the causes of contagion and autointoxication, and the brain as the origin of nerve action. Obstetrician Trotula di Ruggiero of Salerno, Italy, is credited in the mid-1100s with the first description of the physical signs of syphilis and, prior to an understanding of sepsis, for advocating the use of protective pads to prevent fecal contamination during childbirth. Anna Comnena (1083–1148) served as physician-in-chief of an 11,000-bed hospital in Constantinople (Istanbul).

Conflict increased over the next centuries between the learned role of medical men and the widespread denial of education to women. Conflict was reinforced by church decrees in the early 1100s, the development of universities in most of Europe as primarily male preserves, the growth of essentially all-male guilds, and efforts at licensure by the church and state. Women's roles in health care were confined to nurses, midwives, herb gatherers, ecclesiastical and lay village healers, and occasionally empirics, who were lay women apprenticed to university-educated practitioners. Women (along with barber-surgeons) became providers of simple, direct care—treating wounds and infections and setting bones. This dichotomy between learned men and primary care–giving women laid the groundwork for a further division of labor in which women healers were essentially limited to nursing tasks while male practitioners commanded an elite, specialist role.

Jacoba Félicie de Almania's case illustrates the point. Brought to trial in Paris in 1322 for failing to comply with a 1220 licensure law, Jacoba was confronted not with a charge of incompetence but with witnesses and a detailed reading of her medical practices, showing her to be both practical and knowledgeable. She argued that the licensure law of 1220 was made for "idiots and ignorant persons" who knew nothing of the art of medicine and from which groups she was excluded because of her skill and expertise. Her eloquent pleas for the need for women to be treated by other women are recorded in the Charter of Paris, II:

It is better and more honest that a wise and expert woman in this art visit sick women and inquire into the secret nature of their infirmity, than a man to whom it is not permitted to see, inquire of, or touch the hands, breasts, stomach, etc. of a woman; nay rather ought a man shun the secrets of women and their company and flee as far as he can.

Some outstanding midwives and women physicians did survive this period. Important female physicians were still emerging from Italy at a time when England and France were persecuting them. Dorothea Bocchi was appointed professor of medicine and moral philosophy at Bologna in 1390 and taught there for 40 years. A contemporary, Costanza Calenda of Naples, won high honors for her lecturing in medicine.

By the sixteenth century, exclusion of women from most European learning centers was firmly entrenched (Italy was a notable exception). Intense conflicts over women's health raged during the witch-hunts of medieval Europe, when thousands of people were slaughtered. Most of the women were lay women healers or "old wives" who served as midwives. This is an important distinction, because while accusations of witchcraft were also at times leveled at more recognized midwives, some separate provisions were made for them to be licensed. In England in 1587, for example, Eleanor Preade was licensed to perform the functions of midwife, including baptism.

Witchcraft trials had a lasting effect on women's place as healers, as the direct, primary, and often intimate caregiving roles had become so fraught with danger, that few women risked practicing for fear of being accused. The poor lost their village healers, and the professional control by church and state became firmly entrenched. Increasing corruption in the monasteries was matched by decreased interest in the medical and charitable aspects of clerical life, while the exclusion of women from the universities continued to effectively bar the participation of even upper-class women from medical practice. Moreover, by licensing some midwives and not others, stratifications and divisions formed among women healers, preventing a unified protest.

Again, there were exceptions. Outstanding French midwives practiced from the sixteenth to the nineteenth centuries. Louyse Bourgeois (1563–1636) set rules for handling each of the varied fetal positions. Angèlique Marguerite le Boursier du Coudray (1712–89) invented a model of the female torso and was ordered by Louis XVI to travel throughout the provinces, giving free instruction to all "unenlightened midwives." Yet even in France, England, and Germany, where the skills of all highly accomplished midwives were well-rewarded, their discoveries published, and their talents sought after by the noblest and humblest of citizens, conflict still surrounded their licensure and entry into universities. "The midwives of the Academy have no desire of me," mocked Madame Boivin (1773–1847), midwife, decorated by the French crown and awarded an honorary MD degree by Germany in 1827, upon being denied entry into the (male) French Academy of Medicine.

By the end of the eighteenth century, conflicts over female practitioners, particularly midwives, were highly institutionalized throughout Europe. In France and Germany, although the status of some was diminished, the training programs organized led to an overall increase in competence and respect, resulting in the incorporation of the midwife into modern health care systems.

Midwives in England, however, were not only excluded from using rapidly developing technologies such as forceps, but were hampered also by their lack of organization, intragroup competitiveness, their assignment to obstetrics only, and by a wealthy and well-organized onslaught from the male physicians backed by church, state, and licensure laws. The ceaseless struggles of midwives such as Mrs. Elizabeth Nihell, Mrs. Sarah Stone, and Mrs. Elizabeth Cellier are colorful reading. It was not until Rosalind Paget founded the Midwives Institute in 1881 that the midwife once more became an integral part of the English health care system.

In the American colonies several midwives served their communities with great skill. The first midwife of record, Brigett Fuller, as her name is spelled on the land ownership register, reached the Plymouth colony in 1623 on the *Anne* and joined her physician husband Samuel, a *Mayflower* passenger. There was also Anne Hutchinson, a midwife, an organizer of women, and a religious dissident who cofounded a settlement in Rhode Island. We know of a Mrs. Wiat from her epitaph of 1705: "She assisted at ye births of one thousand, one hundred and odd children." The diary of Martha Ballard, midwife, converted to a contemporary book and film, aptly captures the poignant hardships and the joys of the midwife's role in colonial America.

In the United States, too, the midwife gradually lost her status, as did practicing female physicians—generally for the same reasons as in England. Women physicians, such as Dr. Mary Lavinder (1776–1845), who set up a pediatric and midwifery practice in Savannah, Georgia, in 1814, and Dr. Sarah E. Adams (1779–1846), also a practitioner in Georgia, were highly popular and successful even if not given equal status. Similarly, Harriet K. Hunt (1805–75) gained a large following in her Boston practice, even though she had no degree. Oliver Wendell Holmes supported her application to Harvard Medical School, and the faculty could find nothing in the statutes to deny her admission. Nevertheless, Hunt was forced to withdraw her application when the students resolved: "That we object to having the company of any female forced upon us, who is disposed to unsex herself, and to sacrifice her modesty by appearing with men in the lecture room."

The greatest conflicts around women's health care in the United States arose during the popular health movement of the 1830s and 1840s, continuing well into the twentieth century. A current of liberal, democratic thinking hostile to professionalism, fostered the growth of the popular health movement, aided by lax or nonexistent licensing laws, a broad recognition of home cures and synergy between body and mind, and by a generally held belief that anyone who demonstrated healing skills should be permitted to practice medicine. Feminists, women practitioners such as Harriet K. Hunt, and working-class radicals joined together in the popular health movement to reject the perceived arrogance and incompetence of most doctors of the day.

During and following the mid-nineteenth century, women were widely regarded as inherently sickly, as documented by Ben Barker-Benfield in *Horrors of the Half-Known Life*. To help protect themselves, women at Ladies' Physiological Reform Societies, an outgrowth of the popular health movement, lectured on sensible—yet radical—ideas such as personal hygiene and frequent bathing, preventive care, elementary anatomy, loose-fitting female clothing (whalebone corsets worn by women of fashion disastrously cramped their internal organs), temperance, the importance of a healthy diet including whole-grain cereals, sex, and birth control. Birth control, and woman's right to it, continued to be highly controversial even up to the repeal of the last of the Comstock Laws in 1965 in Connecticut. Female sectarian medical colleges established by branches of the popular health movement offered courses to women to improve both their own health and that of their families, while women graduates frequently taught through the societies. Lydia Folger Fowler (1822–79) was one such teacher; in 1851 she was appointed professor of midwifery at the Rochester Eclectic Medical College, becoming the first woman to hold a professorship in a legally authorized medical school in the United States.

These and other topics, including abortion rights, the doctor-patient relationship, and overuse of drugs and surgical intervention, together with many of the historical issues of women's health care such as licensure, sparked the women's health movement of the 1960s and remain central to women's health issues today. We are still struggling over questions of licensure, of whether technological intervention of specialists is superior to the more natural healing methods of general practitioners

and midwives, and while there are now almost as many women as men in medical schools, certain specialties are still dominated by men. Given today's advanced technology, the complexities have changed, but the fundamental conflicts surrounding women's health care—who determines and controls the right to practice and in what manner—remain the same. This sameness does not invalidate today's issues in any way, but shows us there are lessons to be learned from past struggles.

Medicine and Morality in the Nineteenth Century

KRISTIN LUKER

Kristin Luker, excerpt from *Abortion and the Politics of Motherhood*, Berkeley, California: University of California Press, 1984. Reprinted by permission.

Kristin Luker, sociologist at the University of California, San Diego, demonstrates how—beginning in 1859—the American Medical Association launched a successful campaign to ban induced abortions, not for the sake of their patients' health (to the contrary: more women's lives were lost) but to publicize themselves and call attention to their own "moral stature" and "technical expertise."

Surprising as it may seem, the view that abortion is murder is a relatively recent belief in American history. To be sure, there has always been a school of thought, extending back at least to the Pythagoreans of ancient Greece, that holds that abortion is wrong because the embryo is the moral equivalent of the child it will become. Equally ancient, however, is the belief articulated by the Stoics: that although embryos have some of the rights of already-born children (and these rights may increase over the course of the pregnancy), embryos are of a different moral order, and thus to end their existence by an abortion is not tantamount to murder. . . .

In the Roman Empire, abortion was so frequent and widespread that it was remarked upon by a number of authors. Ovid, Juvenal, and Seneca all noted the existence of abortion, and the natural historian Pliny listed prescriptions for drugs that would accomplish it. Legal regulation of abortion in the Roman Empire, however, was virtually non-existent. Roman law explicitly held that the "child in the belly of its mother" was not a person, and hence abortion was not murder. After the beginning of the Christina era, such legal regulation of abortion as existed in the Roman Empire was designed primarily to protect the rights of fathers rather than the rights of embryos. . . .

THE ORIGINS OF THE FIRST RIGHT-TO-LIFE MOVEMENT

At the opening of the nineteenth century, no statute laws governed abortion in America. What minimal legal regulation existed was inherited from English common law tradition that abortion undertaken before quickening was at worst a misdemeanor. *Quickening,* as that term was understood in the nineteenth century, was the period in pregnancy when a woman felt fetal movement; though it varies from woman to woman (and even from pregnancy to pregnancy in the same woman), it generally occurs between the fourth and the sixth month of pregnancy. Consequently in nineteenth-century America, as in medieval Europe, first-trimester abortions, and a goodly number of second-trimester abortions as well, faced little legal regulation. Practically speaking, the difficulty of determining when conception had occurred, combined with the fact that the only person who could reliably tell when the pregnancy had "quickened" was the pregnant woman herself, meant that even this minimal regulation was probably infrequent. In 1809, when the Massachusetts State Supreme Court dismissed an indictment for abortion because the prosecution had not reliably proved that the woman was "quick with child," it was simply reiterating traditional common law standards.

In contrast, by 1900 every state in the Union had passed a law forbidding the use of drugs or instruments to procure abortion at any stage of pregnancy, "unless the same be necessary to save the woman's life." Not only were those who performed an abortion liable for a felony (usually manslaughter or second-degree homicide), but in many states, the aborted woman herself faced the possibility of criminal prosecution, still another departure from the tolerant common law tradition in existence at the beginning of the century.

Many cultural themes and social struggles lie behind the transition from an abortion climate that was remarkably open and unrestricted to one that restricted abortions (at least in principle) to those necessary to save the life of the mother. The second half of the nineteenth century, when the bulk of American abortion laws were written, saw profound changes in the social order, and these provided the foundation for dramatic changes in the status of abortion. Between 1850 and 1900, for example, the population changed from one that was primarily rural and agricultural to one that was urban and industrial, and the birth rates fell accordingly, declining from an estimated average completed fertility for whites of 7.04 births per woman in 1800 to an average of 3.56 births in 1900. The "great wave" of American immigration occurred in this period, as did the first feminist movement.

The intricate relationships between social roles, moral values, and medical technologies that were associated with changing patterns of fertility simultaneously became both the cause and the product of demographic strains—strains between rural and urban dwellers; between native-born "Yankees" and immigrants; between the masses and the elites; and possibly between men and women.

But within this complex background against which the first American debate on abortion emerged, we can trace a more direct social struggle. The most visible interest group agitating for more restrictive abortion laws was composed of elite or "regular" physicians, who actively petitioned state legislatures to pass anti-abortion laws and undertook through popular writings a campaign to change public opinion on abortion. The efforts of these physicians were probably the single most important influence in bringing about nineteenth-century anti-abortion laws. (Ironically, a century later it would be physicians who would play a central role in overturning these same laws.) Even more important is the fact that nineteenth-century physicians opposed abortion as part of an effort to achieve other political and social goals, and this led them to frame their opposition to abortion in particular ways.

PHYSICIANS IN THE NINETEENTH CENTURY

Modern observers accustomed to thinking of the medical profession as prestigious, technically effective, and highly paid are sometimes shocked to learn that it was none of those things in the nineteenth century. On the contrary, much of its history during that century was an uphill struggle to attain just those attributes. Whereas European physicians entered the modern era with at least the legacy of well-defined guild structures—structures that took responsibility for teaching, maintained the right to determine who could practice, and exercised some control over the conduct and craft of the profession—American physicians did not. Because of its history as a colony, the United States attracted few guild-trained physicians, and consequently, a formal guild structure never developed. Healing in this country started out primarily as a domestic rather than a professional skill (women and slaves often developed considerable local reputations as healers), and therefore anyone who claimed medical talent could practice—and for the most part could practice outside of any institutional controls of the sort that existed in Europe.

From the earliest days of the medical profession in this country, therefore, physicians wanted effective licensing laws that would do for them what the guild structures had done for their European colleagues, namely, restrict the competition.

For the first third of the century, physicians had depended on a model of illness that called upon the use of drastic medical treatments such as bleeding or the administration of harsh laxatives and emetics. By the 1850s, a new group of physicians (including such luminaries as Oliver Wendell Holmes) rejected the use of this "heroic armamentarium" and earned for themselves the sobriquet of "therapeutic nihilists" inasmuch as they seemed to argue that anything a physician could do was probably ineffective and might be dangerous as well.

Two other developments in the course of the century kept the social and professional status of medicine low. First, as the effectiveness of "heroic" medicine was called into question by some physicians themselves, there was a proliferation of healers who advocated new models of treatment. Thomsonians, botanics, and homeopaths among others all developed "sects" of healing and claimed the title of doctor for themselves. These nineteenth-century sectarians flourished, perhaps in part because they intended to support relatively mild forms of treatment (baths, natural diets) instead of the "heroic" measures used by many doctors. Thus, regular physicians (those who had some semblance of formal training and who subscribed to the dominant medical model) found themselves in increasing competition with the sectarians, who they considered quacks. . . .

ABORTIONS IN NINETEENTH-CENTURY AMERICA

With respect to abortion, as with respect to physicians, modern-day stereotypes about the nineteenth century can easily lead us astray. Contrary to our assumptions about "Victorian morality," the available evidence suggests that abortions were frequent. To be sure, some of these abortions may have been disguised (or rationalized) by those who sought them. Early in the century, a dominant therapeutic model saw the human body as an "intake-outflow" system and disease as the result of some disturbance in the regular production of secretions. Prominent among medical concerns, therefore, was "blocked" or "obstructed" menstruation, and the nineteenth-century pharmacopoeia contained numerous emmenagogues designed to "bring down the courses," that is, to reestablish menstruation. However, since the primary cause of "menstrual obstruction" in a healthy and sexually active woman was probably pregnancy, at least some of these emmenagogues must have been used with the intent to cause an abortion. Especially in the absence of accurate pregnancy tests, these drugs could be used in good faith by physicians and women alike, but the frequent warnings that these same drugs should not be used by "married ladies" because they would cause miscarriage made their alternative uses quite clear. . . .

PHYSICIANS AND ABORTION

In the second half of the nineteenth century, abortion began to emerge as a social problem: newspapers began to run accounts of women who had died from "criminal abortions," although whether this fact reflects more abortions, more lethal abortions, or simply more awareness is not clear. Most prominently, physicians became involved, arguing that abortion was both morally wrong and medically dangerous.

The membership of the American Medical Association (AMA), founded in 1847 to upgrade and protect the interests of the profession, was deeply divided on many issues. But by 1859, it was able to pass a resolution condemning induced abortion and urging state legislatures to pass laws forbidding it; in 1860, Henry Miller, the president-elect of the association, devoted much of his presidential address to attacking abortion; and in 1864, the AMA established a prize to be awarded to the best anti-abortion book written for the lay public. Slowly, physicians responded to the AMA's call and began to lobby in state legislatures for laws forbidding abortion.

Why should nineteenth-century physicians have become so involved with the question of abortion? The physicians themselves gave two related explanations for their activities, and these explanations have been taken at face value ever since. First, they argued, they were compelled to address the abortion questions because American women were committing a moral crime based on ignorance about the proper value of embryonic life. According to these physicians, women sought abortions because the doctrine of quickening led them to believe that the embryo was not alive, and therefore aborting it was perfectly proper. Second, they argued, they were obliged to act in order to save women from their own ignorance because only physicians were in possession of new scientific evidence which demonstrated beyond a shadow of doubt that the embryo was a child from conception onward.

The physicians were probably right in their belief that American women did not consider abortion—particularly early abortion—to be morally wrong. But the core of the physicians' claim—the assertions that women practiced abortion because they were ignorant of the biological facts of pregnancy and that physicians were opposed to it because they were in possession of new scientific evidence—had no solid basis in fact. . . .

MOTIVES FOR MOBILIZATION

Thus, the question remains: Why, in the middle of the nineteenth century, did some physicians become active anti-abortionists? James Mohr, in a pioneering work on this topic, argues that the proliferation of healers in the nineteenth century created a competition for status and clients. The "regular" physicians, who tended to be both wealthier and better educated than members of other medical sects, therefore sought to distinguish themselves both scientifically and socially from competing practitioners.

Mohr suggests that there were several more practical reasons why regular physicians should have opposed abortion. On the one hand, outlawing abortion would remove a lucrative source of income from competitors they called "quacks" and perhaps remove the temptation from the path of the "regulars" as well. In addition, the "regulars" were predominantly white, upper-income, and native-born; as such, they belonged to precisely the same group that was thought to harbor the primary users of abortion. As a result, they were likely to be concerned both about the depopulation of their group in the face of mounting immigration (and the higher fertility of immigrants) and about "betrayal" by their own women (because abortion required less male control and approval than the other available forms of birth control).

More broadly, Mohr argues that nineteenth-century physicians had a firm ideological belief that abortion was in fact murder. He asserts that they tended to place absolute value on human life and that having established to their own satisfaction that abortion represented the loss of human life, abortion became included in this more general value. The historian Carl Degler has made much the same argument: "Seen against the broad canvas of humanitarian thought and practice in Western society from the seventeenth to the twentieth century, the expansion of the definition of life to include the whole career of the fetus rather than only the months after quickening is quite consistent. It is in line with a number of movements to reduce cruelty and to expand the concept of sanctity of life." . . .

By the middle of the nineteenth century, American physicians had few if any of the formal attributes of a profession. The predominance of proprietary medical schools combined with the virtual absence of any form of licensing meant that the regulars could control neither entry into the profession nor the performance of those who claimed healing capacities. With the possible exceptions of the thermometer, the stethoscope, and the forceps, the technological tools of modern medicine were yet to come; and lacking the means of professional control, regular physicians were hard put to keep even those simple instruments out of the hands of the competition. Because they could offer no direct, easily observable, and dramatic proof of their superiority, regular physicians were forced to make an indirect, *symbolic* claim about their status. By becoming visible activists on an issue such as abortion, they could claim both *moral stature* (as a high-minded, self-regulating group of professionals) and *technical expertise* (derived from their superior training).

Therefore the physicians' choice of abortion as the focus of their moral crusade was carefully calculated. Abortion, and only abortion, could enable them to make symbolic claims about their status. Unlike the other medico-moral issues of the time—alcoholism, slavery, venereal disease, and prostitution—only abortion gave physicians the opportunity to claim to be saving human lives. Given the primitive nature of medical practice, persuading the public that embryos were human lives and then persuading the state legislatures to protect these lives by outlawing abortion may have been one of the few life-saving projects actually available to physicians.

Physicians, therefore, have to exaggerate the differences between themselves and the lay public. Anti-abortion physicians had to claim that women place no value on embryonic life whereas they themselves ranked the embryo as a full human life, namely, as a baby. But these two positions, when combined, created an unresolvable paradox for physicians, a paradox that would haunt the abortion debate until the present day.

Ain't I a Woman?

SOJOURNER TRUTH

Sojourner Truth, "Ain't I a Woman?," speech delivered 1851. Women's Convention, Akron, Ohio.

Sojourner Truth (1797–1883) was born into slavery in New York State. She won her freedom in 1827, when that state emancipated its slaves. After working in New York City as a domestic for some years, she felt called by God to testify to the sins against her people. Dropping her slave name, Isabella, she took the symbolic name of Sojourner Truth. She spoke at camp meetings, private homes, wherever she could gather an audience. By midcentury she was well-known in antislavery circles and a frequent speaker at abolitionist gatherings.

Sojourner Truth consistently and actively identified herself with the cause of women's rights. She was the only black woman present at the First National Woman's Rights Convention in Worcester, Massachusetts, in 1850.

The following year Sojourner Truth spoke at a women's convention at Akron, Ohio, presided over by Frances D. Gage. Since Truth could neither read nor write, all her words have come down through history interpreted by other people, usually white women, all of whom had their own agendas. As Nell Irvin Painter points out in her 1996 book, Sojourner Truth: A Life, a Symbol, *"Truth depended upon disparate amanuenses for the preservation of her identity. They represented her according to their own lights, often in dialect of their own invention."*

The Akron speech was written down by Gage twelve years after it was spoken as a response to an article in The Atlantic Monthly *by Harriet Beecher Stowe. Where Stowe's version of Sojourner Truth emphasizes her religion, Gage emphasizes or invents anger. Specifically, the phrase "ar'nt I a woman?," sometimes written in dialect as "ain't I a woman?," was Gage's invention.*

Well, children, where there is so much racket there must be something out of kilter. I think that 'twixt the Negroes of the South and the women at the North, all talking about rights, the white men will be in a fix pretty soon. But what's all this here talking about?

That man over there says that women need to be helped into carriages, and lifted over ditches, and to have the best place everywhere. Nobody ever helps me into carriages, or over mud puddles, or gives me any best place! And ain't I a woman? Look at me! Look at my arm! I have ploughed and

planted, and gathered into barns, and no man could head me! And ain't I a women? I could work as much and eat as much as a man—when I could get it—and bear the lash as well! And ain't I a woman? I have borne thirteen children, and seen them most all sold off to slavery, and when I cried out with my mother's grief, none but Jesus heard me! And ain't I a woman?

Then they talk about this thing in the head; what's this they call it? [Intellect, someone whispers.] That's it, honey. What's that got to do with women's rights or Negro's rights? If my cup won't hold but a pint, and yours holds a quart, wouldn't you be mean not to let me have my little half-measure full?

Then that little man in black there, he says women can't have as much rights as man, 'cause Christ wasn't a woman! Where did your Christ come from? Where did you Christ come from? From God and a woman! Man had nothing to do with Him.

If the first woman God ever made was strong enough to turn the world upside down all alone, these women together ought to be able to turn it back, and get it right side up again! And now they is asking to do it, the men better let them.

Obliged to you for hearing me, and now old Sojourner ain't got nothing more to say.

On Motherhood

ELIZABETH CADY STANTON

Elizabeth Cady Stanton, excerpt from Alice S. Rossi, ed., *The Feminist Papers: From Adams to de Beauvoir,* New York: Bantam Books, 1973, pp. 399–401. Originally published in *Elizabeth Cady Stanton: As Revealed in Her Letters, Diary, and Reminiscences,* New York: Harper & Bros., 1922. Reprinted by permission.

Her public cause was "votes for women," but her private mission and personal creed was "self-reliance," particularly in matters of health. Elizabeth Cady Stanton—the boldest and most brilliant of nineteenth-century American feminists—was born on November 12, 1815, in upstate New York. The family was prosperous; her father was a judge and her mother was of aristocratic lineage. Of the Cadys' eleven children, only five daughters survived. As a girl Elizabeth studied homeopathy with her brother-in-law, Dr. Edward Bayard. In 1840 she married Henry Stanton—abolitionist, co-founder of Oberlin College, and a follower of Sylvester Graham, a charismatic lecturer, father of the Graham cracker, and, the record suggests, the Gary Null of his era, known for his passionate advocacy of daily excercise combined with a balanced, largely vegetarian diet.

A neighbor, Amelia Bloomer, once wrote on the envelope of a letter she forwarded to Elizabeth, "People have nothing to talk about when you are gone!" That was because Elizabeth usually acted on her beliefs, however unpopular. When her hometown refused to open its tax-supported calisthenics classes to girls, she converted her barn into a gym and subversively offered instruction. Armed with her homeopathic manual and her herbs, she "doctored" her own and her neighbors' children through malaria, whooping cough, mumps, and broken limbs, and even helped deliver some of them.

For more than fifty years, there seemed to be no impediment to women's full equality that Elizabeth did not notice and attempt to rout: besides suffrage, she campaigned for birth control, property rights for wives, custody rights for mothers, equal wages, cooperative nurseries, coeducation, and "deliverance from the tyranny of self-styled medical, religious, and legal authorities." In a famous speech delivered in Rochester, New York, on August 2, 1948, she declared:

> Woman herself must do this work—for woman alone can understand the height, and the depth, the length, and the breadth of her own degradation and woe. Man cannot speak for us—because he has been educated to believe that we differ from him so materially that he cannot judge of our thoughts, feelings, and opinions on his own.

Through it all Elizabeth was a doting, hands-on mother of five sons and two daughters, born between 1842, when she was twenty-six, and 1859, when she was forty-three. It was said that if she wasn't already pregnant or nursing, Elizabeth conceived each time that Henry (a traveling man) came home. She so enjoyed the company of her children (permissively raised, energetic and uppity like their mom) that she moved her writing desk into their nursery.

The acid test of her maternal "self-reliance" occurred when her eldest, Daniel (called "Neil"), was born with a dislocated shoulder. The doctors she consulted set it in restrictive bandages, which made the condition worse. "With my usual conceit," she told Henry, "I removed the bandages and turned surgeon myself."

Here is the story in Stanton's own words, compiled by two of her younger children, Theodore Stanton and Harriot Stanton Blatch, in their old age, and published in 1922, eighty years after their mother first drew her line in the sand to protect and preserve their brother Neil.

Besides the obstinacy of the nurse, I had the ignorance of physicians to contend with. When the child was four days old we discovered that the collarbone was bent. The physician, wishing to get a pressure on the shoulder, braced the bandage round the wrist. "Leave that," he said, "ten days, and then it will be all right." Soon after he left I noticed that the child's hand was blue, showing that the circulation was impeded. "That will never do," said I. "Nurse, take it off." "No, indeed," she answered, "I shall never interfere with the doctor." So I took it off myself, and sent for another doctor, who was said to know more of surgery. He expressed great surprise that the first physician called should have put on so severe a bandage. "That," said he, "would do for a grown man, but ten days of it on a child would make him a cripple." However, he did nearly the same thing, only fastening it round the hand instead of the wrist. I soon saw that the ends of the fingers were all purple, and that to leave that on ten days would be as dangerous as the first. So I took it off.

"What a woman!" exclaimed the nurse. "What do you propose to do?" "Think out something better myself; so brace me up with some pillows and give the baby to me." She looked at me aghast. "Now," I said, talking partly to myself and partly to her, "what we want is a little pressure on that bone; that is what both of those men aimed at. How can we get it without involving the arm, is the question?" "I am sure I don't know," said she, rubbing her hands and taking two or three brisk turns around the room. "Well, bring me three strips of linen, four double." I then folded one, wet in arnica and water, and laid it on the collarbone, put two other bands, like a pair of suspenders over the shoulder, crossing them both in front and behind, pinning the ends to the diaper, which gave the needed pressure without impeding the circulation anywhere. As I finished she gave me a look of budding confidence, and seemed satisfied that all was well. Several times, night and day, we wet the compress and readjusted the bands, until all appearance of inflammation had subsided.

At the end of ten days the two sons of Aesculapius appeared and made their examination, and said all was right, whereupon I told them how badly their bandages worked, and what I had done myself. They smiled at each other, and one said, "Well, after all, a mother's instinct is better than a man's reason." "Thank you, gentlemen, there was no instinct about it. I did some hard thinking before I saw how I could get pressure on the shoulder without impeding the circulation, as you did." Thus, in the supreme moment of a young mother's life, when I needed tender care and support, the whole responsibility of my child's supervision fell upon me; but though uncertain at every step of my own knowledge, I learned another lesson in self-reliance. I trusted neither men nor books absolutely after this, either in regard to the heavens or the earth beneath, but continued to use my "mother's instinct," if "reason" is too dignified a term to apply to a woman's thoughts. My advice to every mother is, above all other arts and sciences, study first what relates to babyhood, as there is no department of human action in which there is such lamentable ignorance.

Why Elizabeth Isn't on Your Silver Dollar

BARBARA SEAMAN

©1999 by Barbara Seaman. Original for this publication.

November 12, 1895, Elizabeth Cady Stanton's eightieth birthday, found her enthroned on the stage of the Metropolitan Opera House, where 6,000 people had gathered to celebrate. Behind her, on the stage, red carnations spelled out her name in a field of white chrysanthemums, while roses banked her red velvet chair. Following three hours of ovations, tributes ("America's Grand Old Woman," "Queen Mother of American Suffragists"), and gifts—including an onyx-and-silver ballot box presented by a delegation of Mormon women from the Utah Territory—Stanton rose and gently reminded her admirers: "I am well aware that all these public demonstrations are not so much tributes to me as an individual as to the great idea I represent—the enfranchisement of women."

Two weeks later, she was in big trouble. Her book, *The Woman's Bible*, was published, and quickly became a best seller, but, according to her biographer Elisabeth Griffith, she was branded as a heretic by a stunned public. *The Woman's Bible* argued that "the chief obstacle in the way of woman's elevation today is the degrading position assigned her in the religion of all countries—an afterthought in creation, the origin of sin, cursed by God, marriage for her a condition of servitude, maternity a degradation, unfit to minister at the altar and in some churches even to sing in the choir." Elizabeth, whose mealtime grace was addressed to "Mother and Father God," proclaimed her belief in an androgynous creator and declared that the story of the expulsion from Eden was a myth. Far from being cursed, woman had been the originator and ruler of Amazonian societies before man seized control and subjugated her.

Humiliated by Elizabeth's "blasphemy," the younger, more "practical" leadership in the suffrage organizations shunned her, convinced that she, their founding mother, had recklessly jeopardized their cause. "They refused to read my letters and resolutions to the conventions; they have denounced *The Woman's Bible* unsparingly," Elizabeth wrote. Susan B. Anthony, Elizabeth's protégé and junior collaborator, was now put forward as the symbol and standard bearer of suffrage. Susan's name, alone, would attach to the 1920 Constitutional amendment; her face, alone, to the commemorative coin and stamp.

Elizabeth died in 1902, eighteen years before women got the vote, fifty-four years after she first demanded it, fifty-one years after she met Susan and recruited her to the cause. In the spirit of androgyny, Elizabeth's funeral service in her New York City apartment was conducted by a man assisted by the Reverend Antoinette Brown Blackwell. Her graveside service was conducted by a woman alone, the Reverend Phebe Hanaford.

Elizabeth was quite content in her old age despite (or perhaps because of) the controversy that her *Woman's Bible* inspired. As her biographer Lois Banner has written: "Politics was not really congenial to her. Independent by nature . . . the political mode of moderation, compromise, and slow progress did not fit her. Rather she preferred to shock her colleagues, to stir them out of complacency, to arouse their passions through introducing issues they had not considered. . . . Since the founding of the women's movement, she had seen her role as that of its radical conscience. . . . She had introduced suffrage in 1848 when the proposal had been new and shocking, [but now it was] accepted by all feminists and actually in force in the territories."

The following selections were written to stir readers out of complacency, to introduce issues they had not considered, and overall, to heighten our consciousness of woman's role in history.

Sylvia Bernstein Seaman (1900–95)

KAREN BEKKER

Karen Bekker, excerpt from Paula Hyman and Deborah Dash Moore, eds., *Jewish Women in America*, vol. 2, New York: Routledge, 1997. Reprinted by permission.

Sharon Batt, founder of Breast Cancer Action Montreal and author of Patient No More: The Politics of Breast Cancer, *remarked in 1999, "Many of the women who spoke out at the beginning . . . had been involved in activist politics before their diagnosis. But [other] women who wrote and spoke and lobbied had no such analysis. They just had breast cancer, and were more vulnerable to co-optation by vested interests."*

In that regard, I close this section in homage to my non-co-optable mother-in-law, Sylvia Seaman, who was born in 1900, played hooky from high school to participate in suffrage demonstrations, and helped introduce breast cancer activism in 1965 with the publication of her book, Always a Woman, *about the mastectomy she'd undergone a decade earlier. It was the first such book by a patient prying open the "closet door," as if in preparation for the transformative 1970s titles,* Why Me? *by Rose Kushner and* First You Cry *by Betty Rollin. Sylvia's book also publicized Reach to Recovery, the first and initially the most radical of breast cancer self-help organizations, which was acquired by the American Cancer Society in 1969 and then tamed down—if not co-opted. She died in 1995 when the breast cancer—diagnosed forty years before—caught up with her as she was preparing her speech for the Diamond Jubilee of the Nineteenth Amendment.*

I like to remind my children that their paternal grandmother may well have been the last living link between the politics of Elizabeth Cady Stanton, and the activist health feminists of today.

I'm still capable of marching. I marched sixty years ago. I just hope my granddaughter doesn't have to march into the next century." So said

Sylvia Bernstein Seaman to a *New York Times* reporter on the occasion of the tenth anniversary of the 1970 Women's Strike for Equality and the coinciding sixtieth anniversary of woman suffrage (Fig. 1). During her long life, she was not only a witness to but a catalyst for the dramatic changes in women's roles and status over the course of this century.

Sylvia Bernstein was born on November 8, 1900, to Nathan Bernstein and Fanny (Bleat) Bernstein. She had one sibling, a younger brother, Steven. She was active in the women's movement from a very young age and first marched for suffrage in 1915. While a student at Cornell University, she marched in the celebratory parades of 1920 when the Nineteenth Amendment was passed and was arrested for publicly wearing riding britches. This was, however, only the beginning of her career as a feminist. After spending several years teaching high school English in New York City, and marrying chemist William Seaman, in 1925, she began writing professionally.

Her first books were novels written in collaboration with her college roommate Frances Schwartz and published under the pen name Francis Sylvin. In 1965, she published *Always a Woman: What Every Woman Should Know about Breast Cancer*, a book based on her own experience of a mastectomy. This was the first book written about breast cancer by someone outside the medical profession. The topic, about which Seaman also wrote magazine and newspaper articles, was rarely discussed publicly in the early 1960s. In a 1980 interview, Seaman recalled, "It was considered daring at the time, but it changed attitudes, I think. . . . As for me, I got so much fan mail on that book, you'd have thought I was a movie star."

How to Be a Jewish Grandmother (1979) is a humorous book of advice and anecdotes. Any topic was fair game for Seaman: vasectomies, daughters-in-law, even her own drinking habits. Besides the discussion of what it meant to be Jewish, a woman, and a grandmother, the book was an indication of the changes American culture

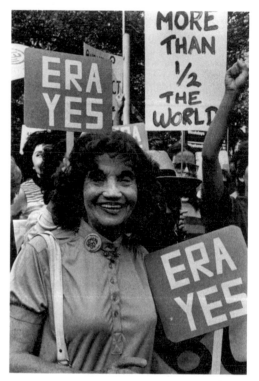

Figure 1: From marching for woman suffrage in 1915 to her groundbreaking book on breast cancer fifty years later to *How to Be a Jewish Grandmother*, Sylvia Seaman candidly and courageously explored a wide range of feminist issues. She is shown here in August 1980 leading a demonstration in celebration of sixty years of women's suffrage. [Carol Halebian]

had undergone in this century. *How to Be a Jewish Grandmother* is a record of the shifting social order of the 1970s, presented from the point of view of one who had herself rebelled against the norms of an earlier generation, but who may have been just a little bit bewildered by the transformations she was witnessing.

Seaman was not the only political activist in her family. Her son, Gideon Seaman, and daughter-in-law Barbara Seaman, coauthored *Women and the Crisis in Sex Hormones* in 1977; Barbara was also a co-founder of the National Women's Health Network. It was she who had encouraged Sylvia to write *Always a Woman*.

It was breast cancer that many years later caused Sylvia Bernstein Seaman's death, on January 8, 1995.

Fanny Burney's Letter to Her Sister, 1812, describing her mastectomy in September of 1811

FANNY BURNEY

Fanny Burney, excerpt from *Selected Letters and Journals*, London: Oxford University Press, 1986. Public Domain.

M. Dubois acted as Commander in Chief. Dr. Larry kept out of sight; M. Dubois ordered a Bed stead into the middle of the room. Astonished, I turned to Dr. Larry, who had promised that an Arm Chair would suffice; but he hung his head, & would not look at me. Two old mattresses M. Dubois then demanded, & an old Sheet. I now began to tremble violently, more with distaste & horror of the preparations even than of the pain. These arranged to his liking, he desired me to mount the Bed stead. I stood suspended, for a moment, whether I should not abruptly escape—I looked at the door, the windows—I felt desperate—but it was only for a moment, my reason then took the command, & my fears & feelings struggled vainly against it. I called to my maid—she was crying, & the two Nurses stood, transfixed, at the door. Let those women all go! cried M. Dubois. This order recovered me my Voice—No, I cried, let them stay! *qu'elles restent!* ("Let them remain!")

This occasioned a little dispute, that re-animated me—the maid, however, & one of the nurses ran off—I charged the other to approach, & she obeyed. M. Dubois now tried to issue his commands *en militaire*, but I resisted all that were resistible—I was compelled, however, to submit to taking off my long robe de Chambre, which I had meant to retain—Ah, then, how did I think of my Sisters!—not one, at so dreadful an instant, at hand, to protect—adjust—guard me—I regretted that I had refused Mile de Maisonneuve—Mile Chastel—no one upon whom I could rely—my departed Angel!—how did I think of her!—how did I long—long for my Esther—my Charlotte! —

My distress was, I suppose, apparent, though not my Wishes, for M. Dubois himself now softened, & spoke soothingly. Can You, I cried, feel for an operation that, to You, must seem so trivial?—Trivial? he repeated—taking up a bit of paper, which he tore, unconsciously, into a million of pieces, *Oui—c'est peu de chose—mais* ("Yes, it is a little thing, but . . .")—he stammered, & could not go on. No one else attempted to speak, but I was softened myself, when I saw even M. Dubois grow agitated, while Dr. Larry kept always aloof, yet a glance showed me he was pale as ashes. I knew not, positively, then, the immediate danger, but every thing convinced me danger was hovering about me, & that this experiment could alone save me from its laws. I mounted, therefore, unbidden, the Bed stead—& M. Dubois placed me upon the mattress, & spread a cambric handkerchief upon my face.

It was transparent, however, & I saw, through it, that the Bedstead was instantly surrounded by the seven men & my nurse. I refused to be held; but when, Bright through the cambric, I saw the glitter of polished Steel—I closed my Eyes. I would not trust to convulsive fear the sight of the terrible incision. A silence the most profound ensued, which lasted for some minutes, during which, I imagine, they took their orders by signs, & made their examination—Oh what a horrible suspension!—I did not breathe—& M. Dubois tried vainly to find any pulse. This pause, at length, was broken by Dr. Larry, who, in a voice of solemn melancholy, said *Qui me tiendra ce sein?* ("Who will hold the center?")—No one answered; at least not verbally; but this aroused me from my passively submissive state, for I feared they imagined the whole breast infected—feared it too justly—for, again through the Cambric, I saw the hand of M. Dubois held up, while his forefinger first described a straight line from top to bottom of the breast, secondly a Cross, & thirdly a Circle; intimating that the WHOLE was to be taken off.

Excited by this idea, I started up, threw off my veil, &, in answer to the demand *Qui me tiendra ce sein?* cried *C'est moi, Monsieur!* & I held my hand under it, & explained the nature of my sufferings, which all sprang from one point, though they darted into every part. I was heard attentively, but in utter silence, & M. Dubois then replaced me as before, &, as before, spread my veil over my face. How vain, alas, my representation! immediately again I saw the fatal finger describe the Cross—& the circle—Hopeless, then, desperate, & self-given up, I closed once more my Eyes, relinquishing all watching, all resistance, all interference, & sadly resolute to be wholly resigned.

My dearest Esther,—& all my dears to whom she communicates this doleful ditty, will rejoice to hear that this resolution once taken, was firmly adhered to, in defiance of a terror that surpasses all description, & the most torturing pain. Yet—when the dreadful steel was plunged into the breast—cutting through veins—arteries—flesh—nerves—I needed no injunctions not to restrain my cries. I began a scream that lasted unremittingly during the whole time of the incision—& I almost marvel that it rings not in my Ears still! so excruciating was the agony. When the wound was made, & the instrument was withdrawn, the pain seemed undiminished, for the air that suddenly rushed into those delicate parts felt like a mass of minute but sharp & forked poniards, that were tearing the edges of the wound—but when again I felt the instrument—describing a curve—cutting against the grain, if I may so say, while the flesh resisted in a manner so forcible as to oppose & tire the hand of the operator, who was forced to change from the right to the left—then, indeed, I thought I must have expired.

I attempted no more to open my Eyes—they felt as if hermetically shut, & so firmly closed, that the Eyelids seemed indented into the Cheeks. The instrument this second time withdrawn, I concluded the operation over—Oh no! presently the terrible cutting was renewed—& worse than ever, to separate the bottom, the foundation of this dreadful gland from the parts to which it adhered—Again all description would be baffled—yet again all was not over—Dr. Larry rested but his own hand, &—Oh Heaven!—I then felt the Knife tackling against the breast bone—scraping it!—This performed, while I yet remained in utterly speechless torture, I heard the Voice of Mr. Larry,—(all others guarded a dead silence) in a tone nearly tragic, desire everyone present to pronounce if anything more remained to be done; the general voice was Yes,—but the finger of Mr. Dubois—which I literally felt elevated over the wound, though I saw nothing, & though he touched nothing, so indescribably sensitive was the spot—pointed to some further requisition—& again began the scraping!—and, after this, Dr Moreau thought he discerned a peccant atom—and still, & still, M. Dubois demanded atom after atom.

My dearest Esther, not for days, not for Weeks, but for Months I could not speak of this terrible business without nearly again going through it! I could not think of it with impunity! I was sick, I was disordered by a single question—even now, nine months after it is over, I have a headache from going on with the account! & this miserable account, which I began three months ago, at least, I dare not revise, nor read, the recollection is still so painful.

To conclude, the evil was so profound, the case so delicate, & the precautions necessary for preventing a return so numerous, that the operation, including the treatment & the dressing, lasted twenty minutes! a time, for sufferings so acute, that was hardly supportable—However, I bore it with all the courage I could exert, & never moved, nor stopt them, nor resisted, nor remonstrated, nor spoke—except once or twice, during the dressings, to say *Ab Messieurs! que je vous plains!*—for indeed I was sensible to the feeling concern with which they all saw what I endured, though my speech was principally—very principally meant for Dr. Larry. Except this, I uttered not a syllable, save, when so often they recommended, calling out *Avertissez moi, Messieurs! avertissez moi!* ("Tell me!")—Twice, I believe, I fainted; at least, I have two total chasms in my memory of this transaction, that impede my tying together what passed.

When all was done, & they lifted me up that I might be put to bed, my strength was so totally annihilated, that I was obliged to be carried, & could not even sustain my hands & arms, which hung as if I had been lifeless; while my face, as the Nurse has told me, was utterly colourless. This removal made me open my Eyes—& I then saw my good Dr Larry, pale nearly as myself, his face streaked with blood, its expression depicting grief, apprehension, & almost horror. When I was in bed,—my poor M. d'Arblay—who ought to write you himself his own history of this Morning—was called to me—& afterwards our Alex.

Women's Health and Government Regulation: 1820–1949

SUZANNE WHITE JUNOD

©1999 by Suzanne White Junod. Reprinted by permission.

Suzanne White Junod, a historian with the Food and Drug Administration, has compiled an original review of health issues over which women consumers organized to obtain government protection. In 1933, Eleanor Roosevelt was so impressed by an FDA "Chamber of Horrors" exhibit of dangerous drugs and cosmetics that she "moved it directly to the White House and showed it to anybody who would look," setting the stage for passage of the 1938 Food, Drugs, and Cosmetics Act.

On the other hand, "the first state statutes regulating abortion were, in fact, poison control laws. The sale of commercial abortifacients was banned but not abortion per se." In 1902, "the editors of the Journal of the American Medical Association *endorsed a policy of denying medical care to a woman who was suffering from abortion complications until she 'confessed.' This practice prevented women from seeking timely medical treatment. By the late 1920s an estimated 15,000 women a year were dying from abortions."*

Women have always taken the lead in protecting themselves and their families from impure foods and dangerous drugs and medical devices. In the last two centuries, largely as a result of pressure from women, government agencies have taken an increasing interest in women's health issues: fertility, childbirth, menopause, geriatrics, and general nutrition and well-being. Following is a chronology of the regulation of products and devices affecting women's health.

THE NINETEENTH CENTURY

ABORTION During the nineteenth century, the abortion business, including the sale of widely advertised abortifacient drugs, was booming. Commercial preparations were so widely available that they inspired their own euphemism: "taking the trade." The first state statutes regulating abortion were in fact poison-control laws. The sale of commercial abortifacients was banned, but not abortion per se.

In June 1895, at the meeting of the Washington DC, Obstetrical and Gynecological Society, Dr. Joseph Taber Johnson encouraged his colleagues to begin a crusade against abortion. They had to convince both women and the medical profession that abortion was wrong. In 1902, the editors of the *Journal of the American Medical Association* endorsed a policy of denying medical care to a woman who was suffering from abortion complications until she "confessed." This practice prevented women from seeking timely treatment. By the late 1920s, an estimated 15,000 women were dying from abortions each year.

DRUGS AND UNSAFE ADDITIVES In 1880, Peter Collier, chief chemist at the US Department of Agriculture, recommended a national food and drug law. Twelve years later, in 1892, the law (known as the Paddock bill) did pass the Senate, but it was not taken up by the House of Representatives.

By the turn of the century, women were actively agitating against the use of opium, morphine, and laudanum in so-called baby-soothing syrups, used to calm colicky babies. Women's groups (most notably the General Federation of Women's Clubs) and muckraking journalists also exposed the high alcohol content of most of the women's proprietary "tonics." Unlike men, who drank openly in saloons, women frequently became addicted to alcohol under the guise of self-medication and nursed their addictions surreptitiously at home.

The Women's National Labor League (later the National Women's Industrial League) decided to take matters into their own hands by putting direct pressure on the National Wholesale Druggists Association at their annual convention in Washington DC. They tried to present the association with a petition that, in effect, called for full disclosure and honesty in advertising.

Since the industrial classes could not always afford adequate medical care, said the league women, it was important that the proprietary remedies on which they depended should be reliable. Therefore, the products should be sold under fully informative labels that would show what was in them but not carry fraudulent claims about their therapeutic value. Furthermore, such products as Mrs. Winslow's Soothing Syrup, which contained morphine and was innocently given to babies, should be taken off the market entirely. Haughtily the druggists told them that unless the reference to Mrs. Winslow's was struck out, they would not entertain the petition.

The women refused. They had drawn up the petition to express their own views, not to please the druggists; now they threatened to move on to Capitol Hill. Thoroughly alarmed, the druggists warned them that if they did anything of the kind and a clause directed against patent medicines found its way into the food and drug bill, the industry would spend half a million dollars to defeat the measure.

Despite the druggists' threat, the women went straight to Capitol Hill and informed members of Congress that it was not enough to prosecute the shippers who violated the law; their adulterated and misbranded merchandise had to be confiscated and destroyed as well. When the Food and Drug Act finally passed in 1906, it contained a provision

for the seizure of illegal foods and drugs, largely as a result of the women's pressure. According to Ruth Lamb, who wrote *American Chamber of Horrors* in the 1930s advocating the need for a new federal food and drug statue:

> The full significance of this provision seems not to have been appreciated by anyone at the time, for it remained in succeeding food and drug bills and was finally enacted into law—to become the most hated and bitterly contested feature of the whole statute. To that perspicacious group of women in the 1890s, and their leader, Charlotte Smith, the public is forever indebted, for this single provision of the Food and Drugs Act has been, beyond all cavil, the government's most powerful weapon against dangerous or fraudulent products.

The drug-labeling provisions of the 1906 act required that the percentages of alcohol and other "dangerous" ingredients be clearly listed on the label. Although this early law did not make such products illegal, it did at least prevent them from being sold as "cures" for alcoholism. As a result, manufacturers generally reduced the amount of alcohol in their products and replaced the opium, laudanum, and morphine with less dangerous ingredients that did not have to be disclosed on the label itself.

THE EARLY TWENTIETH CENTURY

The Nineteenth Amendment granting women's suffrage was ratified on August 18, 1920. This was also a time of important medical discoveries.

➤ In 1922, Banting, Best, Macleod, and Collip at the University of Toronto announced the discovery of insulin as a treatment of diabetes mellitus. Their first patient was a fourteen-year-old girl, who, after initiating injections of insulin, lived to the ripe old age of seventy-seven.

➤ By 1922, radical mastectomy, introduced by

William Halsted, had become the standard "cure" for breast cancer. Lung tissue, but not the soft tissue of the breasts, could be seen on X-rays.

➤ In 1927, Aurel Babes published an article in France discussing the possibility of cancer diagnosis from vaginal smears. His method was substantially different from the one developed later by George Papanicolaou, who published his "New Cancer Diagnosis" a year later in the *Proceedings of the Third Race Betterment Foundation*.

➤ In 1927, Congress enacted the Caustic Poison Act requiring warning labels to protect children from accidental death and injury caused by lye and ten other caustic chemicals. The campaign for passage of the act was led by Dr. Chevalier Jackson and supported by the American Medical Association. The Food and Drug Administration (FDA) was given enforcement responsibilities.

➤ In 1928, Alexander Fleming discovered penicillin (which did not become available for widespread clinical use in civilian populations until 1945). Deaths from childbed or puerpheral fever dropped dramatically as a result of penicillin and other antibiotics.

WOMEN'S PRODUCTS CHAMBER OF HORRORS

During the 1920s, as women became more active outside the home, the cosmetics industry grew out of obscurity into a multimillion-dollar industry. Women's and consumer groups became concerned about the dangers of some of these new cosmetic products, notably hair dyes and rouges, as well as the safety of such devices as womb pessaries, bust enhancers, and nose straighteners; women's "tonics"; and the unrestricted use of amphetamines and other weight reduction drugs.

In the summer of 1933, the FDA set up an exhibit illustrating abuses in the sale of food, drugs, and cosmetics not covered by the Food and Drug Act of 1906. A number of the women's beauty and diet aids in the exhibit—hair dyes, depilatories, pessaries, skin whiteners—contained dangerous poisons such as lead, silver, pyrogallol, mercury, thyroid, thallium acetate, barium sulfide, and paraphenylene diamine. Other products made false or inflated claims.

After viewing the exhibit, Eleanor Roosevelt took up the cause. She had the exhibit moved from the offices of the FDA directly to the White House and showed it to anybody who would look. But, according to a Washington *Star* account, "the politicians paid absolutely no attention to her. They regarded her as a nuisance and didn't think that there were any votes involved in it, and she had no effect at all except as she worked through the women's organizations. And, of course, she did this a lot." She appealed to the nation's women to join the campaign for a new, more all-encompassing law. This set the stage for the passage of the 1938 Food, Drug, and Cosmetics Act.

The new law expanded the FDA's regulatory powers. Under the 1906 act, thyroid preparations were a drug, but because obesity was not considered a disease, the agency could not act against these preparations. But under the new law, the FDA could act against drugs designed *to change the structure of the body* (thyroid increased metabolism). The new law also allowed action against radium waters and radiopharmaceuticals (previously thought to be "natural") as well as nose straighteners and womb pessaries, all of which were now classified as drugs.

The new law also had a direct impact on the quality of prophylactics. The FDA announced that regardless of the nature of the products, or the methods in which they were used, all articles intended as "venereal disease preventives" were subject to the provisions of the act, and that articles depending for their prophylactic effect on preventing contact with infecting organisms should be free from defects. In an extensive survey of rubber and membrane prophylactics, 181 consignments seized from nine manufacturers were found to be defective. As a result, producers withdrew much of their outstanding stocks and made drastic changes in their manufacturing processes.

Another product that had a great impact on women's lives was the tampon. By 1921, there were at least sixteen patents for tampons and one for a tampon applicator. Their use was limited to the treatment of disease. In 1933, Dr. Earle Hass patented the tampon that was introduced three years later in improved form as the Tampax tampon. Doctors and nurses actively promoted disposable sanitary pads and tampons in the increasingly "antiseptic" culture. Women viewed these products as practical and labor-saving. By 1947, 538 gross dozens, with a value of $11,099,000 were shipped to retailers. Tampons had been accepted.

THE 1940S: DIAGNOSING CANCER IN WOMEN

By the 1940s, 26,000 American women were dying of uterine cancer every year. George Papanicolaou and Herbert Traut published "The Diagnostic Value of Vaginal Smears in Carcinoma of the Uterus" in the *American Journal of Obstetrics and Gynecology*. This article presented their technique for obtaining a smear and their theory of exfoliative cytology, which allows the interpretation of the smears and the detection of malignancy. The National Cancer Institute estimates that between 1950 and 1970, deaths from cervical cancer dropped 70 percent. The decrease in cancer deaths was a direct result of the Pap smear.

Realizing the need for better breast imaging, Stafford Warren, a pioneer in radiation at the UCLA School of Medicine, developed a stereoscopic grid system for identifying malignant breast tumors. In 1949, John Wild applied ultrasound to distinguish malignant from healthy tissues. That same year, Paul Leborgne from Uruguay demonstrated the importance of high-contrast breast images in about 30 percent of the cases he examined, and established the value of breast compression in identifying benign and malignant breast tumors.

BRAVE NEW WORLD

In 1937, the *New England Journal of Medicine* carried an anonymous editorial discussing the possibility of conception in a watch glass as a future treatment of dysfunctional fallopian tubes. In 1940, Charles Huggins first reported the value of diethylstilbestrol (DES) in the treatment of prostate tumors. In 1944, after six years of intense experimentation, John Rock, a birth control pioneer, and a colleague claimed in vitro fertilization of a human ovum. The procedure and their results were accompanied with pictures and published in *Science*. In 1949, Barr and his colleagues noted that it was possible to distinguish male and female cells from the presence or absence of a small cellular body. Knowing the sex of the fetus had implications for families with histories of sex-linked diseases.

No one could have predicted where all this would lead in the second half of the twentieth century.

A My Name Is Alice

JENNIFER BAUMGARDNER

Jennifer Baumgardner, excerpt from "My Name Is Alice: The Story of the Feminist Playmate," *MAMM*, October/November 1998. Reprinted by permission.

THE TIME: THE EARLY FIFTIES THE PLACE: NEW YORK CITY'S GREENWICH VILLAGE

Alice Denham, a fiercely independent and dazzling redhead with a master's degree in English and a Phi Beta Kappa from the University of North Carolina, comes to the Big Apple to make it as a writer. From a poor but genteel Southern family, the pert but steely gamine applies for job after job in publishing. Within a few days of pounding the pavement in her pumps, Alice's innocence is shattered: There aren't any jobs for women in publishing in 1953. There might as well be a sign that says "Girls Keep Out!" hanging over the city rather than the promising glitter of the New York skyline at night. "Screw the bastards!" Alice declares as she pours herself a teacup full of whiskey and tries to work out plan B: the one where she can get the respect she deserves in this macho town. Or so Alice Denham's story might begin if it was a novel written by Alice Denham herself. Still petite and red-haired with a drawl that suspends her words in honey and belies her Jacksonville, Florida upbringing, Denham really did move to New York City in the bohemian fifties to find that she couldn't even get interviewed. "All they wanted was secretaries," she says, doll-sized and grinning, dwarfed by the average-sized table of a West Village tea salon. "And I had purposefully not taken shorthand to avoid that fate." Denham decided to focus on writing full-time. No one needed to give her permission to do that. "Writing was the only thing I ever wanted to be or to do, so I decided I would be a writer if it killed me." All she needed in order to get started was a job that paid well and didn't require a lot of time.

CHAPTER 2: ALICE BECOMES A PINUP MODEL

"I was living with a friend who was an actress, and she introduced me to a model. People had asked me to pose for photos from time to time, and soon I started to be sent out for doing romance novel covers," she says, as matter-of-factly as she had mentioned her undeserved reputation as a slut in college (the president of a powerful fraternity sought retribution after she refused to date him) and her breast cancer ten years ago (lying on her back, she noticed her breast was at a 90-degree angle) during the first few moments upon arriving. Modeling a few hours a week to pay the bills, she taught herself to write a novel during the rest of the week by observation, fiction technique books, and "trial and error." Poring over Dostoyevsky in her Village apartment, Denham gleaned the magic of a strong lead, the art of withholding information,

the importance of characterization. Still, "it took me a very long time to write my first novel." She did, indeed, finish her novel, and a few more, but first came a serendipitous piece of fiction called "The Deal." Originally published in the then-prestigious literary magazine *Discovery,* the story centers on a rich man who is so taken with a beautiful woman that he offers her $1,000 to sleep with him once. At that time (the mid-fifties) another magazine was printing serious (read: male) fiction: *Playboy.* Given her day job, our uppity heroine had an idea. "I told my literary agent to say that if *Playboy* would reprint the story, I would be the centerfold." Soon Denham found herself at the Chicago airport, destined to be Miss July 1956, the only playmate to have a piece and be a piece in the same issue. "Hef met me at the airport. I thought he was the limo driver. He was so stiff and formal in his black suit that I got into the backseat of the car. He said, 'Sit up front.' I said, 'What?' He said, 'I'm Hugh Hefner.'" Denham pauses for a moment and then dishes about the man responsible for sexualizing the girl next door. "He was a really silly man, running around in pajamas, and he never grew up," she says, digging into her baked chicken breast. "Ultimately, we had sex," she continues, with a sigh. "It was all right, though he had to watch dirty movies. All of this is in my novel *Amo*— except I changed the names. I called the magazine 'Meat' and I called the Playmates 'Tidbits of the Month' and I called him 'Pelth Pedlar.' 'The Deal' was her break. Still, Denham admits her family was horrified by her national exposure, despite how tame the shots were back in the early days of girlie mags. That is, except for her brother, an Episcopal preacher, who assured Denham that she looked very cute. "The only thing I cared about modeling was would it pay enough to cover my monthly expenses," says the sixty-six-year-old. "The thing is, I wouldn't have to resort to *Playboy* nowadays," says Denham. "I could have been an assistant editor or a freelance writer."

CHAPTER 3: OUR HEROINE DISCOVERS THE WOMEN'S LIBERATION MOVEMENT

"I think all of my work has largely been about discrimination," says Denham. "Social, gender, all that stuff, one way or another." There was a thriving bohemian literary scene at the time of her arrival in New York, and Denham soon found herself amid the swirl. According to a piece in the *New York Observer* by Darius James, she dated James Jones, Philip Roth, spent a couple of "casual" evenings with Norman Mailer, and enjoyed a close "sexual friendship" with that fey icon of early-sixties cool, James Dean. But when it came time to blurb her book, these scribes of the masculine experience made themselves scarce. One assumes that Denham's memoir-in-progress entitled *Sleeping with the Boys* [published in 2006 as *Sleeping with Bad Boys*—Ed.] will do a little toward righting that slight, but it just so happened that she had discovered another downtown intellectual scene—one more interested in her body of work than in her body. As an early second-wave feminist, Denham came to the movement as part of the campaign to legalize abortion (which occurred in 1970 in New York and 1973 nationally) and was part of the original National Organization for Women chapter. As an associate professor at John Jay College at the City University of New York during the seventies, Denham handled an Equal Employment Opportunity Commission discrimination case that was settled in the faculty women's favor for $3.5 million. Always an independent, her work became even more confidently pro-woman. *My Darling from the Lions* concerned a feminist centerfold from outer space, and *Amo* chronicled a feminist's mad passion for her tragically sexist husband. Meanwhile, a movie, *Quizas*, was made from the *Playboy* story.

CHAPTER 4: CANCER

Then, ten years ago, when Denham was fifty-six and married for eight years to an accountant she had met in her part-time home of San Miguel de Allende, Mexico, she discovered breast cancer. "I think diagnosis refocuses your head," she says. "You no longer think so much about physical beauty or the beauty of your breasts. It's whether you're going to live or not." The former model didn't find that the mastectomy changed her body image so much; cancer affected her desire to create. "My work habits were always good, but I started working harder and faster. I wanted to complete all of these things that were halfway done." Her current regimen is an hour of exercise upon waking, breakfast—"If my husband is home and doesn't have work, he makes breakfast, washes the dishes, and then gets out of the house"—and then she writes all day.

CHAPTER 5: THE FUTURE

Alice Denham is working on a family saga called *Shabby Genteel: A Southern Girlhood* and the aforementioned memoir of her days in the Boho/prefeminist fifties and sixties. She spends summers in Mexico and the rest of the year in New York and writes and publishes in both locales. As for her cancer, there is no act two, but her last mammogram showed a burst of calcium which her doctors are watching for bad signs. Typically, Denham is candid about her mammography appointment. "They were going to do something awful called a mammotone where they lay you down on a table with your breast hanging down through a hole and they clamp it like a mammogram," she says, eyes rolling. "After taking my breast photos in about a thousand different ways they decided they couldn't do it because [the calcifications were] too close to the skin." She snorts. "Have you ever had a mammogram?" she inquires, peering across the table with a half smile on her face. "You wait."

CHAPTER 2

Taking Our Bodies Back

THE WOMEN'S HEALTH MOVEMENT

THE WOMAN ON THE COUCH is young, and her expression serious. She is talking about big changes going on in her world and she is passionate about them. Other young women, she says, are learning about their bodies. Learning about the basic landscapes and contours of a woman's most intimate places, about how to gain access to the best health care possible, about how to fight for desired rights and resist attempts to deny women basic health autonomy. This young woman feels she is at the center of a momentous change. She doesn't know, as she gestures and touches her mid-length brown hair in explaining a point, if it is a revolution. But she knows it is bigger than anything she has known in her lifetime. "There are some people who don't really want control over their lives, who prefer to let their doctors do the worrying for them or who are squeamish or whatever," her voice says. "However there's another group of us, and I used to think we were a minority. But now I'm starting to think that maybe we are the majority after all. We want control over our bodies. We want to like our bodies and feel comfortable in them and feel in control over our own lives."

I am that young woman, and I am narrating Margaret Lazarus's groundbreaking documentary, *Taking Our Bodies Back*. Lazarus made the film in 1973, just after she graduated from Vassar. The film depicts a number of topics that you'll read about in these pages: home births, abortion, the insensitivity of many male physicians, racism, self-help gynecology, women of all ages meeting to talk and to confide in each other on the subject of how they really feel about their bodies. We were coming to understand for the first time how numerous our common experiences were. We were acknowledging how many of them had to do with a health care system—and larger cultural outlook on female bodies—that was sexist, over-medicalized and based on preventing us from taking care of ourselves.

The Women's Health Movement, and the larger women's movement, started in deeply personal places—a sick baby, a traumatic birth, a botched abortion—and grew into a massive international phenomenon that changed the world.

In this section we give you some of the classic pieces and players of the movement. Where possible we are including interviews and bits of memoirs of women looking back on their work and looking forward to the challenges they see emerging in this new century of health activism.

The Role of Advocacy Groups in Research on Women's Health

BARBARA SEAMAN AND SUSAN F. WOOD

Barbara Seaman and Susan F. Wood, excerpt from Marlene B. Goldman and Maureen C. Hatch, eds., *Women & Health*, San Diego, Calif.: Academic Press, 2000. Reprinted by permission.

I. INTRODUCTION

Progress in women's health measured at the end of the twentieth century began in the early years of the century and is due to advances in public health, increases in scientific and clinical knowledge, and improved access to care. However, much of the overall improvement in health would not have been targeted to women without the involvement of advocates who worked to ensure that research and policies focused on the health of women. Dating back at least as far as 1913— when a news headline announced that "rich women begin a war on cancer"—medical research, policies, and practices in the twentieth century United States have been profoundly influenced by three distinct waves of women's health advocates: the first spearheaded by progressive wealthy women; the second by feminist activists; and the third by professionals, including doctors, scientists, legislators, lawyers, and corporate executives. Within each wave, key individuals and the organizations they founded or led identified their priority issues and advocated to make them priorities for the nation. They worked not only to

bring women's health to the top of the agenda but also to bring women's voices and input to the development of research initiatives and policies. This chapter reviews some of the key accomplishments of several of these advocates who laid the foundation for future progress in women's health.

II. THE FIRST WAVE: PROGRESSIVE LADIES

Elsie Mead, daughter of a New York gynecologist, and a friend of John D. Rockefeller, whom she enlisted in her cause, epitomizes the wealthy women of her day who took up various diseases as their "charity." Mead helped found, and vigorously chaired, the finance committee of the American Society for the Control of Cancer (ASCC), whose goal—by placing articles in the popular and medical press—was to substitute "a message of hope and early detection" for the fear, denial, secrecy, and despair attached to cancer diagnoses. The organization declined while Mead was in France for the Red Cross during World War I but, on her return, she wrote two thousand letters to people in the New York Social Register and got nearly 690 recruits, of whom many paid considerably more than the $5 membership fee.[1]

The ASCC languished during World War II but was rescued by Mary Woodard Lasker, a philanthropist, advocate, and art collector, who would eventually come to be recognized by insiders as "the most powerful person in modern medicine." She reorganized the ASCC as the American Cancer Society, expanded its budget from $102,000 to $14,000,000 in just five years (1943–48), and established a research program which, over time, would demonstrate the effectiveness of the Pap smear and find cures for childhood leukemia. Lasker modestly described herself as "a self-employed health lobbyist." In fact she was a consummate power broker who exercised unparalleled control over many aspects of health policy, generating tremendous publicity for research into cancer and other diseases, and flogging Congress to boost the budget of the National Institutes of Health (NIH) from $2.8 million in 1945 to $11 billion in 1994—the year she died at age ninety-three.

Lasker's success, according to her colleague, the lobbyist Mike Gorman, "was due to a high class kind of subversion, very high class." For example, she "made her way into the Kennedy White House by writing Jackie the first check—for $10,000—to redecorate the White House." She obtained the then-experimental drug L-dopa for the powerful Senator Lister Hill, whose wife had Parkinson's disease. Like Elsie Mead, Lasker courted influential journalists and leaned on her friends in the media, including Ann Landers, to support her advocacy campaigns. As Landers (herself no shrinking violet) recalls Lasker, "She was intimidating; everything about her was so strong."[2]

Ironically, Lasker's husband, Albert, an advertising genius, had created the slogan "Reach for a Lucky instead of a sweet" which persuaded millions of women to take up cigarette smoking. However, tobacco industry money led to the endowment of the annual Albert Lasker Medical Research Awards, originated in 1946, which have gone to support the work of fifty-two eventual Nobel Prize winners.

III. TRANSITIONAL ADVOCATES/ACTIVISTS OF THE 1950S AND EARLY 1960S

In the era following World War II, reproductive experimentation on women by medical doctors was unchecked such that faculty at prestigious institutions, including Harvard University, the University of Chicago, and Tulane University, fed hormones to healthy pregnant patients, often under the guise that they were vitamins to "grow bigger and better babies." The major hormone used, diethylstilbestrol (DES), was later found to be carcinogenic to both the mothers and their offspring. However, these same years also brought the first eruptions of what would later become a militant and sweeping feminist health movement that would profoundly alter the power relationship between male physicians and their once compliant female patients and transform medicine into a more welcoming profession for women.

Like Mead and Lasker, Doris Haire and Terese Lasser were associated with wealth. Haire's husband, John, managed money for the Vanderbilts, while Lasser's husband, J. K., wrote the perennial bestseller *Your Income Tax*. Each woman was "radicalized" by a hospital experience.

In 1951, at age twenty-six, Haire, part Cherokee, born in Oklahoma from the working class, delivered a healthy daughter in Pittsfield, Massachusetts. Wide awake and with her husband at her side, Haire got permission to follow the precepts of British natural-childbirth proponent Dr. Grantly Dick-Reed because, and only because, Anne Vanderbilt was principal patroness of the hospital and demanded compliance of the reluctant staff. Joyous, yet feeling "miserably over-privileged," Haire pondered why one had to be under Vanderbilt "protection" to be involved in decisions about one's own delivery and birth. Haire soon consecrated her life to study and activism, compiling a record as president of the International Childbirth Education Association (ICEA), the National Women's Health Network (NWHN), the American Foundation for Maternal and Child Health, and author of *The Cultural Warping of Childbirth* (1972), which has inspired, and provided the basis for, many subsequent books and articles and actions restoring birth rights to mothers. It is said that when Doris Haire marched down the halls at the Food and Drug Administration (FDA) the walls trembled, for in overcoming the opposition of both the medical and pharmaceutical industries, she has gotten that agency to withdraw approval for questionable drugs such as oxytocin in the induction of labor. Valuing results more than recognition, Haire has exemplified the activist adage "If you don't demand credit for things you can push them through."[3]

Terese "Ted" Lasser wrote, when recalling her

Halsted radical mastectomy performed following her biopsy at New York's Memorial Hospital in 1952 while she was still unconscious and without prior discussion, "You awake to find yourself wrapped in bandages from midriff to neck—bound like a mummy in surgical gauze, somewhere deep inside you a switch is thrown and your mind goes blank. You do not know what to think, you do not want to guess, you do not want to know."

With good reason, the Halsted radical mastectomy has been called "the greatest standardized surgical error of the twentieth century." Introduced in the 1880s by William Halsted, a surgeon at Johns Hopkins Hospital, it was debilitating, even crippling, and based on Halsted's unproven belief that breast cancer was a local disease that could be fully, if brutally, excised before it spread.

Soignée, energetic, and imperious, Lasser was unaccustomed to being patronized or hustled and was furious at the doctor's failure to state her options prior to her surgery. Later, neither her surgeon nor anyone else at Memorial Hospital would give her the specific information she demanded on treatments or exercises to regain the use of her arm, when or how to resume sexual relations, or even how to shop for a "falsie." Determined not to become a cripple, Lasser herself developed an innovative program of stretch exercises through which she regained her strength; better yet, she concluded, would have been to start exercising right after surgery.

A compulsion came over Lasser to teach what she knew. Founding Reach to Recovery (R2R), Lasser adopted a practice of slipping into the hospital rooms of new "mastectomees," exhorting them to arise from their beds and crawl the fingers of their affected arms up the wall. Lasser personally counseled thousands of patients. Most who had the stamina to do the work showed results that seemed "miraculous" to their doctors, who were ultimately convinced.

Lasser maintained a pretense that her calls were made at the requests of the patients' surgeons or families. In truth, in the early years she was often "escorted out the front door of Memorial Hospital when she was found visiting patients at random and without the consent of the responsible surgeon."[4] In 1969, R2R merged with the American Cancer Society, becoming tame and traditional, activists say, such that they now find it hard to appreciate Lasser's courage or the ground that she first broke.

In 1960, the widespread use of the drug thalidomide in nearly twenty countries set off an epidemic of limbless babies born to mothers whose doctors prescribed a "mild sedative." Evidence of the link was discovered and published in West Germany in November 1961 but was not reported here and was obscured by the US manufacturer, Merrell, who had furnished nearly 1,100 doctors with samples of the drug and who followed up with warning letters to only 10 percent of them. At the FDA, medical officer Dr. Frances Oldham Kelsey, who had resisted pressure to approve thalidomide, was also not informed by her superiors that they had received the West German reports. In 1962, after the *Washington Post* broke the story, Dr. Kelsey received the Presidents Award for Distinguished Federal Civilian Service, but the revelations had come too late for Sherri Finkbine, a thalidomide-exposed pregnant woman whose local hospital refused her request for an abortion following that exposure and whose harrowing well-publicized odyssey took her to Sweden for the procedure. By unflinchingly arguing her case in public, Finkbine aroused new sentiment for abortion law reform, which came to fruition in *Roe v. Wade* eleven years later.[5]

Another key figure in women's reproductive rights was Margaret Sanger, whose long years as an advocate left a mixed legacy. Folk heroine and ever-enlarging mythic figure, Sanger published *The Woman Rebel* in 1914, opened the first US birth control clinic in 1916, and founded the American Birth Control League (later to become Planned Parenthood) in 1921. Her great works notwithstanding, Sanger became an elitist, and in the early 1950s as Lasser and Haire drew their lines in the sand on the rights of women patients, Sanger was writing fund-raising letters to help Gregory Pincus develop the first "universal contraceptive," namely the birth control pill. In a letter to Katharine McCormick, heiress to a farm machinery fortune, Sanger states: "I consider that the world and almost our civilization for the next twenty-five years is going to depend upon a simple, cheap, safe contraceptive to be used in poverty-stricken slums and jungles, and among the most ignorant people . . . I believe that now, immediately, there should be national sterilization for certain dysgenic types of our population who are being encouraged to breed and would die out were the government not feeding them." In the 1920s, Sanger had thrown her lot in with physician advocates of birth control and seems also to have been influenced by "eugenics thinking which contributed to the transformation of the birth control movement, beginning in the 1920s, from a women's rights focus to a more conservative emphasis on family planning, understood as an appeal to responsible motherhood and population control."[6]

IV. PHASE TWO: MILITANT ACTIVISM

Post–World War II feminist advocacy, to combat sex discrimination in all spheres of life (social, political, economic, and psychological), surfaced with the forming of the National Organization of Women (NOW) in 1966. Most of its twenty-nine founders were middle-aged, middle class, Caucasian, and distinguished in areas such as academia and government service. Even Betty Friedan, author of the controversial bestseller *The Feminine Mystique*, was a member of the magazine journalist "establishment." At first, the public response to NOW was limited.

However, some of the issues Friedan and other traditional feminists brought up sparked recognition in radical young women who had been toiling in the activist movements of the 1960s: civil rights, antiwar, pro-student, socialist, and who had therefore had a training, somewhat

unique to late twentieth century women, in civil disobedience, demonstrating, organizing, and making headline news.

By 1969, social control, financial exploitation, and excessive medicalization of women through health care (especially obstetrics/gynecology and psychiatry) were major topics in their consciousness raising (CR) discussions. In May, Bread and Roses, a grassroots, socialist, and feminist group, held a gathering for several hundred women from the Boston area, at which social worker Nancy Miriam Hawley led a workshop called "Women and their Bodies." Participants hoped to come up with a list of good ob-gyn doctors, but, recalls Jane Pincus, "We realized we didn't know what questions to ask to find out if they were good or not." Hawley and Pincus began a study group at which they distributed copies of their research. A year and a half later, the forerunner of the Boston Women's Health Book Collective self-published its work, still called "Women and their Bodies" after Hawley's workshop, in a 138-page newsprint edition of findings, through the New England Free Press. Demand grew and the name changed to *Our Bodies, Ourselves.* They kept printing and expanding the "underground" booklet and had distributed 250,000 copies by 1973 when Simon and Schuster brought out the trade edition. At this point it became an international bestseller, described as "the most powerful revolutionary document since *Das Kapital* because it induced women to seize the means of Reproduction."[7]

Also in 1969, in the nation's capital, Alice Wolfson and other members of Washington, D.C. Women's Liberation were analyzing the "body issues," including specifically their disenchantment with the birth control pill, promoted as a great advance for women but apparently causing many more side effects (some lethal) than manufacturers or most prescribing doctors would acknowledge. They read a review by Victor Cohn in the *Washington Post* of a book by one of the authors of this chapter (Seaman), *The Doctors' Case Against the Pill*, and then they learned that Senate hearings, based on the book and chaired by Wisconsin Senator Gaylord Nelson, were to open on January 14, 1970. At issue was not primarily the safety of the pill, for British studies had established the blood-clotting associated deaths, but rather informed consent.

D.C. Women's Liberation, which was also a "feeder" for the radical feminist newspaper *Off Our Backs*, proved to be another history-bearing group. The very young observers/demonstrators whom Alice Wolfson rounded up to attend the Senate Pill Hearings included such future feminist heavyweights as Charlotte Bunch and Marilyn Salzman Webb. They arrived in "straight-lady" clothes and sat demurely through the first day of testimony, but, on the morning of the second day, as Dr. Roy Hertz, then Associate Medical Director of the Population Council at Rockefeller University, concluded his talk, which included pessimistic analysis of increased cancer risks among pill users, what the record describes as "a disturbance among several women in the audience" occurred. The Wolfson women peppered Hertz and Nelson with insistent questions such as "Why are no patients testifying?" and "Why isn't there a pill for men?" The world press was in attendance and was fascinated by the disruptions, which continued to occur throughout the nine days of hearing, which concluded March 4.[8]

Just one of the scientific experts whose testimony was interrupted was unafraid to declare his support in public. On January 23, Dr. Philip Corfman, Director of the Center for Population Research at NIH and a member of the FDA's Advisory Committee on the Pill, stated after the demonstrators were dragged away, as usual, by the guards, "Incidentally, some of the questions placed by the people who interrupted our hearing were quite important."[9] Corfman would soon prove to be the essential "insider" who, for example, notified advocates when the FDA's Pill Advisory Committee meetings were scheduled so that Alice Wolfson could appear demanding the right to observe because "it's our bodies you're talking about."

Wolfson's demonstrations, with the brilliant strategies and repetitions of deceptively simple questions, were to the women's health movement as the Boston Tea Party was to the American Revolution. As the magazine *Science* pointed out in its special issues on "Women's Health Research," "the dissent helped to launch a political movement focusing on women's health. By 1975, nearly two thousand women's self-help medical projects were scattered across the United States, many of them groups of volunteers without an institution."[10]

Although the NWHN did not formally incorporate until 1975, it grew out of the activist association of Seaman and Wolfson, along with three others who joined with them in the early 1970s. These founders included: Belita Cowan, publisher of *Herself Newspaper* in Ann Arbor, who exposed seriously flawed research on DES as a morning-after contraceptive that had been published in *The Journal of the American Medical Association*; Mary Howell, first woman Dean at Harvard Medical School, who helped force medical schools to abandon their quotas against women through her underground broadside Why Would a Girl Go into Medicine?; and Phyllis Chesler, who held mental health practitioners to a less sexist standard through her classic book *Women and Madness*. Other key activists were Sherry Lebowitz for DES-Action; Helen Rodriguez-Trias, campaigning to curb sterilization abuse of vulnerable women; Byllye Avery, focusing on childbirth and special health problems of black women; Judy Norsigian for *Our Bodies, Ourselves* and a fourteen-year NWHN board member; Rose Kushner, who chaired the NWHN Breast Cancer Task Force; Barbara Ehrenreich, coauthor of *Witches, Midwives, and Nurses*; Anne Kasper, who started the NWHN Clearinghouse; Denise Fuge, the feminist "mole" at Sloan Kettering; Chicago's feminist psychiatrist, Anne Seiden; Doris Haire; Philadelphia health activist JoAnne Fischer Wolf; and a young Dayton, Ohio widower named James Luggen.

Little progress is likely to be made by reformers unless yet more militant advocates appear to threaten at the gates. The radicals of Bread and Roses, D.C. Women's Liberation, Redstockings, and other small groups made NOW seem both more moderate and more relevant, and therefore more mainstream. However, the most original and daring women's health revolutionary was Carol Downer, who initiated self-help gynecology on April 7, 1971 at a Los Angeles bookstore when she jumped on a table, inserted a speculum into her vagina, and invited the other women to observe her cervix. The extent of Downer's radical imagination—bringing menstrual extraction as well as self-examination to laywomen—made those activists involved with the NWHN to appear "respectable." Cynthia Pearson, who became the Executive Director of the NWHN in the 1990s, received her early activist training at Downer's feminist health centers.[11]

Throughout the 1970s, organizations were created that focused on issues of particular concerns to minority women. The issue of sterilization abuse was real, and the activism by women of color led to changes in sterilization regulations at both the state and federal level. Organizations such as the Committee to End Sterilization Abuse, co-founded by Helen Rodriguez-Trias, led the fight. Health disparities, then as now, were apparent, and women of color faced higher mortality and morbidity from diseases such as breast cancer, hypertension, and lupus. They also faced higher infant mortality rates. The National Black Women's Health Project, founded by Byllye Avery in 1981 with the support of the NWHN, stands as the model for other organizations focused on improving minority women's health. Other organizations targeting the health needs of their own constituency formed subsequently, including the National Latina Health Organization and the Native American Women's Health Education Resource Center.

By the early 1980s, activists had made enormous progress in institutionalizing informed consent for both research and treatment, succeeded in getting regulations to restrain sterilization abuse against minority women, and secured the ownership of medical records by patients. They had also opened the FDA to regular consumer participation and had established the custom that patients share an equal voice with scientists and physicians at Congressional hearings. Advocates had popularized natural childbirth, revived midwifery, and reclaimed labor and delivery as a family event. Women were allowed to more freely enroll in medical schools so that female enrollment had tripled.[12] Advocates had effectively challenged the use of radical mastectomies and created an atmosphere where patients could become partners in selecting their treatment plans. Throughout this period, activists played a central role in the legalization and continued availability of abortion, often through underground actions.

V. THE THIRD WAVE: PROFESSIONAL ADVOCATES

In the mid 1980s, the third wave of women's health activism began. Although still not proportional to their overall numbers, women were now becoming established as health professionals, scientists, and policy makers, and therefore advocates began to make their presence known from the inside of government and the halls of Congress. This wave of activism began with a focus on research on women's health and got its momentum from the issue of lack of inclusion of women as research subjects in clinical studies. Advocates from the scientific community partnered with women members of Congress to push through a legislative agenda on women's health research.

A key leader in this movement was Florence Haseltine who, outside of her role as a National Institutes of Health (NIH) scientist, founded along with others the Society for the Advancement of Women's Health Research. Initially, her concern was the lack of research in the areas of contraception and infertility, which had become extremely limited due to the political debates over abortion and to the fears by the pharmaceutical industry of potential lawsuits. The Society was at that time a small group of women scientists who based their activities out of the women-owned political consulting firm Bass and Howes, who in

1989 broadened their focus to include other questions of research ranging from breast cancer and osteoporosis to women in clinical trials.

At that time, they began their discussions with the Congressional Caucus for Women's Issues which was co-chaired by Representatives Patricia Schroeder and Olympia Snowe. Together they worked with Representative Henry Waxman, chair of the House Subcommittee on Health and the Environment, to develop a strategy to bring the issue of research on women's health to the forefront. Key congressional staffers—Lesley Primmer with the Caucus, Andrea Camp from Rep. Schroeder's office, and Ruth Katz from the Subcommittee—developed a request for an investigation by the General Accounting Office (GAO) to examine the implementation by the NIH of its 1986 policy to include women in clinical research studies. Florence Haseltine was later to refer to this investigation as "Lesley's crowbar" because it broke open the issue of women's health research for the public to see.

This policy had been established in 1986 based on a report in 1985 by the Public Health Service's Task Force on Women's Health, which had been led by Ruth Kirschstein, the only woman Institute Director at the NIH. The Task Force report recommended including more women in clinical studies as well as expanding the research portfolio on women's health. The now infamous "GAO report" released in June 1990 found that the policy adopted by the NIH had scarcely been implemented, and, indeed, the NIH could not answer the question regarding how many women were actually included in NIH-funded studies.

Unlike most GAO reports, this one did not gather dust on a shelf but instead served to catalyze action by the public, by Congress, and by the NIH. An enormous amount of press coverage, which had been coordinated by the Society for the Advancement of Women's Health, followed the congressional hearing held in June of 1990. The Congresswomen and Senator Barbara Mikulski introduced the first Women's Health Equity Act, which called for increased focus on women's health through research, services, and prevention activities. Although the research portions of that legislation did not become law until 1993, NIH responded immediately by establishing the Office of Research on Women's Health at the NIH, initially led by Ruth Kirschstein, and by issuing new guidelines requiring the inclusion of women and minorities in all NIH-funded clinical trials.[13]

In the spring of 1991, Bernadine Healy was confirmed as the first woman Director of the NIH and the NIH launched the Women's Health Initiative (WHI) a multiphase, multiyear research study focusing on the major causes of death and disability in older women. The WHI includes the largest clinical trial in the history of the NIH and will assess the impact of dietary fat, hormone replacement therapy, and calcium and vitamin D supplementation on heart disease and cancer in women over the age of fifty. However, Healy and the WHI were also challenged by women's health advocates. The NWHN worked diligently to have the study modified to exclude women with an intact uterus from the part of the trial that included estrogen replacement therapy (ERT). ERT alone is known to cause endometrial cancer and advocates succeeded in convincing the NIH that the study was putting women at unacceptable risk. Questions about the thoroughness of the informed consent form with regard to other cancer risks were also raised by the NWHN, leading to revisions in the consent form. However, these changes in the study did not come easily. As noted in *Science* by Charles Mann, "Bernadine Healy . . . rejected their concerns, arguing that plans to monitor the test subjects with yearly biopsies would protect female subjects."[14] Only in January 1995, after high rates of cellular abnormalities were seen in a related study, "the original plans were quietly dropped."

Meanwhile, other advocates were working on specific women's health issues, the most prominent and most successful being the focus on breast cancer. The National Breast Cancer Coalition, made up of grassroots organizations from around the country, began to make its collective voice heard in Washington and at the NIH. Led by Fran Visco, and once again working with Bass and Howes, funding levels for breast cancer research began to grow. From less than a hundred million dollars in 1990 to over five hundred million in 1998, the level of funding for breast cancer currently more fully reflects the level of concern felt by women around the nation. However, much of this funding did not come by way of the usual channels.

In the early 1990s, funding for areas such as biomedical research was limited by ceilings established by legislation. Therefore, any increase in funding had to be offset by decreases in other areas. To get around this limit, the National Breast Cancer Coalition and others focused on the Defense Department budget. By getting funding from there, not only would there be greater opportunities for increased funding, but advocates also believed that this would create the opportunity for change and innovation in the research process—by allowing consumers and advocates to have a voice in priority setting. Breast cancer advocates were successful in implementing this strategy by working not just with the women in Congress but also with Senator Tom Harkin, chair of the Senate Appropriations Subcommittee on Labor, Health, and Human Services and Education. Senator Harkin had lost two sisters to breast cancer and thus became a champion within the Senate. His amendments to the appropriations bills in 1992 led to the creation of a major breast cancer research program within the Defense Department which broke new ground in the level of consumer and advocate involvement in the funding process. This program now serves as a model for linking the scientific and advocacy communities.

By this time, the "mainstreaming" of women's health had moved to the highest levels. During the campaign for the presidency in 1992, women's health had been identified by the Clinton campaign as a top priority. One of President Clinton's first acts after being sworn in in 1993 was to sign the NIH legislation that mandated the appropriate inclusion of women and minorities in clinical research trials and called for more research on breast and cervical cancer, osteoporosis, contraception, and infertility, and permanently established the NIH Office of Research on Women's Health.[15] He also signed executive orders lifting restrictions on access to information about abortion services and began expansion of the federally funded family planning program.

The National Breast Cancer Coalition did not stop at increasing funding. In October of 1993, they delivered 2.6 million signatures to the White House calling for the establishment of a National Action Plan on Breast Cancer with the goal of eliminating breast cancer. By the end of that year, Secretary of Health and Human Services, Donna Shalala, had convened a conference to identify the critical issues and to establish the Action Plan.[16] Advocates have played the leading role in both the creation and the agenda for this Plan, which has focused on catalyzing efforts in previously overlooked or under-addressed areas, particularly in the research arena. Many of the issues—such as ensuring appropriate informed consent, questions about discrimination based on hereditary susceptibility to breast cancer, and increased advocacy input to the development of research priorities—reflect the earlier issues raised by the advocates of the 1960s and 1970s. Understanding the etiology of breast cancer through increased research continues to be a high priority for breast cancer advocates, who want to take the knowledge gained and target it towards prevention and cure.

The Department of Health and Human Services itself has brought women's health advocacy "inside." Through the establishment of additional women's health offices at the Food and Drug Administration, the Substance Abuse and Mental Health Services Administration, and the Centers for Disease Control and Prevention, as well as the Office on Women's Health within the Office of the Secretary, women's health advocates have increased involvement in the design and implementation of programs and policies, including the research agenda.

Beginning in 1991 with the conference convened by the NIH Office of Research on Women's Health in Hunt Valley, Maryland, and subsequently in 1997 through a conference series known as "Beyond Hunt Valley," the NIH has assessed current research needs in women's health with a view towards ensuring that the research funded by the NIH addresses the key areas identified. The research agenda that has been developed by the NIH Office of Research on Women's Health, now led by Vivian Pinn, drew from women's health advocates as well as from health professionals and biomedical research scientists.

Another trend throughout the nineties was that new issue areas, which previously had had little research, moved to the forefront due to the initiatives of advocates. Areas such as menopause, silicone breast implants, temporomandibular joint disorder (TMJ), autoimmune disorders, interstitial cystitis, ovarian cancer, and the long-term effects of DES, among others, became the focus of both Congressional concern and government-funded research. Each one of these conditions has advocates and organizations focused on their specific topic, and in most cases focused on increasing research in the area. Although some in the scientific community have raised concerns about targeting research funding to specific diseases and about involving nonscientists in priority-setting, patient advocates—modeling after early women's health activists, AIDS activists, and newer organizations such as the Breast Cancer Coalition—have been successful in having their voices heard.

In retrospect, women's health advocates have had a profound impact, particularly in the areas of informed consent and biomedical research. In 1970, Alice Wolfson and the NWHN in formation opened up the FDA to consumer observers, which led, in turn, to consumer representatives on FDA panels and through the 1970s and 1980s to increasing demands for direct consumer participa-

tion in an expanding range of regulatory decisions and taxpayer-funded research. In the 1990s, advocates brought about changes not only in the topic areas under study but also in the study designs to ensure that women's health was addressed. Questions about racial disparities in health status are moving to the front burner. In 1998, the Institute of Medicine published its report "Scientific Opportunities and Public Needs" which endorsed increased consumer participation in priority setting at NIH.[17] However, before their recommendations are implemented, there are crucial issues that require review and discussion, as there is far more at stake than just how much money will be allocated to research on which disease. Issues include ensuring that consumers have a voice in the design and monitoring of studies, improving the clarity and information provided in informed consent forms, and ensuring that clinical research on vulnerable populations is carried out ethically and with appropriate access to care. The future of women's health research will depend on advocates to continue to serve both as watchdogs and also as sources of new ideas and issues to be addressed.

NOTES

1. 1. W. S. Ross, *Crusade—The Official History of the American Cancer Society* (New York: Arbor House, 1987); J. Patterson, *The Dread Disease: Cancer and Modern American Culture* (Boston, MA: Harvard University Press, 1987); and S. Batt, *Patient No More: The Politics of Breast Cancer* (Charlottetown, Prince Edward Island: Gynergy Books, 1994).

2. R. W. Moss, *The Cancer Industry* (New York: Paragon House, 1989); R. A. Rettig, *Cancer Crusade: The Story of the National Cancer Act of 1971* (Princeton, NJ: Princeton University Press, 1977); Institute of Medicine, *Scientific Opportunities and Public Needs* (Washington DC: National Academy Press, 1998); U.S. News Online, "Mary and her 'Little Lambs' Launch a War"; and Albert and Mary Lasker Foundation Online, "About the Lasker Medical Research Awards."

3. *Mothering Magazine*, "Living Treasures, Doris Haire," July–August 1998; and S. B. Ruzek, *The Women's Health Movement, Feminist Alternatives to Medical Control* (New York: Praeger, 1978).

4. S. S. Seaman, *Always a Woman: What Every Woman Should Know about Breast Surgery* (Larchmont, NY: Argonaut Books, 1965); T. Laser and W. K. Clarke, *Reach to Recovery* (New York: Simon and Schuster, 1972); and B. Seaman, "Beyond the Halsted Radical," *On the Issues*, Fall 1997.

5. B. Seaman, "Thalidomide," in *The Reader's Companion to U.S. Women's History*, eds. W. Mankiller, G. Mink, M. Navarro, B. Smith, and G. Steinem (Boston: Houghton Mifflin, 1998).

6. C. S. Weisman, *Women's Health Care: Activist Traditions and Institutional Change* (Baltimore, MD: John Hopkins University Press, 1998); and B. Seaman and G. Seaman, *Women and the Crisis in Sex Hormones* (New York: Bantam Books, 1978), 79.

7. Ruzek, *The Women's Health Movement, Feminist Alternatives to Medical Control*; and S. Rimer, "Women's Health: A Special Section," *New York Times*, June 22, 1997, 27.

8. Anonymous, *Competitive Problems in the Drug Industry* (Washington DC: US Gov. Printing Office), part 15, 6053.

9. Ibid., 6395.

10. Ruzek, *The Women's Health Movement, Feminist Alternatives to Medical Control*; C. Mann, "Women's Health Research Blossoms," *Science* 269 (1995): 766–70; E. S. Watkins, "Oral Contraceptives and Informed Consent," in *On the Pill: A Social History of Contraceptives, 1950–1970* (Baltimore, MD: John Hopkins University Press, 1998), 103–31; A. J. Wolfson, "Clenched Fist, Open Heart," in *The Feminist Project Memoir, Voices from Women's Liberation*, eds. R. B. Du-Plessis and A. Snitow (New York: Three Rivers Press, 1998), 268–83; and B. Seaman, *The Doctors' Case Against the Pill*, 25th anniversary updated ed. (Alameda, CA: Hunter House, 1995), 222–26.

11. Ruzek, *The Women's Health Movement, Feminist Alternatives to Medical Control*, 1–2, 53, 54–58, 60, 145–155, 167–169, 173, 195, 203, 214; Carol Downer, "Snapshot," *Ms. Magazine*, 1996. M. A. Campbell (aka Mary Howell), *Why Would a Girl go into Medicine* (Old Westbury, NY: The Feminist Press, 1973). W. Saxon, "Mary Howell, a Leader in Medicine, Dies at 65," *New York Times*, February 6, 1998, lead obituary; Figures on medical school admissions, American Medical Association compilations; Boston Women's Health Book Collective, *Our Bodies, Ourselves* (Boston: New England Free Press, 1970); Boston Women's Health Book Collective, *Our Bodies, Ourselves* (New York: Simon and Schuster, 1973); Boston Women's Health Book Collective, *Our Bodies, Ourselves*, rev. ed. (New York: Simon and Schuster, 1976); Boston Women's Health Book Collective, *Our Bodies, Ourselves*, rev. ed. (New York: Touchstone, 1979); Boston Women's Health Book Collective, *The New Our Bodies, Ourselves* (1984); Boston Women's Health Book Collective, *The New Our Bodies, Ourselves*, rev., updated (New York: Simon and Schuster, 1992); and Boston Women's Health Book Collective, *Our Bodies, Ourselves for the New Century* (New York: Simon and Schuster, 1998).

12. U.S. Department of Health and Human Services (US-DHHS), Public Health Service (PHS), Health Resources and Services Administration, Council on Graduate Medical Education, Fifth Report: Women and Medicine, Part II, 1995.

13. USDHHS, "Women's Health: Report of the Public Health Service Task Force on Women's Health Issues," *Public Health Reports* 100, no. 1 (Jan–Feb 1985): 73–106; and U.S. General Accounting Office (GAO), "Problems in Implementing Policy on Women in Study Populations, or, Statement of Mark V. Nadel," before the Subcommittee on Health and the Environment Committee on Energy and Commerce, House of Representatives, 1990.

14. C. Mann, "Women's Health Research Blossoms," 770.

15. NIH, Office of Research on Women's Health, Office of the Director, "Report of the National Institutes of Health: Opportunities for Research on Women's Health," 1991.

16. National Institutes of Health (NIH), "Proceedings, Secretary's Conference to Establish a National Action Plan on Breast Cancer," 1993.

17. Institute of Medicine, *Scientific Opportunities and Public Needs* (Washington DC: National Academy Press, 1998).

Inside and Out: Two Stories of the Rumblings Beneath the Quiet

COMPILED BY SUZANNE CLORES

The Halsted radical mastectomy has been called "the greatest standardized surgical error of the twentieth century." Introduced in the 1880s by William Halsted, a surgeon at Johns Hopkins, it was debilitating, even crippling, and based on Halsted's unproven conviction that breast cancer was a local disease that could be fully—if brutally—excised. The Halsted radical was exacting. The woman was anesthetized and the doctor performed a "quick-section" biopsy. If the biopsy was positive, the doctor, without waking the patient, began his incision at the shoulder and removed the breast as well as the lymph glands, the muscles of the chest wall, and all the fat under the skin. The patient was left with a loss of feeling on that side of her body, a sunken chest, restricted movement, and probably some degree of "milk arm," the chronic and painful condition in which lymph fluid can no longer circulate properly and thus accumulates.

In 1954, Terese ("Ted") Lasser, founder of Reach to Recovery, became the first militant advocate for radical mastectomy patients. Recalling the Halsted radical she had in 1952, she said, "You awake to find yourself wrapped in bandages from midriff to neck—bound like a mummy in surgical gauze, somewhere deep inside you a switch is thrown and your mind goes blank. You do not know what to think, you do not want to guess, you do not want to know." Lasser, the soignée, energetic (and imperious) matriarch in an affluent and well-connected family (J. K. Lasser, her husband, was author of the perennially popular *Your Income Tax*), was not accustomed to being patronized or hustled and had not been prepared for this drastic result. Nor did her surgeon (whom she described as a "brilliant but very busy man"), or anyone else at Memorial Hospital, give her the specific advice she craved on arm exercises, if, when, or how to resume sex relations with her husband, what to tell her children, or even how to shop for a prosthesis. Her epiphany occurred when she showed up at the department store where she normally bought brassieres, and the saleswoman screamed and fled, crying "People like us shouldn't have to wait on people like you."

As soon as Lasser discovered how to cope with these matters, a compulsion came over her to teach what she knew. She slipped into the hospital rooms of "mastectomees," bearing gift boxes with (1) a starter "falsie" for them to pin on the inside of their nightgowns; (2) a ball, a string, and instructions, which she demonstrated, for the painful but effective arm-restoring exercises that she herself had devised out of her desperation and genius; and (3) perhaps most daring, her famous "Letter to Husbands" about sex. Lasser maintained

a pretense that she made these calls only at the request of the patient's doctor or family. However, she was often escorted out of the front door of Memorial Hospital when she was found visiting patients at random and without the consent of the responsible surgeon.

One consistent message from breast cancer activists has been that when cancer cells are "growing wild" inside, some sense of outer autonomy becomes imperative, even life-saving, for the woman. Dr. M. Vera Peters thought so, and is said to have treated her patients accordingly from the time she graduated medical school in Toronto in 1934. A world-class radiotherapist and oncologist before she reached the age of forty, she'd made a major contribution to the treatment of Hodgkin's disease. She argued for an aggressive approach; but regarding her second major interest, breast cancer, the evidence led her in the opposite direction.

Peters worked at a Toronto facility that admitted 7,261 patients for treatment of breast cancer between 1935 and 1960. On April 10, 1967, she published a paper in the *Journal of the American Medical Association* that reported the outcome for 825 of these women, including 200 who had only lumpectomies with radiation. All of the patients in the three other treatment groups had had some combination of mastectomy and radiation, but in only one group was the mastectomy performed immediately after a "quick-section" biopsy, eliminating patient choice.

Lumpectomy patients with stages one and two breast cancer survived fully as well, at five years, as those who had had mastectomies. With the chance to present evidence against the scourge of quick-section biopsies, she writes,

> It behooves us as cancer therapists to [find methods] which will not harm the self respect and good will of the patient. With quick section biopsy . . . the patients feel that they have been deprived of an opportunity to think positively about their treatment because the diagnosis had not been confirmed preoperatively. . . . If a preliminary

local incision had been carried out routinely, the more radical treatment could then be discussed with the patient and the final decision in favor of either surgery or irradiation could safely be influenced by the patient's "special" fears.

Upon her retirement in 1976, Vera Peters was appointed to the Order of Canada, in recognition of her extraordinary contributions to the treatment of Hodgkin's disease and breast cancer, just as patents all over the world were beginning to seize their newfound opportunities to "think positively" for themselves.

In 1960, the judgment of Food and Drug Administration medical officer Dr. Frances Oldham Kelsey brought the widespread use of the drug thalidomide to a stop, but not before an epidemic of limbless babies were born to thousands of mothers who were sampling the pills purported to be mild sedatives. Kelsey refused to approve the drug, despite early news of the drug's success and pressure from the manufacturer, the Merrell Company, to distribute in the United States. While thalidomide's effects on animals tested negative to malformation, Dr. Kelsey mistrusted the sleeping pill that did not cause sleepiness in animals.

In 1961, West Germany reported to the FDA that thalidomide had been associated with birth defects. The Merrell Company, who had furnished nearly 1,100 doctors (almost 250 obstetricians and gynecologists) with samples of the drug, merely issued a letter of warning to just 10 percent of those physicians, hoping still for FDA approval and promising prescription sales. Thalidomide's danger to pregnant women was not made public in the United States until 1962. For her role in preventing distribution, Dr. Kelsey received the President's Award for Distinguished Federal Civilian Service in 1962.

The same year, Sherri Finkbine, a thalidomide-exposed pregnant woman, was denied the abortion she sought for medical reasons in the US. Finkbine was not an abortion radical, believing an abortion should be undertaken only when absolutely necessary, but she thought herself the exception. She was disturbed that she had been given a drug that had destroyed her pregnancy, so the day before her scheduled abortion, she called a friend in the press and told her story. When the paper's headlines screamed of thalidomide's mutagenic effects, her scheduled abortion was canceled. She eventually did obtain one in Sweden, and her harrowing, well-publicized odyssey ultimately helped arouse sentiment for abortion law reform. Underneath her disclosure of the danger of the drug is the same vision for consumer well-being that prompted Dr. Kelsey's judgment. These two women acted in order to protect future female patients from medical industry politics—those of the FDA, pharmaceutical companies, or the medical community—which may not have the health and interest of the patient in mind.

Women's Health and Government Regulation: 1950–1980

SUZANNE WHITE JUNOD

Many of the medical discoveries that were made in the first half of the twentieth century came to fruition in the second half. New techniques for detecting cancer and fetal abnormalities were developed. A number of new products were introduced into the market—not always with happy results. And women's struggle to make informed decisions about their own bodies often led to clashes with both the government and private industry. Some of these clashes took place in the courts; others, in the streets.

FETAL STUDIES

By 1955, four different research groups were credited with discovering that the sex of the fetus could be predicted through analysis of fetal cells in amniotic fluid. This information was important in cases of genetically transmitted sex-linked diseases.

In 1959, French cytogeneticist Jerome LeJeune discovered that one form of Down's syndrome was caused by trisomy of the twenty-first chromosome; this paved the way for a wider use of amniocentesis in diagnosing fetal genetic abnormalities. By 1966, the problems in culturing fetal cells obtained through amniocentesis were solved, and two years later, the first abortions after mid-trimester amniocentesis and karyotyping were performed.

A cooperative registry was set up in 1971 to ascertain the safety of amniocentesis. By 1976, amniocentesis was shown to have favorable results in clinical trials. By the late 1970s, there were a number of successful lawsuits against obstetricians who had failed to refer a patient over the age of thirty-five for amniocentesis. As a result, amniocentesis came in to greatly expanded use.

Ultrasound, which Lars Leksell had used successfully in 1953 to diagnose a hematoma in an infant's brain, became a routine part of obstetrical practice after 1975, when improvements in gray-scale and real-time imaging made it commercially successful.

IN VITRO FERTILIZATION

The first successful use of follicle-stimulating hormone for ovulation induction was reported in 1958. The first pregnancy after treatment with human pituitary gonadotropin was reported in 1960; this led to studies of the hypothalamic-releasing factors that enable or block ovulation.

In 1969, Patrick Steptoe and Robert Edwards began collaboration on the human IVF project. Steptoe had improved the laparoscopy instrument in the 1950s and used it to operate on the fallopian tubes and to extract ova.

In 1973, Landrum Settles of Columbia University extracted an ovum from a patient with dysfunctional fallopian tubes, fertilized it with her husband's sperm, and incubated it in his lab in preparation for implantation in her womb. Horrified, the chairman of the Department of Obstetrics and Gynecology deliberately destroyed Settles' experiment, claiming that it was both unethical and a risk to the woman's health.

On July 25, 1978, Steptoe and Edwards reported the birth of the first "test-tube" (IVF) baby in England.

CANCER DETECTION AND TREATMENT

PAP SMEAR During the 1950s, cytology laboratories were established in the United States, signifying the medical community's growing acceptance of the Pap smear as a means of detecting cervical cancer, as well women's increasing demand for the test. The American Cancer Society was instrumental in educating physicians on its use. By the 1960s, the Pap smear was part of regular gynecology practice. Pap Check, a do-it-yourself test that had never received FDA approval was finally recalled in 1973.

MAMMOGRAPHY In 1960, Robert Egan at M. D. Anderson Hospital in Houston revolutionized breast imaging when he adapted a high-resolution industrial film to a mammographic technique. In 1962, Egan reported the discovery of unsuspected "occult carcinomas."

In 1963, Health Insurance Plan of New York tested Egan's breast-imaging technique and, in 1964, organized the first randomized controlled study to evaluate the effect of screening on mortality. Women who were screened were a third less likely to die from breast cancer than those who received physical examination only. This study served as a model for a national study sponsored by the American Cancer Society and the National Cancer Institute that included 250,000 women. In 1965, the American College of Radiology held its first conference on mammography.

Throughout the 1970s, however, there was concern about the side effects from mammography, especially in women who had undergone radiation treatment. Xerox Corporation replaced the film of the traditional x-ray with a selenium-coated aluminum plate prepared for exposure after being electrically charged. Xeroradiology reduced exposure and produced better quality images. Magnification mammography, which allowed better analysis of suspicious areas, was also introduced.

TAMOXIFEN Paclitaxel (Taxol) was first isolated from the Pacific yew in 1966. Dr. Craig Jordan, professor of cancer pharmacology and director of the breast cancer research program at the Lurie Comprehensive Cancer Center at Northwestern University Medical School in Chicago began studying tamoxifen as a graduate student in 1969. "It was the age of making love and not war, and everybody was looking for more contraceptives." Tamoxifen was a great postcoital contraceptive in rats, but it proved totally ineffective in women, so it went back on the shelf, at least temporarily.

But then Dr. Jordan found that tamoxifen could prevent breast cancer in animals, so in 1974 he began testing it in American women with breast cancer. In 1977, Tamoxifen was approved for patients with advanced breast cancer, and in June 1990, it was approved for node-negative patients.

NEW TREATMENTS, NEW PRODUCTS, NEW THREATS

DES In 1940, Charles Huggins first reported the value of a potent hormone, diethylstilbestrol (DES), in the treatment of prostate tumors. Over the next three decades, DES was prescribed to pregnant women, supposedly to improve the chances of a healthy delivery. A generation later physicians found that it caused adenosis (abnormal gland development) and vaginal adenocarcinoma (a form of cancer) in the daughters of women who took the drug. Genitourinary defects have also been found in sons, and more recent lawsuits allege harm to grandchildren as well. Since the 1970s, several thousand DES victims have sued pharmaceutical companies nationwide.

ENOVID In 1959, the FDA approved Enovid (produced by G. D. Searle) as an oral contraceptive. This profoundly altered the scope of the FDA's authority and established what evolved into a long-term interest in women's health issues. As FDA commissioner George Larrick pointed out, pregnancy was not a "disease." The agency had no experience in either approving or regulating a drug for such a purpose, and although the efficacy of the pill was not in doubt, its safety was soon rendered suspect when reports of associated thromboemolic problems began to surface. In 1967, British epidemiological studies confirmed the statistical link between thromboembolism and oral contraceptives. In 1968, the FDA instituted an Adverse Reaction Data Reporting Program on oral contraceptive drugs.

SILICONE IMPLANTS The first breast implant was in 1962. In 1963, Dow Corning launched a national advertising campaign for Dow Corning Medical Fluid 360, a liquid silicone preparation that could be injected into the body "for removing facial wrinkles, recontouring women's breasts, and reshaping other parts of the body." FDA agents seized some of the product in the office of an osteopath and in the offices of two California cosmetic surgeons. The agents discovered that the California physicians had not only used the Dow silicone "360" in their medical practice, but also a laboratory-grade silicone and an industrial-grade silicone, which the physicians had ordered through a furniture dealer.

In 1968, Dow defendants move to dismiss the government's criminal indictment against them, arguing that the product that they had shipped, silicone fluid, was not a "drug" or a "new drug" under the law. The court ruled that it could not make such a determination until the evidence was heard at trial. The defendants also charged that the statutory definitions of "drug," "device," "cosmetic," and "new drug" were unconstitutionally vague in regard to their product. The court also rejected this argument, saying "the choice of the proper classification is not as difficult as defendants make it out to be. With the guidance of the avowed Congressional policy of protecting the public health, when an item is capable of coming within two definitions, there is really only one answer, namely, that which affords the public the greater protection."

In 1971, Dow Corning and S. W. Rhode, former director of Dow's Medical Products Division, entered pleas of no contest to charges that they had sold a silicone product for rejuvenating middle-aged women in violation of the federal Food, Drug, and Cosmetic Act. The company acknowledged that it had failed to obtain premarket clearance for their product as a drug. Rhodes and Dow were subject to maximum fines of $8,000 and eight years in prison.

Four years later Dow Corning modified its original breast implant product. The FDA responded in a Talk Paper that it had "never approved injectable liquid silicone for breast augmentation or enlargement. Serious injury and at least four known deaths have been attributed to this procedure," and warned against medical use of nonsterile industrial-grade silicone. The FDA further noted that "there is another method of breast augmentation which is performed in the United States. It involves the use of silicone in a pliable plastic bag placed over the chest muscles. None of the problems connected with liquid silicone have been reported for this procedure."

On March 24, and July 6, 1978, the General and Plastic Surgery Devices Panel recommended that the silicone inflatable breast prosthesis be given a class II designation, but identified certain risks to health presented by the device.

DALKON SHIELD The Dalkon Shield, marketed by A. H. Robins Pharmaceutical Company, was developed before passage of the 1976 Medical Devices Amendment and therefore did not go through a premarketing screening. Regulators had concerns about the device from the beginning, however, and it was targeted for investigation when reports of injury began to emerge.

Litigation began in 1974 and ultimately involved hundreds of thousands of claimants from among the 2.2 million women who had had the Shield implanted. By 1980, clear evidence of corporate wrongdoing and fraud had emerged, and juries routinely began awarding multimillion-dollar punitive damages. As a result, Robins entered bankruptcy court voluntarily in 1985, and in 1989 a plan was implemented to permit injured women to choose an administrative compensation scheme instead of litigation.

TOXIC SHOCK SYNDROME Toxic shock syndrome (TSS) was first identified in 1989. The earliest reported cases occurred among seven children; all were linked to the presence of staphylococcus aureus. Symptoms of the disease include vomiting, diarrhea, high fever, and a sunburnlike rash.

Before 1977 all tampon products were made of rayon or a rayon-cotton blend. Since 1977, 40 percent of tampon products have contained more absorbent synthetic material. In 1979, the FDA listed tampons as a class II device under the 1976 Medical Device Amendments and ruled that they must not contain drugs or antimicrobial agents. Today, 70 percent of menstruating women use vaginal tampons.

In 1978, TSS was identified as a distinct disease. A dramatic upsurge in cases reported to CDC occurred in 1980, when 890 cases were reported, 812 among women whose illness coincided with the start of their menstrual periods. The fatality rate among early TSS patients was around 8 percent. This striking association of TSS with menstruating women stimulated careful epidemiological analysis. When information collected by the Utah Department of Health suggested that a particular tampon brand, Rely, had been sued by many women with TSS, a detailed study was devised by the Centers for Disease Control in September 1980 to examine tampon brand use. This study found that 71 percent of a recent group of women with TSS had used Rely tampons.

On September 22, 1980, Procter and Gamble recalled all Rely tampons on the market, and all tampon manufacturers subsequently lowered the absorbency of their tampons. The FDA began requiring that all tampon packages carry information on TSS and advise women to use tampons with the minimum absorbency needed to control menstrual flow.

In 1980, the American Society for Testing and Materials organized a task force to develop uniform absorbency testing and labeling at the FDA's request.

Although cases of menstrually related TSS fell off dramatically after 1984, the overall number of cases is suspected to have risen as the staphylococcal bacteria that produces the deadly toxin has spread to more people. Today, only about half of the cases of staphylococcal toxic shock syndrome are connected with menstruating women. TSS has been reported in men, children, and older women, and in conjunction with surgery, a wound, influenza, sinusitis, childbirth, use of a contraceptive sponge, cervical cap, or diaphragm, intravenous drug abuse, an abscess, boil, cut, or even an insect bite.

THE WOMEN'S HEALTH MOVEMENT TAKES OFF

➤ 1969: Journalist Barbara Seaman publishes *The Doctors' Case Against the Pill*, charging that women were not being adequately informed about dangerous side effects from the pill, including stroke, heart disease, diabetes, depression, and other ailments.

➤ 1970: Senate hearings on the pill; activist Alice Wolfson demanded to know why no women were being allowed to testify. TV cameras recorded the disruption as Seaman and other women joined the protest. The dissent helped to launch a political movement focusing on women's health.

➤ 1975: Seaman, Wolfson, and three other women activists went on to found the National Women's Health Network as an umbrella institution for nearly two thousand women's self-help medical

projects. The movement centered on the overuse of medical technology, insufficiently rigorous drug testing, and refusal to listen to patients (paternalism).

➤ 1970: Alice Wolfson took the first critical steps to open a dialogue between the FDA Obstetrics and Gynecology Advisory Committee and the FDA. The meetings were closed to the public, but Wolfson and several colleagues persisted in attending anyway. "What are you discussing that women shouldn't hear?" she asked. This was the occasion of the first sit-in at the FDA.

➤ 1970: The AMA House of Delegates passed a resolution opposing the patient package insert (PPI) on the grounds that it would "confuse and alarm many patients." A compromise was reached wherein a modified version was mailed to physicians to hand out with every pill prescription. Over the next five years, the AMA distributed only four million copies, although an estimated ten million US women per annum were taking the pill. In time, the FDA went back to its original concept—distributing the PPI in the pill packet through pharmacists. Again there was opposition from doctors and the drug industry. This time the consumer groups were more successful. It is likely that the PPI has contributed to the subsequent decline in pill use.

➤ 1971: Self-help gynecology helped transform women's health and body issues into a separate social movement. The movement was born on April 7, 1971, at the Everywoman's Bookstore in Los Angeles. For some time feminists had met there to discuss health and abortion issues. After exhausting "book learning," Carol Downer, a member of the group, suggested empirical observation. After inserting a speculum in her own vagina, she invited other women present to observe her cervix.

➤ 1972: Police officers arrested Carol Downer and Coleen Wilson on charges of practicing medicine without a license. Margaret Mead observed that "men began taking over obstetrics and they invented a tool that allowed them to look inside women. You could call this progress—except that when women tried to look inside themselves, this was called 'practicing medicine without a license.'" (*Los Angeles Times*, February 5, 1974). Several months later, Downer was acquitted after two days of deliberation by the jury.

➤ 1972: Boston women organized Speakoutrage, a public hearing for women to testify about their experiences with abortion, forced sterilization, unnecessary surgery, and other forms of exploitation and mistreatment. Conditions at the Boston City Hospital OB-GYN clinic were especially decried. As evidence of medical abuse came to light in city after city and hospital after hospital generated a broader-based women's health movement.

Carol Downer, the "mother" of self-help gynecology, was arrested for using yogurt to treat yeast infections and for using a device called the Del-Em for menstrual extraction, also called "self-abortion." Her defense was eloquent and long-quoted as a cornerstone of the concerns of the women's health movement:

> In what has been described as "rape of the pelvis," our uteri and ovaries are removed, often needlessly. Our breasts and all supporting muscular tissue are carved out brutally in radical mastectomy. Abortion and preventive birth control methods are denied us unless we are a certain age, or married, or perhaps they are denied us completely. Hospital committees decide whether or not we can have our tubes tied. Unless our uterus has "done its duty," we're often denied. We give birth in hospitals run for the convenience of the staff. We're drugged, strapped, cut, ignored, enemaed, probed, shaved—all in the name of "superior care." How can we rescue ourselves from the dilemma that male supremacy has landed us in? The answer is simple. We women must taken women's medicine back into our own capable hands.

MEN, WOMEN, WHAT'S THE DIFFERENCE?

In 1961, news that the hypnotic drug thalidomide had been linked with an epidemic of malformed infants in Europe focused attention on women and pregnancy. Worldwide concern about thalidomide led to the passage of drug reform legislation in the United States which shut women out of the early phases of clinical drug testing and virtually orphaned clinical studies of pediatric drug efficacy and safety.

In the 1970s it was discovered that women taking the prescription drug Premarin to treat menopausal symptoms showed a lower risk of cardiovascular illness. As a result, in 1975 Rush-Cook County undertook a hormone therapy study—on men—to see what effects estrogen drugs had on heart disease. This study remains the only randomized, controlled scientific study about estrogen therapy and heart disease.

In 1977, the FDA published research guidelines that officially excluded women of reproductive age from early phases of clinical drug trials. As a result, drugs were routinely approved for general use that had not been tested on women. "Nobody was thinking much about how drugs might act differently in men and women," said Dr. Lainie Friedman Ross, assistant director of the MacLean Center for Clinical Medical Ethics at the University of Chicago. "Men are steady-state subjects. The problem is, about half of the people eventually taking the tested drugs were women with monthly hormonal changes."

The scratch-your-head logic of using men to test women's treatments helped garnish important support for the Women's Health Initiative in the 1980s.

Sisterhood

GLORIA STEINEM

Gloria Steinem, "Sisterhood," *Ms.*, Spring 1972. Reprinted by permission.

A very, very long time ago (about three or four years), I took a certain secure and righteous pleasure in saying the things that women are supposed to say.

I remember with pain—

"My work won't interfere with marriage. After all, I can always keep my typewriter at home." Or:

"I don't want to write about women's stuff. I want to write about foreign policy." Or:

"Black families were forced into matriarchy, so I see why black women have to step back and let their men get ahead." Or:

"I know we're helping chicano groups that are tough on women, but that's their culture." Or:

"Who would want to join a women's group? I've never been a joiner, have you?" Or (when bragging):

"He says I write about abstract ideas like a man."

I suppose it's obvious from the kinds of statements I chose that I was secretly nonconforming. (I wasn't married, I was earning a living at a profession I cared about, and I had basically—if quietly—opted out of the "feminine" role.) But that made it all the more necessary to repeat some Conventional Wisdom, even to look as conventional as I could manage, if I was to avoid the punishments reserved by society for women who don't do as society says. I therefore learned to Uncle Tom with subtlety, logic, and humor. Sometimes I even believed it myself. If it weren't for the women's movement, I might still be dissembling away. But the ideas of this great sea change in women's view of ourselves are contagious and irresistible. They hit women like a revelation, as if we had left a small dark room and walked into the sun.

At first my discoveries seemed complex and personal. In fact, they were the same ones so many millions of women have made and are making. Greatly simplified, they went like this: Women are human beings first, with minor differences from men that apply largely to the act of reproduction. We share the dreams, capabilities, and weaknesses of all human beings, but our occasional pregnancies and other visible differences have been used—even more pervasively, if less brutally, than racial differences have been used—to mark us for an elaborate division of labor that may once have been practical but has since become cruel and false. The division is continued for clear reason, consciously or not: the economic and social profit of men as a group.

Once this feminist realization dawned, I reacted in what turned out to be predictable ways. First, I was amazed at the simplicity and obviousness of a realization that made sense, at last, of my life experience: I couldn't figure out why I hadn't seen it before. Second, I realized, painfully, how far that new vision of life was from the system around us, and how tough it would be to explain the feminist realization at all, much less to get people (especially, though not only, men) to accept so drastic a change.

But I tried to explain. God knows (*she* knows) that women try. We make analogies with other groups that have been marked for subservient roles in order to assist blocked imaginations. We supply endless facts and statistics of injustice, reeling them off until we feel like human information retrieval machines. We lean heavily on the device of reversal. (If there is a male reader to whom all my prerealization statements seem perfectly logical, for instance, let him substitute "men" for "women" or himself for me in each sentence, and see how he feels. "My work won't interfere with marriage. . . ." "Chicana groups that are tough on men. . . ." You get the idea.)

We even use logic. If a woman spends a year bearing and nursing a child, for instance, she is supposed to have the primary responsibility for raising that child to adulthood. That's logic by the male definition, but it often makes women feel children are their only function or discourages them from being mothers at all. Wouldn't it be just as logical to say that the child has two parents, both equally responsible for child-rearing, and that therefore the father should compensate for that extra year by spending *more* than his half of the time with the child? Now *that's* logic.

Occasionally, these efforts at expelling succeed. More often, I get the feeling that we are speaking Urdu and the men are speaking Pali. As for logic, it's in the eye of the logician.

Painful or not, both stages of reaction to our discovery have a great reward. They give birth to sisterhood.

First, we share with each other the exhilaration of growth and self-discovery, the sensation of having the scales fall from our eyes. Whether we are giving other women this new knowledge or receiving it from them, the pleasure for all concerned is enormous. And very moving.

In the second stage, when we're exhausted from dredging up facts and arguments for the men whom we had previously thought advanced and intelligent, we make jokes, paint pictures, and describe humiliations that mean nothing to men, but *women understand.*

The odd thing about these deep and personal connections of women is that they often ignore barriers of age, economics, worldly experience, race, culture—all the barriers that, in male or mixed society, had seemed so difficult to cross.

I remember meeting with a group of women in Missouri who, because they had come in equal numbers from the small town and from its nearby campus, seemed to be split between wives with white gloves welded to their wrists and students with boots who talked about "imperialism" and "oppression." Planning for a child care center had brought them together, but the meeting seemed hopeless until three of the booted young women began to argue among themselves about a young male professor, the leader of the radicals on campus, who accused all women unwilling to run mimeograph machines of not being sufficiently devoted to the cause. As for child care centers, he felt their effect of allowing women to compete with men for jobs was part of the "feminization" of the American male and American culture.

"He sounds just like my husband," said one of the white-gloved women, "only he wants me to have bake sales and collect door-to-door for his Republican Party."

The young women had sense enough to take it from there. What did boots or white gloves matter if they were all getting treated like servants and children? Before they broke up, they were discussing the myth of the vaginal orgasm and planning to meet every week. "Men think we're whatever it is we do for men," explained one of the housewives. "It's only by getting together with other women that we'll ever find out who we are."

Even racial differences become a little less hopeless once we discover this mutuality of our life experience as women. At a meeting run by black women domestics who had formed a job cooperative in Alabama, a white housewife asked me about the consciousness-raising sessions or "rap groups" that are the basic unit of the women's movement. I explained that while men, even minority men, usually had someplace where they could get together every day and be themselves, women were isolated in their houses; isolated from each other. We had no street corners, no bars, no offices, no territory that was recognized as ours. Rap groups were an effort to create that free place: an occasional chance for total honesty and support form our sisters.

As I talked about isolation, the feeling that there must be something wrong with us if we weren't content to be housekeepers and mothers, tears began to stream down the cheeks of this dignified woman—clearly as much of a surprise to her as to us. For the black women, some barrier was broken down by seeing her cry.

"He does it to us both, honey," said the black woman next to her, putting an arm around her shoulders. "If it's your own kitchen or somebody else's, you still don't get treated like people. Women's work just doesn't count."

The meeting ended with the housewife organizing a support group of white women who would extract from their husbands a living wage for domestic workers and help them fight the local hierarchy: a support group without which the domestic workers felt their small and brave cooperative could not survive.

As for the "matriarchal" argument that I swallowed in prefeminist days, I now understand why many black women resent it and feel that it's the white sociologist's way of encouraging the black community to imitate a white suburban lifestyle. ("If I end up cooking grits for revolutionaries," explained a black woman poet from Chicago, "it isn't my revolution. Black men and women need to work together for partnership, not patriarchy. You can't have liberation for half a race.") In fact, some black women wonder if criticism of the strength they were forced to develop isn't a way to keep half the black community working at lowered capacity and lowered pay, as well as to attribute some of black men's sufferings to black women, instead of to their real source—white racism. I wonder with them.

Looking back at all those male-approved things I used to say, the basic hang-up seems to be clear: a lack of esteem for women—black women, Chicana women, white women—and for myself.

This is the most tragic punishment that society inflicts on any second-class group. Ultimately, the brainwashing works, and we ourselves come to believe our group is inferior. Even if we achieve a little success in the world and think of ourselves as "different," we don't want to associate with our group. We want to identify up, not down (clearly my problem in not wanting to write about women, and not wanting to join women's groups). We want to be the only woman in the office, or the only black family on the block, or the only Jew in the club.

The pain of looking back at wasted, imitative years is enormous. Trying to write like men. Valuing myself and other women according to the degree of our acceptance by men—socially, in politics, and in our professions. It's as painful as it is now to hear two grown-up female human beings competing with each other on the basis of their husbands' status, like servants whose identity rests on the wealth or accomplishments of their employers.

And this lack of esteem that makes us put each other down is still the major enemy of sisterhood. Women who are conforming to society's expectations view the nonconformists with justifiable alarm. "Those noisy, unfeminine women," they say to themselves. "They will only make trouble for us all." Women who are quietly nonconforming, hoping nobody will notice, are even more alarmed because they have more to lose. And that makes sense, too.

Because the status quo protects itself by punishing all challengers, especially women whose rebellion strikes at the most fundamental social organization: the sex roles that convince half the population its identity depends on being first in work or in war, and the other half that it must serve as docile ("feminine") unpaid or underpaid labor. There seems to be no punishment inside the white male club that quite equals the ridicule and personal viciousness reserved for women who rebel. Attractive or young women who act forcefully are assumed to be male-controlled. If they succeed, it could only have been sexually, through men. Old women or women considered unattractive by male standards are accused of acting only out of bitterness, because they could not get a man. Any woman who chooses to behave like a full human being should be warned that the armies of the status quo will treat her as something of a dirty joke; that's their natural and first weapon. She will *need* sisterhood.

All of that is meant to be a warning but not a discouragement. There are so many more rewards than punishments.

For myself, I can now admit anger, and use it constructively, where once I would have submerged it and let it fester into guilt or collect for some destructive explosion.

I have met brave women who are exploring the outer edge of human possibility, with no history to guide them, and with a courage to make themselves vulnerable that I find moving beyond the words to express it.

I no longer think that I do not exist, which was my version of that lack of self-esteem afflicting many women. (If male standards weren't natural to me, and they were the only standards, how could I exist?) This means that I am less likely to need male values to identify myself with and am less vulnerable to classic arguments. ("If you don't like me, you're not a Real Woman"—said by a man who is Coming On. "If you don't like me, you're not a Real Person, and you can't relate to other people"—said by anyone who understands blackmail as an art.)

I can sometimes deal with men as equals and therefore can afford to like them for the first time.

I have discovered politics that are not intellectual or superimposed. They are organic, because I finally understand why I for years inexplicably identified with "out" groups. I belong to one, too. It will take a coalition of such groups to achieve a society in which, at a minimum, no one is born into a second-class role because of visible difference, because of race or of sex.

I no longer feel strange by myself, or with a group of women in public. I feel just fine.

I am continually moved to discover I have sisters.

I am beginning, just beginning, to find out who I am.

Dear Injurious Physician

BARBARA SEAMAN

Barbara Seaman, "Dear Injurious Physician," *New York Times*, December 2, 1972. Reprinted by permission.

In 1957, pregnant with my first child, I told my doctor that I planned to breast-feed. "You wouldn't make a good cow," he said. To his mind that settled the matter, for he gave me a laxative that went straight to the milk and almost finished off my son.

In 1960, my oldest daughter was born "by appointment." All went well. In 1962, pregnant again, I chanced to fall into conversation with a public health pediatrician.

"When do you expect the baby?" she asked.

"My doctor is inducing her on October 15."

"Why?"

"Why not?"

"Because it's dangerous," she explained. "Go back and ask him why he's doing it—and he better have a good reason."

I went back and asked him. He was hoping to go on a cruise in late October.

If I had known then what I know now, having babies would have been a lot more enjoyable. Having miscarriages—and abortions—would have been a lot less terrifying. Some women want to let their doctors "do the worrying for them," but for those of us who don't, it has been extremely difficult to get honest health information.

Women are making a valiant effort to correct the situation. In recent months, several important health books by women have appeared, and there are more to come. I am thinking, for example, of *The Nature and Evolution of Female Sexuality*, by Dr. Mary Jane Sherfey; *Why Natural Childbirth*, by Dr. Deborah Tanzer and Jean Libman Block; *Vaginal Politics*, by Ellen Frankfort; *Our Bodies, Ourselves*, by the Boston Women's Health Book Collective; *Women and Madness*, by Dr. Phyllis Chesler. There will even be a book telling women that radical mastectomy is not necessarily the treatment of choice for breast cancer.

These books have been and will be misunderstood in many quarters. We do not expect men to be endlessly fascinated by the ins and outs of feminine plumbing, but it hurts when our sisters reject us. A reporter for the *New York Times* complained that she was tired of hearing feminists badmouth their gynecologists. Why don't they go to a woman doctor? she asked. She might as well have said, "Let them eat cake." According to the American College of Obstetrics and Gynecology, only 3 percent of its members are female. Furthermore, there are some male chauvinists among women doctors too.

Let those who doubt that women have cause to be angry at their doctors leaf through the ads in almost any medical journal. One of the worst offenders sells a widely and often irresponsibly used tranquilizer. A shrewish-looking woman is depicted, and the message seems to say: "Doctor, get her off your back. . . . Get her off her husband's back. . . . Shoot her up and shut her up with our product."

And let the skeptics, please, when the time comes, look up the January 1973 issue of the *American Journal of Sociology*. It will contain a study by Diana Scully and Pauline Bart on the images of women in gynecology textbooks. Even if the medical student starts out as a nice kid, he is bound to be a screwed-up sexist by the time he finishes memorizing these gems:

➤ "The traits that compose the core of the female personality are feminine narcissism, masochism and passivity." —Dr. James Robert Willson, 1971

➤ "The frequency of intercourse depends entirely upon the male sex drive. . . . The bride should be advised to allow her husband's sex drive to set their pace and she should attempt to gear hers satisfactorily to his." —Dr. Edmund R. Novak et al., 1970

➤ "If like all human beings, he [the gynecologist] is made in the image of the Almighty, and if he is kind, then his kindness and concern for his patient may provide her with a glimpse of God's image." —Dr. C. Russell Scott, 1968

Amen.

The Ultimate Revolution

SHULAMITH FIRESTONE

Shulamith Firestone, *The Dialectic of Sex: The Case for Feminist Revolution*, New York: Bantam Books, 1971. Reprinted by permission.

We have seen how women, biologically distinguished from men, are culturally distinguished from "human." Nature produced the fundamental inequality—half the human race must bear and rear the children of all of them—which was later consolidated, institutionalized, in the interests of men. Reproduction of the species cost women dearly, not only emotionally, psychologically, culturally but even in strictly material (physical) terms: before recent methods of contraception, continuous childbirth led to constant "female trouble," early aging, and death. Women were the slave class that maintained the species in order to free the other half for the business of the world—admittedly often its drudge aspects, but certainly all its creative aspects as well.

This natural division of labor was continued only at great cultural sacrifice: men and women developed only half of themselves, at the expense of the other half. The division of the psyche into male and female to better reinforce the reproductive division was tragic: the hypertrophy in men of rationalism, aggressive drive, the atrophy of their emotional sensitivity was a physical (war) as well as a cultural disaster. The emotionalism and passivity of women increased their suffering (we cannot speak of them in a symmetrical way, since they were victimized as a class by the division). Sexually, men and women were channeled into a highly ordered—time, place, procedure, even dialogue—heterosexuality restricted to the genitals, rather than diffused over the entire physical being.

I submit, then, that the first demand for any alternative system be:

1. THE FREEING OF WOMEN FROM THE TYRANNY OF THEIR REPRODUCTIVE BIOLOGY BY EVERY MEANS AVAILABLE, AND THE DIFFUSION OF THE CHILDBEARING AND CHILD-REARING ROLE TO THE SOCIETY AS A WHOLE, MEN AS WELL AS WOMEN. There are many degrees of this. Already we have a (hard-won) acceptance of "family planning," if not contraception for its own sake. Proposals are imminent for day-care centers, perhaps even 24-hour child-care centers staffed by men as well as women. But this, in my opinion, is timid if not entirely worthless as a transition. We're talking about *radical* change. And though indeed it cannot come all at once, radical goals must be kept in sight at all times. Day-care centers buy women off. They ease the immediate pressure without asking why that pressure is on *women*.

At the other extreme there are the more distant solutions based on the potentials of modern embryology, that is, artificial reproduction, possibilities still so frightening that they are seldom discussed seriously. We have seen that the fear is to some extent justified: in the hands of our current society and under the direction of current scientists (few of whom are female or even feminist), any attempted used of technology to "free" anybody is suspect. But we are speculating about postrevolutionary systems, and for the purposes of our discussion we shall assume flexibility and good intentions in those working out the change.

To thus free women from their biology would be to threaten the *social* unit that is organized around biological reproduction and the subjection of women to their biological destiny, the family. Our second demand will come also as a basic contradiction to the family, this time the family as an *economic* unit:

2. **THE FULL SELF-DETERMINATION, INCLUDING ECONOMIC INDEPENDENCE, OF BOTH WOMEN AND CHILDREN.** To achieve this goal would require fundamental changes in our social and economic structure. This is why we must talk about a feminist socialism: in the immediate future, under capitalism, there could be at best a token integration of women into the labor force. For women have been found exceedingly useful and cheap as a transient, often highly skilled labor supply,* not to mention the economic value of their traditional function, the reproduction and rearing of the next generation of children, a job for which they are now patronized (literally and thus figuratively) rather than paid. But whether or not officially recognized, these are essential economic functions. Women, in this present capacity, are the very foundation of the economic superstructure, vital to its existence.** The paeans to self-sacrificing motherhood have a basis in reality: Mom *is* vital to the American way of life, considerably more than apple pie. She is an institution without which the system really *would* fall apart. In official capitalist terms, the bill for her economic services*** might run as high as one fifth of the gross national product. But payment is not the answer. To pay her, as is often discussed seriously in Sweden, is a reform that does not challenge the basic division of labor and thus could never eradicate the disastrous psychological and cultural consequences of that division of labor.

As for the economic independence of children, that is really a pipe dream, realized as yet nowhere in the world. And, in the case of children too, we are talking about more than a fair integration into the labor force; we are talking about the abolition of the labor force itself under a cybernetic socialism, the radical restructuring of the economy to make "work," i.e., wage labor, no longer necessary. In our postrevolutionary society adults as well as

---

*Most bosses would fail badly had they to take over their secretaries' job, or do without them. I know several secretaries who sign without a thought their bosses' names to their own (often brilliant) solutions. The skills of college women especially would cost a fortune reckoned in material terms of male labor.

**The Chase Manhattan Bank estimates a woman's overall domestic workweek at 99.6 hours. Margaret Benston gives her minimal estimate for a *childless* married woman at sixteen hours, close to half of a regular workweek; a *mother* must spend at least six or seven days a week working close to twelve hours.

***Margaret Benston ("The Political Economy of Women's Liberation," *Monthly Review*, September 1969), in attempting to show that women's oppression is indeed economic—though previous economic analysis has been incorrect—distinguishes between the male superstructure economy based on *commodity* production (capitalist ownership of the means of production, and wage labor), and the preindustrial reduplicative economy of the family, production for immediate *use*. Because the latter is not part of the *official* contemporary economy, its function at the basis of that economy is often overlooked. Talk of drafting women into the superstructure commodity economy fails to deal with the tremendous amount of necessary production of the traditional kind now performed by women without pay: Who will do it?

children would be provided for—irrespective of their social contributions—in the first equal distribution of wealth in history.

We have now attacked the family on a double front, challenging that around which it is organized: reproduction of the species by females and its outgrowth, the physical dependence of women and children. To eliminate these would be enough to destroy the family, which breeds the power psychology. However, we will break it down still further.

3. THE TOTAL INTEGRATION OF WOMEN AND CHILDREN INTO ALL ASPECTS OF THE LARGER SOCIETY. ALL INSTITUTIONS THAT SEGREGATE THE SEXES, OR BAR CHILDREN FROM ADULT SOCIETY, E.G., THE ELEMENTARY SCHOOL, MUST BE DESTROYED. DOWN WITH SCHOOL! These three demands predicate a feminist revolution based on advanced technology. And if the male-female and the adult-child cultural distinctions are destroyed, we will no longer need the sexual repression that maintains these unequal classes, allowing for the first time a "natural" sexual freedom. Thus we arrive at:

4. THE FREEDOM OF ALL WOMEN AND CHILDREN TO DO WHATEVER THEY WISH TO DO SEXUALLY. There will no longer be any reason *not* to. (Past reasons: Full sexuality threatened the continuous reproduction necessary for human survival, and thus, through religion and other cultural institutions, sexuality had to be restricted to reproductive purposes, all nonreproductive sex pleasure considered deviation or worse. The sexual freedom of women would call into question the fatherhood of the child, thus threatening patrimony. Child sexuality had to be repressed because it was a threat to the precarious internal balance of the family. These sexual repressions increased proportionately to the degree of cultural exaggeration of the biological family.) In our new society, humanity could finally revert to its natural polymorphous sexuality—all forms of sexuality would be allowed and indulged. The fully sexuate mind, realized in the past in only a few individuals (survivors), would become universal. Artificial cultural achievement would no longer be the only avenue to sexuate self-realization: one could now realize oneself fully, simply in the process of being and acting.

Our Bodies, Ourselves: Remembering the Dignity

EDITED BY MEI HWEI ASTELLA SAW AND SARAH J. SHEY

Excerpts from *Our Bodies, Ourselves*, New York: New England Free Press, 1971; New York: Simon & Schuster, 1973, 1998); selections from Joanna Perlman's interview with Judy Norsigian, March 1999. Reprinted by permission.

> *Remember the dignity of your womanhood.*
> *Do not appeal, do not beg, do not grovel.*
> *Take courage, join hands, stand beside us.*
> *Fight with us . . .*
> *—Christabel Pankhurst, English suffragette, 1880–1958*

In May 1969, Bread and Roses, a grassroots socialist-feminist collective in Boston, organized a one-day conference that included a workshop on "Women and Their Bodies." At the workshop, according to *Our Bodies, Ourselves* program director Judy Norsigian in a 1999 interview with Barnard College senior Joanna Perlman, the women were "struck by their level of ignorance about their own bodies." They decided to take action, and *Our Bodies, Ourselves* grew from there.

"The women decided to collect basic information about health care issues that concerned them—childbirth, pregnancy, contraception, abortion," Norsigian recalls. "They ended up drafting term papers and sharing them with one another. And they discovered that it was electrifying to share their own experiences. Women, in general, were not assertive and did not feel entitled to ask questions in the medical care setting. They realized that the key to getting good health care was to get as well-informed as possible."

Our Bodies, Ourselves was revolutionary on several counts. At the time, books on women's health issues were not easy to find. From the very first self-published issue of *OBOS*, in 1971, the Boston Women's Health Course Collective worked to make it accessible to all women who sought health information. Between 1971 and 1973, the collective paid for eleven printings altogether. When Simon & Schuster started publishing the book in 1973, the collective arranged for a special "clinic copy discount" of 70 percent off the cover price for nonprofit agencies. The collective also gave away free books to women in prison, and to others who couldn't afford to buy it, especially women in developing countries. This free book distribution continues to this day.

Existing texts tended to be "written in technical language that didn't really appeal or relate to women's lay experiences," says Norsigian. *Our Bodies, Ourselves* put information into language that was accessible. As Norma Swenson, a founding member of the Boston Women's Health Book Collective, pointed out in a *New York Times* article in 1997, "what was groundbreaking was the candor and honesty of women speaking about their experiences." The editors of the 1971 edition urged readers to "make suggestions, write up your own experience, or otherwise work on the course," reminding readers of a central fact of *OBOS*'s existence: "The course is what all of us make it."

In one of the early zine-like issues, the candor and honesty of *Our Bodies, Ourselves* is clear:

> A few years ago an American woman with an unwanted pregnancy was doomed to a lonely and dangerous trip underground for an illegal abortion. Although things aren't perfect today, enough attitudes and state laws have changed so that *you can get a legal abortion.* If there is no chance of getting a legal abortion in your state, you can go elsewhere, probably to New York. *Do not risk your life by going to an illegal*

> *abortionist!* You don't have to do that anymore. Remember—early abortion (before 12 weeks since your last menstrual period) is safer and it is easier to obtain. So if you think you're pregnant and you don't want to be, don't delay in consulting one of the agencies mentioned below. And if you're pregnant and don't know how you feel about it, counselors at many of these agencies can help you think it out.[1]

Our Bodies, Ourselves dealt firmly and honestly with prickly issues like abortion, birth control, and sexuality, and also took it upon itself to bring to attention the troubling relationship between women and their doctors. "The feminist principles that were developing in the women's movement sort of collided with the dismay and distress women had with their medical and health encounters," Norsigian says.

"We looked at women's health and medical care, and saw how badly physicians were being trained," she says. "At that point, most of the physicians were men. Women were encouraged to think of their physicians as gods. In the period when *OBOS* was created, women were still reluctant to move out of the role of the passive obedient female in the presence of doctors. Women learned quickly that when they didn't ask questions and think 'What about me?' 'What are the side effects?' 'What are the risks?' they ended up having unnecessary surgery, and taking drugs they didn't know about, and wishing they hadn't done what they had done. That sense of entitlement I think *OBOS* has helped to facilitate in women—as well as the larger women's movement—was a great contribution."

Looking back today, one cannot help but notice the changes that *Our Bodies, Ourselves* has helped bring about in this area. Look at this account of the doctor-patient relationship in the 1971 edition . . .

> Perhaps the most obvious indication of this ideology is the way that doctors treat us as women patients. We are considered

stupid, mindless creatures, unable to follow instructions (known as orders). While men patients may also be treated this way, we are worse because women are thought to be incapable of understanding or dealing with our own situation.

It is important for us to understand that mystification is the primary process here. It is *mystification* that makes us postpone going to the doctor for "that little pain," since he's such a "busy man." It is *mystification* that prevents us from demanding a precise explanation of what is the matter and how exactly he is going to treat it. It is *mystification* that causes us to become passive objects who submit to his control and supposed expertise.[2]

Now consider this woman's statement, from the 1998 edition.

Friends now marvel at my close relationship with my current doctor and my ability to talk back, question, and disagree with him and his colleagues. He respects me and trusts me to tell him what is going on, and I in turn trust him to listen, make suggestions, and consult with me before any action is taken. When I don't want a procedure done or feel the psychological burden of making yet another trip to the lab or to his office is just too much for me on an occasion, I will tell him and he understands me most of the time. I have finally after many, many years found someone willing to take into account my whole medical history and apply it to my current situation.[3]

The 1973 edition included a chapter on sexually transmitted diseases, something that "had never been seen before," according to Norsigian. "We were among the first to talk about the fact that women were largely asymptomatic when we have STDs [sexually transmitted diseases]. We encouraged safer-sex practices before the term had even

been coined. We saw the transition from when STDs couldn't be talked about to now when they're everywhere." In a manner that was now characteristic of *Our Bodies, Ourselves,* the writers conveyed medical advice and sound practical information, all the time urging women to take their health into their own hands.

PROTECT YOURSELF— PROTECT OTHERS

If you notice any symptoms of venereal disease (VD) in yourself, no matter how mild, you should go to a doctor or a clinic at once.

➤ Don't panic or feel guilty or embarrassed.

➤ Don't depend on one test only. If the first test for gonorrhea or syphilis doesn't show anything, make sure the doctor takes another one to be safe. Women should make sure the doctor takes smears from at least the cervix and the anus or urethra. Don't just accept what he says. Some doctors aren't careful enough—and it's your life, not his.

➤ Even if you are sure that you have had no contact with someone infected with VD, you may be saving other women's lives by demanding that your doctor routinely give you and every other woman tests for VD without attached moral judgment.[4]

The 1979 edition proved that *Our Bodies, Ourselves* was not only a book that broke taboos but also a much needed medical reference and guide for women. The comprehensive chapter on venereal diseases revealed serious gaps in educating doctors about VDs and taught women how to recognize their own symptoms.

THE MEDICAL SYSTEM

VD education for doctors has been ignored by medical schools for the past 25 years and is only now being reinstated. Doctors who got their medical education during that period may not know enough about diagnosing and treating VD. Since doctors and health workers in clinics that regularly serve VD patients learn on the job, they probably have the best and most up-to-date VD information. Unfortunately, they are rarely informed about the preventive methods that women can use.[5]

This edition, and later ones as well, included a detailed drawing of a woman's body, illustrating sites where VD symptoms occur. A page-long table full of information about venereal diseases ("How you catch it"; "How to tell you have it"; "How to find out for sure"; and so on) enabled women to do a quick self-diagnosis before rushing to the doctor, thus putting vital medical information—and power—into their own hands.

As a tribute on its twenty-fifth anniversary, Vivian Pinn, director of the Office of Research on Women's Health at the National Institutes of Health, wrote to the Boston Women's Health Book Collective, "Your visionary call to action has inspired many women to take greater control of their lives, their bodies, and their health. . . . Women have come a long way from the time when they were afraid to ask their doctors questions concerning their health." Norsigian agrees, pointing out one of the main reasons for the early and continued success of *Our Bodies, Ourselves*: "The book meets many women where they are at. It doesn't preach. It doesn't say that something is wrong with you because you don't agree with what it says. The book tries to point out ways in which women are shortchanged and the ways in which women could be more fulfilled human beings."

In the 1970s, women certainly felt shortchanged, and found their way to *Our Bodies, Ourselves*, which took the role of wise and trusted friend for many a curious woman. It spoke honestly and openly about women's issues, many of which were strictly taboo. It was filled with first-person anecdotes. As the writers of the 1971 edition article on sexuality noted: "We felt that our own voices, our own histories, rang the clearest and truest and helped us reclaim the mysterious topic of sexuality." The effect was to normalize women's experiences. Here's one such example: a girl discovering masturbation.

> I was 14 or 15 years old, and a virgin. I was sitting cross-legged on my bed one day, and became aroused by memories of petting with my boyfriend, and having orgasms. I was also aroused by the sex smell I was exuding. I suddenly realized that I could do to my clitoris what he had done. I masturbated for the first time, had an orgasm, and wasn't so sure that what I had done was right.[6]

The writers followed with instructions on how to masturbate and achieve an orgasm—this at a time when doctors told many frustrated women that not all women had orgasms and that they would be better off forgetting about it.

One of the most famous pieces was published in the 1973 edition: an article entitled "In Amerika They Call Us Dykes" by the Boston Gay Collective. Their paper was made up of personal anecdotes that helped women begin to understand their own complicated sexuality. In this excerpt, a woman describes her gradual change in attitude about lesbianism.

> We had dancing classes in junior high. One night between dances a cold breeze started blowing through the open window. I reached over and touched Margaret's knee and asked her if she was getting cold too. She shrank back in mock horror and said, "What's the matter, Diana, are you a lesbian?" Everyone nearby started snickering. I didn't know what a lesbian was, but I knew I didn't want to be one. Later I found out; there was a lot of joking and taunting

among girls in my class about lesbianism, which they viewed as sick and disgusting. . . .

I got into the women's movement, and felt an enormous relief that I would no longer have to play roles with men and act feminine and sweet, dress in skirts and heels, and do all the things I'd done on dates. Then I began to feel hatred for men for having forced me into these roles. During this time . . . I began to hang out with gay women, who turned out to be regular people, not the stereotypes I had imagined. On a gut level I was beginning to realize that gayness was not a sickness. One night I went out for a long walk, and when I got home I had decided that I was a lesbian. For me it was not a decision to become a lesbian. It was a question of accepting and becoming comfortable with feelings I had always had.[7]

Twenty-five years later, *Our Bodies, Ourselves* includes articles on lesbians, transsexuals, bisexuals, and transgendered people. It still retains its personal approach, incorporating individual voices into the essays.

Since 1971, *Our Bodies, Ourselves* has grown from a quasi-underground, 138-page newsprint edition selling for forty cents a copy to an 800-page tome the size of the Manhattan phone book. It is truly a historical, social, and cultural icon. According to a recent article in the *Journal of the American Medical Women's Association*, OBOS became a best-seller within five years of its first publication, in both the United States and internationally. More that 4 million copies have been sold to date; there are editions in Japanese, Russian, Chinese, Spanish, French, Italian, German, and a dozen other languages, including an edition in Braille. From a one-day conference in 1969, a movement was born. Just a group of women sharing their experiences forever changed the course of women's health care.

NOTES

1. Boston Women's Health Book Collective, *Our Bodies, Ourselves* (Boston: New England Free Press, 1971), 66.
2. Ibid., 134.
3. Boston Women's Health Book Collective, *Our Bodies, Ourselves for the New Century* (New York: Touchstone, 1998), 686.
4. Boston Women's Health Book Collective, *Our Bodies, Ourselves: A Book by and for Women* (New York: Simon & Schuster, 1973), 104–05.
5. Boston Women's Health Book Collective, *Our Bodies, Ourselves* (New York: Touchstone, 1979), 171–72.
6. Boston Women's Health Book Collective, *Our Bodies, Ourselves* (1971).
7. Boston Women's Health Book Collective, *Our Bodies, Ourselves: A Book by and for Women* (1973).

Looking Back on *Our Bodies, Ourselves*

EDITED BY JOANNA PERLMAN AND SARAH J. SHEY

Excerpts from Joanna Perlman's interview with Judy Norsigian, conducted in March 1999; and *Our Bodies, Ourselves for the New Century*, New York: Simon & Schuster, 1998. Reprinted by permission.

JP: What are some of the early issues *OBOS* picked up on that are now taken for granted?

JN: We included a chapter on sexually transmitted diseases in the 1973 edition, and we were among the first to talk about the fact that women were largely asymptomatic when we had STDs. We encouraged safer-sex practices before the term had even been coined. We saw the transition from when STDs couldn't be talked about to now when they're more frequently addressed.

Another issue we raised early on was out-of-hospital birth, home birth and greater utilization of midwives. We raised questions about . . . the best place for birth and . . . the best caregivers. We now know that out-of-hospital birth can be as safe as hospital birth, and sometimes even safer.

JP: What are some of the issues that *OBOS* has not been able to overcome or tackle?

JN: From our very earliest editions we did mention violence in women's lives as a major threat to women's health. When we first began, we talked about rape. Subsequent editions add other forms of violence against women: for example, incest, domestic partner abuse, sexual harrassment. Although there are many more resources like shelters and rape programs, this is the one area where statistics seem to get worse year by year.

JP: When the collective first set out, were there any unanticipated roadblocks?

JN: I don't think we gave much attention to the profound effect of technology, especially reproductive technology, on women's lives—for example, the possibility of women giving birth well past menopause. There are women who have undergone repeated attempts at in vitro fertilization who say they wish they had never done it because it made their lives so miserable for so long. Very small percentages of women actually succeed with these methods in having biological children of their own. We hear about the successes but we don't often hear about the failures and the emotional struggle that women and their partners feel. These technologies have brought limited benefits and serious drawbacks.

CHANGING DIAGNOSIS AND TREATMENTS

New causes of infertility will be discovered as our environment becomes more toxic. Names and kinds of drugs change rapidly. New techniques and treatments appear regularly; few are studied in a controlled, randomized fashion. . . . You have a right to know whether your treatment is new, or part of an experimental study.[1]

JP: How have women's economic situations played into the quality of medical and health care they receive?

JN: In a climate where profit looms large and companies want to make a fast buck, we see advertising and the promotion of products that have not been adequately assessed from a scientific point of view. A recent example is the promotion of tamoxifen, which in some studies has been shown to reduce breast cancer risk. We saw a very misleading advertising campaign by Zeneca, which produces and distributes tamoxifen under a brand name. The National Women's Health Network successfully protested the misleading nature of Zeneca's ads, and as a result the FDA sent Zeneca a very strongly worded letter to remove these ads from magazines. Because pharmaceutical companies can now advertise prescription products directly to consumers, consumers must be more wary than ever. Silicone breast implants represent a good example of putting profit before safety. We still don't know whether the silicone implants are really and truly safe. But we do know that for thirty years no good quality data were collected by plastic surgeons or the implant manufacturers, despite repeated requests by the FDA. Is this a statement on how we, as a society, have valued women's health? There shouldn't be products on the market not adequately tested. . . . If we don't have a strong FDA and strong government controls we will see unethical behavior time and time again.

JP: Another economic concern is funding for women's health research. In recent years, the amount of funding for breast cancer research has increased a great deal. Do you think there's a particular reason breast cancer is getting so much of the attention, and do you think we'll see a spillover into increased funding and research for other areas of women's health—or does breast cancer stand out for a particular reason?

JN: In this country, the squeaky wheel gets the grease more often than not. There are a number of women with breast cancer who are articulate, middle-class, and able to organize around this issue. . . . For example, they gathered 600,000 signatures to pressure Congress for more research. We can learn a lot from both the breast cancer and AIDS activists of the past decade or so.

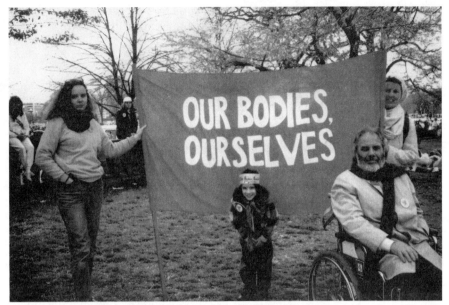

Left to right: Boston Women's Health Book Collective staff member and co-founder Sally Whelan; Kyra Zola Norsigian; Irving Kenneth Zola, longtime friend and contributor to *OBOS*; Cynthia Pearson, now executive director of the National Women's Health Network. [Courtesy of Judy Norsigian]

JP: With all the funding going toward breast cancer and the attention women's health issues have been getting because of the squeaky wheel, do you think we could see a backlash against the women's health movement or women's health activists, who might be perceived as somewhat leftist or radical?

JN: I don't think so. What has happened is that the pharmaceutical companies have begun defining the women's health terrain, and they want to promote drugs for prevention as well as therapy because of the potential market and profits. They don't necessarily want to emphasize lifestyle practices that promote prevention. Take our sexual experiences, for example. Drug companies are pursuing Viagra-like drugs for women to go along with their increasingly medicalized view of female sexual "dysfunction." For women without particular medical problems, we could just as well promote greater knowledge of our sexuality—how to masturbate, for example—as another approach to improving our sexual experience.

Ironically, it is because of Viagra and the way it allowed us to expose a double standard, that we finally were able to obtain insurance and HMO coverage for prescription contraceptives. If having sexual experiences wasn't considered essential to women's health and well-being, then how could it be argued that having erections was essential for men's health?

JP: Since you mention not having basic contraceptive coverage and women's limited access to primary health care, do you think that somehow that detracts from or downplays the progress the women's health movement has made over the past thirty years?

JN: We've made a lot progress in many areas but many women still don't have access to health and medical care, don't have even the most basic insurance or HMO coverage. That problem has only been exacerbated as we've seen the profit motive become a dominant force in health and medical care. It doesn't belong there, and we've long advocated strongly for a government-funded model.

There should be universal coverage that is not tied to employment. Health care is a right, not a privilege. We liken it to the police department and fire department—essential services in our communities.

JP: Barbara Seaman says that *OBOS* became one of the most powerful debriefing documents of patriarchy. What is your response to that?

JN: Feminism is about creating a society that recognizes capabilities in everyone and opportunities for everyone. . . . The book tries to point out the ways in which women are shortchanged and the ways in which women could be more fulfilled human beings. *OBOS* tries to create a picture, a critique, that isn't so adversarial, and that doesn't portray men as necessarily being the enemy. We challenge institutions and traditional patriarchal values, and even invite men to join up in this effort—ultimately everyone benefits from eliminating sexism and other forms of oppression.

JP: Why hasn't the collective come out with a book that is more accessible and more friendly to men so that men can start to be incorporated into this movement of women's health?

JN: The point of *OBOS* is to reach *women* and help *women* to think about the particulars of our lives. We have encouraged men to do a similar book for men, and in fact there have been some books like *OBOS* for men. Many men have found *OBOS* to be helpful, especially in better understanding the issues their women partners face.

JP: Do you think that some women might not find the book very accessible because of its leftist position?

JN: It might be a deterrent. However, the practical information is so accessible and so well-written that most women who disagree with the politics simply decide to put the politics aside and concentrate on the material they find most useful. Hopefully, we are able to reach those unconnected with the women's movement to adopt a more feminist perspective.

JP: What do you see coming to the foreground of the women's health movement in the next few years?

JN: Because there are now so many places where you can get women's information, it will become increasingly important to identify sources and distinguish quality information from material that is largely commercial hype.

JP: With all the rapid changes in the medical and health fields as well as the increasing amount of new information, how does *OBOS* keep up to date?

JN: It's extremely difficult. In the book we included information on Web sites that are constantly updated with new information and at our own Web site we constantly offer updated resources.

JP: How could you measure the impact of *OBOS*?

JN: We know from the tremendous amount of mail we get that the book is relevant and useful to many women. In other countries women have translated and adapted the book to suit their own needs, maintaining the essential feminist perspective that has become a universal theme in so many parts of the world. We are committed to updating this book and keeping it alive as a tool for social change.

THE IMPACT OF OBOS ON ONE WOMAN'S LIFE

I think you would have been proud of the way I handled the situation with the surgeon. Despite a fair amount of crying on my part, I was able to demand a second opinion for my diverticulosis treatment and the most conservative treatment possible. My surgeon was appalled when I balked at surgery . . . without what I felt was adequate time to discuss the situation or get another opinion. I really think that if it wasn't for my experience with the Women's Health Collective and the support of my friends and family, I would have a temporary colostomy right now.[2]

JP: When the Boston collective celebrates the book's fiftieth anniversary, in 2020, what would you have to see as its greatest accomplishment?

JN: With over 3.5 million copies in print, the book has heightened awareness among so many women and even pushed the health and medical care system to be more responsive to women's needs. At our fiftieth anniversary, maybe we will be able to say that health and medical care has become less driven by profits, and more science-based and accessible to all. Maybe we will be able to say that we are finally rid of the sexism, racism, and other forms of discrimination that are still so common today. I think these are things we would be very happy to say have happened.

NOTES

1. Boston Women's Health Book Collective, *Our Bodies, Ourselves for the New Century* (New York: Touchstone, 1998), 533.
2. Ibid., 681.

The Boston Women's Health Book Collective and *Our Bodies, Ourselves*

Excerpt from Judy Norsigian et al., "The Boston Women's Health Book Collective and *Our Body, Ourselves*," edited by Joanna Perlman and Sarah J. Shey, *Journal of American Medical Women's Association*, Winter 1999. Reprinted by permission.

RECENT GROWTH AND DEVELOPMENT

Over the nearly three decades since the first edition of *OBOS*, we have continued to develop our awareness of the injustices that prevent women from experiencing full and healthy lives. As we approach the millennium, such causes of poor health as poverty, racism, hunger, and homelessness continue to disproportionately affect nonwhite populations in this country and around the world.

We continue to believe that effective strategies for mitigating these problems require all of us to reject the assumptions that so often have hurt women of color and women who are poor. Over the years we have collaborated with women's groups both in the United States and abroad to ensure that the priorities for the women's health movement reflect the needs and concerns of all women. We also recognize the importance of supporting the leadership of women of color and low-income women within our own organization as well as in the larger women's health movements. Although this is a difficult challenge for many groups founded originally by white women, we believe that our ultimate success as a movement depends on respectful collaboration at many levels.

The structure of the Boston Women's Health Book Collective (BWHBC) has evolved over the years. We began as a collective, a circle of twelve women. . . . We took no profits from sales of the books, using the royalties to support women's health projects and eventually to start our own WHIC and advocacy work. As soon as we hired staff who were not authors of the book, the BWHBC was not formally a collective any more, although the board (mostly original authors for many hears) and the paid staff each worked in a largely collaborative manner.

BWHBC'S ROLE IN THE GLOBAL WOMEN'S HEALTH MOVEMENT

Over the years, we have developed a number of fruitful collaborations with women's groups in different countries and have attended almost all the international women and health meetings that have been convened since the first International Conference on Woman and Health held in Rome in 1977. At the 1995 NGO Women's Forum in Beijing, many of the women working on these translation/adaptation projects came together to compare notes and to share strategies for dealing with problems such as government censorship and fundraising.

One continuing concern of the current global women's health movement has been the growing trend, especially among environmental groups, to label population growth as a primary cause of environmental degradation. It would be a serious step back if this trend were to lead to more overly zealous family planning programs' driven by demographic goals rather than by women's reproductive health needs. We believe that the unethical and growing use of quinacrine, a sclerosing agent, as a means of nonsurgical sterilization in countries such as Indonesia, India, Pakistan, and Vietnam, represents the very "population control" mentality that has so often been destructive to women's health. Thus, we have joined activists around the globe in protesting the use of quinacrine.

We also collaborated with such other groups as the Women's Global Network for Reproductive Rights (Amsterdam), the International Reproductive Rights and Research Action Group (IRRRAG), and WomanHealth Philippines to sponsor "The Double Challenge," a well-attended workshop series at the Beijing NGO Forum in September 1995. The brochure for this series stated: "Women from around the world face a formidable challenge. On one side are the fundamentalists led by the Vatican; on the other is the population establishment. Both are vying for control over women's sexual and reproductive lives. While the fundamentalists outlaw contraception and abortion, the populationists push new reproductive and contraceptive technologies."

THE CONTINUED NEED FOR A WOMEN'S HEALTH MOVEMENT

The concerns that brought women together several decades ago to form women-controlled health centers, advocacy groups, and other educational and activist organizations largely remain. Women are still the major users of health and medical services, for example, seeking care for themselves even when essentially healthy (birth control, pregnancy and childbearing, and menopausal discomforts). Because women live longer than men, we have more problems with chronic diseases and functional impairment, and thus require more community and home-based services. Women usually act as the family "health broker": arranging

care for children, the elderly, spouses, or relatives, and are also the major unpaid caregivers for those around them.

Although women represent the great majority of health workers, we still have a relatively small role in policy making in all arenas. Despite increases in the number of women physicians, we also have a limited leadership role in US medical schools, where women represent less than 10 percent of all tenured faculty. Women face discrimination on the basis of sex, class, race, age, sexual orientation, and disability in most medical settings. Many continue to experience condescending, paternalistic, and culturally insensitive treatment. Older women, women of color, fat women, women with disabilities, and lesbians routinely confront discriminatory attitudes and practices, and even outright abuse.

Women usually find it difficult to obtain the good health and medical information necessary to ensure informed decision making, especially for alternatives to conventional forms of treatment. This problem is intensified for poor women and for those who do not speak English, in part because their class, race, and culture increasingly differ markedly from those of their health care providers.

Many women are subjected to inappropriate medical interventions, such as overmedication with psychotropic drugs (especially tranquilizers and antidepressants), questionable hormone therapy, and unnecessary cesarean sections and hysterectomies, although managed care has reduced the rates of unnecessary surgery in some places.

Despite enormous advances for women over the past two decades, ongoing gender bias in public and private settings continues to relegate women to a separate and unequal place in society. We must have a strong community of women's organizations to assist women individually, to articulate women's needs, to advocate for policy reform, and to resist the more destructive aspects of corporate medicine. Organizations such as the National Women's Health Network, the National Black Women's Health Project, the National Latina Health

Organization, the National Asian Women's Health Organization, and the Native American Women's Health Education Resource Center, to name just a few, could play a key role in ensuring that lay and consumer voices are part of any larger women's health debate. The inclusion of such groups by the Office of Women's Health Research at the National Institutes of Health already has enriched discussions concerning research affecting women.

Ironically, except in a handful of states, poor women on Medicaid can obtain a federally funded sterilization but not a federally funded abortion. This limitation has led some women to "choose" sterilization because we have so few options. As the women's health movement continues to emphasize, without access to all reproductive health services, there can be no real choice in matters of childbearing.

Over the years, the BWHBC has collaborated with physicians who have shared the feminist perspective represented in *OBOS*. One such colleague, Mary Howell, MD (more recently known as Mary Raugust), died from breast cancer in February 1998. The author of a popular 1972 book entitled *Why Would a Girl Go into Medicine?* and the first woman dean at Harvard Medical School, Mary contributed to the research that resulted in a legal ruling forcing medical schools to eliminate female quotas. These informal quotas had kept the female presence in medical schools no more than 8 percent of the total number of students since the turn of the century. She remains for us one of the finest role models for women in medicine, and we hope that her speeches and writings will be published to inspire the younger generations of female physicians. Another physician, Alice Rothchild, MD, has written and spoken eloquently about her experience as a feminist obstetrician-gynecologist, and we have made her 1998 AMWA speech available at our website (www.ourbodiesourselves.org).

Members of the media often ask us if we think that progress has been made in addressing the concerns women have had about medicine. We believe that physician awareness of condescending and paternalistic behaviors that are now generally regarded as disrespectful elsewhere in society has been heightened. It also appears that more women feel that their physicians take their concerns seriously, rather than dismissing complaints with, "It's all in your head." But other problems have been exacerbated, and although not unique to women, women's more frequent contact with the medical care system means that women confront these issues much more regularly than men do. Many managed care plans have contributed to reductions in access to care, especially good quality care, for some women. They have, for example, not allowed some physicians to provide needed treatments. Sometimes, physicians have not had the time to adequately assess the plethora of new drugs and medical technologies that they regularly recommend to patients. Cutbacks in local community services and public health programs make it harder to sustain an emphasis on preventive health care.

The BWHBC has a special interest in such problems as the increasing influence of right-wing organizations over public policies affecting women's health, the explosion of health and medical technologies marketed primarily to women, the objectification of women's bodies in the media, the exclusion of consumers from policy setting and oversight functions in many managed care plans, and the relatively few sources of noncommercial information about women and health, especially with a well-informed consumer perspective. We recognize institutional racism as a continuing problem exacerbated by the fact that most caregivers and health care administrators come from economic, social, racial, and ethnic backgrounds quite different from those of the people they are serving. Finally, we believe it is critical to challenge the tendency to overmedicalize women's lives and turn normal events such as childbearing and menopause into disabling conditions requiring medical intervention.

As the women's health movement moves into

the next century, the ability to build broad coalitions will largely determine the political effectiveness of women's health care advocates. We can learn much, for example, from the passage of the Americans with Disabilities Act, which succeeded in large part because of the disability rights community reached out to form broad alliances with other groups not initially aware of the universal impact of this legislation. Finding common ground and ways to bridge racial, ethnic, and class differences in particular, will be among the great challenges we face.

Alice Wolfson

INTERVIEW BY TANIA KETENJIAN

Alice Wolfson is a founding member of the National Women's Health Network. This interview was conducted in May 1999.

TK: What gave you the confidence, in 1969, to stand up in such a male-dominated arena as a Senate committee to protest the lack of women's involvement in the birth control pill hearings?

AW: When we first stood up at the Senate hearings we really had no idea that we were doing something that was going to have so much importance. We went as five women from a small group in Washington DC concerned with health issues. Someone told us that there were going to be hearings on the Hill about the birth control pill. After we heard about the hearings we all sat around and talked about our own experiences with the pill. It turned out that all of us in this small group had had some side effect or another. None of us had been warned that there might be side effects. Not only that, but half of the time, when you complained of a side effect to doctors, the doctors themselves didn't know that the pill caused side effects. For instance, in my case, when I stopped taking the pill, I started to lose a lot of hair. I went to a dermatologist who didn't know anything about the connection of hair loss to the pill, and my gynecologist didn't connect it at all. I was terrified that I was going bald and I

had no idea why. So we went to the hearings where we started to hear some very frightening information about the pill. We were also shocked to see that there wasn't a single woman testifying, no women researchers, no women who had taken the pill. We had so many questions that we just started to raise our hands asking to be called on, wanting to be heard. It was such an outrageous thing to do that the TV cameras and the newspaper photographers all swiveled around from the senators to focus on the women in the audience!

We really had not planned a demonstration but then, when we saw the kind of reception we got, we understood that the most important issue was not the fact that the pill had been recklessly marketed and had been approved way before there was enough information about safety, but that women who were taking it, who were dying from a "safe and effective" contraceptive, weren't told anything about the side effects. So the issue grew from our individual outrage at what was happening to an understanding of how important our outrage was, and how much we—meaning all women— had suffered from not having had informed consent when we were given the pill.

TK: What were some of the more serious known side effects that you had not been told about?

AW: It was hard for us to believe that the FDA was not on the side of women. They held secret meetings about the birth control pill and its side effects. There was data coming over from research done in England; which they were trying to keep secret. We were getting fed different pieces of information by Barbara Seaman, who was in New York. I was in Washington DC, and Barbara would call and say, "They're meeting today, they're at the FDA"; and we would go there with some excuse or other, and break into the meeting room. We felt very powerful, like, "Alright, fine, arrest us. We're the people taking the pill, and if that's what you want, fine, you can arrest us." We were fearless; we would put ten dollars in our boots and go off. If we were arrested, we'd bail ourselves out. They never did, actually, arrest any of us but they threatened us a lot. Senator Dole had us into his office and basically begged us to stop the demonstrations:

"We can't continue if you don't stop." He said something like that. It's not an exact quote. I think we made some kind of deal with him at that point. We agreed that we would stop the demonstrations if they would stop the hearings and bring women back into the next round of hearings.

TK: Tell me about the April 1, 1970 secret FDA meeting. How did you get in?
How did Barbara Seaman find out about it and let you know?

AW: Barbara was a health writer in New York. She had many mainstream contacts, and she was very interested in the side effects of the pill; so she became aware, through her own contacts, of things that were happening in Washington. There was a meeting that was held in secret. Barbara told me who to ask for at the meeting, so I knocked on the door. I think there were three of us there. We were told, "Sorry, this meeting is private; you can't come in." So we pushed open the door, and said to them, "Alright, call the police. We'll call the paper, you call the police."

So doctors were sitting around discussing whether or not to tell women to call them if they got a headache and they were on the birth control pill. There was an argument between a short patient package insert and a longer, more informative patient package insert, and the doctors sat around and said things like, "If you tell a woman she's going to get a headache, she'll get the headache. I'll be beleaguered by calls; my wife will kill me; people will be calling me in the middle of the night about all of these side effects; we can't do it."

Meanwhile, they had data that was definitely showing that women were dying from taking these pills. It's important to remember that it was healthy women who were taking the pill. This wasn't a pill that was being given to somebody who was sick to make them better, this was something that was being given to women who started out healthy and who were dying. I think one of our signs once said, "Must we die for love?" along with "Feed your pills to the rats at the FDA."

TK: Did you find that you had to hide your radical appearance to be effective in the hearings?

AW: For the first pill hearing, we dressed for the occasion. We knew we were going to the Senate, so all of us dressed to fit in, not to stand out. We wore dresses, skirts, high heels, and felt that it would be much more important to have our message heard for what it is, than to be judged for something that would create an immediate kind of knee-jerk reaction to who we were. So for every demonstration that I ever participated in, I dressed up. Just like I do for court today.

TK: What was the D.C. Women's Liberation?

AW: D.C. Women's Liberation coalesced at a particular moment in history. There were a lot of great women who were living in Washington, DC at that time—around 1969—early feminists who managed to obtain enough money to actually open an office. We had a humming, vibrant movement. We had daycare and a health group, and we had a newspaper, and the office was active. It seemed like, day and night, we had retreats; we had demonstrations at the drop of a hat. I think people don't know much about what birth control pills were like at the time. Abortion was still illegal, so it was very radical to say that the safest method of birth control was a barrier method followed up by safe, legal abortion. That was basically what the feminists were saying in those days, and it just wasn't said.

Another thing that people don't know much about is that there was a very large population control movement headed by the biggest names in the ruling class—the Duponts, the Mellons, and the Rockefellers—who had a vested interest in marketing population control abroad, and the pill was one of the tools with which it was marketed. I remember one guerilla theater event where we went into a very large population control meeting of maybe 500 people. There was something called the Women's International Terrorist Conspiracy from Hell (WITCH). We had our hats and our capes stuffed into our purses and at a certain point, we jumped up, put on our hats and capes, ran to the stage, grabbed the microphone, and did a skit, and—I don't remember the skit—but I remember the refrain was, "You think you can cure all the world's ills / by making poor women take your unhealthy pills." And then we would throw the pills out into the audience. We were really making connections to very large issues after starting with small issues—or what we thought was small at the time—that was the birth control pill.

There is a difference between a single issue and a broad spectrum of issues. If the birth control pill or abortion as a single issue are broadened out, they become a whole spectrum of issues called reproductive rights or reproductive choice. Part of being able to choose to have a child is to have the systems in place that make it possible: day care, after-school care. When my kids were little, after school care was awful, you couldn't find it anywhere, and it was really hard to figure out what to do with your kids when school was out. Today we're seeing all sorts of cuts in welfare, but we're not seeing a growth in the kinds of systems that we need to support working parents. So, no true choice.

TK: What was the Hyde Amendment and how was it discriminatory?

AW: The Hyde Amendment was the first congressional effort to cut off public funding for abortions for poor women: it actually discontinued Medicaid funding for abortions, discriminating against poor women by not allowing them to have access to the same kind of health care as middle-class women. A group that I belonged to in California, called the Committee to Defend Reproductive Rights, was successful in bringing a law suit and in maintaining MediCal funding for abortion, even though there wasn't any federal funding. The Com-

mittee to Defend Reproductive Rights was successful in maintaining MediCal funding, which is California's public funding, on an issue of equal access. The California Supreme Court could be convinced in a way that obviously Congress could not, that poor women had to have equal access to every kind of health care. If, for instance, no health plans offered abortion, it would be acceptable in the eyes of the law for MediCal not to offer it. But if other health plans offered abortion, then MediCal had to.

TK: Can you tell me about the Vancouver conference?

AW: That convened during the Vietnam war and it had two parts. There was one meeting in Vancouver, British Columbia, and one in Toronto. I was still on the East Coast at the time, so I was one of the planners of the Toronto conference. In addition to being on the two coasts, there were two parts to each conference. One was for women's liberation, and one was led, I think, by Women's Strike for Peace. They were held back to back; first the one, then the other. The women's liberation movement at that time, around 1971, was beginning to be pulled apart by its own internal politics, forces that we didn't realize we had set in motion because of a faulty or an incomplete analysis. I don't know what allowed some of the things that happened to emerge, but there was a great rift between lesbian women and straight women. This was very apparent at the Toronto conference, where there were groups of lesbian women who were interrupting meetings and basically scolding the Vietnamese, Laotian, and Cambodian women who were there and telling them that the war was their fault because they were heterosexual and slept with men. It was truly bizarre. Some of the women had walked weeks and weeks to meet the plane to take them to the conference. Their countries were being blown apart, their children killed—it was too much for me. That was around the time that I moved away from that part of the feminist movement.

TK: Because?

AW: Because I don't think that you can make a rev-olution by leaving out half the world, and—as it happened—I then went on to have boy children. I didn't know at the time that my children were going to be boys, but I felt, thank goodness, in my gut, that you cannot expect to build a women's movement which makes men its victims. Instead of a woman being valued for giving birth to boys, suddenly having girls was what was important, but it was the same thing. It was oppression based on your body, whether focused on boys or girls, and I just felt that was a mistake.

TK: I know that you became a radical because of anti-war protests and related issues, and then, as a feminist, you began to focus on health. Was it specifically the birth control pill hearings that caused you to focus on health?

AW: I began to focus on health when I began to focus on legalizing abortion. Part of my analysis was that as women, we weren't really going to be able to talk about being free if we couldn't control our own bodies. I saw abortion as a keystone issue for the whole women's movement. I lived in Wash-ington DC at the time, and Washington DC is a ma-jority black city; back then, it was 76 percent black, and you couldn't really talk about abortion without talking about sterilization abuse. So we very early on had an analysis that said you had to think of abortion as larger than a single issue. I always saw the health care system as a microcosm of what was happening in the larger world, and I saw it from the top down. I saw the doctor as the ruling class, which we could put next to a senator, and you could just go right on down to the woman who was the pa-tient.

TK: What was the focus of pre-movement feminist health groups?

AW: I always saw the women's health movement as having two wings: a service-oriented, clinic-based wing, which was composed of the feminist women's health centers and other clinics that women would set up to try and receive the kind of care they wanted:

birth control counseling, abortion, humane and re-spectful medical care, which was so hard to obtain; and the other wing being the community-based, more legislative impact–oriented wing of the women's health movement. There were, of course, many oc-casions on which they would join together to change a system. There were often times when feminist women's health center issues would end up in court. I always found the work that I did was in what I call the impact-based groups, but many times—for in-stance, in the early days of the National Women's Health Network— the feminist women's health centers were an integral part of all of that.

TK: So after D.C. Women's Liberation you became one of the founders of the National Women's Health Network.

AW: Yes, that was a direct outgrowth of the pill hearings. With Barbara Seaman, Belita Cowan, Mary Howell, Phyllis Chesler, we started a little group, which grew into the National Women's Health Network. The purpose of the network was to bring a feminist voice to health issues in Con-gress.

TK: Tell me more about the founding of the National Women's Health Network.

AW: In 1975, this small group that I talked of before, Barbara Seaman, Mary Howell, Phyllis Chesler, Belita Cowan, and I led a kick-off demonstration for what then became the National Women's Health Network. Lots more women were involved as well, women like Judy Norsigian and Norma Swensen from Boston and Joanne Fisher from Philadelphia. We were in touch with James Luggen, whose wife, Dona Jean Walter, had died from a pulmonary em-bolism associated with the pill. We had a demon-stration in honor of her memory outside of the FDA and it got a lot of press coverage. By then, most of the things we did seemed to get a lot of press coverage. But I remember my house in Wash-ington DC was filled with women the night before, making signs such as "Feed your pills to the rats at the FDA" and "Must we die for love?"

You can now see it in history books, which is hard to believe. I remember Barbara's children carrying my baby Eric, in their arms, and from there the National Women's Health Network has become a major and powerful political organization.

Belita Cowan

INTERVIEW BY TANIA KETENJIAN

Belita Cowan is president of the Lymphoma Foundation of America and a founder and former executive director (1978–83) of the National Women's Health Network. This interview was conducted in September 1999.

TK: What made you decide to start the National Women's Health Network?

BC: In 1974, women had very little say when it came to making medical care decisions. Everyone but the patient herself made decisions—doctors, drug companies, hospitals, law makers. I wanted to change that. I envisioned a lobby in Washington to serve as a counter-force to the AMA and the drug industry, a strong voice for women's health rights. I telephoned my friend Barbara Seaman in September of that year to tell her about my idea. I will never forget the encouragement and support she gave. It meant a lot to me. By the end of our conversation, the Women's Health Lobby was born. (We changed the name from Lobby to Network when the organization was incorporated in 1976.)

TK: What were you doing before that?

BC: I was on the faculty of the local community college in Ann Arbor, Michigan, teaching three courses in women's health care, and writing a book on the women's health movement. I worked part-time at the University of Michigan [U of M] Hospital, a big teaching research facility; I volunteered as a crisis counselor for the largest teen runaway shelter in the midwest, and served as a patient advocate for the local free clinic. In 1970 my lawsuit against the city of Ann Arbor opened up the city's sports programs to girls. I later joined a group of faculty at the U of M and did research on labor law and sex discrimination, which helped us file the first affirmative action complaint in the United States against an institution of higher learning. I credit those early years in Ann Arbor with giving me the experience and confidence to later challenge the health care system.

TK: In Ann Arbor, you uncovered a medical experiment on campus. Tell me about that.

BC: I'd come to the university as a graduate student in 1969 and at orientation we were told about a "morning-after pill." Actually it was ten pills. You could take them for five days to prevent a pregnancy after having unprotected sex. I had friends who took the "morning-after pill." I listened to their stories how they were so nauseous, they were vomiting, then quitting the pills after only two days. I wondered at that time: How can these pills be effective? How can they work if they make you so sick that you stop taking them?

After I earned my degree, I started a newspaper in 1972 called *her-self.* There were other feminist papers of course, in Denver, Los Angeles, New York. But none reported primarily on health news. So I published *her-self* to meet this need. In September, I asked one of our reporters, Kay Weiss, to write an article on what was then an obscure drug—DES diethylstilbestrol, a synthetic estrogen. Earlier, Kay's husband Rick had come across an alarming report in the *New England Journal of Medicine* describing eight cases of a very rare form of cancer in young , otherwise healthy women. All eight were exposed to the drug DES when their mothers were pregnant. This was shocking news. The "morning-after pill" dispensed by The U of M student health service was the very same drug—DES. A cancer-causing drug was being given to college students and the student health service wasn't warning students about the potential danger. So you can imagine what a bombshell it was when I published Kay's article in *her-self* newspaper.

TK: Why was the university dispensing DES?

BC: A gynecologist at the university, Lucille Kuchera, was testing DES as a "morning-after" contraceptive, and published her results in the *Journal of the American Medical Association* (*JAMA*) in 1971. She claimed one hundred percent effectiveness in preventing pregnancy among one thousand students, and that the side effects were minimal and insignificant. Common sense told me that this could not be right. I was working at the University of Michigan Hospital then and mentioned this to others. I suspected that with a thousand people, you can't get one hundred percent efficacy, no matter what drug you're testing. I was concerned because the DES had not been approved by the Food and Drug Administration as a contraceptive, and yet it was being tested on students, some of whom were friends of mine. And they had no idea they were participating in an experiment. I had to get to the bottom of this.

TK: How did you do that?

BC: I started a student organization called Advocates for Medical Information, and placed an ad in the University of Michigan student newspaper, asking anyone who took the "morning-after pill" to contact me. I developed a survey and interviewed by telephone more than a hundred students: what they took, the side effects, how they got the pills, the results, and the circumstance for which they took the DES. I found more than minor side effects, and virtually all of the responders were unaware that they had been involved in an experiment.

I organized the survey results and Kay and I flew to Washington to meet with Ralph Nader, Harrison Welford, Dr. Sidney Wolfe (who headed Ralph Nader's Health Research Group), and attorney Anita Johnson. I explained the DES survey and told them what was happening at the University of Michigan. I said we had information that contradicted the *JAMA* article on DES.

TK: Why Ralph Nader?

BC: We needed national publicity, and who better than Ralph Nader to get it? He was Mr. Consumer, and so well respected. This was two years before

we started the Network. The women's health movement had no national voice. So we went to Washington to see if Ralph Nader could help.

Nader's Health Research Group had a press conference and they got a lot of publicity. They also sent a letter to every major college in the United States, informing them that if DES was used on campus, it was not an FDA-approved contraceptive and there might be risks associated with it. Both Sidney Wolfe and Anita Johnson did a superb job with the media.

TK: What lessons did you learn from the Nader group?

BC: The clout and effectiveness of the Nader organization made a strong impression on me. I thought, if Ralph Nader can do this, so can I. I felt that we needed a woman's voice to speak out and stand up for our health rights. That's another reason why starting the National Women's Health Network was so important to me—I needed a strong feminist organization to back up my DES efforts.

TK: Did you meet Dr. Kuchera?

BC: In 1973, Kay and I went on a syndicated TV talk show with Dr. Kuchera and confronted her with the survey results. I said that her research couldn't be true because there must have been some drug failures. If the morning-after pill didn't work in all cases, then children might be born who were at risk for cancer. A surprising thing happened. Some time after the show, Dr. Kuchera wrote a letter to the editor of *JAMA*, a short letter, retracting her claim of one hundred percent efficacy and admitting that there had been some pregnancies after all.

TK: Was that the end of it or did national interest keep growing?

BC: We convinced reporter Harry Reasoner at NBC to come to the U of M campus to do an exposé on DES for the evening news. That segment helped a lot. Almost instantly, my work became easier because people now took the DES issue seriously.

Then, in 1974 I was asked by Senator Ted Kennedy to testify as an expert witness at his Senate subcommittee hearings on DES and the morning-after pill. I flew to Washington in February 1975 to present my survey results, to expose the DES experiment that had recruited unsuspecting students at the U of M, and to say that there were no reliable safety and efficacy studies on DES. I testified that FDA approval of DES would be a mistake because there was no adequate evidence of safety. I said that DES was being dispensed to young, healthy women at college campuses all over the country, and I asked the senator to stop the FDA from moving forward with its plan to approve the DES as a contraceptive.

A number of cancer experts, including Dr. Peter Greenwald, testified that DES should be banned for use in pregnancy because it had caused an epidemic of cancer in the offspring. [By 1975, there were more than 3,000 documented cases of cancer in DES daughters.] The commissioner of the FDA and two FDA medical officers were brought before the subcommittee, under subpoena. The medical officers said that they had never before seen such a circumvention of FDA procedures as in this case [approval of DES as a contraceptive].

In December 1975, I testified before the US House of Representatives, and arranged for Doris Haire, a childbirth advocate, and two DES daughters to tell their story to Congress. That same month, I helped organize a public demonstration on the doorstep of the FDA, to protest the indiscriminate use of DES, birth control bills, and estrogen replacement therapy in menopause—drugs known to cause cancer, blood clots, and death. This demonstration resulted in publicity for the National Women's Health Network, and we gained many new supporters.

I spent the next eight years fighting the FDA, and also publicizing the need for DES children, both male and female, to seek medical attention because of their increased risk of vaginal and tes-ticular cancer. Years later, it became evident that mothers who took DES during pregnancy had higher rates of breast cancer.

To this day, the FDA has never approved DES as a morning-after pill, and I am very happy for that. I have always believed that one person, acting with passion, can make a difference.

TK: How did you recruit the Network's first members?

BC: In my mind, we needed not only a strong lobby in Washington to influence public health polic, but a large, grassroots constituency. So I used the *her-self* newspaper mailing list to get the Network off the ground. There were 2,000 community-based women' health groups, consumer organizations, and individual artists who were subscribers. I sent them each a letter announcing the new organization. The first 1,000 members of the National Women's Health Network came directly from my newspaper's mailing list.

TK: How did the other co-founders come to join you?

BC: Barbara Seaman suggested that the visibility and credibility of the Women's Health Lobby would be enhanced if a doctor was on board. She suggested feminist physician Mary Howell, Dean of Students at Harvard Medical School. Barbara also felt it was important that we include the mental health side of medicine, and suggested psychologist Phyllis Chesler who had written *Women and Madness.* By the beginning of 1975, there were four of us listed as co-founders.

But I was in Michigan, Mary was in Massachusetts, and Barbara and Phyllis were in New York City. How could we keep on top of laws and regulations in Washington when none of us lived there? Barbara had been talking with Alice Wolfson, who lived in DC and had been involved in the birth control pill hearings years earlier. When I went to Senator Kennedy's hearings in 1975 to testify on DES, I met Alice and felt we could work together, so she joined us. I continued to oversee the Network's activities and provide direction to the many volunteers until 1977, when I moved to Washington DC to become the Network's first executive director (1978–1983).

TK: What were some of the other issues the Network was dealing with at the beginning—aside from DES?

BC: ➤ Menopause. We participated in a lawsuit on estrogen replacement therapy that resulted in the FDA requiring all companies making estrogen drugs to print patient warning labels about the link between those drugs and endometrial cancer.

➤ Childbirth. We participated in a Congressional effort that successfully expanded Medicaid coverage to include nurse-midwives.

➤ Sterilization (NWHN helped publicize the problem of forced sterilization of poor and minority women, and worked with other groups to help draft federal rules to prohibit this practice).

➤ Birth Control. We pressured the FDA to approve the cervical cap as a barrier method of birth control and led a successful campaign from 1979–81 to block approval of the controversial birth control shot, Depo-provera.

➤ Abortion. We participated in Congressional letter-writing campaigns and statewide marches to keep abortions safe and legal.

➤ Self-help. We supported the formation of local, autonomous self-help groups around the country, as well as feminist women's health centers.

➤ Sterilization. We worked closely with the Breast Cancer Advisory Center to end the radical mastectomy and give women more humane options for breast cancer treatment.

One of the most difficult issues the Network faced in the beginning was its own survival. When I was hired as executive director, we had no office, not even a telephone, and very little money. My job included fundraising, and during my five-year tenure, I raised from direct mail and foundation grants more than one million dollars.

TK: What was Anita Johnson's role in your work?

BC: She introduced me to Senator Kennedy and his staff, making it possible for me to be invited to testify as an expert witness at the senator's DES hearings. As chair of the Network's board and later as executive director, I consulted with Sidney Wolfe and Anita Johnson on many health issues, and our two organizations often joined with other consumer groups to file petitions or take legal action.

TK: Can you tell me about the case you were involved in with Marcia Greenberger?

BC: Marcia Greenberger was a lawyer with the Center for Law and Social Policy in Washington DC. She asked me if I would agree to have the Network become an intervenor in a lawsuit brought by the Pharmaceutical Manufacturers Association (PMA) against the Food and Drug Administration. At issue was FDA's regulatory authority to require drug companies to provide patients with written cancer groups who intervened (including the Network) against the PMA and the American College of Obstetricians and Gynecologists. The Court's ruling set a precedent for requiring drug companies to print patient warning labeling for all estrogen drugs.

A Mother's Story

HELEN RODRIGUEZ-TRIAS

Helen Rodriguez-Trias, excerpt from *The Conversation Begins*, Christina Looper Baker and Christina Baker Kline, eds., New York: Bantam Books, 1996. Reprinted by permission.

When I was born in 1929 in New York City, my parents' marriage was already going downhill. My father, a prosperous businessman, squandered his gains on alcohol. When he drank, his urbanity disappeared and he threatened violence in a booming, rough voice. My mother returned with us to Puerto Rico before I was a year old and finally divorced him in 1939, when I was ten. When she returned to New York, seeking a better life, like many Puerto Ricans, she brought me with her but left my fourteen-year-old sister with Aunt Estela, my childhood nurturer. When we left Puerto Rico, I did not cry. My mother denied her feelings of loss, too. I did not see Aunt Estela again until I returned to study at the university.

The year of my return to Puerto Rico, 1947, was highly charged politically. University authorities refused to allow Nationalist Party leader Pedro Albizu Campos, just released from federal prison, to speak on campus. Students went on strike and the university shut down. I was peripheral to the student movement but began to identify with the political struggles of the island. After a year I quit school and joined a leftist youth organization. I returned to New York, where I met my first husband in the office of a left-wing Columbia University student publication. Dave, twenty-three, was an editor; I was nineteen, author of an article on Puerto Rican student activists.

As suited to two young leftists, we were married in 1949 in a nontraditional ceremony. Ten months later Jo Ellen was born. I followed Dave to Lorain, Ohio, when Jo was three months old. In Lorain we were asked to vacate our furnished room after a black couple who were our friends visited us. Finding no place that allowed children, we sent six-month-old Jo back with my mother to New York while we bought and restored a house. When my mother brought her back to Lorain five months later, Jo acted fearful, as if we were strangers. I felt guilty and pained. It was a month before her first birthday, seven weeks before her first Christmas, and I was seven months pregnant.

Laura, born in January, thrived during the bitter Ohio winter. Eighteen months later David arrived. Having three children in two and a half years was horrendous. I felt inadequate and frightened. Dave tried to help, but he worked three rotation shifts as a machinist's apprentice and was president of his local union. When he was home, he got impatient with the babies. I feel compassion now toward the naïve neophytes we once were, but back then I was dying of loneliness and isolation.

My mother stayed with us on and off for two years. In Lorain she discovered a lump in her breast and had a radical mastectomy. When she left for Puerto Rico, I said, "I am not going to be alone here anymore," and went with her. Jo Ellen was three, Laura not quite two, and David only five months old. My decision arose out of sheer desperation and pain. At twenty-five I was embarrassed to need my mother so desperately. I did not want to admit it to Dave or myself, but I think I knew then that I would not be back.

Dave came to Puerto Rico in an attempt at reconciliation, but I already had a lover, whom I later married. My lover, X, was divorced, with two sons. My mother urged me to stay with Dave. "He may not be the ideal person," she said. "He has a bad temper, but he's sober and decent and the father of these three children. That counts for a great deal." I felt guilty, but X was seductive and passion got in the way of reason. Furthermore, he seemed devoted to me. When I told him I wanted to study medicine, he suggested I stop working after we got married and start school right away. I trusted him because he seemed unconditionally supportive. He helped us financially during the divorce from Dave and became my lifeline. I grew more dependent on him each day.

My mother vehemently opposed my marrying X. We quarreled bitterly, and she left for New York. X and I married in the summer of 1954. In September I enrolled in the university's premedical course. I loved school and discovered my capacity to concentrate and do well. A year later my mother died of breast cancer in New York City. We made peace in her bare hospital room and I told her that I loved her, always had. She expressed her happiness that I had gone back to school. Sadly, considering what X turned out to be, she apologized for her opposition to him, saying, "I was mistaken."

In 1956 I entered medical school. I was twenty-seven and on top of the world. In all honesty, I was not a great mom when I was in training. During the premedical years I had more time with the kids, but with the pressures of medical school I had no time or energy to spare. Jo, Laura, and

David attended a nursery school run by a Canadian missionary, and I had irregular hired help. But my husband was the present parent. He came from a large and apparently close family, with a mother considered by everyone a saint. Ashamed of the broken family I grew up in, I trusted his ways with children more than my own.

I suspected him of sexual abuse only once. During my third year of medical school, I arrived home one evening to find seven-year-old Laura in our bed. Irritated with her, which I deeply regret, I said sharply, "To your bed. You know I don't like children in adult beds." At the time X feigned deep sleep. The next day he said, "Last night you pulled a fast one on me, accusing me of something improper with Laura. She was just sleeping here and so was I." He attacked me as disturbed and evil-minded, and I cried and apologized, convinced that my view of men was distorted. I never suspected again. I wish I had been able to say to Laura, "Come here, baby. I won't be angry at you, and I will always love you, no matter what you tell me is happening."

We had a son together. Professionally I kept advancing. After medical school and pediatric training, I began teaching. I received increasing acknowledgment from my peers, but my husband's resentment grew. "You can't get a raise," he would say. "I don't want a wife who earns more than I do"; or, "You doctors are such bores at parties. I have never met people like you, always talking about your work." He told friends that I had fooled him into believing that once training was completed I would be more of a homebody.

Ironically, the more active I became as a parent, voicing opinions about his harsh discipline of the kids, the angrier he became. I was "the other rebellious adolescent," he moaned, "as if three weren't enough!" Interspersed with his complaints were romantic interludes of intense wooing, now recognizable as the cycle of abuse. At the time our problems seemed mainly my fault—for wanting a career, for choosing one so demanding and rewarding, for succeeding, for speaking out, for laughing too much, for weeping

when hurt, for having three difficult adolescents from a first marriage, for having a little boy not masculine enough, for not being a good mother.

By 1970 Jo, Laura, and David had left home, and I felt the enormous void in my marriage. Sessions with a woman psychiatrist marked the beginning of my understanding of my situation.

Within three months we were divorced. In early September, Daniel and I moved to New York with Maria, our housekeeper of seven years and our security and support. Before me lay the challenging job of chief of pediatrics at Lincoln Hospital in the South Bronx.

When X announced his forthcoming marriage a few months later, I refused to send Daniel, still pained over the divorce, back to Puerto Rico. I doubted my decision, however, and consulted with Jo Ellen, in New York for Thanksgiving. She gazed at me steadily for a long moment and said, "Mami, he is very bad for children."

"Why do you say that?"

"Because he molested us regularly when we were little."

I questioned her perceptions. "Children often fantasize. Is it possible?"

"This is no fantasy, there is no misinterpreting what happened; it went on for years," Jo Ellen said. "I intended never to tell you, but I have to protect Daniel."

I was shattered. For weeks I hardly stopped crying. I had known and loved X for eighteen years, been his wife for sixteen, borne his son, praised him as a good, if strict, father. Even after the divorce, I felt guilty that I was taking his son to New York. If I had been so wrong about this man, how could I ever trust my senses again?

In January 1971 I used the occasion of a trip to Puerto Rico to recruit house officers for Lincoln Hospital as an opportunity to meet with all three kids and Anita, who would later become David's wife. During our days at the remote country house of a friend, we spoke of things long hidden, many of them painful and frightening. We wept and shouted, understood and misunderstood one another, but for the first time we spoke about our feelings without pretense.

On Monday I called to arrange an appointment with X at his office after work, ostensibly to speak about Daniel's visit. As we one by one entered his office, X's expression changed from surprise to fear. "I am not here to talk about your visitation rights with Daniel," I said quickly. "I came to talk about your abuse of the girls."

He rose and began to push past us, but Jo Ellen and David pushed him back down, saying, "Sit down. You are going to hear what we have to say."

"Who said so?" he said defiantly.

"We said so," we responded in unison.

Screaming, "Police, police, help!" he attempted to flee. Jo and David thrust him back into his chair, but the moment they relaxed their hold, he turned, kicked in the window, and jumped out, screaming, "Police! I am being attacked!" I last saw him cowed and shaken, sitting on a grassy knoll ten feet below the window, a small crowd gathering. The man who had terrorized my children had become a nothing. Throughout the melee, Laura had stood in front of the desk, her hands in her skirt pockets. Later she said, "I could only see cut-glass ashtrays to hit him with; I feared I might do him great injury." He may have harmed her the most, shy little girl that she was when he started molesting her. Her anger must have frightened her greatly that afternoon of our confrontation.

The following day a news article billed X as a prominent businessman and former governor's aide, attacked by unknown assailants. A second news article identified the assailants as family members and cited X's former wife as having seriously wounded him with high-heeled shoes. Three days later, Jo Ellen, Laura, and I were arrested at the airport. Our arrest made headlines, and we were charged with assault, battery, and attempted murder. Meanwhile the "intended victim" stayed home, virtually unharmed.

A friend posted bail, and Jo and I returned to New York; Laura and David remained in Puerto Rico. After putting us through a lawyer's expense and several trips to Puerto Rico for hearings never held, X dropped all charges. True to type and guarding appearances above all, he stated that in the interest of restoring the proper father-son relationship, he would forgive our actions. Of the family, only Daniel has a relationship with him now, and it is superficial.

In 1981 I met Eddie, a nurturing man, who has helped me heal and brought peaceful joy. Eddie taught labor studies at Cornell. Our marriage works because he lets me be me, as I let him be himself. I am in a new phase of my life—much more creative and secure. Being older gives me great freedom, and I am less self-conscious than I ever was. I say what I think or feel without getting terribly upset about the way I am perceived.

I want to leave my children and grandchildren with a sense of life-long growth and survivorship, a sense of joy in life and joy in struggle. The women's movement is about survival, about finding our strength and using it to help other women. We reach out to each other to build a different kind of society—one where women are equal in power to men and where children are truly prized.

Helen Rodriguez-Trias

INTERVIEW BY TANIA KETENJIAN

Helen Rodriguez-Trias, M.D., was a board member of the National Women's Health Network and became the first latina president of the American Public Health Association in 1993. This interview was conducted in June 1999.

TK: What are the most serious and prevalent health problems facing latina women today?

HRT: Latinas, like African-American women and all ethnic groups we tend to lump together are very diverse. Here in California there are many latino nationalities, organizations and groups. I am on the Policy Committee of one called the Latino Coalition for a Healthy California, a public policy advocacy organization. One of its projects was put together by latinas organizing around better health. Their report on health access for latinas reveals that of seven million uninsured Californians, 1.4 million are latina. That is a serious health issue. But apart from that terrible reality we need to address, I try not to talk just in terms of narrow health issues or, just about health care and lack of access to health care. I try to emphasize the need to improve health conditions: where we work, where we live, what our environment is like, what are the chances of you or someone in your family being victimized by violence, traumatized by violence? What are your chances of tranquillity unless your kids are safe in school and at home? All of these elements in life are determinants and definers of our health. Yes, we have some groups of latinos who are better off than others in all of the above and their health indicators such as life expectancy and infant mortality are very good. But the fact is that, overall latinas are among the ranks of the working poor and therefore less likely to have health coverage, more likely to be living poor quality housing and environments and to be working in hazardous conditions. Basically, it all goes together. Having low-income means living in poor environments and reduced access to life's necessities.

TK: What would you suggest to latina women who want to improve the condition of their health care? Should they go to a local clinic, should they turn to larger institutions? Should they connect with patient's rights and women's organizations?

HRT: Be informed, read all you can, talk to others, know your rights, and speak up. We all need better health information, particularly for folks who have low literacy levels who are not going to read these pamphlets made for college graduates or above. We need to have more commitment on the part of the media that reaches latina women— radio, television—to give appropriate health messages, to be very proactive about the rights people have to certain services. The previous governor of California, Pete Wilson, was loudly anti-immigrant. He became very aggressive in denying services to immigrants and a lead in denying prenatal care to undocumented women, a right secured by law in California. Public Advocates, the Latino Coalition for a Healthy California and others immediately challenged the denial in the courts. In effect, he could not implement his policies. Nevertheless, the impression that immigrants are not entitled to care still remains and many are afraid. Many, who clearly have a right to enter clinics and receive care, are afraid they are going to be deported or afraid they won't get citizenship. The fear that has been created is keeping people away. People need information; they need to know about their rights; they need to know about available services; they need to know about what in California is known as the Healthy Families Program and nationally as the Child Health Insurance Program (CHIP) so that they can register their kids. They need to have information about how to keep themselves healthy. But I also think that people have to know that they need to organize and that they need to actually advocate for coverage. The California Senate is going to debate a proposal introduced by Senator Hilda Solis to come up with a plan for California to cover all uninsured people. We need to look at how we can move the richest state in the Union to provide universal access to health care. We need to look at what's happening to peoples' working conditions. These are issues that I think latinos and latinas need to get involved in. Above all, getting people to vote, getting people together and getting out the vote.

TK: As I was reading through the Reid Memorial lecture, a speech you presented to Barnard students in 1976, I learned that, during the late 1950s, while you were in medical school as a student, you realized that there was a very powerful dual system of health care. Do you feel that any of this has changed since more women have entered the health care profession?

HRT: Yes, I think there have been some changes because the health care profession has recognized the value of primary care—the care that people access immediately. I also think there's been more recognition of people skills in the health professions. Women have had a lot to do with that. Nevertheless there are still major gaps. Although, since the 1960s, there have been more government programs and more support for public health, the fact of the matter is that we still have a system that excludes, underserves, and even mis-serves all too many people. The latest census tells us that there are over 44 million Americans without health insurance. That is inexcusable!

TK: Would you agree that the majority of this disservice occurs with low-income women rather than with higher status groups?

HRT: Most certainly! There is no doubt that money can buy you good things, good medicine included, although good medicine requires more than money; it also takes a system that has quality controls and well trained people who are compassionate; it takes more than just money but definitely, money does buy better services.

TK: One issue that really came to the fore in your speech was the sterilization abuse of low-income women. Can you discuss the different ways and forms in which coerced sterilization has shown up among different ethnic groups?

HRT: You have to take an historical perspective to understand the phenomena. Sterilization has now become very popular as a means for people to end their fertility and their worries. Sterilization now is not the same as sterilization in the early '60s or late '50s in Puerto Rico, or even in the early '70s in the United States, which was the period I was speaking of. During those earlier decades we already had a procedure—vasectomy—for men that was never very popular among them. Men did not go in any large numbers to get vasectomies although the surgery itself was relatively simple. Prior to 1970 in the United States

sterilization of women was relatively infrequent. Voluntary sterilization for women was pretty much restricted by the "rule of 120." That is, if a woman went to an OB-GYN and wanted a sterilization, she would be asked how old she was and how many children she had and the rule was that, unless her age multiplied by the number of children was 120 or more, a woman was not a good candidate for sterilization. In other words, a thirty-year-old woman would have to have four children to be a candidate. So this meant that sterilization as a voluntary procedure was restricted for certain women, but perversely it was being promoted, if not downright pushed or coerced, for others—women of low income, women of color, women whom, for whatever reason, the provider decided should not have more children. I think that is the context that we talked about when describing how sterilization abuse manifested itself in many places in the world. And in many places, such as India and Bangladesh, it was the only birth control offered to women

But the point is that now sterilization has become something relatively common among married couples and among couples and individuals who may not be married but have decided they have as many children as they want or that they don't want any children at all. So now we're talking about the more subtle kinds of incentives or coercion for sterilization that may operate in the context of women's lives. For instance, take welfare reform and the pressure not to have additional children. That is a not-so-subtle coercion for women to be sterilized saying, "Let me get this over and done with"—whether or not that's really what they want to do—because it gives them the security that they won't get pregnant. Lack of access to abortion services may also push women to get sterilized. Restrictions on abortions have been going on ever since the 1973 *Roe v. Wade* decision. After a few years of burgeoning services, a backlash has created tremendous hardship for women in accessing abortion services. Currently over 80 percent of the counties in the United States don't have abortion clinics and there are all kinds of restrictions at state levels. We stopped funding abortion services for low-income women recipients of Medicaid. I think there are only five or six states that still use public funds to fund abortion services. All the others stopped funding them in the '70s following the Hyde amendment to the appropriations bill. All of this means that sterilization is a more contextual and complex phenomenon as it now applies to lower-income women and women of color. We always have to look at things in an historical perspective. By the way, the guidelines on sterilization and informed consent that we succeeded in getting into HEW in 1976 applied only to sterilizations funded by public money. They were not necessarily accepted guidelines within private practice.

TK: You are one of the pioneers who initiated an end of sterilization abuse for latina women. . . .

HRT: I have worked within a collective context from the very beginning. In the early '70s the Committee for Puerto Rican De-Colonization was holding an event at NYU where they were showing the movie Blood of the Condor. It presented a fictionalized version of a Quechua Indian uprising in Bolivia because the women were being sterilized without their knowledge. The organizers of the event asked me to give a talk about how this applied to Puerto Rico. I wasn't sure how it applied to Puerto Rico, so I read some books and talked to people to prepare. That was when I first personally began to understand what had been happening in Puerto Rico during the time I was there as a medical student, as a young mother, and as a practicing pediatrician. During those years of 1956 to 1970 I had been totally oblivious to the campaign to sterilize women that was social policy. I began to understand that social policy could creep up on you without it being explicit public policy. The example today of nonexplicit social policy is welfare reform. No one has actually said that women were going to be thrown off welfare and wouldn't have any health insurance, nor that they were going to be put into low-income jobs, be without child care,

and there would be pressure on them not to have more children. Yet when we begin to examine the effects on women, it certainly seems that much of this happens to them. It is just that the policies are not explicit in their intent and implementation.

TK: So how did you start things going as an activist and organizer?

HRT: During the question and answer period following my talk on what had happened in Puerto Rico mainly in the '50s and '60s, several people in the audience spoke about similar things going on in the United States. One was a psychiatrist working in a Brooklyn hospital who said that he saw all kinds of things—such as people having unnecessary operations, and women being sterilized without first being told about other kinds of contraception. A young woman, a writer for one of the left Puerto Rican papers, also became very interested and we formed a small group along with several people who started talking after that meeting. Later we met and created the Committee to End Sterilization Abuse. That was in 1974 when a series of abuses were being exposed. The Relf case, about the two black girls in Alabama—two sisters, one twelve and the other fourteen, who were surgically, irrevocably, and illegally sterilized—had come to light at the end of 1973. There was a huge outcry in the African-American press and some organization around issues raised by the Relf case and eventually a court suit. There were others among them ten women in Los Angeles who were suing the County Hospital. The suit, known as the Madrigal case, was brought by women who were mainly not English- but Spanish-speaking, who had been coerced into sterilization in some way, or lied to.

For me, telling this story as a story of individuals and their organizations is important. I think that individuals and leadership are crucial, but we should never deny the need for organizations and movements because they shape individuals. Some of the distress we of the progressive communities feel comes from the fact that we don't currently have a unifying movement.

TK: What do you think it takes to have a unified movement?

HRT: I think it takes a lot of hard work and organization but it requires other conditions too. There has to be a climate or event that wakes people up to an issue and gives them a vision of change. For health care reform, I think we were closer to having these conditions at the beginning of the Clinton administration. But, having lost those opportunities, to put it mildly, it is now a lot more difficult to regroup around universal health care. It takes a lot of hard work and organization and some force driving people to move toward a vision to get us to a better place.

TK: What are the steps that an individual should take to become an effective activist?

HRT: I think you have to have the heart to say, "I care a lot about this issue." That's the first thing: feeling committed. The second thing is to look around to see who else feels like you do and thinks like you do, or if there's something going on already that you can become part of. I would say single-issue activism more than anything else has united people effectively. Let's take MADD, Mothers Against Drunk Driving, an organization that I really like and that I think is really effective. Mothers anguished by their kids getting killed created it. Or take the women who felt strongly about breast cancer and breast cancer visibility because they had it or someone in their family did. I do think that, for me, the feeling of outrage comes first.

TK: While challenging these sterilization abuses, you experienced obstacles both at local and national, or federal levels. Could you compare the two?

HRT: I saw several things: one was just the capacity that we all have to organize locally. By and large, you're talking about organizing people who are working—most of us actually working full time. For us, local organization is more doable. Another is that whenever you start organizing around a given issue, you will find people out there who are very affected by the issue you are addressing. If you are working locally it is easier to help them find resources and to recruit them for continuing work. In our case, the moment we started doing public things—speaking to colleagues, in churches, organizing workshops in youth clubs, reaching out to social groups, we started hearing from people who wanted direct help. In those years there was some very effective organizing by women's groups at the community level. We did a number of radio shows and, invariably, people called in and wanted help. It wasn't about political analysis. Someone would call in and say, "Three years ago, I was told I had something wrong with my uterus and they took it out and I don't have any children and I'm only twenty two years old and I don't know what's happening." They wanted something concrete, they wanted help, and they wanted information. What I learned is that when you are organizing around an issue, you should be prepared to have some concrete services available for people. You need to know where people can get help. Do not assume that all others will be interested in your issue as you may be, as a political issue, or as an issue of public policy, or as human rights or whatever it is that is your driving ideal. I remember one radio show, when we had at least twenty calls and at least half of them were people calling for help, and we weren't ready for it. It was a painful experience for me.

TK: How about the challenges of organizing nationally?

HRT: Whether organizing locally or nationally, the organizers always have to let people know what they can concretely do. But national organizing does create new challenges. As example, we had a strange hearing in one of those organizing drives around the national guidelines on informed consent for sterilization procedures for HEW, Health and Human Services, now HHS, Health and Human Services. Joseph Califano was the head of it at that time. He was basically anti-choice. And there were some other anti-choice people who were very much in favor of restrictions if not downright prohibitions against sterilization. Many also did not like contraception and opposed any measures that made contraception more accessible. Going national created these kinds of contradictions because in that larger arena we found people who would take up our cause for very different reasons. At the local level it was much easier to keep focused on one issue and work with people whose thinking was somewhat more alike. There are greater hazards of forced compromises and undesirable partners when we go national.

TK: You worked at Lincoln Hospital.

HRT: Yes, from 1970 to 1978. I graduated from medical school in 1960, and I did my residency at the University Hospital in Puerto Rico. Then in 1970 I relocated to New York and became the Director of Pediatrics at Lincoln Hospital.

It was very interesting and maybe more exciting than I had wished. It was a sanctuary of fascinating people, who tried to work together in some way. It was a challenge to try and run a department comprised mainly of young people who supported things I thought were innovative, progressive, and worthy of support while at the same time trying to tone down some of the wilder manifestations of individuals wanting to dress as they wished, even though the community didn't like it, or who wanted to wear their hair or beards long when the community found that disrespectful. It was challenging and there was a lot of opposition from the medical school staff about all that was going on. There were periods when people would organize demonstrations to protest about those uptown institutions, meaning the medical school. Once, the police came into the department of pediatrics conference room because there had been an injunction against the Young Lords and I had allowed some to show a film there. They even arrested one of our doctors for protesting the police violence. Working there was fascinating and complex.

TK: You were also a board member of the National Women's Health Network and the president of the American Public Health Association in 1993. How did it feel to be the first latina president of the American Public Health Association?

HRT: I enjoyed it tremendously. There is a wonderful latino leadership in the American Public Health Association, the result of a Latino Caucus formed in the early '70s. I was at the birth of that Latino Caucus, so I remember the contributions to its organization of my wonderful colleagues, great researchers, teachers, activists for public health many of whom who are still active. The Latino Caucus has become a very important structure that young latino public health folks attach to and where they have an opportunity to grow in leadership skills. It felt very good to preside over the great organization that APHA is for a year.

TK: So you never felt you had to compromise your beliefs or "tone it down?"

HRT: I have toned it down, I think; we all tone it down as we get older. First of all, I realized that a lot of times I wasn't communicating well when I wouldn't tone it down. I just wasn't communicating. I had more than a bit of a confrontational style in those days when it wasn't always worthwhile to be confrontational. There were times you could actually find better points of unity when you were less confrontational and more reasonable and actually listened to other people more and not just see them as being off the deep end, or evil. That was part of what I learned that toned me down. It is less about compromise than it is about being effective. Even with the issue of sterilization abuse that seemed so clear cut to us we needed to use analysis and be more self-critical. When we first devised the draft guidelines for the Health and Hospitals Corporation, we got to every single hospital in the system, there were fifteen of them, each with an OB-GYN department director. I recall that there was not one of the directors who was willing to listen about the guidelines. In part their antagonism was because the document we prepared trying to justify why guidelines were needed actually started out with a list of all the abuses. If you tell people that under their service, their command, their watch, these terrible things are going on, they stop listening right there. You just are not going to make your point, and so we ended up with this infuriated bunch of doctors. After reflection, we realized that we could have said things differently and gotten a more attentive audience. We might have started by stating that there have been a series of lawsuits around issues of inadequate consent processes and here are the guidelines to guard against lawsuits and ensure that patients' rights are being respected. It would have gone much better. As it was, we won anyway, but after a longer and bitterer struggle than was necessary. I certainly have calmed down. But its not been as much about consciously saying, "Well let me compromise on this or on that." It's more about saying, "How can I be more effective in getting from point A to point B? How can I be more effective about persuading this group of people to look at what the outcome of their health care should be, or that they want to be including others at this table. How can I be more effective?"

A Is for Activism

BYLLYE AVERY

Byllye Avery, excerpt from *An Altar of Words: Wisdom, Comfort and Inspiration for African American Women*, New York: Broadway Books, 1998. Reprinted by permission.

Just when does one decide to devote her life or some part of her life to activism? I can't recall ever hearing a child say, "I want to be an activist when I grow up." What transforms regular, hardworking citizens into dedicated, passionate activists? Perhaps it is anger fuming in the blood that makes us resist the injustices hurled at members of society. Perhaps it is the high standards of excellence that we hold for our society, to be better than the best, with integrity and respect for everyone. Whatever the cause, we never know when the moment will come that an issue emerges as a burning passion and we commit ourselves to mak-

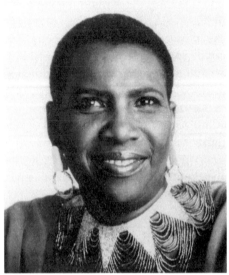

Byllye Avery

ing sure the world knows about "our" issue.

Activists help make the world a better place. Many important changes have been made because something clicked and made people see the picture more clearly, focusing on the vision of what could be, and how changes can lead to a better society. We must celebrate our activists. They are trailblazers who are not afraid to speak out, stand up, and challenge the status quo. They do their work today, and create a place for volunteers later. Activism leads and inspires change. The activist's passion provides a driving force for the rest of us.

I became an activist in the early '70s. The women's health movement was in full swing, making us all think about health in terms of personal involvement and control. My husband had a massive heart attack and died in 1970, and I realized that as an educated black person I knew very little about health and taking care of myself.

I began to educate myself, and I dedicated more and more time to working on women's health issues. Before I knew it, health had become my issue and my full-time job.

We all have some parts of activism within us. Very few people don't have strong feelings about something. Some of us are quiet activists, keeping our feelings to ourselves and using our quiet strength and resources to advance our issues. We all need to seek ways to be activists and support activism.

As you add activism to your altar, think about and feel the passion of an issue that is important to you.

My actions are important and are inherently powerful.

"Dissension is healthy, even when it gets loud."
—Jennifer Lawson

Byllye Avery

INTERVIEW BY TANIA KETENJIAN

Byllye Avery is the founder of the National Black Women's Health Project. This interview was conducted in April 1999.

TK: How did you come to join the National Women's Health Network?

BA: Back in the 1970s we were all working at the Gainesville Women's Health Center, and I remember they sent a letter around saying they were looking for people to serve on their board. So I joined and applied to be on their board and became a member.

TK: When did you decide that a black women's health project needed to be started?

BA: The project first became an idea in my head in 1980, when I had been at the network for about five years. Black women were not attending the conferences and programs that the network was putting on. They were all good programs with good information, but there were very few black women participating. So I became concerned with how we could increase participation of black women in the organization.

TK: Why do you think the NWHN was so dominated by white middle-class women?

BA: It doesn't really have anything to do with

"domination." It's just that those were the women on the board and that was the perspective they were teaching. What you have to understand is the way racism affects us. Unless something speaks specifically to black women, Asian women, Native American women, if you just say "women," then the assumption is "white women." That's what that was about. It wasn't that people were not interested in having black women be in the organization, that they weren't trying to reach out. They just were not the ones to do it.

TK: What was your vision for the NWHN? What did you want it to accomplish? What were the many problems black women were facing at the time?

BA: The way I came to understand the NWHN—which might not be the NWHN's vision of itself—was that I saw it as a place where women of all ethnic groups could come together to work collectively for the health of all women. For instance, maybe the board would have an Asian woman organizing Asian women, a Native American organizing Native American women, so that you'd have representatives of hundreds of thousands of women organizing around ethnicity and health issues. I understood that black women needed to come together to decide what our health issues were. We could look at health statistics and see what we were dying from, but more important to me was what other things we were living with, and that needed to come from a black women's perspective. That's what was missing for me in the NWHN—the black woman's perspective. Later I came to understand that all women down that color line, due to class and other such factors, develop their own perspective about their health. Some of the health problems we identified, once we came together, had to do with psychological well-being—not mental illness, but psychological well-being: What are the things that get in the way of your life every day? A lot of people live in a lot of psychological distress. How will we come together and talk about this? A lot of it comes from painful experiences. Women would talk about being victims of domestic violence, rape, incest—all these things kind of gnaw, they really rob us of our power and keep us from being all of who we are. So back in the early 1980s when women really started coming together, we declared that violence was the number one health issue for black women, just before the CDC [Centers for Disease Control and Prevention] and all the rest of them determined that violence was a health issue. Once you got this psychological stuff straight, and got the message that you are a good and whole person just because you were born, then you could start to deal with some of the other issues. Cardiovascular diseases, heart problems, hypertension, cancer, diabetes are all things people are living with, but sometimes they really can't get to them until they become chronic.

TK: The pamphlet *Our Voices, Our Choices* talks about the reproductive and sexual diseases that black women were facing then and are still facing relative to white women.

BA: Yes, women still have trouble getting prenatal care. Lack of access can mean many things. It could be the bad clinic in my neighborhood or my head telling me not to go in and get the care. A lot of women aren't getting prenatal care early enough. Many are denying their pregnancies because of their situations. In this country we have such a high level of technologically advanced health care systems, but there are very basic things that don't get to all of the people. See, I think they're using the wrong yardstick. We say our health care system is special because we have all these technological advances, but if you can't get them to the people, you really don't have them as far as I'm concerned. There are 47 million people right now without health insurance, and health insurance is your entree. A lot of people get left out of a lot of preventive services, so they get things that could be avoided. Then you see black women not having preventive care, not having an attitude that every year you need to get your breasts examined, get a mammogram, get a Pap smear, that there are certain routine things that

you need to do every single year. And people go for years without doing these things even when they are available. To me that's one of the greatest factors that leads to us having a disproportionate amount of disease. So we work on the access and on the mind: certainly you are worthy of these things, certainly you are good enough for them, certainly you deserve to have them. Most of what we're trying to do is educate women about health.

Overall health means psychological well-being as well as physical and spiritual well-being, and it's the combination of these three that make a whole and healthy being. We're not telling women, "You should weigh 125 pounds," and laying that guilt trip on, because black women don't have those self-esteem issues around weight. As a matter of fact, it's pretty much the opposite in the black community, so that strategy doesn't work. We don't have great numbers of women feeling guilty that they wear a size 10. So we try to stress to people to think more about their health problems: What's your blood pressure? What's your cholesterol count? How are your indicators that you're a healthy person?

TK: The other point you're making, if I understand you correctly, is that self-worth is the major issue, because if you feel like you deserve it, you'll make yourself go. How much has the past affected women's feelings about themselves today?

BA: We all come with our history, and it takes a long time to get rid of it, but you have to always examine the history so as to know what's happened. Then you know how to think about things. We can't be too trusting, we must get information ourselves. I know people are tired of hearing about slavery and they're tired of hearing about the Holocaust, but these were horrendous things that happened to people. They not only scarred that generation, they scarred generations to come because they became a part of people's inherent past. The history of slavery told you that you were nothing but a workhorse, from the moment you opened your eyes until, for many people, the moment you died. These things take a long time to overcome. They become ingrained and are passed on as part of our social differences, and different ethnic groups act upon them, so they don't just go away. Then you see bits of them being repeated, such as sterilizations done on poor women and retarded women and women of color. And the sterilization abuse of Puerto Rican women. The history of what we do to each other, the legacy that comes from those actions, lasts many years, for many generations.

TK: What are some of the techniques or skills or attitudes that the National Black Women's Health Project tries to infuse in its members?

BA: We have what we call self-help, which is akin to the consciousness-raising that white women did. Through these self-help groups, we bring the women together to talk about the realities of their lives, to do the analysis, to share, because mostly when you hear the story of someone else's life, you sort of relive your own life and you come to understand why you made decisions or why other people made decisions. You get to claim what was yours and understand the process of discarding that which is not yours. You learn how to discard the pain from the internalized oppression and how to move these oppressive elements out of the midst of your life. We bring women together to sit in a circle to talk openly about their lives and what's going on with them. Through that talking and self-examination, people are able to then make decisions about where they want to go with their lives and get direction and support while they do it. That's the crux of our whole work. People come to understand that no matter what the problem is, somebody else has had that problem and has solved it before them.

TK: What are the main problems a black woman faces now when she's going out to seek health care as compared to a white woman?

BA: First she has to have the resources—not only the financial resources, she has to have insurance. Only about 38 percent of people have really good coverage or have access to discretionary funds that can pay for things their insurance won't pay for. Then there's a bunch of us who use HMOs, who don't necessarily get doctors we want to see or have to wait a long time. The black woman's plight is being part of those who are excluded, which means people on Medicaid and all the uninsured and the working poor. They absolutely don't get the best care, they get whatever they can get. So a woman with breast cancer, for instance, needs an advocate with her, someone to help her navigate the system. I have a friend who got breast cancer, and—as much as we all know—it took every single little thing we had to make sure she actually got the three or four opinions, and when they didn't make sense, to find out where else to go to get information. It's very difficult to navigate the system. So you get Ms. Jones who goes right to the clinic, she does whatever the doctor says, and things don't necessarily get better. But she plugs along with it, considering it her lot in life. Whereas if a white woman doesn't like the care, she's got means, so she goes to somebody else and then somebody else until she gets someone who makes sense and who can give her a level of care that she knows she needs to have.

TK: How do doctors affect the process of childbirth for women now and before?

BA: Sometimes they make decisions—not based on information and certainly not based on consultation with their clients—about what treatment people should get, and these decisions are forced on women. Unempowered patients are very accepting, for there are just so many other difficulties in their lives. Take a pregnant woman who's among the "working poor." She works on a line in a factory where there might not be any health insurance. She knows she needs to go in for care, but she doesn't have the ability to take off half a day to go to a doctor appointment. If she leaves for half a day she might lose her job, 'cause there's somebody waiting to take it over, and missing half a day definitely means she'll miss the money from the job. So that's one way women are discriminated against right from the beginning around childbirthing. The women get blamed for not being compliant, not coming in for care, but nobody is looking at the reasons behind that. If doctors had night hours, if employers were required to give pregnant women paid time off to get health care and prenatal care, if we valued our women and our children—there are many ways, with the new laws, to make sure women get what they need. Those are just the simple ways.

TK: What are some of the most prominent health issues facing black women today?

BA: High blood pressure and cardiovascular disease. A lot of black women have heart problems. Something like 42 or 43 percent of women over 40 have hypertension. When I'm speaking to audiences and I ask how many people have breast cancer, I might get a few hands. When I ask how many people have problems with their heart, I get so many hands, all the time. Diabetes is another problem. A lot of this stems from being hypertensive, and that has a lot to do with weight and with inactivity. You know how difficult it is to keep yourself active. People have the attitude that they don't have time to go to the gym, they look at it as playing or leisure. Our whole mindset is: that's what you do when you play basketball or football. Breast cancer is maybe third or fourth on the list, even though most women don't die from breast cancer; they die from cardiovascular diseases. Another issue, for a lot of women, is lack of access to abortions. These are women who feel disempowered, who are left out, who are on Medicare and can't have their abortions paid for and are forced to have children that they can't really afford.

TK: So you wouldn't put sexually transmitted diseases up there?

BA: I would put sexual *activity* there. A lot of women are having problems with AIDS, HIV, STDs. Unprotected sex is an issue and leads to a lot of diseases.

TK: Do you think the problem is lack of information or resources to get protection?

BA: I think it's both, but it's also not having a way to present this issue to the man. A lot of women out there are desperate to have men in their lives, desperate to be held, desperate for male companionship, so they'll risk almost anything to have that, and this is the basis for many other problems.

TK: What role have men played in the movement and the project?

BA: They didn't have a presence because we didn't allow them to, but there were men who supported our work all the way from the beginning. Men supported their wives, who came to our meetings—a lot of the women wouldn't have been able to just take off from home and leave their children unless someone was supportive at home. And most of the women, once they found they could see, didn't stop seeing. They took the work home and were able to convince the men in their lives to start to make changes.

TK: What changes have you seen since 1981 when the project started?

BA: Oh, lots! Black women have just absolutely blossomed in the nineties. We first changed our attitude about ourselves, which is probably the most important, how we see ourselves. We see ourselves very differently in the world and a lot of things came together to make that happen. Then we changed our attitude toward each other and once we started doing that, we could start being in the world in a very different way, and being more accepting of our peers in a different way. What I mean is that they're accepting our questioning, forging new horizons, doing different things, being all of who we want to be. A lot of barriers have been removed.

The Female Eunuch

GERMAINE GREER

Germaine Greer, *The Female Eunuch*, New York: Bantam Books, 1972. Originally published in 1970 by MacGibbon and Kee in Great Britain. Reprinted by permission.

THE WICKED WOMB

Women who adhere to the Moslem, Hindu, or Mosaic faiths must regard themselves as unclean in their time of menstruation and seclude themselves for a period. Medieval Catholicism made the stipulation that menstruating women were not to come into the church. Although enlightenment is creeping into this field at its usual pace, we still have a marked revulsion for menstruation, principally evinced by our efforts to keep it secret. The success of the tampon is partly due to the fact that it is hidden. The arrival of the menarche is more significant than any birthday, but in the Anglo-Saxon households it is ignored and carefully concealed from general awareness. For six months while I was waiting for my first menstruation I toted a paper bag with diapers and pins in my school satchel. When it finally came, I suffered agonies lest anyone should guess or smell it or anything. My diapers were made of harsh toweling, and I used to creep into the laundry and crouch over a bucket of foul rags, hoping that my brother would not catch me at my revolting labors. It is not surprising that well-bred, dainty little girls find it difficult to adapt to menstruation, when our society does no more than explain it and leave them to get on with it. Among the aborigines who lived along the Pennefather river in Queensland the little girl used to be buried up to her waist in warm sand to aid the first contractions, and fed and cared for by her mother in a secret place, to be led in triumph to the camp where she joined a feast to celebrate her entry into the company of marriage-able maidens; it seems likely that menstruation was much less traumatic. Women still buy sanitary towels with enormous discretion, and carry their handbags to the loo when they only need to carry a napkin. They still recoil at the idea of intercourse during menstruation and feel that the blood they shed is a special kind, although perhaps not so special as was thought when it was the liquid presented to the devil in witches' loving cups. If you think you are emancipated, you might consider the idea of tasting your menstrual blood—if it makes you sick, you've a long way to go, baby.

Menstruation, we are told, is unique among the natural bodily processes in that it involves a loss of blood. It is assumed that nature is a triumph of design and that none of her processes is wasteful or in need of reversal, especially when it only inconveniences women, and therefore it is thought extremely unlikely that there is any "real" pain associated with menstruation. In fact, no little girl who finds herself bleeding from an organ which she didn't know she had until it began to incommode her feels that nature is a triumph of design and that whatever is, is right. When she discovers that the pain attending this horror is in some way her *fault,* the result of improper adaptation to her female role, she really feels like the victim of a bad joke. Doctors admit that most women suffer "discomfort" during menstruation, but disagree very much about what proportion of women suffer "real" pain. Whether the contractions of the women are painful in some absolute sense or could be rendered comfortable by some psychotherapy or other is immaterial. The fact is that no woman would menstruate if she did not have to. Why should women not resent an inconvenience which causes tension before, after, and during; unpleas-antness, odor, staining; which takes up anything from a seventh to a fifth of her adult life until the menopause; which makes her fertile thirteen times a year when she only expects to bear twice in a lifetime; when the cessation of menstruation may mean several years of endocrine derangement and the gradual atrophy of her sexual organs? The fact is that nature is not a triumph of design, and every battle against illness is an interference with her design, so that there is no rational ground for assuming that menstruation as we know it must be or ought to be irreversible.

The contradiction in the attitude that regards menstruation as divinely ordained and yet unmentionable leads to the intensification of the female revolt against it, which can be traced in all the common words for it, like the *curse,* and male disgust expressed in terms like *having the rag on.* We have only the choice of three kinds of expression: the vulgar resentful, the genteel ("I've got my period," "I am indisposed"), and the scientific jargon of the *menses.* Girls are irrepressible though: in our Sydney girls' school napkins are affectionately referred to as *daisies*; Italian girls call their periods *il marchese* and German girls *der rote König.* One might envy the means adopted by *La Dame aux Camélias* to signify her condition to her gentlemen friends, but if it were adopted on a large scale it might look like a mark of proscription, a sort of leper's bell. There have been some moves to bring menstruation out into the open in an unprejudiced way, like Sylvia Plath's menstruation poem. Perhaps we need a film to be made by an artist about the onset of menstruation, in which the implications emerge in some nonacademic way, if we cannot manage a public celebration of a child's entry into womanhood by any other means.

Menstruation has been used a good deal in argument about women's fitness to undertake certain jobs: where women's comfort is concerned the effects are minimized—where the convenience of our masters is threatened they are magnified. Women are not more incapacitated by menstruation than men are by their drinking habits, their hypertension, their ulcers, and their virility fears. It is not necessary to give menstruation holidays. It may be that women commit crimes during the premenstrual and menstrual period, but it is still true that women commit far fewer crimes than men. Women must be aware of this enlistment of menstruation in the antifeminist argument, and counteract it by their own statements of the situation. Menstruation does not turn us into raving maniacs or complete invalids; it is just that we would rather do without it.

FAMILY

If women could regard childbearing not as a duty or an inescapable destiny but as a privilege to be worked for, the way a man might work for the right to have a family, children might grow up without the burden of gratitude for the gift of life which they never asked for. Brilliant women are not reproducing themselves because childbearing has been regarded as a full-time job; genetically they might be thought to be being bred out. In a situation where a woman might contribute a child to a household which engages her attention for part of the time while leaving her free to frequent other spheres of influence, brilliant women might be more inclined to reproduce. For some time now I have pondered the problem of having a child which would not suffer from my neuroses and the difficulties I would have in adjusting to a husband and the demands of domesticity. A plan, by no means a blueprint, evolved which has become a sort of dream. No child ought, I opine, to grow up in the claustrophobic atmosphere of a city flat, where he has little chance of exercising his limbs or his lungs; I must work in a city where the materials for my work and its market are available. No child ought to grow up alone with a single resentful girl who is struggling to work hard enough to provide for herself and him. I . . . hit upon the plan to buy, with the help of some friends with similar problems, a farmhouse in Italy where we could stay when circumstances permitted, and where our children would be born. Their fathers and other people would also visit the house as often as they could, to rest and enjoy the children and even work a bit. Perhaps some of us might live there for quite long periods, as long as we wanted to. The house and garden would be worked by a local family who lived in the house. The children would have a region to explore and dominate, and different skills to learn from all of us. It would not be paradise, but it would be a little community with a chance of survival, with parents of both sexes and a multitude of roles to choose from. The worst aspect of kibbutz living could be avoided, especially as the children would not have to be strictly persuaded out of sexual experimentation with their peers, an unnatural restriction which has had serious consequences for the children of kibbutzim. Being able to be with my child and his friends would be a privilege and a delight that I could work for. If necessary the child need not even know that I was his womb mother and I could have relationships with the other children as well. If my child expressed a wish to try London and New York or go to formal school somewhere, that could also be tried without committal.

Any new arrangement which a woman might devise will have the disadvantage of being peculiar: the children would not have been brought up like other children in an age of uniformity. There are the problems of legitimacy and nationality to be faced. Our society has created the myth of the *broken home* which is the source of so many ills, and yet the unbroken home which ought to have broken is an even greater source of tension as I can attest from bitter experience. The rambling organic structure of my ersatz household would have the advantage of being an unbreakable home in that it did not rest on the frail shoulders of two bewildered individuals trying to apply a contradictory blueprint. This little society would confer its own normality, and other contacts with civilization would be encouraged, but it may well be that such children would find it impossible to integrate with society and become dropouts or schizophrenics. As such they would not be very different from other children I have known. The notion of integrating with society as if society were in some way homogeneous is itself a false one. There are enough eccentrics carving out various lifestyles for my children to feel that they are no more isolated than any other minority group within the fictitious majority. In the computer age disintegration may well appear to be a higher value than integration. Cynics might argue that the children of my household would be anxious to set up "normal" families as part of the natural counterreaction. Perhaps. When faced with such dubious possibilities, there is only empiricism to fall back on. I could not, physically, have a child any other way, except by accident and under protest in a hand-to-mouth sort of way in which case I could not accept any responsibility for the consequences. I should like to be able to think that I had done my best.

The point of an organic family is to release the children from the disadvantages of being the extensions of their parents so that they can belong primarily to themselves. They may accept the services that adults perform for them naturally without establishing dependencies. There could be scope for them to initiate their own activities and define the mode and extent of their own learning. They might come to resent their own strangeness, but in other circumstances they might resent normality; faced with difficulties of adjustment, children seize upon their parents and their upbringing to serve as scapegoats. Parents have no option but to enjoy their children if they want to avoid the cycle of exploitation and recrimination. If they want to enjoy them, they must construct a situation in which such enjoyment is possible.

The Hite Report on Shere Hite: Voice of a Daughter in Exile

SHERE HITE

Shere Hite, excerpt from *The Hite Report on Shere Hite*, n.p.: Arcadia Books, 2003. Reprinted by permission.

Designing a Questionnare for Women: My Research Career

THE AMERICAN DREAM AND ME: A NEW DEFINITION OF WOMEN'S SEXUALITY

While virtually every other issue was being debated in the women's movement in 1970, sexuality was not—though there were a few early queries. Barbara Seaman published a book called *Free and Female*, based on the sexual descriptions of the women in her women's group, as early as 1969. Masters and Johnson's second book was in our group's library, but it claimed that although clitoral stimulus was important for women's orgasms, this should happen automatically during intercourse (coitus). Mary

Jane Sherfey in her book, *The Nature and Evolution of Female Sexuality*, and Anne Koedt, in her pamphlet *The Myth of Female Orgasm*, differed with them. Koedt stated that there was no such thing as a vaginal orgasm: Albert Ellis, too, had questioned this even earlier.

Who was right—this pamphlet by Koedt, or Masters and Johnson? No woman did have orgasm during coitus, or all women "should?" We wondered, but we were not debating this. Not us, we were devoted to issues like "equal pay for equal work," health issues related to the birth-control pill, sexist depictions of women in advertising and so on. But the pressure on women to have vaginal orgasm, or be deemed frigid, "psychologically immature," or "fucked up," was everywhere.

I suggested we have a weekend conference open to women from all over the city to try to discuss this. My friends in the group looked at me in horror: "Well, who's going to speak out? Not me! You think I'm going to stand up and tell everybody about how I have orgasms?! You've got to be kidding!" So I decided an anonymous questionnaire was the only way to go forward. I would distribute it, then read some of the answers at the conference.

I went home and wrote my questions. When I brought them to the next meeting to ask for suggestions, looks of shock and even outrage filled some faces after just the first few questions. One woman later wrote me a condescendingly patient letter explaining that, "It would be better to ask 'If you masturbate, how do you do it?' rather than 'How do you masturbate?'" since, she said, she did not masturbate! I was amazed that she needed to tell me this! However I merely wrote back that it was better to imply that it was normal and acceptable for people to do this, rather than the reverse, i.e., reinforcing the assumption that "nice girls don't," would make it doubly difficult for women to answer or describe how they did it. This information was crucial, in light of stereotypes that women had "problems" having orgasm; women's ability to masturbate to orgasm contradicted this stereotype.

I began this project riding around on the back of my friend Mike Wilson's motorcycle, distributing questionnaires all over New York City. This soon expanded into distribution by mail all over the United States.

I distributed my questionnaires (supported in name by the New York chapter of the National Organization for Women—and supported financially by myself) from 1972–76. During this time, sexuality discussion groups of all kinds began to form within the movement and Betty Dodson began her famous masturbation seminars; the New York Radical Feminists, another group, held an evening to debate "What Is Good Sex?" Two women who worked in publishing had advised me to publish the material I was receiving as a book, so it could be seen by as many women as possible everywhere so, soon, armed with a minimalist $20,000 advance, I stopped modeling, distributed thousands of questionnaires for four years, borrowed money from friends, and analyzed and wrote my conclusions about the answers. My editor came up with the name *The Hite Report*, and the book was published in 1976.

During these four—really five—years, I took what little money I had, and went into overdrive, working seven days a week. Every day I would work twelve or more hours. What was I doing? Reading questionnaire replies, sorting them, and making huge charts (this was before personal computers), placing all the 3,000 essay answers to one of the questions (there were over one hundred questions) on first one chart, then another, and so on.

I was totally committed. I didn't even have time for meetings of the women's movement now, since I hardly had money to pay the rent, never mind the astronomic cost of postage to mail all those heavy, five-page questionnaires. The paper cost a fortune and I used to buy it at end-of-stock warehouses that sold it ridiculously cheap, in interesting colors. In order to get the thousands of responses I wanted, with this kind of unsolicited distribution, I had to print hundreds of thousands of questionnaires. This involved a major outlay of cash in terms of paper, ink, and printing press.

To save money, I learned to run a printing press myself. Fortunately, there was a radical collective in New York at the time, which grew out of a Quaker organization, making it possible for people to print posters for their "alternative" events. I'm glad they believed in what I was doing and let me work there. I had to pay for ink and electricity, and bring food and paper. (This was a hippie commune, with no door on the bathroom, because that would represent unnecessary privacy and be elitist!)

My editor's doorman loaned me money to continue when things got difficult. My editor lived in a big building across the street. The doorman, Virgilio del Toro, used to say hello to me during the night when, after working, I would take my dog Rusty out for a short break. This was in the middle of the night, or sometimes in the day. He was a gentle person, originally from Puerto Rico, full of a poetic love of the calm night. He said he was surprised he always saw my light at all times of the day and night, that I never went out. (It was his job to stand in front of the building across the way, so he knew what everyone did.) And why didn't I go out more? What was I doing? Little by little, I got to know him, and told him about my project, and how I had to rush because soon I would run out of money, and so on. He had three daughters, he told me. One day he said, "Say, look I've saved up some money, and I could loan it to you." I didn't pay any attention until he kept saying it over a few weeks. I felt that I shouldn't borrow it, but it saved the project.

I continued to distribute questionnaires for years, first in New York, then all over the US. I mailed batches to organizations and student centers, also church and health groups, with a letter explaining their purpose, asking the president or whoever received the letter to put the questionnaires out for members to take, if they wanted one. Then, the respondent would mail them back to me (these were long, often handwritten responses to essay questions) without signing them, so she

could have absolute confidence that she could say anything she wanted, without fear. This made utter and absolute honesty possible. From 1972–76, I hardly went out. My best friends were my editor, Regina Ryan, Veronica di Napoli, who was helping me stamp envelopes and open mail—and Rusty!

I lived then in a tiny basement apartment for which I paid about $450 a month (very cheap). It had two rooms and a small backyard, in which I planted ivy and paved the concrete yard with beautiful rusty old red bricks I found on a walk with Virgilio, passing by a building that was being torn down. He helped me carry them home, carefully laying the beautiful old red bricks over the existing grey concrete.

To do a nationwide study of female sexuality for almost five years—how much money does this take? Answer: a lot! But I didn't have a lot. I was living on very little money—plus paying for the questionnaires, mailings, paper, postage, telephone—everything with a budget of about $1,000 a month.

With the total advance payment I received for *The Hite Report* ($20,000 in installments) and another $35,000 I borrowed bit by bit from banks and friends, I lived and worked for five years, paid quite a few assistants (slave wages), and printed and mailed over 100,000 questionnaires all over the United States. And as I've mentioned the printing was done inexpensively with the help of a collective, Come! Unity Press in New York City, which asked only for donations, as long as the item printed was not to be sold, and you learned to run the printing press yourself.

$55,000 is a very small amount of money to live on for over four or five years, plus produce an elaborate piece of research. The government often pays for similar research, with a cost in the six- or seven-figure range. But it was a wonderfully happy period of my life, because I felt I was doing something worthwhile, and the women working on it with me seemed to feel the same way. Nothing like it had ever been done before: recording women's voices on these personal topics, on sexuality—an area previously always defined by men—this was new and important. Discussing what female sexuality was really all about, underneath the clichés and pressures. I loved receiving the answers to my questions from women, and knowing that together we would redefine some part of ourselves—forever.

On the day of publication, over one hundred people came to the press conference: all women but one man (the invitation had said this was a press conference for women). We presented our information, and the debate and questions were great. All the major newspapers and magazines were there. I have tapes of our statements made that day, and the question and answer period which followed. What a day—the first time anyone had publicly declared, on the basis of a large sample of women, that most women do not orgasm from simple coitus. And that this was no disaster, since they could orgasm easily from other stimulation—so that there was nothing wrong with women, it was just the definition of sex which society should change! And thanks to Barbara Seaman, Ti-Grace Atkinson, Anne Koedt, and 3,019 women, there I was saying it.

The reaction was something else! Something I never expected and more than I had ever dreamed. I had thought that this would be a book seen by academics and feminists, I never dreamed it would turn into what is called a bestseller. The press rush was fun, it was great, it was terrifying, and it was fantastic. Everyone seemed to get the message.

In Defense of Shere Hite

SARAH J. SHEY

©1999 by Sarah J. Shey. Original for this publication.

In 1987, cultural historian and researcher Shere Hite presented results of a groundbreaking survey, *Women and Love: A Cultural Revolution in Progress,* to great animosity. It was her third of a trilogy, the first two being *The Hite Report on Female Sexuality* (1976) and *The Hite Report on Male Sexuality* (1981). Commenting on Hite's wide-spread influence, Naomi Weisstein, scientist and author of *How Psychology Constructs the Female*, wrote: "These books comprise complex and fascinating portraits of a crucial fifteen-year period in American culture—a period in which society came into an extraordinary confrontation with the traditional ideas of home and family."

The media scrutinized Hite's training, her methodology, her penmanship, her ringlet hair, but dismissed quite easily her findings collected from 4,500 women, who, by and large, yearned for independence, emotionally satisfying relationships with men, and equality at work and at home. In the following excerpt from *Backlash*, Pulitzer Prize-winning journalist Susan Faludi explores Hite's struggle with the press.

"The picture that has emerged of Shere Hite in recent weeks is that of a pop-culture demagogue," the November 23, 1987, issue of *Newsweek* informed its readers, under the headline "Men Aren't Her Only Problem." Shere Hite had just published the last installment of her national survey on sexuality and relationships, *Women and Love: A Cultural Revolution in Progress*, a 922-page compendium. The report's main findings: Most women are distressed and despairing over the continued resistance from the men in their lives to treat them as equals. Four-fifths of them said they still had to fight for rights and respect at home, and only 20 percent felt they had achieved equal status in their men's eyes. Their quest for more independence, they reported, had triggered mounting rancor from their mates.

This was not, however, the aspect of the book that the press chose to highlight. The media were too busy attacking Hite personally. Most of the evidence they marshaled against her involved tales, that as *Newsweek* let slip, "only tangentially involve her work." Hite was rumored to have punched a cab driver for calling her "dear" and phoned reporters claiming to be Diana Gregory, Hite's assistant. Curious behavior, if true, but one that suggests a personality more eccentric than demagogic. Nonetheless, the nation's major publications pursued tips on the feminist researcher's peculiarities with uncharacteristic ardor. The *Washington Post* even brought in a handwriting expert to compare the signatures of Hite and Gregory.

Certainly, Hite's work deserved scrutiny; many valid questions could be raised about her statistical approach. But Hite's findings were largely held up for ridicule, not inspection. "Characteristically grandiose in scope," "highly improbable," "dubious," and "of limited value" was how *Time* dismissed Hite's report in its October 12, 1987, article "Back Off, Buddy"—leading one to wonder why, if the editors felt this way, they devoted the magazine's cover and six inside pages to the subject. The book is full of "extreme views" from "strident" women who are probably just "malcontents," the magazine asserted. Whether their views were actually extreme, however, was impossible to determine from *Time's* account: the lengthy story squeezed in only two two-sentence quotes from the thousands of women that Hite had polled and quoted extensively. The same article, however, gave plenty of space to Hite's critics—far more than to Hite herself.

When the media did actually criticize Hite's statistical methods, their accusations were often wrong or hypocritical. Hite's findings were "biased" because she distributed her questionnaires through women's right groups, some articles complained. But Hite sent her surveys through a wide range of women's groups, including church societies, social clubs, and senior citizens' centers. The press charged that she used a small and unrepresentative sample. Yet the results of many psychological and social science studies that journalists uncritically report are based on much smaller and nonrandom samples. And Hite specifically states in the book that the numbers are not meant to be representative; her goal, she writes, is simply to give as many women as possible a public forum to voice their intimate, and generally silenced, thoughts. The book is actually more a collection of quotations than numbers.

The reason for the cold shoulder turned toward Shere Hite by the press becomes further clouded when we consider that in the same year Hite's findings were being publicly trashed, psychologist Srully Blotnick quickly became the darling of the news media. Susan Faludi considers the connection:

In 1987, the media had the opportunity to critique the work of two social scientists. One of them had exposed hostility to women's independence; the other had endorsed it. . . .

At the same time the press was pillorying Hite for suggesting that male resistance might be partly responsible for women's grief, it was applauding another social scientist whose theory—that women's equality was to blame for contemporary women's anguish—was more consonant with backlash thinking. Psychologist Srully Blotnick, a *Forbes* magazine columnist and much quoted media "expert" on women's career travails, had directed what he called "the largest long-term study of working women ever done in the United States." His conclusion: success at work "poisons both the professional and personal lives of women." In his 1985 book, *Otherwise Engaged: The Private Lives of Successful Women*, Blotnick asserted that his twenty-five-year study of 3,466 women proved that achieving careerwomen are likely to end up without love, and their spinsterly misery would eventually undermine their careers as well. "In fact," he wrote, "we found that the anxiety, which steadily grows, is the single greatest underlying cause of firing for women in the age range of thirty-five to fifty-five." He took some swipes at the women's movement, too, which he called a "smoke screen behind which most of those who were afraid of being labeled egomaniacally grasping and ambitious hid."

The media received his findings warmly—he was a fixture everywhere from the *New York Times* to "Donahue"—and national magazines like *Forbes* and *Savvy* paid him hundreds of thousands of dollars to produce still more studies about these anxiety-ridden careerists. None doubted his methodology—even though there were some fairly obvious grounds for skepticism. . . .

In the mid-'80s, Dan Collins, a reporter at *U.S.*

News & World Report, was assigned to a story on that currently all-popular media subject: the misery of the unwed. His editors suggested he call the ever-quotable Blotnick, who had just appeared in a similar story on the woes of singles in the *Washington Post.* After his interview, Collins recalls, he began to wonder why Blotnick had seemed so nervous when he asked for his academic credentials. The reporter looked further into Blotnick's background and found what he thought was a better story: the career of this national authority was built on sand. Not only was Blotnick not a licensed psychologist, almost nothing on his résumé checked out; even the professor cited as his current mentor had been dead for fifteen years.

But Collins's editors at *U.S. News* had no interest in that story . . . and the article was never published. Finally, a year later, after Collins had moved to the *New York Daily News* in 1987, he persuaded his new employer to print the piece. Collins's account prompted the state to launch a criminal fraud investigation against Blotnick, and *Forbes* discontinued Blotnick's column the very next day. But the news of Blotnick's improprieties and implausibilities made few waves in the press; it inspired only a brief news item in *Time,* nothing in *Newsweek.* And Blotnick's publisher, Viking Penguin, went ahead with plans to print a paperback edition of his latest book anyway. As Gerald Howard, then Viking's executive editor, explained at the time, "Blotnick has some very good insights into the behavior of people in business that I continue to believe have an empirical basis."

Since then, professors and scholars—men and women—have come out in support of Hite's innovative essay methodology, which depends on thousands of anonymous responses. To quote Barbara Seaman, "Even if the survey was not representative, it was probably representative of what was coming down the turnpike. The rest of the culture is in the process of catching up with the forerunners and pioneers who responded to Hite's questionnaires." Below are some examples of those who lauded this forward-thinker.

When analyzing emotions and attitudes in depth, it has been customary in the social/psychological sciences to use extremely small samples; indeed, Freud based whole books on a handful of subjects. Thus for Hite to have used the small samples typical of psychological studies would have been quite legitimate. However, she took on the more difficult goal of trying to develop a larger and more representative sample, while still retaining the in-depth qualities of smaller studies. She does the latter by allowing thousands of people to speak freely instead of forcing them to choose from preselected categories—in essence, predefining them and prepackaging them, as with so many studies. It is a method that is hard on the researcher, requiring analysis of thousands of individual replies to hundreds of open-ended questions, an analysis that involves many steps.

—Gladys Engel Lang, professor of communications, political science and sociology, University of Washington

To call Shere Hite's monumental work "surveys" is to use an inadequate label. The ground-breaking questionnaires she designed . . . became the underpinnings of a new and most illuminating frame of reference for analyzing power and the relationship between the sexes. . . . Until the modern women's movement it was accepted practice for men to speak for women in everything from marriage ceremonies to anthropological studies and research findings. No questions were asked about the validity of the "male only" opinions. But when Shere Hite presented women speaking for themselves, she was denounced for use of flawed methodology!

—Dale Spender, feminist theorist and writer

The Hite Reports are a medium that has

made it possible for a large number of human beings to speak openly and candidly about needs the expression of which society has tended to censor or limit, and the satisfaction of which society has often condemned and punished. . . . *The Hite Reports* are essays in knowledge of others and also in knowledge of ourselves. In them we have a classic example of how science and morality go hand in hand: they offer a knowledge of human beings directed at a future in which we may better fulfill each other because we better understand each other.

—Joseph P. Fell, presidential professor of philosophy, Bucknell University

Hite's 127 questions that sparked fury ranged from "Do you have a daughter? How do you feel about her? Have you talked to her about menstruation and sexuality? What did you say? What did she say?" (#120) to "What is the biggest problem in your relationship? How would you like to change things, if you could?" (#31) From the thousands of women's answers, Hite culled data about women's attitudes toward relationships, marriage, and monogamy:

➤ *On Affairs:* The majority of women having affairs say they feel alienated, emotionally closed out, or harassed in their marriages; for 60 percent, having an affair is a way of enjoying oneself, reasserting one's identity, having one person appreciate you in a way that another doesn't. . . . "I am a homemaker, raising two children going back to school at fifty-five. Do I believe in monogamy? Yes, but I am not monogamous. The reason for my affair for three years now has been hunger for affection. I told my husband several times I could not live without affection. But I plan to stay married."

➤ *On Love in Marriages:* Most of the women in this study do not marry the men they have most deeply loved. . . . Women, as seen here, hope that by avoiding the highs and lows of being "in love," they can make a relationship more secure, if not inspired,

and a better setting for living and raising children.

➤ *On Marriage and Divorce:* Fifty percent of women leave their marriages, 50 percent stay, even if not emotionally satisfied. We are clearly at a turning point, half in and half out of a new time. The picture is striking—almost as if women were pausing, stopping a moment for reflection, halfway out of a door, still turning to look back, bidding goodbye to the past, before setting out on a journey.

➤ *On Gender:* Gender may be the basic, original split that needs to be healed to alter society, to lessen aggression as a way of life. Women are reintegrating "female" identity, leaving behind the double-standard split that began at the beginning of patriarchy, with Eve, followed by Mary as her opposite—and beyond this, trying to end/overcome the opposition between "male" and "female" emphasized by our culture.

➤ *On Relationships:* Ninety-eight percent of the women in this study say they want to make basic changes in their relationships and marriages and improve the emotional relationships they have with men.

"Our biggest problem is not being able to talk. He talks at me, and what he says is law.". . .

As women think about [why relationships are so difficult]—first asking themselves if there is something wrong with them, then trying to decipher the personal history of the man they love, asking themselves about his childhood, his family, why he is silent, why he behaves the way he does—when women are asking themselves these things, they frequently go on to question the whole system that has made relationships the way they are, and ask, "Why does it have to be this way?"

At least 88 percent of the women in this study, whether married or single, are now asking themselves these questions on a more or less daily basis. . . . [Women are,] unavoidably, changing who they are—and the more distant they are (ironically) becoming from the very men they want to be closer to—the men with whom they can't even discuss these questions.

Sifting through the women's responses to Shere Hite's questions in *The Hite Report*, Susan Faludi found little to scorn. In her book, *Backlash*, she wrote:

> While the media widely characterized these women's stories about their husbands and lovers as "man-bashing diatribes," the voices in Hite's book are far more forlorn than vengeful: "I have given heart and soul of everything I am and have . . . leaving me with nothing and lonely and hurt, and he is still requesting more of me. I am tired, so tired." "He hides behind a silent wall." "Most of the time I just feel left out—not his best friend." "At this point, I doubt that he loves me or wants me. . . . I try to wear more feminine nightgowns and do things to please him." "In daily life he criticizes me for trivial things, cupboards and doors left open. . . . I don't like him angry. So I just close the cupboards, close the drawers, switch off the lights, pick up after him, etc., etc., and say nothing." . . .

That the media find this data so threatening to men is a sign of how easily hysteria about female "aggression" ignites under an antifeminist backlash. For instance, should the press really have been infuriated—or even surprised—that the women's number-one grievance about their men is that they "don't listen"?

If anything, the media seemed to be bearing out the women's plaint by turning a deaf ear to their words. Maybe it was easier to flip through Hite's numerical tables at the back of the book than to digest the hundreds of pages of rich and disturbing personal stories. Or perhaps some journalists just couldn't stand to hear what these women had to say; the overheated denunciations of Hite's book suggest an emotion closer to fear than fury—as do the illustrations accompanying *Time*'s story, which included a woman standing on the chest of a collapsed man, a woman dropping a shark in a man's bathwater, and a woman wagging a viperish tongue in a frightened male face.

The impact of Hite's research is evident not only in the voluminous, heartfelt responses to her questionnaires but in the transformation of traditional psychology and of women's perceptions about their lives.

"We seem to be living in a time of a radical shift: we are in the midst of a very real revolution," wrote Naomi Weisstein in her introduction to Shere Hite's 1993 book, *Women as Revolutionary Agents of Change*. "Despite the cultural backlash, despite the media blitz and the mocking feminism, what the modern women's movement started continues its explosive growth. Women all over the United States have come to some very important conclusions; indeed, their whole perspective on the world seems to be changing. What we see in *Women and Love* (*The Hite Report on Love, Passion, and Emotional Violence*) is women defining themselves emotionally, defining themselves on their own terms, leaving behind a 'male' view of the world, saying good-bye to an allegiance to 'male' cultural values which define women as second-class emotionally or any other way, and which insist that competition and aggression are the basic realities of 'human nature.'"

Dale Spender agrees: "The chorus of women whom Shere Hite has brought together is taking on a new role and insisting on new words. They are voicing ideas, possibilities, and criticisms that many men (and some women) do not want to hear. Their speaking out is one reason that Shere Hite and her reports have received a backlash press over the years. Disliking the message, some individuals have tried to shoot the messenger. . . . Shere Hite's essays have broken the silence so that women now know what's happening in relationships other than their own. They are beginning to appreciate that they are not alone with their 'problems.'"

The climate of the late 1980s had been such that the "messenger"—Hite—chose to sell her New York apartment. Having undoubtedly inspired generations of American women, Shere Hite moved to Paris with her husband in 1989, and has continued to publish books and articles in Europe and other parts of the world, actively campaigning for women's rights in many areas.

Susan Brownmiller: Memoir of a Revolutionary

CARRIE CARMICHAEL

Susan Brownmiller's most recent book is *In Our Time: Memoir of a Revolution*, New York: Dial Press, 1999. This interview was conducted in May 1999. ©1999 by Carrie Carmichael. Reprinted by permission.

Anti-rape activist and feminist author Susan Brown-miller shares her thoughts with writer and stand-up comic Carrie Carmichael about women's progress since the heady days of the 1970s women's movement, and about her life as a feminist today.

CC: When did you get into the movement?

SB: In 1968. By 1970, I was full-time. But the feeling was that there would be a revolution within five years. Whatever the feeling was then was that revolution wouldn't take more than five years. And I never felt that way. You know, I was older. Most of the public space people and leaders of the movement were older than that group of twenty-somethings that made the revolution. So I knew it wasn't going to happen in five years. They got very upset at the institutionalization of our ideas. For example, we were talking about rapists, political crimes against women, you had to stop the rapists. And then it became a social work strategy with the rape crisis centers. That's something else. Same thing with battered women. The whole idea was to stop the batterers, and to help the women too, of course. But now it's become institutionalized with the battered women's shelters, which were an idea from the movement. But the taking over of radical causes, and then dropping the feminist politics and just going with the social concern, is inevitable. Although a lot of people would say that

it has made them unhappy. I mean, where is the politics in all this anymore? I don't know. But what does bother me is that we have lived through enormous changes, and young people don't seem to know that all these changes were hard-won; that people fought for them, that a whole generation of women fought for these changes. They don't know about it. They just know this is the way the world is now. So that makes me sad. But the changes have been enormous, particularly the transformation of the workplace. It's absolutely enormous.

CC: I feel that tinge of sadness when I see the huge changes in the workplace. Women aren't Fortune 500 CEOs yet, but there are these short-skirted executives, throwing out their IPOs, who are now multizillionaires, who have absolutely no sense of historical perspective—who they owe or who helped get them there. Do I expect something from them? Not that I was that active in the movement that way, but as a generation member, as a political supporter, I would expect them to at least know the history and to acknowledge it. And it saddens me. Is that vanity on my part or is it that I'm so afraid that women's power and rights will just get sucked away again?

SB: It's possible because there are certainly those out there who would like that to happen. But I guess they haven't known the history because they haven't been given the history *as history*. While it was happening, there was no need to say anything. We were all doing it. Everybody knew. Then there was that decade or so when people just said, "Shut up, already, would you?" Nobody wanted to talk about it. And now we're all starting to write our books and try to get our programs on television and say, "Hey, look—this was a revolution! We did it; We ought to know about it."

CC: I wanted to talk about aging and taking care of our aging bodies both as political women and as—

SB: It's tough. It's tough to see the changes to your

body and know that they are not attractive. Being attractive is so important to a woman's sense of identity. It's not pleasant.

CC: Do you think it's easier to be aging and older and still attractive as a woman now?

SB: Yes. For sure. We don't have to wear old-lady clothes.

CC: And it's a function of . . . ?

SB: It's a function of the women's movement. And it's a function of the whole loosening up of conformity, which led to so much rigidity in attire and clothing. You can be in your sixties and wear jeans, and people don't think you're weird. You can wear a T-shirt. You don't have to look like what they always used to say, "A little old lady in tennis shoes," which was such a hostile image. You don't have to look that way anymore. . . .

CC: When you were in your twenties and you thought about someone in her sixties, what did she look like in your mind's eye? Was she healthy? I mean, she certainly wasn't in jeans.

SB: Well, it seemed like it was the end of the line. But it's not now, because we all are living longer and we all are healthier.... There are all sorts of problems that our parents' generation and our grandparents' generation faced in terms of health that we do not face in terms of health. So our problems now include face lifts. Because people feel, "Hey, I'm still alive and I'm still sexual, and I can look a little better."

CC: There's a terrible pressure to maintain a false sense of youth.

SB: You know, it's funny. I read a section from my book out loud and it was from our *Ladies' Home Journal* sit-in. And one of our demands was, "We demand that the magazine stop publishing all articles geared to the preservation of youth, implying that age has no graces of its own"—something that young women could say. Now I'm trying to figure out, what are the graces, I don't know any. I

got so upset a few years ago. . . . I hadn't done anything athletic in years. And also I noticed all of these terrible things happening to my body that I know can be fixed by plastic surgery: A little liposuction here, a little moving the breasts back up to where they used to be here. And when I began to realize I was thinking of these things, I was terrified. I was absolutely horrified that even I had fallen into a consideration of these procedures. And then I remembered that . . . if I wanted to do something positive for my body at this stage of my life, I should find a sport and do it. So I took up competitive Ping-Pong. And it's wonderful. It didn't take away those problems, but I'm thinking about other things. I'm thinking about how to whop that ball, really wallop it.

CC: How different are we now from the way we were thirty years ago and—for young women—in terms of seeing ourselves as the world sees us . . . choosing to extend the time of aging, and changing our appearance to be more beautiful?

SB: I don't know, because aging is a whole other thing. You can't just ask that generation that was militant in the 1970s, you can't ask them in the 1990s if they have reevaluated some of the things they thought they'd never do, because they would say yes. But it's not fair. You have to talk to young women and find out if things are different for them. And I don't think they are so different—I think that no one ever thinks they're going to age. And certainly our movement was a Peter Pan and Wendy movement. I don't think we ever thought we'd age. And I don't think we ever thought that we would have to deal with these problems. But you notice how many women who were feminists, or who still are feminists, write a final book about aging. It's no accident that the list includes Beauvoir, Friedan, Germaine Greer. There you are. If you are a person who has been dissatisfied in life with the condition of women, and then you find that you are an old woman, you're going to be latching on to that issue. But it is a slightly different issue.

CC: Your second class status is now compounded

by your elderly status. When men may, for the first time in their lives, maybe upon retirement or infirmity, suddenly get a sense of "I'm not as powerful as I was before."

SB: Getting older has certainly made me understand why older men choose younger women. It gives them that illusion that they are young again. It must be wonderful for them.

CC: Does it make you want to take up with a younger man?

SB: I did.

CC: And did it do the same thing for you?

SB: At the time. Yes, it did. I still see him a bit. But I'm too realistic. I can't delude myself into thinking I'm that age. And also it's not what I need. I need that, yes. You can't think of that as a life partnership for the rest of your life.

CC: My own personal theory is that older men take up with bimbos that they would never take home to Mom because, by the time they are older, mothers are dead.

SB: Now they can literally play.

CC: I think that in the last ten years, menopause has come out of the closet.

SB: I don't know, has it?

CC: I think people talk about it. I think women who were feminists learned how to fight in the medical women's movement field, and I think they fought in the menopause area pretty well too. What's your take on that, or your experience with friends who've gone through menopause and the hormonal replacement issue?

SB: But hormonal replacement is so debatable. I don't know. I had such an easy menopause that it wasn't a concern. Friends who had a tougher one and chose to do estrogen replacement, I wish they hadn't chosen that. That's just my feeling, that it's not a good thing. And we haven't talked at all about breast cancer.

CC: That's totally out of the closet. We don't even refer to it as "the big C" anymore. We're very clear about it: there are pink ribbons, there are marches.

SB: That was fascinating because it seemed to be the result of all the AIDS activism. Women with breast cancer said, "Hey, what about us?" There are a lot more women with breast cancer than men with AIDS. Once they became militant, now there's this movement of men with prostate cancer. It's all very positive.

CC: What all these movements tell me, as a mortal person subject to disease, is that you've got to be in a constant state of diligence and advocacy for yourself because the model of the medical community is not going to help you out unless you scream. It's the squeaky wheel syndrome. And I think that women learned that early on and now various diseases in groups have taken that up. Abortion rights wouldn't have changed if it hadn't been for the screaming. Breast cancer treatment wouldn't have changed if it hadn't been for the screaming. We'd like to think that the medical community could help us out. One of the things that I think that is difficult for the unsophisticated and the non-insiders to figure out is what health experts to pay attention to. Which ones are really being paid by the drug companies to promote something. Do you have any sense of how we can judge who we should listen to? I can't find a doctor who is not trying to push hormone replacement on me. It's almost like brainwashing. I do not believe in it. I think if you have bad symptoms, short-term hormonal replacement is okay to get you through. . . . How do you judge a health expert's independence? How can you trust them?

SB: I don't know. I don't know what job the women's magazines are doing in sorting it all out. There are so many kooks out there with health regimens for people.

CC: Herbal colonics.

SB: Right. It's hard to know. You just have to go with what sounds right to you and what sounds very wrong to you is wrong. . . .

CC: I have a friend who is really smart, and she self-diagnosed a couple of conditions and she took a copy of *Harvard Women's Health Watch* [a health newsletter] to her internist. And she has a fairly young female internist who is of a different mind who said, "You know, you're right." This is a sea change in a medical practitioner who, because of youth, or experience, or gender, could see herself in a partnership with the patient. That's an enormous difference.

SB: And also they're not first-naming you and treating you like a child anymore either.

CC: What about abortion? How do we evaluate the direction we're going in?

SB: There's a problem with abortion rights. Because when abortion was illegal, the movement could speak with one voice and say, "We demand our right, we demand access to good and legal medical attention. We need the procedure. We need the right to abortion." And it was a very simple articulation. And as soon as abortion became legal, unfortunately, in a movement led largely by women—people like Lynda Bird Franke and others—they began to express their doubts, they began to talk about the trauma of having an abortion, they began to say, "Oh God, I really wish I didn't have to. It's a memory I'm going to have to live with for the rest of my life." I think that's been very, very negative. And it's not anything that I've ever thought. I've had three abortions and I never had a moment of doubt that what I was doing was anything but absolutely right and necessary. So in a strange way, the success of *Roe v. Wade* opened a whole new dialogue. There was another reason for it, and that was that reproductive technology itself became much more sophisticated so that you could save the life of the fetus outside the womb earlier than you could before. But it's almost impossible now to say "I had an abortion, and you know what, I didn't suffer any ambivalence or any emotional trauma here, I was just very glad that I was unpregnant." It's impossible to say that aloud

now. Because the conventional discourse says that you must suffer in some way. It has to have been an agonizing decision. And I can tell you that for a lot of us, it wasn't. By putting that new element into the public dialogue, it has prevented a lot of women from having an abortion. They're not so afraid of the physical procedure, it's that they have been conditioned to expect emotional repercussions. And I think that's nonsense. I really do.

CC: Do you think that that is a sadistic or manipulative plot from those who fight choice?

SB: Well, it becomes that. . . . The right to abortion is such a fundamental right for women that the anti-abortion movement is fueled by those who wish that women would not have equal rights in society. They convince themselves that they are so obsessed about saving lives. There are lots of lives out there to save if they want to save lives. But they know that it's the crucial issue to women's evolving. They must have the right to an abortion.

CC: Where do you think we are in terms of maintaining the security of that right? Is it threatened if women take it for granted?

SB: They take it for granted until it happens to them and then they don't take it for granted any more. It's hard.

CC: You've done a lot with not only the way we move our bodies around, but with how they are invaded and assaulted against our will in your study of rape. Where are we now as a society in terms of dealing with rape, the medical consequences of it for the victims?

SB: There have been enormous changes. When we started talking about rape, it was shrouded in silence, it was the subject of frightening, hysterical rumors, and also giggles. It was not a subject you could talk about without nervous laughter. And that has certainly disappeared. And I think more women than ever before in history are aware of their right not to be violated physically. And if they are, they get much more sympathetic treatment by the police, by the hospitals, and in the courts. There have been famous cases. Like the Tupac Shakur case, [which] was extraordinary, and Mike Tyson. That's just amazing.

CC: On a scale from 0 to 100 percent, where are we in terms of removing the victim as blame object?

SB: That still crops up from time to time, because you've still got defense lawyers out there who want to win at any cost. So they'll keep bringing it up. And if it's an interracial case, people are still afraid to challenge a defense that tries to play with it. That's a tough area, because you're pitting race against sex. I do think we are not blaming the victim so much, but we're still not so far along in terms of ending the assaults. Someone once said to me, "Well, if your book was that successful, why aren't there fewer rapes? Why are men still raping us?" Well, they're not the ones who are reading the book.

A Mother's Story

PATSY MINK

Adapted from Patsy Mink, "A Mother's Story," excerpt from Christina Looper Baker and Christina Baker Kline, eds., *The Conversation Begins*, New York: Bantam Books, 1996. Reprinted by permission.

While I was pregnant with my daughter, Wendy, in 1951 and 1952, I was administered a drug that dramatically affected both our lives. My doctor was participating in a University of Chicago experiment to test whether diethylstilbestrol (DES), a form of estrogen, prevents miscarriages. Years later, dust-covered records in a Chicago basement revealed that the blind study had created tremendous health hazards for one thousand women involved in the experiment and their offspring. For years Wendy had puzzling physical symptoms, the cause of which remained a mystery. In 1976, on her twenty-fourth birthday, I received a letter

saying, "You were in this test, and our records show that you were given DES. Are you alive? Are you sick? What happened to your child?" They even requested we participate in a follow-up experiment to track the effects of the drug on offspring.

In 1978, I and two others won a significant settlement from the University of Chicago and DES manufacturer Eli Lilly because they had not informed us that we were part of an experiment. Our daughters have been less successful in court. Wendy sued, but since she didn't have cancer at the time, she was awarded nothing. A two-year statute of limitations prevented her from recovering for any DES-related medical problems that developed since 1976.

There was no women's movement in the mid-1950s, when the DES experiment took place, nor when I first entered politics. In my youth I didn't understand that there was such a thing as discrimination against women. I lived my life as I felt inclined, never considering myself a lesser being because I was female. I attribute this to the influence of my parents, who treated me and my brother with absolute equality.

From childhood I had been preoccupied with the idea of becoming a doctor. All my studies were directed toward that end, and in 1948 I graduated from the University of Hawaii with a major in zoology and chemistry and a minor in physics. At the appropriate time I applied to twenty-five medical schools—my parents willingly paying the application fees. But my dream never materialized. Had I been male I would have been accepted because of good grades, but medical schools across the country simply were not accepting women. The reasons may have been ethnic as well. In any case, I was shattered, and I was left with nothing to do. The jobs I qualified for were unrelated to my goal.

One day my boss said, "Don't be so depressed; life doesn't end just because you didn't go to medical school. Surely there are other ways to express your individuality and your desire to serve people." I asked, "What can I do?" and she enumerated possible careers. "Why don't you go to law school?" she said. "You like to talk." I had no idea what the study of law entailed, but I took her up on it, and in 1950 the University of Chicago accepted me as a "foreign student." I didn't bother to say they were wrong to think me foreign.

I became interested in Democratic politics through friends who pulled me into party workshops and seminars. One thing led to another, and soon I was elected to the state legislature. Campaigning took a lot of time, and much of my political activity in those early years I did alone. Equal pay for equal work was one of my early achievements. Male legislators got up on the floor and ridiculed the legislation ("Equal pay?"), but in 1957 they voted for it. We took pleasure in the fact that Hawaii adopted the bill six years sooner than the nation. As a representative, I helped open up state government after noticing that it was always the same people who served on important commissions. "A lot of talented people want to serve," I said. "Give them an opportunity." In all, I served three terms in the Hawaii legislature.

When I first ran for national office in 1959, I lost by 8 percent. Losing felt awful. It's terrible enough to be rejected by just one person, but to be rejected by thousands you thought were in love with you is devastating. That's why most people don't run for office. You can run again only if you believe strongly that you have something to contribute. After losing I said, "Never again," but soon I reentered local politics and was elected to the Hawaii state senate in 1962.

In 1964 a seat opened in the US House of Representatives, and I decided to seek national office. This time I campaigned for federal aid to education, which became law my first year in Congress. As a representative, I pushed for equity in education. We held hearings to determine how textbooks were demeaning to black people and looked at gender discrimination in the handling of federal funding. When we wrote Title IX, out of a belief that federally funded institutions should treat girls and boys equally, I had no idea how far-reaching it would be and how it would withstand all the court tests. Though just twenty words long, Title IX has produced stunning results in prohibiting sex discrimination.

I am a feminist—one who cares about the role of women in society—but I do not believe the women's movement is broadly enough based. In limiting itself to a certain segment of society, it leaves out the rest. Millions of women, such as those on welfare, are not connected to it, but I don't see the feminist movement getting involved in welfare reform; women of color are the only ones who care about this issue. I would like to see preschool child care become part of the official educational program so that child care workers' pay is comparable to that of teachers. Child care workers are currently paid less than animal shelter employees. Why aren't feminists campaigning for better salaries for childcare workers? Is an animal more precious than a child?

The women's movement still focuses on middle-class white women, which I don't see changing. The "glass ceiling" is an upper-class ceiling for those aspiring to be bank presidents and executives, not those who can never rise above the minimum wage. The majority of people working at minimum-wage jobs in the United States are women. That's the glass ceiling I am committed to doing something about. American women must stand up and be counted. The new women in Congress have absolutely made a difference—forty-nine is better than twenty-nine—but to get more women into office, it must be easier for women to run. If we could just persuade women to support more women candidates, more would win.

HOW WE WON TITLE IX

When I came to Congress in 1965, I was on the Education and Labor Committee chaired by Adam Clayton Powell. From the moment I sat in my chair as a freshman member down in the lower tier, he began hearings on discrimination and textbooks, and we hauled in all the textbooks to show that women were really being discarded. We hauled in the Department of Education because they were issuing films on vocational education which showed women as nurses, teachers, social workers, but not of occupations like scientist, doctor, or engineer or anything of that kind. Finally, with the enactment of Public Law 8910, which was the first federal aid to elementary and secondary schools, we wanted to make sure that women and girls would have an equal opportunity and that was all we were trying to say.

Edith Green, chairperson of the Higher Education Committee, convened a hearing in June of 1970 to add protections for women to the Civil Rights Act. This was all going on at the same time that women in the country were getting excited about the Equal Rights Amendment. But the Justice Department intervened and said we cannot support an amendment of the Civil Rights Act; why not put this measure in the education bill? When the education amendments came up in November of 1971, we were able to argue all of this.

In 1975, opponents tried to exclude college and university athletics from Title IX regulation. They paraded a number of college and professional athletes to testify that Title IX hurt men's sports. The only well-known woman athlete we had to testify was Billie Jean King. The fact that there were virtually no prominent women athletes in our country was a testament in itself of the necessity of the legislation.

Just a minute or so before the critical vote, I got word that my daughter had gotten into a car accident. I rushed off to Ithaca to see how she was. In my absence, the devastating amendment passed by one vote. The newspapers reported that I had left the floor "crying" in the face of defeat. But in reality I was facing a tremendous family crisis. The next day, the Speaker explained the circumstances of my departure and a new vote was taken, preserving the regulations and Title IX's application to athletes.

On July 26, 1999, the Congressional Record recorded that: no person in the United States shall, on the basis of sex, be excluded from participation in, be denied the benefits of, or be subjected to discrimination under any educational program or activity receiving Federal financial assistance. These are the achievements of Title IX:

➤ When President Nixon signed this bill, about 31,000 women were involved in college sports. Today that number has more than tripled.
➤ Spending on athletic scholarships for women has grown from less than $100,000 to almost $200 million.
➤ In 1972, women received 9 percent of the medical degrees and 7 percent of the law degrees in this country; in 1994, the numbers were 38 percent and 43 percent, respectively.
➤ In 1994, 44 percent of all doctoral degrees were granted to women.

On July 10, 1999, the American team's victory in the Women's World Cup soccer competition reminded us how important it is to have the protections for women that we now have. These young women are the products of Title IX. But this victory was about more than the game and the win. It was about female athletes, sports, and equality.

DES Litigation

SYBIL SHAINWALD

Sybil Shainwaild, "DES Litigation," 2008. Original for this publication.

I was pregnant with my second child in 1953. I stained during my pregnancy but I was not able to afford a gynecologist and my general practitioner did not keep up with the latest developments. Fortunately for my daughter, I did not receive DES. Additionally, I had read *Childbirth Without Fear*, the bible of the alternative birth movement and I doubt whether I would have taken DES because I wanted natural childbirth.

Six million women in the United States were given the drug. Among them was Dorothy Bichler, who had DES prescribed to her by Dr. Abraham Fleischer, whom Dorothy trusted implicitly. The DES was prescribed in its generic form and Dorothy purchased the prescription at the Willing Pharmacy across the street from her home. When Dorothy's unborn daughter was exposed in 1953, not a single drug producer had done any testing before marketing it to pregnant women.

Dorothy gave birth that year to her daughter, who seemed to be a healthy baby girl. At age seventeen, however, Joyce developed adenocarcinoma of the cervix and vagina caused by the DES her mother had ingested to "save" her pregnancy.[1] As a result, Joyce was required to undergo a radical hysterectomy, oopherectomy, salpingtectomy and vaginectomy, effectively removing all of her reproductive organs and the greater part of her sex organs.

Joyce's doctors unequivocally stated that her cancer was caused by the DES administered to Dorothy Bichler. This was totally preventable.

DES, diethylstilbestrol, is a powerful synthetic estrogen. It is 2.5 times more potent than natural estrogen. In 1937, Sir Charles Dodds was successful in discovering this new "miracle" drug that he never patented. The lack of a patent meant that every manufacturer made generic, fungible DES or supplied its raw powder to others. Dodds thought that the drug was useful for other purposes, and said that it did not save pregnancies but instead caused miscarriage or abortions.[2] The dose initially was 5 mg. It is a transplacental teratogen and a carcinogen according to the Food and Drug Administration (FDA), World Health Organization, and every major writer in the field.[3]

The United States believes there is a causal connection between DES and cancer. *The Consolidated List of Hazardous Products* issued by the United Nations lists DES as a carcinogen. The National Institutes of Health supports a causal relationship between DES exposure in utero and DES changes such as adenosis, cervical ridge, T-shaped uterus, and other teratologic DES non-cancerous changes, which affect almost all women exposed. "Non-cancerous changes appear in the vagina in about one-third and in the cervix in nearly every DES-exposed daughter."[4] In European countries where DES was never used, there is a complete absence of clear cell cancer (e.g., Denmark, Norway, and West Germany).

By 1947, when the supplemental filings with the FDA were approved for use in pregnancy, it was well known that DES produced cancer in rats and mice; that DES was a teratogenic agent in humans; that cancer-producing agents could cross the placenta and insult the fetus; and that DES applied to a portion of an animal produced cancer of the uterus.

FAILURE TO TEST

Since at least 1936, researchers knew that breast cancer could be produced in male mice by giving them estrogen injections, and that sex hormones could produce cancer in laboratory animals in strains not usually susceptible.

DES was the first drug that was designed to reach the fetus through the placenta. In 1939, a Northwestern University study was performed to determine if DES, when given during pregnancy, crossed the placenta. The results of the study showed that it did and that it acted as a malforming agent on the fetus. Researchers found "an alarming number" of the offspring of pregnant rats that were fed DES had reproductive tract abnormalities: misshapen uterus, ovaries, and vaginas in the females, and tiny and malformed penises in the male. Consistent with these findings, more than forty articles documenting carcinogenic effects of material and synthetic estrogens, including DES, had been published in medical journals before initial FDA approval of the drug in 1941.

Dr. Allan Goldman, the head of pharmacology at the University of Pennsylvania, and one of the ten leading experts on teratology in the world, said, "if a fetus or embryo were exposed to a cancer-producing agent it was more likely to get cancer than a similar tissue of an adult."

Dr. Goldman later testified that the failure to test this drug for its effect on the fetus was irresponsible. He said:

> I think that it is inconceivable to me that this drug, which was so potent and could, and was intended to the use in the fetus, was not tested on the fetus to establish safety before or during its first submission to the market. I find that—I'm at a total loss to explain why that was not done. I think it is the responsibility of the drug house to assure safety.

Dr. Goldman said the failure to perform a test on mice to ascertain the effect of DES on the fetus was a departure from proper practice and "was below the standard of research science as it existed in 1947."

There was also a 1942 study done by Sklow which examined estrogen transfer through the placenta. According to the study, results would appear in the vaginal areas of female offspring. Other articles in the medical community considered the dangers and delayed effects of DES.

In order to get DES approved, in 1941 Eli Lilly & Co. (Lilly) spearheaded a consortium of manufacturers, known as the Small Committee, to pool data on DES for submission to the FDA. Lilly's first application and those of other producers had been rejected because they were based on foreign studies. Lilly's campaign to achieve acceptance of DES created a climate of favorable medical opinion. This campaign, however, disregarded the unpleasant truths about DES, i.e., it was never subjected to any testing, even though it was a transplacental carcinogen and teratogen, with no therapeutic benefits.

The Small Committee consisted of Lilly, Squibb, Upjohn, and Winthrop. A master file was created containing all the clinical data and testing performed by all of the drug companies jointly and was submitted to the FDA.[5]

Whether twelve drug manufacturers thereafter worked together at the direction of the government, as they claim, or did so of their own accord, really makes no difference. The point is that they *did* work together through the Small Committee, chaired by Lilly's representative, Dr. Don Carlos Hines. Dr. Hines testified that he represented all twelve companies seeking to market DES. Uniform labels, descriptions, and warning labels had been prepared by Lilly and agreed to and adopted by all the others.

The FDA relied solely upon the material furnished by the drug companies, and in 1941, DES was approved for purposes other than prevention of miscarriages during pregnancy such as treatment of menopausal disorders, gonorrheal vaginitis, and unwanted lactation with a maximum dose of 5 mg.

In 1947, Lilly and several other companies submitted supplemental drug applications to be permitted to provide DES for the purpose of "preserving pregnancies." The indicated dose for the new use was 25 mg, five times the dose on the original application.[6]

By its terms, the supplemental New Drug Application was permitted to rely upon the data used for the original joint application.

In 1947, the very year that the drug companies obtained approval to market DES to pregnant women, the standard listing for pharmacological drugs in the United States, the *Dispensatory of the United States of America*, stated with regard to DES:

> To date no national catastrophe [sic] has been recognized but it is perhaps too early for any deleterious effect on the incidence of carcinoma of the female genital tract or breast to appear.[7]

Thus, by the time the 1941 filings were amended to permit DES manufacturers to market a 25 mg tablet for use in "accidents of pregnancy," the potential for harm was self-evident.

Yet none of the adverse literature was filed with the FDA in the original 1941 filing or in the supplemental filings in 1947. Before 1947, Dr. Don Carlos Hines, Lilly's medical director, who prepared Lilly's supplemental application, said that he had read everything about DES at that time and knew that it caused cancer in animals. He also knew that it crossed the placenta and that every new drug should be tested on animals.[8]

It is incontrovertible that prior to marketing DES for this use in the so-called preservation of pregnancy in 1947, Lilly and other drug companies who had filed the original New Drug Application in 1941 had never tested DES to determine if it would have any effect on the offspring of the mothers who ingested it. Admittedly, not one manufacturer had ever conducted a test of the potential for harm of this drug in use in pregnancy. As Lilly's lawyer, Russell H. Beatie Jr., stated in his summation at Joyce Bichler's trial,

Now there was no testing on pregnant animals. Nobody did that. Nobody ever thought of it. No testing for cancer.[9]

In 1950, Eli Lilly began the first double-blind controlled study of DES. The so-called Dieckmann study,[10] using Lilly's own pills, was conducted on two thousand unsuspecting women at the University of Chicago, starting in 1950 and completed in 1952. The study showed that the incidence of miscarriage in DES mothers was twice that in mothers not given DES, and similar studies were conducted elsewhere.[11] DES did not save a single baby.

In 1952, the FDA declared that DES was no longer a new drug and marketing for DES peaked. By 1953, the year Dorothy Bichler filled her prescription, Lilly knew that this generic drug made by it and other producers was being used to fill prescriptions for "accidents of pregnancy." Lilly was also providing the drug in bulk to other producers to market under their names. In 1962, after the Kefauver Amendments, the FDA changed its requirements by establishing a rating system for efficacy of all pharmaceuticals. The National Academy of Sciences did not even rate DES as "probably effective," and no drug company ever appealed that rating.

Through aggressive marketing and various exclusivity agreements, Lilly created the demand for their DES by requiring wholesalers to carry and provide Lilly's brand of "Stilbestrol," or DES, whenever ordered on the threat of canceling the entire Lilly line of pharmaceuticals it provided to the wholesalers.

In addition to covering the wholesale end of the sales, Lilly also created the demand for their DES through its detail men and its advertising campaigns by providing physicians with periodic literature such as the "De Re Medica" (DRM) brochures, prescription blanks, which hawked their DES among other Lilly products. As such, Lilly made the following claims on behalf of DES:

1. Effective to stop uterine bleeding (DRM 204)
2. Preventing ovulation and the pains and cramps of dysmenorrheal (DRM 205)
3. Benefit to ovarian functions, irritation, and vaginitis (DRM 206)
4. Prescribed dosage 25 mg plus 5 mg every fifteen minutes in threatened miscarriage (DRM 211)
5. The "most effective" agent for preventing miscarriage
   (a) Start treatment even "before" bleeding (DRM 212)
6. DES is more effective than progesterone
7. Daily dosage up to 125 mg per day is safe
8. Use whenever estrogenic therapy is indicated (DRM 467)
9. Present evidence suggests "DES is the most effective therapy for functional uterine bleeding" (PB 9/10/44)
10. "Will not initiate human cancer"

Yet, although Lilly was the primary manufacturer of DES and essentially created the demand for its product through tremendous marketing efforts, when it came time for trial, Lilly"s lawyers claimed, and continue to claim, that they are not in possession of any marketing, sales, and distribution records. This enhanced the already prevalent problem of product identification for plaintiffs.

On December 10, 1959, the Secretary of Health, Education, and Welfare (HEW) announced that the use of DES in the poultry industry had led him to the conclusion that there was a potential cancer hazard to the public "occasioned by the use of Stilbestrol-treated poultry." On December 15, 1961, Deputy Food and Drug Commissioner (FDC) Harvey ordered a blanket ban on the use of diethylstilbestrol as a poultry additive, saying, "There is substantial evidence that this drug may be expected to produce, incite, or stimulate cancer growth in human beings."

This action was the culmination of two years of battling with the manufacturers of DES. Indeed, "Hearing Examiner Leonard D. Hardy's decision ended the long first round of a battle that began in Dec. 1959 when former HEW Secretary Arthur S. Flemming pulled the plug regarding Stilbestrol in chickens on the basis of FDA and NIH judgment that chicken liver and skin residues of the drug are potential carcinogens."[12]

In fact, in *Helmrich v. Eli Lilly & Co.*, a case where the prescribing doctor denied prescribing DES and the plaintiff had clear cell cancer, the Court stated, "Maybe the mother ate Stilbestrol-fattened poultry."[13]

Lilly's own records of 1961 contain the following statement: "It must be admitted that other studies fail to confirm the effectiveness of DES for accidents of pregnancy."[14]

In 1966 the Court found in *Bell v. Goddard* that "the effects of DES . . . on either humans or animals are identical, however administered," and that DES had:

> been shown to cause cancers of the breast, endometrium, uterine cervix, pituitary, testes, ovaries, adrenals, and kidneys, and leukemia, in mice, rats, rabbits, hamsters and dogs; often more than one of those cancers appear in a particular species or strain. In addition, fibroid tumors have been produced in guinea pigs. In humans, chronic estrogic stimulation of the uterus, whether due to excessive ovarian pro-

duction or abnormalities of the reproductive cycle, results in increased cancer of the endometrium. Such cancer has also been observed to develop in women during or following estrogen therapy.[15]

Lilly admits this connection in its literature published before the withdrawal of 1971.

Lilly's advertisement in the 1967 *Physician's Desk Reference* (*PDR*) states:

> CONTRAINDICATIONS: The contraindications to diethylstilbestrol administration are the same as to estrogen therapy in general. Estrogens should not be administered in the absence of a positive indication, and they should be avoided in women who have cancerous or precancerous lesions of the breast or cervix or who have a family history of high incidence of breast or genital malignancy.[16]

Not coincidentally, two years later, Lilly abandoned its promotion of DES for use by pregnant women altogether and deleted that indication from its *PDR*, adding the caveat:

> Warning: Because of the possible adverse reactions of the fetus, the risk of estrogen therapy should be weighed against the possible benefit for use in a known pregnancy.

Finally, in 1971, in an article entitled "Adenocarcinoma of the vagina. Association of maternal stilbestrol therapy with tumor appearance in young women,"[17] Drs. A. L. Herbst, H. Ulfelder, and D. C. Poskanzer publicized the relationship between DES ingestion by pregnant women and clear cell adenocarcinoma of the cervix and vagina in their offspring. After this report, the National Institute of Cancer funded the Registry for Research on Hormonal Transplacental Carcinogenesis, and six months later DES was forced off the US market. During that time, over two thousand prescriptions were written for DES and the drug companies did not advise pregnant women who had been exposed to DES while pregnant that they should have immediate check-ups. Not until 1973 did Lilly send "Dear Doctor" letters warning doctors of the adverse effects of DES exposure to their patients.[18] Additionally, the drug companies continue to brazenly claim that there is no causal connection shown between cancer and DES.

The pharmaceutical industry should have immediately been held accountable and required to advise women who had been exposed to DES while pregnant that their children should have immediate check-ups.

At approximately the same time that Drs. Herbst, Ulfelder, and Poskanzer publicized the relationship between DES exposure and clear cell adenocarcinoma of the cervix and vagina, Joyce Bichler was diagnosed with her tragic injuries.

OVERCOMING PROCEDURAL HURDLES

TIMELINESS

Each state has a statute of limitations that limits the period of time during which a plaintiff may successfully bring a cause of action against another party. In the state of New York, for example, prior to adoption of a "tort reform" package in 1986, the general limitations period for bringing a claim resulting from exposure to DES would begin at birth and run until the DES-exposed daughter or son reached age twenty-one. Thus, the biggest hurdle for DES litigants was the statute of limitations. This posed a significant dilemma as it related to DES litigation, and consequently, prior to 1986 numerous plaintiffs, including two of my own young clients, Susan Helmrich and Linda Fleishman, were left without remedies.

Because of the latent deleterious effects of DES (and certain other toxic substances), justice necessitated a different method for determining the limitations period for women and men to bring their cases for severe injuries. After years of aggressive advocacy inside and outside of the courtroom, New York adopted a discovery rule and a special one-year statute giving new life to previously time-barred actions called the "Revival Statute" in 1986.[19] Under the discovery rule, where a plaintiff claimed that a substance was toxic, she could bring an action against its manufacturer once she "knew or should have known" that she had suffered an injury arising from the toxic substance. Despite the supposed leniency of this model, the rule posed a number of complications as it related to DES litigation, given the unique circumstances surrounding DES exposure.

First, because of the pharmaceutical industry's failure to warn its consumers about the extreme risks associated with DES exposure, DES-exposed women (and their offspring) had no reason to expect that any health problems they developed were a result of the drug. Second, given the latent effects of DES, often a plaintiff's injuries would not manifest themselves until long after the exposure. Third, in many cases, the DES daughters and sons were unaware that they had been exposed to DES. The DES daughters and sons did not voluntarily expose themselves since they were exposed in utero, and having no warning from the pharmaceutical industry that DES was dangerous, their mothers often had no reason to tell them that they had ingested DES.[20]

In making this legal change the legislature adopted the eloquent admonition expressed by Chief Judge Cooke in his dissent in *Fleishman v. Eli Lilly*.

A grave injustice—to victims of DES as well as to past and future victims of identified and unidentified substances which do not immediately make known their harmful effect upon the body but have a "time-bomb" effect—is causes of action to be brought before a plaintiff could reasonably know of their existence and very likely before any medically cognizable injury has occurred. It is time to abandon that inequitable rule as a mistake of the past that we have a duty to correct . . . The current rule is unreasonable and the Statute of Limitations should not be construed in such a manner.[21]

What did the pharmaceutical companies do in response? They immediately filed briefs full of misstatements that the Revival Statute was unconstitutional and unreasonable. Their records were a mélange of material that carefully excluded the records in *Bichler* and *Helmrich*, the two cases tried in New York under a concert of action theory.[22]

At the time, there were approximately five hundred cases in New York County. Justice Ira Gammerman was appointed to preside over the New York County cases. Judge Jack B. Weinstein of the Eastern District of New York was appointed to preside over the federal cases and he appointed Kenneth R. Feinberg as Special Master for settlement purposes. To compensate the victims would hardly bankrupt the corporations who benefited from the marketing of DES nor would it impede the marketing of pharmaceuticals.

Seeking to foreclose a remedy at the threshold, and screaming that recovery without identification was unprecedented, the drug industry urged that all the complaints be dismissed if they failed to identify the specific manufacturer of the DES ingested.

Lilly and its friends howled that disaster would overtake the drug industry. Actually, all the *Bichler* case stands for is an unusual fact pattern, meaning the ruling wouldn't be easily applicable to other cases. The likelihood of that happening again with a generation-skipping harmful drug is remote. No huge floodgate of liability can follow because the direct exposure to DES is now at an end. Its use is forbidden, and the statute of limitations has thus far been sustained against claims instituted more than three years after the DES daughter's majority.[23]

As Lilly's attorney, Russell H. Beatie Jr. said succinctly,

Eli Lilly is like any other company ladies and gentlemen. I would be a dummy to stand up here and say it is not in business to make money. It is in business to make money, of course it is.

PRODUCT IDENTIFICATION

As a general rule, a drug company that possessed an exclusive right to a given product would identify that product with a trade name. A generic name, on the other hand, is one used generally to designate the nature of the chemical composition of the drug. In the case of DES, no drug company had exclusive rights and the companies elected a marketing pattern wherein DES was promoted generically. All the involved manufacturers had full knowledge of this and their individual efforts would benefit the entire group. In effect the very use of the generic name concealed the identity of the specific manufacturer. The concealment, however, does not shield a manufacturer from liability.

To recover damages for injuries resulting from a defective product or toxic substance, a plaintiff must usually show product identification. In other words, a plaintiff must show who caused her injury and by what acts or omissions that injury was caused. This creates a unique problem for DES victims because, although the woman might be able to trace the cause of her injuries to DES exposure, she may have no way of identifying the specific manufacturer of the DES to which she was exposed.[24] Without pharmacy or medical records, or someone able to attest to the physical appearance of the DES ingested, ascertaining the specific manufacturer of the DES to which one woman was exposed from among the two hundred and sixty-seven manufacturers of DES is akin to finding a needle in the proverbial haystack.[25]

Imagine trying to identify an aspirin ingested in 1954 without a lead from the prescription, the drugstore, or the physician. To find a way out of the quagmire of dead or amnesiac pharmacists, burned or abandoned pharmacies, lost or destroyed doctor's records, faded memories, and obstructive defense tactics, courts have resorted to various theories: enterprise, concert of action, or alternative liability theories, such as market share liability.

Bichler v. Eli Lilly & Co.[26]

Lilly and its friends complained that the essence of the DES daughters' and sons' argument was that the drug companies failed to test the drugs on humans. Plaintiffs say they did test DES on humans—on their mothers and on them. Joyce Bichler's mother was a test subject because not a single producer ever conducted tests of DES on pregnant animals. Lilly's counsel admitted this fact, although Lilly's medical officer, Dr. Don Carlos Hines, testified that the supplemental drug application included safety and efficacy as basic considerations.

Lilly complained that Mrs. Bichler's medication could have been made by any one of 147 producers. However, it was one of eleven other manufacturers who formed the committee that was run and managed by the Small Committee, under the leadership of Lilly. There were only four brands in Mr. Willing's[27] pharmacy, where Joyce Bichler's mother purchased the drug. Although DES was sold under approximately 222 labels in 1953, Lilly had the largest share of the market. In Joyce Bichler's case, the pharmacist first stated that he carried only the best in his small Bronx store. When he testified at the trial, he changed his story and stated that he carried four brands: Lilly, Squibb, Upjohn, and APC. Squibb had to be prescribed by its trade name Stilbetin. And in all the years I have been doing DES litigation, I have only seen one prescription for it. Upjohn made perles, soft capsules with a liquid center, and Dorothy Bichler testified that she had taken tablets, therefore Squibb and Upjohn could be immediately eliminated as the manufacturer of the pill that Dorothy had taken. That left only Lilly and APC, who both made white pills. In fact, Lilly supplied the powder to APC and Dorothy Bichler remembered taking Lilly's pill.

Lilly was not being sued for someone else's product. As Lilly said, "No one knows who did" manufacture it.[28] It was being sued as a company that led the joint campaign to bring the drug to the market and be tested on the innocent public, including Joyce's mother, in its generic form. It is not who directly caused the injury, it is who created the risk.

It must be remembered that Eli Lilly led the Small Committee, had an army of detail men, was instrumental in the approval of DES, and should be held responsible because of its promotional efforts. No matter who tabletized or bottled the drug, Lilly supplied the powders to many of the companies and under strict liability law, is responsible for the manufacture, sale, and testing of the drug. At a congressional hearing in 1960, Robert Carney, Lilly's president, testified, in response to Congressman Moss's question, that Eli Lilly produces as much as 75 percent of the DES consumed in the US.

At the end of Joyce Bichler's trial, Lilly offered $100,000 in a settlement while the jury was deliberating. The offer was good until noon of that day. Joyce and I walked around the Bronx courthouse rotunda as she was being urged by members of the firm to take the settlement. I told her that if money was not essential, and that if she could hold out for a jury verdict, it would be a victory for women everywhere.

After seven weeks of trial before Justice Arnold G. Fraiman in the Bronx, Joyce Bichler was awarded $500,000.[29] In addition to a unanimous general verdict for Joyce, the jury answered seven specific interrogatories:

(1) Was DES reasonably safe in the treatment of accidents of pregnancy when it was ingested by the plaintiff's mother in 1953?

(2) If not, was DES a proximate cause of the plaintiff's cancer?

(3) If so, in 1953 when the plaintiff's mother ingested DES should the defendant, as a reasonably prudent drug manufacturer, have foreseen that DES might cause cancer in the offspring of pregnant women who took it?

(4) If so, foreseeing that DES might cause cancer in the offspring of pregnant women who took it, would a reasonably prudent drug manufacturer test it on pregnant mice before marketing it?

(5) If so, if DES had been tested on pregnant mice, would the tests have shown that DES causes cancer in their offspring?

(6) If so, would a reasonably prudent drug manufacturer have marketed DES for use in treating accidents of pregnancy at the time it was ingested

by the plaintiff's mother, if it had known that DES causes cancer in the offspring of pregnant mice?

(7) If not, did the defendant and other drug manufacturers act in concert with each other in the testing and marketing of DES for use in treating accidents of pregnancy?

The jury's judgment was affirmed unanimously in the Appellate Division's First Department, where a twenty-page opinion detailed every issue of fact and law.

It was far better that the judgment against Lilly be affirmed than that it be left to a cancer victim, Joyce Bichler, to singly meet the horror and the damage done by the manufacturers' race to the market. According to Mr. Beatie (in his summation), the defendant's expert, Dr. Wilson, said that the human is the best test animal. If this is so, then the human being who was used is entitled to her compensation.

Remedies

Judge Jack B. Weinstein provided an additional form of closure for DES sons and daughters whose cases were heard in his courtroom. After the conclusion of their cases, Judge Weinstein listened to the DES daughters and sons. He spoke with them and provided plaintiffs with an official transcript of their story. One client of mine, a pharmacist and DES son, told me that after his conference with Judge Weinstein, he did not need to go to therapy anymore. He was done, he had closure.

The Emergency Fund

In 1996, I brought a class action lawsuit[30] against the pharmaceutical companies to establish a court-supervised program funded by all the pharmaceutical companies that manufactured DES. As a result, a fund managed by the Special Master was established to pay in whole or part for the costs incurred by those suffering from DES exposure including, but not limited to: increased costs of DES-related medical expenses not reimbursed by insurance policies, the denial of insurance coverage due to DES-related conditions, or the payment of higher insurance rates due to DES-related "pre-existing" conditions; increased costs of raising children born to Plaintiffs prematurely as a result of Plaintiffs' DES exposure; costs of adopting children due to infertility resulting from DES exposure; psychological counseling to alleviate the emotional distress imposed by Plaintiffs' knowledge of her DES exposure and its consequences; maintenance and expansion of support groups to share concerns and vital DES-related information as well as to alleviate their emotional distress; maintenance and expansion of networks to share vital medical information about the dangers and harms caused by DES exposure; ongoing research into the dangers of DES and the harms caused by exposure to it; a DES education and outreach campaign directed at health professionals; and a DES education and outreach campaign aimed at the general public.

There is no way to put a dollar amount on the injuries caused by DES, which range from infertility to death. No court will charge a jury with instructions that punitive damages may be awarded. This is the only way that these wrongdoers would be adequately punished for their corporate misconduct. Contrary to Lilly's claim that if the *Bichler* verdict was allowed to stand, the bloom would be off the pharmaceutical industry, the industry continues its enormous profit margin even today. The litigation has helped the women, but unfortunately, it has not hurt the industry.

CONTINUED HEALTH CONCERNS: DES TODAY AND TOMORROW

Today, wrongs continue to occur as a result of the DES catastrophe. For example, many DES daughters and sons have developed various forms of cancer as a result of their exposure to DES. In addition, numerous DES-exposed daughters and sons remain infertile as a result of their DES exposure. An increase in the amount of research, supported by government funding, has uncovered new developments with regard to DES. Recent studies link in utero DES exposure to breast cancer, endometriosis, paraovarian cysts, mucinous cancer, and uterine fibroids. Furthermore, since 2002, studies have linked DES to breast cancer. A study published in June 2000, conducted at the Netherlands Cancer Institute, analyzed questions answered by the 5,421 DES daughters. Overall, the study determined that DES daughters had an increased risk of breast cancer of 40 percent, but for those women over the age of forty, the increased risk was 250 percent.[31]

In addition, DES daughters are at risk for endometriosis. Endometriosis is a painful, chronic disease occurring when the endometrial tissue is found outside the uterus.[32] The misplaced tissue develops into growths or lesions that respond to the menstrual cycle in the same way that the tissue of the uterine lining does. As a result, internal bleeding and inflammation may occur, which can cause pain and infertility.[33]

The Nurses Health Study II, which is a collection of data from September 1989 to June 1, 1999, found that the rate of endometriosis was 80 percent greater among women exposed to DES in utero compared with unexposed women.[34]

DES exposure is associated with paraovarian cysts. Paraovarian cysts are non-cancerous fluid-filled sacks, adjacent to but not part of the ovary.[35] According to the American Society for Investigative Pathology, in comparing a human with a mouse model, six women exposed prenatally to DES had paraovarian cysts during routine gynecological surgery. Four of the twenty-five unexposed and eight of the nine exposed women who were undergoing infertility surgery had paraovarian cysts.[36]

According to the *Journal of Gynecological Oncology*, the association of in utero DES exposure and the development of clear cell adenocarcinoma of the vagina and the cervix has been well established. Recently, however, in addition to these well-known DES related injuries, there have been cases of non-clear-cell mucinous adenocarcinoma in women having a history of DES exposure.[37]

Uterine leimyomata, commonly referred to as fibroids, are benign tumors that can cause pain, bleeding, infertility, and pregnancy complications. In adult mice, exposure to DES causes uterine fibroids.[38] The National Institute of Environmental Health Sciences Uterine Fibroid Study, designed to estimate uterine fibroid prevalence, found that there is an increased risk of uterine fibroids in women prenatally exposed to DES, and that DES-exposed women tended to have larger fibroids than did unexposed women.[39] According to the researchers of this study, uterine fibroids should be added to the list of long-term health problems experienced by DES daughters.

It must be remembered that women and women's groups have been at the forefront of DES advocacy throughout the history of this litigation. The first epidemiological study of the effects of DES was conducted by a group of women in 1969, sitting together in Dr. Herbst's office, trying to uncover why their young daughters had clear cell adenocarcinoma by questioning each other to see what they had in common. These women realized that their ingestion of DES during pregnancy was the commonality. Women's groups such as DES Action and the National Women's Health Network were essential to the advocacy process. They picketed the courthouse, gave out leaflets, marched, spoke to the media, and some even filed briefs with the court in support of plaintiffs such as Joyce Bichler.

I recall my first acquaintance with DES Action was at Fran Fishbane's kitchen table. Under the leadership of Pat Cody, it has become a worldwide organization that acquaints women with the effects of DES and has forced the government to fund further research. Clients have come from England, Spain, Scotland, France, and Italy, among other countries, as a result of their efforts. A recent clear cell cancer client was exposed in 1977 in England, well after the drug was taken off the market in the United States. Unfortunately, there is still DES litigation: both individual cases and a medical monitoring class action brought on behalf of DES daughters for their increased risk of breast cancer. It is believed that DES litigation will last until 2011, forty years after it was taken off the market by the FDA.

NOTES

1. Bichler Record on Appeal, 1608.
2. *Bichler v. Eli Lilly & Co.*, 436 NE2d. 182 (NY 1982), *State of New York Court of Appeals Brief for Plaintiff-Respondent*, 22–23.
3. A. L. Herbst, H. Ulfeder, and D. C. Poskanzer, "Adenocarcinoma of the Vagina: Association of Maternal Stilbestrol Therapy with Tumor Appearance in Young Women," *New England Journal of Medicine* 284, no. 15 (1971): 878–81; United States Department of Health, Education, and Welfare, "Certain Estrogens for Oral or Parental Use," *Federal Register* 16 (November 10, 1971): 217; International Agency for Research on Cancer, *Monograph on the Evaluation of Carcinogenic Risk of Chemicals to Man—Sex Hormones* 4 (n.p.: Lyon, 1974).
4. "Prenatal DES Exposure: Recommendations of the DESAD Project", US HEW, *National Institutes of Health Publication* (March 1981): 81–2049.
5. Bichler Record on Appeal, 2031.
6. Bichler Record on Appeal, 8111.
7. *Bichler v. Eli Lilly Co.*, Ex. 31, 6984 of Appellate Division record.
8. Bichler Record on Appeal, A776.
9. Bichler Record on Appeal, 6212.
10. See W. J. Dieckmann, M. E. Davis, L. M. Rynkiewicz, and R. E. Pottinger, "Does the administration of diethylstilbestrol during pregnancy have therapeutic value?" *American Journal of Obstetrics and Gynecology* 66, no. 5 (November 1953): 1062–81.
11. See *Mink v. University of Chicago*, 460 F. Supp. 713 (1978). As early as 1961 Lilly's records indicate, "It must be admitted that other studies fail to confirm the effectiveness of DES in accidents of pregnancies." Bichler Record on Appeal, 4892.
12. See *FDC Report* 23, no. 12 (March 20, 1961): 23.
13. In the matter of New York County DES Litigation, *Helmrich v. Eli Lilly*, 195 AD2d 415, 601 NYS2d 796 (1st Dept. 1993).
14. Bichler Record on Appeal, 4892.
15. 366 F2d 177, 179 (7th Cir. 1966).
16. *Physician's Desk Reference* (1967): 750.
17. Herbst et al., "Adenocarcinoma of the vagina. Association of maternal stilbestrol therapy with tumor appearance in young women," 878–81.
18. If the brakes fail on your Ford car, it is recalled as defective. DES, on the other hand, continued to be marketed to pregnant women.
19. With the help of DES Action, the White Lung Association, and the New York Public Interest Research Group, after five years the legislature passed a general "tort reform" package, encompassing the discovery rule and the "Revival Statute." Susan Helmrich's case was the first to be filed under the statute.
20. Furthermore, in many cases, although a DES mother may have told her exposed daughter or son that she or he had been exposed, the details were unclear because of the mother's faulty memory or guilt associated with her decision to ingest the drug.
21. See *Fleishman v. Eli Lilly & Co.*, NY2d 888, Cert. denied 459 US 1192.
22. Concert of action theory holds that those who act together, or in concert, are jointly and severally liable for any damages that occur. Where DES had been involved, drug companies that had collaborated in the manufacture, market, and sales of DES were each responsible for every woman injured, even if they did not produce the specific DES to which she was exposed.
23. J. Kasoff, "*Fleishman v. Lilly & Co.*," *New York Law Journal* 121 (December 24, 1981), 15.
24. When Charles Dodds synthesized DES in 1938, he did so pursuant to a grant, the provisions of which barred him from patenting the drug. Consequently, any interested drug manufacturer was free to replicate the drug's formula and submit an application to the FDA to manufacture and sell DES. This resulted in a large number of DES manufacturers who did manufacture the drug and thus could be held liable.
25. Robert Meyers, *D.E.S., the Bitter Pill* (New York: Seaview/Putnam, 1983), quoted in Anita Bernstein, "*Hymowitz v. Eli Lilly and Co.: Markets of Mothers*," in Robert L. Rabin and Stephen D. Sugarman, eds., *Torts Stories* (New York: Foundation Press, 2003), 151–78.
26. While most of the highest courts of the states have remained silent on the issues in DES litigation, a few of the highest state courts and the New York Court of Appeals have issued rulings in addition to the Bichler decision, e.g., *Smith v. Eli Lilly & Co., et al.*, 137 Ill. 2d 222, 560 NE2d 324 (1990); *Collins, et al. v. Eli Lilly & Co., et al.*, 116 Wis. 2d 166, 342 NW2d 37 (1984); *Pardey v. Abbott Laboratories, et al.*, 988 F2d 1217 (US App. 1993); *Martin v. Abbott Laboratories, et al.*, 102 Wn 2d 581, 689 P2d 368 (Wash. 1984).
27. Mr. Willing, coincidentally, was represented by Eli Lilly's counsel. Mrs. Bichler got up in front of Mr. Willing at the trial and Lilly's counsel asked Mr. Willing if he recognized Joyce's mother. He said he never saw her before, when in fact, the Bichlers lived across the street and brought all their prescriptions in his pharmacy.
28. Page 13, appellant's brief.
29. In 1980, Joyce Bichler started a registry for DES daughters through the National Women's Health Network.
30. See *Abbaticchio, et al. v. Abbott Laboratories, et al.* Clients have this fund for adoption, surgery, colostomy bags, and many of the tragedies that befall DES daughters and sons.

31. Evelyn Pringle, "DES Miscarriage Drug Linked to More Cancer," *Lawyers and Settlements: Justice for Everyone* (August 20, 2006), http://www.lawyersandsettlements.com/articles/DES_Miscarriage_Cancer.html (accessed November 13, 2006).

32. DES Action UK, "DES Daughters at Increased Risk for Endometriosis," *Newsletter* 25 (November 2005).

33. Ibid.

34. Stacey Missmer, "In Utero Exposures and the Incidence of Endometriosis," *Fertility and Sterility* 82, no. 6 (December 2004).

35. *DES Action Annual Report 2005*, www.desaction.org/pdfs/2005%20Annual%20Report.pdf.

36. DES Action UK "DES Exposure Positively Associated with Paraovarian Cysts," *Newsletter 25* (November 2005).

37. Leslie R. DeMars, MD, Linda Van Le, MD, Irving Huang, MD, and Wesley C. Fowler, MD, "Primary Non-Clear-Cell Adenocarcinomas of the Vagina in Older DES-Exposed Women," *Gynecologic Oncology* 58 no. 3 (September 1995).

38. Donna Baird and Retha Newbold, "Prenatal Diethylstilbestrol (DES) Exposure is Associated with Uterine Leiomyoma Development," *Reproductive Toxicology* 20, no. 1 (May–June 2005): 81–4.

39. Ibid.

CHAPTER 3

Birth Control

ACCESS TO BIRTH CONTROL is one issue in women's lives that has changed completely in the last one hundred years. Where women were once limited by social stigma, laws that limited access, and science that hadn't developed efficient methodology for preventing pregnancy, now we are inundated with options.

Scholar and medical historian Andrea Tone has demonstrated that women always had birth control devices—including IUD's, vaginal pessaries, douching syringes, suppositories, foaming tablets, and sponges. However, access and social attitudes had yet to change enough to let birth control go "mainstream."

Birth control is also a topic that demonstrates how complex the concerns of the women's health movement can be. When Margaret Sanger's protégé, Dr. Gregory Pincus, set out to develop oral contraceptives in the early 1950s, he faced some daunting obstacles. The first was scientific—although women had been taking estrogen to treat menopausal symptoms for over a decade, and tests of the drug in the 1930s showed that it would suppress ovulation in rabbits, scientists (outside Nazi Germany) had always considered it unethical to perform human trials. Another problem was cultural—would the notoriously sex-wary American public be ready for such a drug? A final problem—one that to my mind has never really been resolved—had to do with safety. Even if such a pill could be made efficacious, how could serious and even fatal side effects be prevented?

Pincus's trial of the drug on women in Puerto Rico yielded some troubling results: The majority dropped out and three (who were never autopsied) died. How much Pincus himself wavered is evident in his papers, now available at the Library of Congress. They comprise approximately 44,000 items on 85.2 feet of shelf space and reveal an awesome scientific and entrepreneurial brinkmanship, making one wonder why Pincus didn't burn the evidence. Among the questionable aspects of the trial: the "control" group was falsified using files from women who had dropped out when the drug was still significantly different in chemical makeup than the pill that hit the market in 1960.

Many women saw the approval of the pill as a great step forward for women, and in some ways it was. Certainly it provided a serious option for women who wanted to be sexually active but for a variety of reasons didn't want to have babies. However, as a young journalist in the early '60s, I began to receive letters from readers who shared stories that were alternately terrifying and heartbreaking. Side effects ranged from the inconvenient—hair loss, weight gain, mood swings—to the deadly—blood clots in women too young for such problems. I was sufficiently scared about the pill to write my first book, *The Doctors' Case Against the Pill*, as a warning to women everywhere.

The book prompted senate hearings about the safety of the drug. It was there that I witnessed the most amazing display of activism I have seen in my now nearly fifty-year career. A group of young women from Washington D.C. Women's Liberation—all veterans of the antiwar, civil rights, and student movements—disrupted the hearings, asking questions like "Why isn't there a pill for men?" and "Why are ten million women being used as guinea pigs?" The group, led by a young Barnard graduate named Alice Wolfson, was taken out of the hearing, but continued its protests. The TV cameras were there, and soon their message was traveling around the world. Eventually the hearings led to patient package inserts in the pill—the first such consumer warning.

The pill is much safer now than it was. It should be: it has one-tenth the hormones. Still, safety questions persist, particularly around new delivery systems. The disaster of Norplant in the 1990s—within ten years the method went from new pharmaceutical darling to being pulled from the market for safety concerns—shows the danger of being the first kid on the block to try a method that has yet to be tested by time. In the end, while women seemingly have more options, the truth is that most of the new "breakthroughs" are all reconfig-

urations of the original estrogen and progestin or progestin-only methods. And as far as I'm concerned, the jury is still out on the relationship of the pill to breast cancer and high blood pressure, and we are only beginning to learn about some of its potentially dangerous interactions with other common drugs, like some antidepressants. In the end, there is still much activism to be done for birth control—making sure it stays safe and continuing to search for safer and even nonpharmaceutical alternatives.

In the Matter of Rosemarie Lewis: Women and the Corporatization of Contraception

ANDREA TONE

Andrea Tone, excerpt from *Devices and Desires: A History of Contraceptives in America*, New York: Hill & Wang, 2001. Reprinted by permission.

In the late 1930s, the Federal Trade Commission (FTC) began to crack down on the over-the-counter contraceptive trade, issuing dozens of cease-and-desist orders to manufacturers. The FTC's actions, designed to stop misleading advertising claims and to promote fair commerce, did much to promote consumers' contraceptive health. But the regulatory assault occurred at the expense of small-business people, who had neither the financial muscle nor the political clout to repel it. Theirs was not always the best birth control available, but it was often no worse than what large firms and "ethical" outfits made.

One businessperson adversely affected was Rosemarie Lewis, the founder and president of Certane Company, a Los Angeles firm that specialized in contraceptives for women. Her tale is not the usual subject of pharmaceutical history, which has favored captains of industry over those who failed or just made do. Yet it is precisely what Lewis lost rather than what she gained that reveals the dynamics of the birth control business in an era of flux. Behind the seemingly faceless forces of regulation, technological innovation, and modernization, women and men fought to hold on to their livelihoods during an era of profound social, political, and industrial transformation.

Lewis's story begins in Los Angeles. The city was home to 1.2 million people when Lewis founded Lewis Laboratories in the fall of 1929 and began selling tubes of contraceptive jelly.[1] The move was bold and potentially risky. California law frowned on medical quackery, and its restrictions on birth control and abortion, passed in 1874 and not revised until 1931, were among the toughest in the country. Merely advertising contraceptives was a felony.

But paper laws were no match for the droves of lay health practitioners who called LA home. In this mecca of proselytism, Lewis set up shop, upholding a long tradition of female contraceptive entrepreneurship. The 1873 Comstock Act, which banned the distribution and manufacture of contraceptives, had nurtured a rich entrepreneurial culture in bootleg birth control. Women, especially immigrants, Jews, and other minorities, had been central to its operation. In an economic milieu that restricted opportunities for female entrepreneurship and branded businesswomen deviant, the contraceptive business (like prostitution and abortion, two kindred illicit trades) was more welcoming of female proprietors than other commercial enterprises. Lewis was her own breadwinner. Recently divorced, she remained friends with her ex-husband and, in 1934, entrusted him with the management of a branch office she opened in Chicago. The business was her doing, her initiative. She had never run one before. But in late 1929 the Depression had begun, and like so many other single women, she needed a job to survive.[2]

Lewis was one of hundreds of newcomers to the contraceptive business. The economics of austerity attracted small-business people to the industry where, as *Fortune* magazine put it, they "discovered that birth control products could be produced at a quick and enormous profit with very little capital investment."[3] Of the four hundred known businesses making female contraceptives in 1938, most were founded in the early Depression. Aided by a local chemist, Lewis began manufacturing antiseptic jellies and powders. She had no formal schooling but was not uneducated. "I get a lot of different books and read up and try to be intelligent about it," she told the FTC.[4] In 1930, she renamed her business, of which she remained sole owner, the Certane Company—a good name for a firm that pledged to put women's minds at ease about pregnancy prevention.

By 1935, Certane had added suppositories, douching syringes, a one-size cervical cap, and diaphragms of varying sizes to its product list. The company made douching powder and jelly at its LA headquarters and diaphragms in its Chicago office. The Certane diaphragm—retailed as the Dia-Dome—came in sizes 47.5 to 100 millimeters. "We have a form and a mold for each," Charles Luntz, the company manager, explained, "and that form is dipped into liquid latex."[5] Other products were manufactured through outsourcing and then repackaged. Vaginal cones came from a local drug compounder, cervical caps from an LA rubber company. B. F. Goodrich made the rubber tubing on the douche shields, Kensington Glass Works the glass applicators used with the douching powders, and the Seamless Rubber Company of New Haven, Connecticut, the rubber bulb that attached to the glass applicators.[6]

By the time the FTC investigated Certane in 1938, Lewis had carved out a birth control empire whose annual sales were between fifty-five thousand and sixty thousand dollars (at a time when few women earned over five thousand dollars).[7] Her company was not the leading distributor of feminine hygiene products and rubber pessaries, but it was probably among the top twenty. Lewis herself felt she had made it to the big leagues. She identified her primary competitors as Lanteen, Johnson & Johnson, and Holland-Rantos, not the smaller outfits that, according to one Planned Parenthood report, were plentiful and "buzzing [around] like bees."[8]

FTC records do not identify who filed a complaint against Certane. The FTC was established in 1914 by an act of Congress to promote competitive interstate commerce by investigating persons, partnerships, or corporations accused of practicing "unfair methods of competition," such as false or misleading advertising. Businesses the FTC determined to be in violation of the act were issued cease-and-desist orders.[9] In theory, the FTC promoted fair play and restored competition to an economy increasingly marked by concentrated power. In practice, it often functioned as corporate capitalism's handmaiden, censoring the practices of smaller businesses that established firms considered threats.[10]

The FTC did not subject contraceptive companies to investigation until after the 1936 ruling *United States v. One Package* permitted doctors in every state (unless forbidden by local laws) to acquire contraceptive information and articles through the mail. *One Package* exempted physicians from prosecution and asserted the legality of contraceptive commerce operated by and for doctors. The decision liberated the birth control business from its most oppressive legal shackles even as it excluded nonmedical professionals, like Lewis, from participation.[11]

The FTC complaint against Lewis charged her with circulating advertisements that were "false and misleading and in truth and in fact said products do not form or constitute safe and competent remedies against contraception and are not a guarantee against pregnancy." If Certane's products were found to be ineffective, the company was competing unfairly against those who made reliable birth control.[12]

Lewis denied the charges. The FTC hearing began on November 18, 1938, in a hotel in downtown Los Angeles. The commission called to testify three expert witnesses, "three of the most prominent gynecologists and obstetricians on the West Coast," each of whom disputed the safety and reliability of Lewis's products. One physician, discussing the Certane douche, warned that "if not accompanied by proper instructions and properly handled [it] would be a very dangerous instrument to place in the hands of a woman." He condemned Certane's diaphragms and refuted the company's assurances of pregnancy prevention by insisting that "there is no guarantee of any description against pregnancy except absolute continence from intercourse."[13] He failed to mention that doctor-recommended douches and contraceptives were a common, albeit not universally endorsed, facet of American medical practice.

Lewis's defense was a familiar one. Her advertising practices, she argued, were identical to those of other, more established firms—she mentioned Holland-Rantos as an example—whose actions went unnoticed. "While I realize that the mere fact that my competitors use certain phrases is not in itself sufficient reason to permit me to use similar phrases or make similar statements," she pleaded, "if I am to remain in competition, you can appreciate how vital it is that I should be granted the same latitude as my competitors."[14]

Lewis was right, but the FTC dismissed her claims as "being entirely without merit" and ordered her to stop "representing . . . that the Certane preparations or appliances . . . are safe, competent, or effective preventatives against contraception."[15] Lewis was not so easily deterred. Complying with the FTC order she edited out references to birth control in Certane's promotional literature. But she continued to sell her products to druggists, jobbers, and mail-order consumers.

It was not enough to save her. In a 1942 case initiated by the US Post Office, she was charged with conducting an unlawful business through the mail. This prosecution was not business as usual. It was personal. By the 1940s, Post Office investigations of contraceptive purveyors had become extremely rare. Moreover, the new charge contradicted the FTC's previous findings that Certane's wares were too ineffective to be considered contraceptives. It was a lose-lose situation: reprimanded for selling products not good enough to be considered birth control, Lewis was now being charged for selling identical products that were.

Because Lewis had revised Certane ads to comply with the FTC's order, Post Office inspectors resorted to cloak-and-dagger techniques to exact even moderately damning evidence. Posing as contraceptive consumers, they sent Lewis thirteen unsolicited letters. All masqueraded as letters from laypersons, signaled by the deliberate and condescending use of ungrammatical language. One letter, allegedly sent from a Van G. Okie, Dampton, Kentucky, read:

> Mom and I gest got back from a visit with our boy Fred what lives on Lawndale Ave. Mebe youse no where that is. Fred married a city girl about 3 yr. ago & they ain't got no childs. Mom turns out one ever year and ever time she says that the last. We got 9 now and 7 at home. Fred is the olest. So I ask Fred how they aint got no childs . . . and [he] shows me all that stuff he got from youse to keep from having children. I don't know offen I can get mom to where that rubber thing but I ken shoot that stuff up her. Youse let me no what it costs, so I can git sum.

Van sent Lewis a money order for a three-dollar Dia-Cap jelly kit and a request:

> if that [kit is] what mom needs to keep her from gittin pregnant youse send it.[16]

Lewis sent Van the kit.

But did that act make Lewis a lawbreaker? Lewis had not called the kit birth control, and as she told those at her hearing, Certane Jelly, the Dia-Cap, and the Dia-Dome were retailed as "pharmaceutical[s] and not for contraception." When asked whether they possessed contraceptive attributes, she referred to the testimony of the FTC's expert witnesses to assert her innocence. "According to the FTC [they do] not," she insisted, "and according to their physicians. They had the finest and best in Los Angeles, and they said no."[17]

The Post Office decided otherwise. It suspended Lewis's right to conduct business through the mail. It was a lethal blow. Although Certane products are listed in a 1945 Consumer Union report, no mention of Rosemarie Lewis or the company appears in contraceptive literature after 1950. Like so many other contraceptive entrepreneurs in this age of federal regulation and business consolidation, Lewis just disappeared from the corporate map.

The government continued its campaign against feminine hygiene manufacturers, but the results were mixed. The FDA's insistence that contraceptives were not drugs, and thus not subject to its jurisdiction, left the FTC in charge of regulating contraceptive commerce. But the FTC's authority was limited, confined to the elimination of false and misleading advertising. The regulatory vacuum encouraged companies to resurrect euphemistic language to obfuscate the intended contraceptive use of their products. Punished for daring to label its products birth control, Lewis's business was eclipsed by established firms such as Lehn & Fink, manufacturers of the popular Lysol douche, which profited from keeping women uninformed about how bad a contraceptive the Lysol douche was.[18] For too many women in the 1930s and 1940s, the freedom, pleasure, and security pledged by reputable manufacturers and protected by government regulations amounted to nothing more than empty promises.

NOTES

1. "Pocket Book Los Angeles," *Southern California Business* 16 (November 1937): 21.
2. United States of America before Federal Trade Commission, Docket no. 3846, In the Matter of: Rosemarie Lewis, Trading as Certane Company, et al., Complaint [hereafter *In the Matter of Rosemarie Lewis*], box 2590, Docketed case files 1915–1943, Records of the Federal Trade Commission, RG 122, National Archives.
3. "Accident of Birth," *Fortune* (February 1938): 208.
4. *In the Matter of Rosemarie Lewis*, 9.
5. Ibid., 5–7, 55–56, 86.
6. Ibid., 8–15, 27–28, 34, 36; Commission's Exhibit 2.
7. Ibid., 9, 13, 58–61, 238.

8. Ibid., 10–11; Lewis to Federal Trade Commission, December 9, 1937 (also in FTC Transcript); PPFA 1943 study, 38, Planned Parenthood Federation of America Papers, Sophia Smith Collection.

9. Henry Miller, *Statutes and Decisions Pertaining to the Federal Trade Commission*, 1914–29 (Washington, DC: Government Printing Office, 1930): 1, 5–7.

10. Gabriel Kolko, *The Triumph of Conservatism* (New York: Free Press, 1963).

11. *United States v. One Package*, 13 F. Supp. 334; James Reed, *From Private Vice to Public Virtue: The Birth Control Movement and American Society since 1830* (New York: Basic Books, 1978), 121; Kennedy, *Birth Control in America*, 242–52.

12. *In the Matter of Rosemarie Lewis*, Brief of Counsel for the Commission, 7.

13. *In the Matter of Rosemarie Lewis*, 81–104; Brief of Counsel for the Commission, 6–9.

14. *In the Matter of Rosemarie Lewis*, Exhibit 26A.

15. *In the Matter of Rosemarie Lewis*, Brief of Counsel for the Commission; "Official Actions against the Misrepresentation of Contraceptive Products," *Human Fertility* (June 1941): 90–91.

16. *In the Matter of Charges against Rosemarie Lewis, Charles Luntz, and Max Lewis*, 2–3, 7–31, box 159, Transcripts of Hearings on Fraud Cases, 1913–1945, Records of the Post Office Department.

17. Ibid., 50.

18. Elizabeth H. Garrett, "Birth Control's Business Baby," *New Republic* (January 1934): 270–71; "Accident of Birth," *Fortune*, 108, 110, 112; Dorothy Dunbar Bromley, "Birth Control and the Depression," *Harper's Magazine* (October 1934): 572; Reed, *From Private Vice to Public Virtue*, 114, 244–46; Kennedy, *Birth Control in America*, 183; Rachel Lynn Palmer and Sarah K. Greenberg, *Facts and Frauds in Woman's Hygiene: A Medical Guide Against Misleading Claims and Dangerous Products*, New York: Vanguard Press, 1936, 21–24; Grace Naismith, "The Racket in Contraceptives," *American Mercury* 71 (July 1950): 4, 9.

Racism, Birth Control and Reproductive Rights

ANGELA DAVIS

Angela Davis, adapted from "Racism, Birth Control and Reproductive Rights," in *Women, Race & Class,* New York: Vintage Books, 1983, 202–221. Originally published in 1981 by Random House. Reprinted by permission.

Birth control—individual choice, safe contraceptive methods, as well as abortions when necessary—is a fundamental prerequisite for the emancipation of women. Since the right of birth control is obviously advantageous to women of all classes and races, it would appear that even vastly dissimilar women's groups would have attempted to unite around this issue. In reality, however, the birth control movement has seldom succeeded in uniting women of different social backgrounds, and the movement's leaders have rarely popularized the genuine concerns of working-class women. Moreover, arguments advanced by birth control advocates have sometimes been based on blatantly racist premises. The progressive potential of birth control remains indisputable. But in actuality, the historical record of this movement leaves much to be desired in the realm of challenges to racism and class exploitation.

The most important victory of the contemporary birth control movement was won during the early 1970s, when abortions were at last declared legal. . . . But in 1973 when the US Supreme Court ruled in *Roe v. Wade* (410 US) and *Doe v. Bolton* (410 US) that a woman's right to personal privacy implied her right to decide whether or not to have an abortion, the ranks of the abortion rights campaign did not include substantial numbers of women of color. Given the racial composition of the larger women's liberation movement, this was not at all surprising. When questions were raised about the absence of racially oppressed women, in both the larger movement and in the abortion rights campaign, two explanations were commonly proposed: women of color were overburdened by their people's fight against racism; and/or they had not yet become conscious of the centrality of sexism. But the real meaning of the almost lily-white complexion of the abortion rights campaign was not to be found in an ostensibly myopic or underdeveloped consciousness among women of color. The truth lay buried in the ideological underpinnings of the birth control movement itself.

The failure of the abortion rights campaign to

conduct a historical self-evaluation led to a dangerously superficial appraisal of black people's [generally] suspicious attitudes toward birth control. . . . Granted, when some black people unhesitatingly equated birth control with genocide, it did appear to be an exaggerated, even paranoiac, reaction. Yet white abortion rights activists missed a profound message, for underlying these cries of genocide were important clues about the history of the birth control movement, [which includes] for example, [the advocacy of] . . . involuntary sterilization—a racist form of mass "birth control."

. . . As for the abortion rights campaign itself, . . . women of color [certainly did not] fail to grasp its urgency. They were far more familiar than their white sisters with the murderously clumsy scalpels of inept abortionists seeking profit in illegality. In New York, for instance, during the several years preceding the decriminalization of abortions in that state, some 80 percent of the deaths caused by illegal abortions involved black and Puerto Rican women. Immediately afterward, women of color received close to half of all the legal abortions. . . . When black and latina women resort to abortions in such large numbers, the stories they tell are not so much about their desire to be free of their pregnancy, but rather about the miserable social conditions which dissuade them from bringing new lives into the world. They were in favor of *abortion rights*, which did not mean that they were proponents of abortion, a distinction missed by those within the abortion rights campaign.

Black women have been aborting themselves since the earliest days of slavery. Many slave women refused to bring children into a world of interminable forced labor, where chains and floggings and sexual abuse for women were the everyday conditions of life. A doctor practicing in Georgia around the middle of the last century noticed that abortions and miscarriages were far more common among his slave patients than among the white women he treated. According to the physician, either black women worked too hard, or

. . . As the planters believe, the blacks are

possessed of a secret by which they destroy the fetus at an early stage of gestation. . . . All country practitioners are aware of the frequent complaints of planters (about the) . . . unnatural tendency in the African female to destroy her offspring.[1]

Expressing shock that ". . . whole families of women fail to have any children,"[2] this doctor never considered how "unnatural" it was to raise children under the slave system. The [position taken by] Margaret Garner, a fugitive slave who killed her own daughter and attempted suicide herself when she was captured by slave catchers, is a case in point:

> She rejoiced that the girl was dead—"now she would never know what a woman suffers as a slave"—and pleaded to be tried for murder. "I will go singing to the gallows rather than be returned to slavery!"[3]

Why were self-imposed abortions and reluctant acts of infanticide such common occurrences during slavery? Not because black women had discovered solutions to their predicament, but rather because abortions and infanticides were acts of desperation, motivated not by the biological birth process but by the oppressive conditions of slavery. Most of these women, no doubt, would have expressed their deepest resentment had someone hailed their abortions as a stepping stone toward freedom.

During the early abortion rights campaign it was too frequently assumed that legal abortions provided a viable alternative to the myriad problems posed by poverty, as if having fewer children could create more jobs, higher wages, better schools, etc., etc. This assumption reflected the tendency to blur the distinction between *abortion rights* and the general advocacy of *abortions*. The campaign often failed to provide a voice for women who wanted the *right* to legal abortions while deploring the social conditions that prohibited them from bearing more children.

. . . It was not until the issue of women's rights

in general became the focus of an organized movement that reproductive rights . . . emerge[d] as a legitimate demand. In an essay entitled "Marriage," written during the 1850s, Sarah Grimke argued for a ". . . right on the part of a woman to decide when she shall become a mother, how often and under what circumstances." But, as she insists, "the right to decide this matter has been almost wholly denied to women."[4]

. . . Grimke advocated women's right to sexual abstinence. Around the same time the well-known "emancipated marriage" of Lucy Stone and Henry Blackwell took place. These abolitionists and women's rights activists were married in a ceremony that protested women's traditional relinquishment of their rights to their persons, names, and property. In agreeing that as husband, he had no right to the "custody of the wife's person," Blackwell promised that he would not attempt to impose the dictates of his sexual desires upon his wife.

The notion that women could refuse to submit to their husbands' sexual demands eventually became the central idea of the call for "voluntary motherhood." By the 1870s, when the woman suffrage movement had reached its peak, feminists were publicly advocating voluntary motherhood. . . . It was not a coincidence that women's consciousness of their reproductive rights was born within the organized movement for women's political equality. Indeed, if women remained forever burdened by incessant childbirths and frequent miscarriages, they would hardly be able to exercise the political rights they might win. Moreover, women's new dreams of pursuing careers and other paths of self-development outside marriage and motherhood could only be realized if they could limit and plan their pregnancies.

In this sense, the slogan "voluntary motherhood" contained a new and genuinely progressive vision of womanhood. At the same time, however, this vision was rigidly bound to the lifestyle enjoyed by the middle classes and the bourgeoisie. The aspirations underlying the demand for "voluntary motherhood" did not reflect the conditions of working-class women, engaged as they were in a far more fundamental fight for economic survival. Since this first call for birth control was associated with goals that could only be achieved by women possessing material wealth, vast numbers of poor and working-class women would find it rather difficult to identify with the embryonic birth control movement.

Toward the end of the nineteenth century the white birth rate in the United States suffered a significant decline. Since no contraceptive innovations had been publicly introduced, the drop in the birth rate implied that women were substantially curtailing their sexual activity. By 1890 the typical native-born white woman was bearing no more than four children. Since US society was becoming increasingly urban, this new birth pattern should not have been a surprise. While farm life demanded large families, they became dysfunctional within the context of city life. Yet this phenomenon was publicly interpreted in a racist and anti-working-class fashion by the ideologues of rising monopoly capitalism. Since native-born white women were bearing fewer children, the specter of "race suicide" was raised in official circles.

In 1905 President Theodore Roosevelt concluded his Lincoln Day Dinner speech with the proclamation that "race purity must be maintained."[5] By 1906 he blatantly equated the falling birth rate among native-born whites with the impending threat of "race suicide." In his State of the Union message that year, Roosevelt admonished the well-born white women who engaged in "willful sterility—the one sin for which the penalty is national death, race suicide."[6] These comments were made during a period of accelerating racist ideology and of great waves of race riots and lynchings on the domestic scene. Moreover, President Roosevelt himself was attempting to muster support for the US seizure of the Philippines, the country's most recent imperialist venture.

How did the birth control movement respond to Roosevelt's accusation that their cause was promoting race suicide? . . . Linda Gordon maintains that this controversy ". . . brought to the forefront those issues that most separated feminists from the working class and the poor."[7]

. . . In the context of the whole feminist movement, the race suicide episode was an additional factor identifying feminism almost exclusively with the aspirations of the more privileged women of the society. First, the feminists were increasingly emphasizing birth control as a route to careers and higher education—goals out of reach of the poor with or without birth control. Second, the pro–birth control feminists began to popularize the idea that poor people had a moral obligation to restrict the size of their families, because large families create a drain on the taxes and charity expenditures of the wealthy and because poor children were less likely to be "superior."

The acceptance of the race suicide thesis, to a greater or lesser extent, by women such as Julia Ward Howe and Ida Husted Harper reflected the suffrage movement's capitulation to the racist posture of Southern women. If the suffragists acquiesced to arguments invoking the extension of the ballot to women as the saving grace of white supremacy, then birth control advocates either acquiesced to or supported the new arguments invoking birth control as a means of preventing the proliferation of the "lower classes" and as an antidote to race suicide. Race suicide could be prevented by the introduction of birth control among black people, immigrants, and the poor in general. In this way, the prosperous whites of solid Yankee stock could maintain their superior numbers within the population. Thus class bias and racism crept into the birth control movement when it was still in its infancy. More and more, it was assumed within birth control circles that poor women, black and immigrant alike, had a "moral obligation to restrict the size of their families."[8] What was demanded as a "right" for the privileged came to be interpreted as a "duty" for the poor.

When Margaret Sanger embarked upon her lifelong crusade for birth control—a term she coined and popularized—it appeared as though the racist and anti-working-class overtones of the previous period might be overcome. For Sanger came from a working-class background herself and was well acquainted with the devastating pressures of poverty. When her mother died, at the age of forty-eight, she had borne no less than eleven children. Sanger's later memories of her own family's troubles would confirm her belief that working-class women had a special need for the right to plan and space their pregnancies autonomously. Her affiliation, as an adult, with the socialist movement was a further cause for hope that the birth control campaign would move in a more progressive direction.

When Sanger joined the Socialist Party in 1912, she assumed the responsibility of recruiting women from New York's working women's clubs into the party. *The Call*—the party's paper—carried her articles on the women's page. She wrote a series entitled "What Every Mother Should Know," another called "What Every Girl Should Know," and she did on-the-spot coverage of strikes involving women. Sanger's familiarity with New York's working-class districts was a result of her numerous visits as a trained nurse to the poor sections of the city. During these visits, she points out in her autobiography, she met countless numbers of women who desperately desired knowledge about birth control.

According to Sanger's autobiographical reflections, one of the many visits she made as a nurse to New York's Lower East Side convinced her to undertake a personal crusade for birth control. Answering one of her routine calls, she discovered that twenty-eight-year-old Sadie Sachs had attempted to abort herself. Once the crisis had passed, the young woman asked the attending physician to give her advice on birth prevention. As Sanger relates the story, the doctor recommended that she "tell (her husband) Jake to sleep on the roof."[9]

. . . Three months later Sadie Sachs died from another self-induced abortion. That night, Sanger says, she vowed to devote all her energy toward the acquisition and dissemination of contraceptive measures. . . .

During the first phase of Sanger's birth control crusade, she maintained her affiliation with the Socialist Party—and the campaign itself was closely associated with the rising militancy of the working class. . . . Personally, she continued to march on picket lines with striking workers and publicly condemned the outrageous assaults on striking workers. In 1914, for example, when the National Guard massacred scores of chicano miners in Ludlow, Colorado, Sanger joined the labor movement in exposing John D. Rockefeller's role in this attack.

Unfortunately, the alliance between the birth control campaign and the radical labor movement did not enjoy a long life. While Socialists and other working-class activists continued to support the demand for birth control, it did not occupy a central place in their overall strategy. And Sanger herself began to underestimate the centrality of capitalist exploitation in her analysis of poverty, arguing that too many children caused workers to fall into their miserable predicament. Moreover, "women were inadvertently perpetuating the exploitation of the working class," she believed, "by continually flooding the labor market with new workers."[10] Ironically, Sanger may have been encouraged to adopt this position by the neo-Malthusian ideas embraced in some socialist circles. Such outstanding figures of the European socialist movement as Anatole France and Rosa Luxemburg had proposed a "birth strike" to prevent the continued flow of labor into the capitalist market.

When Margaret Sanger severed her ties with the Socialist Party for the purpose of building an independent birth control campaign, she and her followers became more susceptible than ever before to the anti-black and anti-immigrant propaganda of the times. Like their predecessors, who had been deceived by the "race suicide" propaganda, the advocates of birth control began to embrace the prevailing racist ideology. The fatal influence of the eugenics movement would soon destroy the progressive potential of the birth control campaign. . . .

Eugenic ideas were perfectly suited to the ideological needs of the young monopoly capitalists. Imperialist incursions in Latin America and in the Pacific needed to be justified, as did the intensified exploitation of black workers in the South and immigrant workers in the North and West. The pseudo-scientific racial theories associated with the eugenics campaign furnished dramatic apologies for the conduct of the young monopolies. As a result, this movement won the unhesitating support of such leading capitalists as the Carnegies, the Harrimans, and the Kelloggs.

By 1919 the eugenic influence on the birth control movement was unmistakably clear. In an article published by Margaret Sanger in the American Birth Control League's journal, she defined "the chief issue of birth control" as "more children from the fit, less from the unfit."[11] Around this time the ABCL offered Lothrop Stoddard, Harvard professor and the author of *The Rising Tide of Color Against White World Supremacy*, a seat on [its] board of directors. In the pages of the ABCL's journal, articles by Guy Irving Birch, director of the American Eugenics Society, began to appear. Birch advocated birth control as a weapon to "prevent the American people from being replaced by alien or Negro stock, whether it be by immigration or by overly high birth rates among others in this country."[12]

By 1932 the Eugenics Society could boast that at least twenty-six states had passed compulsory sterilization laws and that thousands of "unfit" persons had already been surgically prevented from reproducing. Margaret Sanger offered her public approval of this development. "Morons, mental defectives, epileptics, illiterates, paupers, unemployables, criminals, prostitutes, and dope fiends," ought to be surgically sterilized, she argued in a radio talk.[13] She did not wish to be so intransigent as to leave them with no choice in the matter; if they wished, she said, they should be able to choose a lifelong segregated existence in labor camps.

Within the American Birth Control League, the call for birth control among black people acquired the same racist edge as the call for compulsory sterilization. In 1939 its successor, the Birth Control Federation of America, planned a "Negro project." In the federation's words,

> The mass of Negroes, particularly in the South, still breed carelessly and disastrously, with the result that the increase among Negroes, even more than among whites, is from that portion of the population least fit, and least able, to rear children properly.[14]

Calling for the recruitment of black ministers to lead local birth control committees. . . . Margaret Sanger wrote in a letter to a colleague, "We do not want word to get out,"

> . . . that we want to exterminate the Negro population and the minister is the man who can straighten out that idea if it ever occurs to any of their more rebellious members.[15]

This episode in the birth control movement confirmed the ideological victory of the racism associated with eugenic ideas. It had been robbed of its progressive potential, advocating for people of color not the individual right to *birth control,* but rather the racist strategy of *population control.* The birth control campaign would be called upon to serve in an essential capacity in the execution of the US government's imperialist and racist population policy.

The abortion rights activists of the early 1970s should have examined the history of their movement. Had they done so, they might have understood why so many of their black sisters adopted a posture of suspicion toward their cause. They might have understood how important it was to undo the racist deeds of their predecessors, who had advocated

birth control as well as compulsory sterilization as a means of eliminating the "unfit" sectors of the population. Consequently, the young white feminists might have been more receptive to the suggestion that their campaign for abortion rights include a vigorous condemnation of sterilization abuse, which had become more widespread than ever.

It was not until the media decided that the casual sterilization of two black girls in Montgomery, Alabama, was a scandal worth reporting that the Pandora's box of sterilization abuse was finally flung open. But by the time the case of the Relf sisters broke, it was practically too late to influence the politics of the abortion rights movement. It was the summer of 1973 and the Supreme Court decision legalizing abortions had already been announced in January. Nevertheless, the urgent need for mass opposition to sterilization abuse became tragically clear. The facts surrounding the Relf sisters' story were horrifyingly simple. Minnie Lee, who was twelve years old, and Mary Alice, who was 14, had been unsuspectingly carted into an operating room, where surgeons irrevocably robbed them of their capacity to bear children. The surgery had been ordered by the Health, Education, and Welfare (HEW)–funded Montgomery Community Action Committee after it was discovered that Depo-Provera, a drug previously administered to the girls as a birth prevention measure, caused cancer in test animals.

After the Southern Poverty Law Center filed suit on behalf of the Relf sisters, the girls' mother revealed that she had unknowingly "consented" to the operation, having been deceived by the social workers that handled her daughters' case. They had asked Mrs. Relf, who was unable to read, to put her "X" on a document, the contents of which were not described to her. She assumed, she said, that it authorized the continued Depo-Provera injections. As she subsequently learned, she had authorized the surgical sterilization of her daughters.

In the aftermath of the publicity exposing the Relf sisters' case, similar episodes were brought to light. In Montgomery alone, eleven girls, also in their teens, had been similarly sterilized. HEW-funded birth control clinics in other states, as it turned out, had also subjected young girls to sterilization abuse. Moreover, individual women came forth with equally outrageous stories. Nial Ruth Cox, for example, filed suit against the state of North Carolina. At the age of eighteen—eight years before the suit—officials had threatened to discontinue her family's welfare payments if she refused to submit to surgical sterilization. Before she assented to the operation, she was assured that her infertility would be temporary.

Nial Ruth Cox's lawsuit was aimed at a state that had diligently practiced the theory of eugenics. Under the auspices of the Eugenics Commission of North Carolina, 7,686 sterilizations had been carried out since 1933. Although the operations were justified as measures to prevent the reproduction of "mentally deficient persons," about 5,000 of the sterilized persons had been black.

. . . As the flurry of publicity exposing sterilization abuse revealed, the neighboring state of South Carolina had been the site of further atrocities. Eighteen women from Aiken, South Carolina, charged that a Dr. Clovis Pierce had sterilized them during the early 1970s. The sole obstetrician in that small town, Pierce had consistently sterilized Medicaid recipients with two or more children. According to a nurse in his office, Dr. Pierce insisted that pregnant welfare women "will have to submit (sic) to voluntary sterilization,"[16] if they wanted him to deliver their babies. While he was ". . . tired of people running around and having babies and paying for them with my taxes,"[17] Dr. Pierce received some $60,000 in taxpayers' money for the sterilizations he performed. During his trial he was supported by the South Carolina Medical Association, whose members declared that doctors ". . . have a moral and legal right to insist on sterilization permission before accepting a patient, if it is done on the initial visit."[18]

Revelations of sterilization abuse during that time exposed the complicity of the federal government. At first the Department of Health, Education, and Welfare claimed that approximately 16,000 women and 8,000 men had been sterilized in 1972 under the auspices of federal programs. Later, however, these figures underwent a drastic revision. Carl Shultz, director of HEW's Population Affairs Office, estimated that between 100,000 and 200,000 sterilizations had actually been funded that year by the federal government. During Hitler's Germany, incidentally, 250,000 sterilizations were carried out under the Nazis' Hereditary Health Law. Is it possible that the record of the Nazis, throughout the years of their reign, may have been almost equaled by the US government-funded sterilizations in the space of a single year?

Given the historical genocide inflicted on the native population of the United States, one would assume that Native American Indians would be exempted from the government's sterilization campaign. But according to Dr. Connie Uri's testimony in the Senate committee hearing, by 1976 some 24 percent of all Indian women of childbearing age had been sterilized. "Our blood lines are being stopped," the Choctaw physician told the Senate committee, "our unborn will not be born. . . . This is genocidal to our people."[19] According to Dr. Uri, the Indian Health Services Hospital in Claremore, Oklahoma, had been sterilizing one out of every four women giving birth in that federal facility.

. . . The domestic population policy of the US government has an undeniably racist edge. Native American, Chicana, Puerto Rican, and black women continue to be sterilized in disproportionate numbers. According to a national fertility study conducted in 1970 by Princeton University's Office of Population Control, 20 percent of all married black women have been permanently sterilized. Approximately the same percentage of Chicana women had been rendered surgically infertile. Moreover, 43 percent of the women sterilized through federally subsidized programs were black.

The astonishing number of Puerto Rican women who have been sterilized reflects a special government policy that can be traced back to 1939. In that year President Roosevelt's Interdepartmental

Committee on Puerto Rico issued a statement attributing the island's economic problems to the phenomenon of overpopulation. This committee proposed that efforts be undertaken to reduce the birth rate to no more than the level of the death rate. Soon afterward an experimental sterilization campaign was undertaken in Puerto Rico. Although the Catholic Church initially opposed this experiment and forced the cessation of the program in 1946, it was converted during the early 1950s to the teachings and practice of population control. In this period over 150 birth control clinics were opened, resulting in a 20 percent decline in population growth by the mid-1960s. By the 1970s, over 35 percent of all Puerto Rican women of childbearing age had been surgically sterilized.

. . . During the 1970s, the devastating implications of the Puerto Rican experiment began to emerge with unmistakable clarity. In Puerto Rico the presence of corporations in the highly automated metallurgical and pharmaceutical industries had exacerbated the problem of unemployment. The prospect of an ever-larger army of unemployed workers was one of the main incentives for the mass sterilization program. Inside the United States today, enormous numbers of people of color—and especially racially oppressed youth—have become part of a pool of permanently unemployed workers. It is hardly coincidental, considering the Puerto Rican example, that the increasing incidence of sterilization has kept pace with the high rates of unemployment. As growing numbers of white people suffer the brutal consequences of unemployment, they can also expect to become targets of the official sterilization propaganda.

. . . The 1977 Hyde Amendment has added yet another dimension to coercive sterilization practices. As a result of this law passed by Congress, federal funds for abortions were eliminated in all cases but those involving rape and the risk of death or severe illness, and many state legislatures followed suit. Black, Puerto Rican, Chicana, and Native American Indian women, together with their impoverished white sisters, were thus effectively divested of the right to legal abortions. Since surgical sterilizations, funded by the Department of Health, Education, and Welfare, remained free on demand, more and more poor women have been forced to opt for permanent infertility. According to Sandra Salazar of the California Department of Public Health, the first victim of the Hyde Amendment was a twenty-seven-year-old Chicana woman from Texas. She died as a result of an illegal abortion in Mexico shortly after Texas discontinued government-funded abortions. There have been many more victims—women for whom sterilization has become the only alternative to abortions, which are currently beyond their reach.

. . . Over the last decade the struggle against sterilization abuse has been waged primarily by Puerto Rican, black, Chicana, and Native American women. Their cause has not yet been embraced by the women's movement as a whole. Within organizations representing the interests of middle-class white women, there has been a certain reluctance to support the demands of the campaign against sterilization abuse. . . . While women of color are urged, at every turn, to become permanently infertile, white women enjoying prosperous economic conditions are urged, by the same forces, to reproduce themselves. They therefore sometimes consider the "waiting period" and other details of the demand for "informed consent" to sterilization as further inconveniences for women like themselves. Yet whatever the inconveniences for white middle-class women, a fundamental reproductive right of racially oppressed and poor women is at stake. . . . What is urgently required is a broad campaign to defend the reproductive rights of all women—and especially those women whose economic circumstances often compel them to relinquish the right to reproduction itself.

NOTES

1. Herbert Gutman, *The Black Family in Slavery and Freedom, 1750–1925*, New York, Pantheon, 1976, 80–81 (note).
2. Ibid.

3. Herbert Aptheker, "The Negro Woman," *Masses and Mainstream*, 11(2): 12, 1948.

4. Gerda Lerner, *The Female Experience*, Indianapolis, Bobbs-Merrill, 1977, 91.

5. Melvin Steinfeld, *Our Racist Presidents*, San Ramon, Calif., Consensus Publishers, 1972, 212.

6. Bonnie Mass, *Population Target: The Political Economy of Population Control in Latin America*, Toronto, Women's Educational Press, 1977, 20.

7. Linda Gordon, *Woman's Body, Woman's Right: Birth Control in America*, New York, Penguin, 1976, 157.

8. Ibid., 158.

9. Margaret Sanger, *An Autobiography*, New York, Dover Press, 1971, 75.

10. Bruce Dancis, "Socialism and Women in the United States, 1900–1912," *Socialist Revolution*, No. 27, 6(1): 96, 1976.

11. Gordon, op. cit., 281.

12. Ibid., 283.

13. Gena Corea, *The Hidden Malpractice*, New York, A Jove/HBJ Book, 1977, 149.

14. Gordon, op. cit., 332.

15. Ibid.

16. Les Payne, "Forced Sterilization for the Poor?" *San Francisco Chronicle*, February 26, 1974.

17. Ibid.

18. Ibid.

19. Arlene Eisen, "They're Trying to Take Our Future: Native American Women and Sterilization," *The Guardian*, March 23, 1972.

Informed Consent

ELIZABETH SIEGEL WATKINS

Elizabeth Siegel Watkins, excerpted from "Oral Contraceptives and I.C.," in *On the Pill: A Social History of Oral Contraceptives, 1950–1970*, Baltimore: Johns Hopkins University Press, 1998. Reprinted by permission.

In September 1969, the head of the information and education department of Planned Parenthood sent memos to the directors of the medical department and to the president of Planned Parenthood about the imminent publication of a book called *The Doctors' Case Against the Pill* by Barbara Seaman. The memos warned that "the effect of the book . . . will be to destroy consumer faith in the efficacy of the pill" and advised the Planned Parenthood lead-ership to "put balance and background in the hands of reviewers to offset the impact of this book in all media before the bomb hits." The following month, days before the scheduled release of Seaman's book, Planned Parenthood sent a memo to all of its affiliates' executive directors and medical directors to alert them to "books attacking the pill." The memo contrasted portions of text from *The Doctors' Case Against the Pill* with sections of the 1969 FDA Advisory Committee's *Second Report on the Oral Contraceptives* to illustrate the "distorted picture" presented by Seaman. It urged the affiliates to respond to queries from local media by "report[ing] your own clinic[']s experience to add the very impressive positive side of oral contraception." What did this book say to elicit such a strong reaction from the nation's largest family planning organization?

The Doctors' Case Against the Pill presented a wealth of evidence against the safety of oral contraceptives. Barbara Seaman had written dozens of articles during the 1960s about issues related to women's health for magazines such as *Brides* and *Ladies' Home Journal*. Her book marshalled the testimony of physicians, medical researchers, and women who had used oral contraceptives to build her case against the pill and to indict the medical-pharmaceutical establishment that developed and marketed it.

Seaman's critique of hormonal birth control in particular and the medical-pharmaceutical complex in general lent support to the two renascent social movements of consumerism and feminism. The consumer movement, which originated in the United States with efforts to regulate the manufacture of food and drugs in the late nineteenth century, entered a new phase in the 1960's with the publication of books such as Rachel Carson's *Silent Spring* (1962), Jessica Mitford's *The American Way of Death* (1963), and Ralph Nader's *Unsafe at Any Speed* (1965).

Whereas Carson took on the chemical industry, Mitford the funeral industry, and Nader the automobile industry, Seaman challenged the pharmaceutical industry and the closely allied medical profession. She demanded that pill manufacturers and physicians share all available information about the health risks of oral contraception with patients, so that the women themselves could make informed decisions about birth control. This demand for full disclosure represented an extension of the relatively new concept of informed consent in medicine beyond the operating room to include all doctor-patient interactions.

Seaman's charge that women received inadequate care from their physicians, particularly obstetrician-gynecologists, mirrored a growing concern among feminists about women's health issues. *The Doctors' Case Against the Pill* inspired feminists to vocalize the shared perception that the medical profession was "condescending, paternalistic, judgmental and noninformative." In part owing to the publication of this book, the controversy over the safety of the pill galvanized the women's health movement of the 1970s.

The book created little stir when it was released in 1969. Seaman recalls that "it didn't make a big splash when it came out, not in the first few weeks." When the *New York Times* finally got around to reviewing the book, two months after its release, the reviewer dismissed it as "disorganized" and "scatterbrained." However, the publisher, Peter Wyden, believed that the message deserved a wider audience. He hired a publicist in Washington who passed along a copy of *The Doctors' Case Against the Pill* to US Senator Gaylord Nelson.

HEARINGS ON COMPETITIVE PROBLEMS IN THE DRUG INDUSTRY

By the time Nelson received Seaman's book, he had already led his Subcommittee on Monopoly of the Select Committee on Small Business through sixty-four days of hearings over two and a half years on a broad range of topics, including drug pricing, testing, and advertising; brand name versus generic drugs; the relationship between the drug industry and the medical profession; and investigations into the use and misuse of spe-

cific kinds of drugs. One year earlier, the US Congress had approved the Medicaid and Medicare amendments to the Social Security Act, which used federal tax dollars to provide health care for the poor and the elderly. Since the federal government spent more than half a billion dollars annually to purchase prescription drugs, Nelson, as a member of the legislative branch, felt it was his duty to expose the pharmaceutical industry to public scrutiny.

After the first year of hearings, Nelson concluded that since both the medical profession and the Food and Drug Administration (FDA) depended on pharmaceutical companies for information about drugs, neither doctors nor government officials could rely on promotional literature to be completely objective. The industry, not the FDA, was responsible for conducting and/or arranging for tests and clinical trials of new drugs. Since pharmaceutical firms wanted to earn FDA approval quickly for their products, to reach the market as soon as possible, they often compromised the quality of new drug evaluations. Nelson also questioned the professional and ethical implications of close relations between medicine and the drug industry as in, for example, industry-sponsored medical publications and physician-stockholders in drug companies. Since doctors relied in part on drug detailmen, promotional literature, and free samples provided by drug companies for their continuing education in pharmacology, Nelson worried that physicians could not make intelligent decisions about prescription drugs because of the commercially biased information they received.

Thus when a book describing the hazards of a drug taken by millions of women each day landed on his desk, the senator took notice. He and the staff economist for the Senate Committee on Small Business, Ben Gordon, interviewed Barbara Seaman several times during the fall of 1969. She passed the test, and on December 22, 1969, Nelson released a statement to the press announcing his intention to hold public hearings on the oral contraceptives, to "present for the general public's benefit the best and most objective information available about these drugs. First, whether they are dangerous for the human body, and, second, whether patients taking them have sufficient information about possible dangers in order to make an intelligent judgment whether they wish to assume the risks."

THE PILL HEARINGS, PART I

The two issues of oral contraceptive safety and informed consent corresponded closely to Senator Nelson's larger concerns about medicine and the pharmaceutical industry. The adverse health effects of oral contraceptives cast doubts on the merit of the drug tests and clinical trials conducted prior to FDA approval, and thus deepened his suspicions about the integrity of the drug manufacturers. The question of whether women could make informed decisions about using the birth control pill reflected Senator Nelson's misgivings about the ability of physicians to obtain objective information from the pill manufacturers and in turn to pass that information on to their patients.

To evaluate the alleged health risks of oral contraceptives, Nelson and Gordon assembled a group of expert witnesses to testify about the biochemical, physiological, and psychological effects of the pill. Many of the scientists and physicians who appeared before the committee had also appeared on the pages of Seaman's book, and their testimony provided little, if any, new information about the biological effects of oral contraceptives. However, as a result of the intense media coverage of the hearings, the medical controversy over the safety of the pill reached a much wider audience.

Although Gordon relied heavily on Barbara Seaman for advice in choosing witnesses, he did not invite her to appear before the committee, "because she wasn't a primary source." Nor were any women who had experienced pill-related adverse health effects asked to testify. Seaman, by contrast, recognized the importance of women's voices and experiences in the pill debate, and included in her book heartrending stories of women

who had died or suffered serious consequences as a result of taking oral contraceptives.

In a way, Seaman and Nelson represented the ambivalence toward science and medicine in American society at the end of the 1960s. On the one hand, they questioned the merit and safety of the pill, a product of medical science and technology, and criticized scientists and physicians for their incursion into family planning. On the other had, they relied on scientists and physicians for evidence on which to base their critique. Nelson never acknowledged this inconsistency, at least not in public. Seaman, however, underwent a significant transformation after the publication of *The Doctors' Case Against the Pill*. She had written the book as a "reformist" feminist, hoping to influence changes within the existing system of medical care. Later, after coming in contact with more radical feminists, she became critical of the medical establishment and its (mis)treatment of women's health care needs.

Seaman's enlightenment began on the first day of the Nelson hearings. Although not invited to testify, she attended the hearings as a press correspondent. In the middle of testimony from the second witness, some women in the audience interrupted the hearings. Seaman vividly recalled the disturbance:

> All of a sudden, these women started standing up and yelling. . . . I heard my name, "Why isn't Barbara Seaman testifying?" And then somebody else was saying, "Why isn't there a pill for men?" And someone else was saying, "Why aren't there any patients testifying?" . . . Then they were cleared out of the room. . . . So, I went outside. I followed them out. This was my story. What these guys were saying that I'd been writing about for years wasn't my story. . . . So I went out and introduce myself to them. . . . When I said that I was Barbara Seaman, they fell all over themselves. . . . It turned out that it was my book that had inspired them to demonstrate.

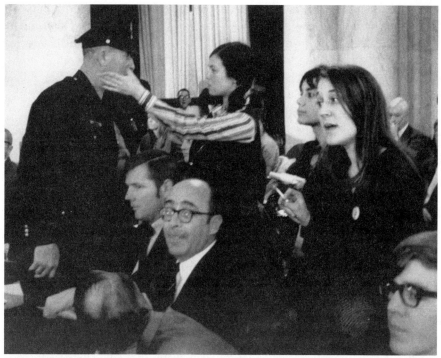

A pregnant Marilyn Webb (slapping the police officer) is one of a group of women who disrupted the 1970 Senate monopoly subcommittee hearings on the birth control pill, protesting the fact that no women had been called as witnesses. [AP/Wide World Photos]

The demonstrators belonged to a group called D.C. Women's Liberation, which had come together in 1969 to protest illegal abortion; their work soon led to a broader interest in women's health care. Alice Wolfson, a member of D.C. Women's Liberation and later one of the founders of the National Women's Health Network, explained how the demonstration got started:

> We were sitting at a meeting—which we did all the time in those days, nobody worked, I don't know what we did for money!—in the middle of the afternoon, and we had heard that there were going to be these hearings on the birth control pill on the Hill, so about seven of us went. . . . When we got there, we were both frightened, really frightened, by the content and appalled by the fact that all of the senators were men [and] all of the people testifying were men.

> They did not have a single woman who had taken the pill and no women scientists. We were hearing the most cut-and-dried scientific evidence about the dangers of the pill. . . . Remember all of us had taken the pill, so we were there as activists but also as concerned women. . . . So while we were hearing this, we suddenly said, "My God," and we—because in those days you did things like that—raised our hands and asked questions.

The women quickly organized themselves and held militant demonstrations at every subsequent hearing. A group of twenty women arrived early each day and strategically placed themselves at the end and in the middle of every other row of seats. They came prepared with questions to interrupt the hearings and with bail money tucked inside their boots.

Ironically, both the feminists and Senator Nelson agreed on most issues. They believed that the FDA had allowed the drug companies to market the pill without adequate tests of its long-term safety. Neither the feminists nor Nelson advocated a ban on the oral contraceptives; both argued that women needed access to all available information so that they could make intelligent decisions about birth control. They agreed that the lack of informed consent stemmed from the problem of poor communication between doctors and patients.

At this point, the opinions of the senator and the feminists diverged. For Nelson, the issue of informed consent could be solved by improving the channels of communication among the manufacturers, the FDA, physicians, and patients. The more radical feminists saw the pill as the tip of the iceberg of much larger problems in women's health care; they doubted that these problems could be solved within the context of the contemporary system of male-dominated medicine.

The members of D.C. Women's Liberation took umbrage at the absence of female witnesses. Nelson's attempt to placate the demonstrators after the first interruption—in which he referred to them as "girls" and counseled them against disruptive behavior—only exacerbated the women's anger and increased their resolve to protest. Although they supported increasing public awareness of the health risks of oral contraceptives, they could not tolerate the established format of the Senate hearings.

Nelson also faced criticism from within his Senate subcommittee, mainly from a freshman senator from Kansas named Bob Dole. Dole professed concern that women would be unduly alarmed by public hearings of medical testimony regarding the safety of the pill. In his opening statement (read in his absence by the minority counsel), Dole warned: "We must not frighten millions of women into disregarding the considered judgments of their physicians about the use of oral contraceptives. . . . Let us show some sympathy for the beleaguered physician who must weigh not only the efficacy and safety of alternative methods for a particular woman, but the emotional reactions of that woman which have been generated by sensational publicity and rumored medical advi[c]e." As a conservative Republican, Dole's ulterior interests probably agreed with those of the pharmaceutical industry, as well as the "beleaguered physician." When he joined the hearings on the third day, he remarked: "I think we probably have terrified a number of women around the country. . . . I would guess they may be taking two pills now—first a tranquilizer and then the regular pill—because of our erudite investigation."

The controversial nature of the pill hearings did not go unnoticed by the media. All three national television networks covered them on evening news broadcasts in January 1970. Of the eight witnesses who testified during the first two days, seven voiced serious concerns about the safety of oral contraceptives, and excerpts from their testimony were televised to the American public. On ABC, Sam Donaldson reported, "Doctors do not agree on the relative safety of the pill. But on this first day of Senator Gaylord Nelson's hearings, the emphasis was on the dangers." On CBS, Walter Cronkite reported, "Almost nine million women in America, and ten million elsewhere, are taking the pill each day, in the words of one expert, 'as automatically as chickens eating corn.'" NBC's Chet Huntley led that network's evening news: "The pills have been on the market for ten years, but today was the first time Congress has seen fit to investigate them." The television cameras also captured the disturbance created by D.C. Women's Liberation as well as the impromptu news conference held by the women after the hearings.

Despite repeated invitations from Nelson, no industry representative ever appeared before the committee. G. D. Searle & Company chose to defend the pill by allowing one of its spokesmen, Dr. Irwin Winter, to be interviewed on television in his office at Searle's headquarters in Skokie, Illinois. Dr. Winter complained, "I thought when we brought out the pill several years ago that we were doing mankind [sic] a great favor and that this is a thing that women had been wanting from time immemorial. Now, from the headlines and the way this is being reported, or being presented . . . one would think we had unleashed a monster on the world." Nelson's invitations to the drug companies contrasted dramatically with his disregard of the feminists who had asked to testify. On January 23, D.C. Women's Liberation again interrupted the hearings, demanding to be allowed to appear. All three networks featured the protest on the evening news, in which different women in the audience shouted:

> Why have you assured the drug companies that they could testify? Why have you told them they will get top priority? They're not taking the pills, we are!

> Why is it that scientists and drug companies are perfectly willing to use women as guinea pigs in experiments to test the high estrogen/low estrogen content of the pill, but as soon as a woman gets pregnant in one of these experiments she's treated like a common criminal! She can't get an abortion!

> Women are not going to stay quiet any longer! You are murdering us for your profit and convenience!

ABC reported that after Senator Nelson ordered the room to be cleared, he readmitted the press, but "the public and its virago element were not welcomed back." The other networks were more generous in their characterizations of the demonstrators and their intentions.

By the end of the first round of hearings, the television-viewing public knew a great deal more about the controversy surrounding the safety of the pill, but no more about whether the pill was safe to take. The *Washington Daily News* captured this uncertainty in a cartoon of a woman in a Hamlet pose holding in one hand a birth control pill and in the other a newspaper headlined, "Sci-

entists say pill is unsafe but safe enough." The cartoon's caption read: "To take or not to take . . ." On February 9, *Newsweek* reported the results of a Gallup poll of women between the ages of twenty-one and forty-five. News of the hearings reached an extremely wide audience; 87 percent of American women had heard or read about them. The survey found that 18 percent of the eight and a half million women with pill prescriptions had stopped taking the pills in recent months, and another 23 percent were considering stopping. One-third of those who had quit or thought about quitting directly attributed their recent or imminent abandonment of oral contraceptives to the Nelson hearings; another one-fourth cited side effects—experienced personally or by friends—as the reason for their doubts about the pill.

Perhaps the most disturbing finding of the survey addressed one of Senator Nelson's initial questions in the pill hearing: Were women being adequately informed by their doctors about the adverse health effects of the pill? The answer was a resounding "no." The poll revealed that two-thirds of women on the pill were never told by their physicians about the potential health risks of oral contraception. Millions of women chose to take birth control pills without knowing the whole story; the lack of communication between doctor and patient precluded informed consent in decision-making about birth control. This discrepancy between their doctors' actions and the expectations of the Senate committee heightened women's concerns about the wisdom of taking birth control pills in particular and about the quality of their medical care in general.

Data from Planned Parenthood clinics mirrored the trend away from the pill identified by the *Newsweek* Gallup poll. In Detroit, during the month from January 14 to February 13, the clinic reported a tenfold increase in diaphragm requests, a doubling of requests for IUDs, and an "astounding increase" in requests for tubal ligations and vasectomies, all resulting from patients discontinuing the pill. At the New York City clinic, almost one-fifth of oral contraceptive users switched to either the IUD or the diaphragm. *Business Week* reported an "almost hysterical cry for diaphragms" in January and February, resulting in a five-fold increase in sales of the device. A urologist in Rhode Island reported that vasectomy requests had tripled since the hearings began. Women all over the country telephoned their physicians demanding information on whether they should continue to take the pill.

Some doctors regretted the public forum of the hearings because of the alarm generated. An article in the *New York Times,* written by a physician, described the results of the hearings as "an epidemic of anxiety that has spread like wildfire." The author likened the scientific debate in the Senate Caucus Room to medical rounds in a hospital: "Unless the physician explains to the patient in words of one syllable and with understanding and sensitivity the facts in simple lay language, the consequences are anxiety and often real fear."

By 1970, fewer patients were willing to accept that kind of paternalistic treatment. As consumer advocates turned their attention to professional services, such as medicine, they criticized the unequal balance of power in the doctor-patient relationship. Friction between doctors and female patients was further compounded by emerging feminist critiques of the male-dominated medical profession and of male-dominated society in general.

THE PILL HEARINGS, PART II

The second round of hearings presented testimony from witnesses both in favor of and opposed to the birth control pill. Many witnesses devoted their testimony to bemoaning the results of the first round of hearings held a month earlier. These experts generally approved of the pill as a valuable means of fertility control, and they lamented the anxiety and alarm produced by the hearings and concomitant media coverage. Not coincidentally, several of the pill advocates were affiliated with large-scale family planning agencies, such as the Margaret Sanger Research Bureau, or population control organizations, such as the Population Crisis Committee and Planned Parenthood/World Population. One witness, Phyllis Piotrow, formerly of the Population Crisis Committee, anticipated that one hundred thousand unwanted "Nelson babies" would be born in the coming year as a result of women discontinuing the pill because of fear generated by the hearings. In an article for the *Progressive,* journalist Morton Mintz ridiculed this eponymy and its supporters (notably Senator Dole) by suggesting pill-related diseases be called "Piotrow strokes" or "Dole thromboembolisms." The media immediately reported the concern about more unplanned pregnancies. In one of its articles on the Nelson hearings, *Time* printed a cartoon that showed one pregnant woman greeting another in an obstetrician's waiting room with the caption, "Corinne . . . You didn't tell me you gave up the pill, too?"

Once again, Senator Nelson found himself in unexpected opposition to his usual allies. Nelson prided himself on being an environmentalist; he helped to originate the idea of Earth Day (which took place just two months after the pill hearings). He worried about the effects of overpopulation and supported most fertility control programs. However, his doubts about the safety of oral contraceptives and his leadership of the public hearings on the pill alienated him from the population control community.

By the last days of the hearings, the central issue had boiled down to informed consent. Most physicians and scientists agreed that no new biomedical evidence had been presented; the debate over whether the pill caused cancer, for example, would have to wait for more data in order to be resolved. They disagreed, however, on how much of this information should be presented to patients. Some concurred with Nelson, who insisted that women should be given all available information so that they could make up their own minds. Others sided with the witness who testified: "A patient cannot reasonably be expected to make a profound professional judgment—she is not a doctor."

The issue of informed consent crystallized on the final day of the hearings, when FDA Commissioner Edwards announced that his agency planned to require pill manufacturers to include information for patients in every package of birth control pills. This pamphlet, written in lay language and directed to the patient, would outline the health risks associated with taking the medication. Dr. Edwards explained that the insert was "designed to reinforce the information provided the patient by her physician." In the absence of good doctor-patient communication (which, according to the *Newsweek* Gallup poll, characterized two out of every three women's experiences), the leaflet would supply the patient with the facts necessary to make an informed choice.

The hearings in February brought the first female witnesses to appear before the subcommittee. In total, four women testified: three physicians and the immediate past executive director of the Population Crises Committee (Ms. Piotrow). All of the women strongly advocated the use of the pill under a physician's supervision; none of them acknowledged the concerns expressed by the D.C. Women's Liberation protesters.

Dr. Elizabeth Connell, unlike many others, could afford the simultaneous luxury of a large family and a professional career. Given Connell's generously sized family, her interest in overpopulation and pollution could be interpreted as classist. However, she also felt concern and sympathy for women with unwanted pregnancies, and annoyance with a system that did not allow women to make their own reproductive choices. Connell argued for legalized abortion and relaxed sterilization laws, as well as for the availability of a wide variety of contraceptive options, so that every individual could be free to decide how many babies to have and when to have them. Connell offered powerful rhetoric, in a style reminiscent of that of Margaret Sanger, to make her case for oral contraceptives:

> As a physician who began practice before the advent of the pill, I am constantly aware of the immense difference it has made to the lives of women, their families, and to society as a whole. The look of horror on the face of a twelve-year-old girl when you confirm her fears of pregnancy, the sound of a woman's voice cursing her newborn and unwanted child as she lies on the delivery table, the helpless feeling that comes over you as you watch women die following criminal abortion, the hideous responsibility of informing a husband and children that their wife and mother has just died in childbirth—all these situations are deeply engraved in our memories, never to be forgotten. With the advent of more effective means of contraception, the recurrence of these nightmares was becoming blessedly less frequent.

It would be inaccurate to dismiss Connell as insensitive to women. Her distance from the younger generation of activists pointed instead to their differing agendas, which precluded consensus on the best way to fight for women's reproductive rights.

In February 1970, D.C. Women's Liberation held a press conference to announce their intention to hold their own hearings. They specifically invited women who had suffered ill effects on the pill to testify. The women's hearings took place in March, three days after the Senate hearings ended, in a church in Washington, with child care provided. Flyers advertising the hearings read, "The Pill: Is It a Menace, A No-No, or a Girl's Best Friend?" About a hundred people turned out to hear testimony from Barbara Seaman; Sarah Lewit Tietze, a research associate at the Population Council (and wife of Dr. Christopher Tietze, also affiliated with the Population Council); Elaine Archer, a women's health care advocate; Etta Horn, a welfare rights leader; and others.

In their opening statement, the women of D.C. Liberation made their position clear:

> We are not opposed to oral contraceptives for men or for women. We are opposed to

unsafe contraceptives foisted on uninformed women for the profit of the drug and medical industries and for the convenience of men. It is not our mission to have all women of the pill discard it and change to another form of contraception. Our mission, if such it can be called, is to rise up, as women, and demand our human rights. We will no longer let doctors treat us as objects to be manipulated at will. Together we will ask for and demand explanations and humane treatment by our doctors and if they are too busy to give this to us we will insist that the medical profession must meet our needs. We will no longer tolerate intimidation by white coated gods, antiseptically directing our lives.

Doctors did not have to be male to fit the model of "white-coated gods." Women doctors, such as Elizabeth Connell, who did not disclose all information to patients about the side effects of the pill, were subjected to the same sort of criticism from the new health feminists. Connell set her sights on the more reformist goal of helping women to achieve reproductive control as a means to greater economic stability and personal fulfillment; she viewed the pill as a beneficial—but not perfect—technological solution to family planning. The members of D.C. Women's Liberation, by contrast, rejected reformist feminism because it did not address what they perceived as the underling ills of a patriarchal system. Their objective was nothing less than the redistribution of power in society. In the realm of medicine, these feminists wanted women to participate as equal partners in their health care, which included the necessary prerogative of informed consent.

Thus, when FDA Commissioner Edwards announced the requirement for package inserts, many feminists regarded this as an important victory. After all, such an insert was a novel idea; oral contraceptives would be the first orally administered drug to carry a detailed warning directed at patients. However, as feminists and other advocates of the package insert soon found out, the road from promise to reality was not easily navigated.

FDA AND THE PATIENT PACKAGE INSERT

In 1938 the federal Food, Drug, and Cosmetic Act obliged pharmaceutical manufacturers to make information about the safety of drugs available to physicians. In 1961, an amended version of the law required this information to be listed on the label of the package in the interest of "full disclosure," and within a few years most prescription drugs included a detailed package insert directed to physicians. These pamphlets contained instructions for using the medications, as well as information on indications, contraindications, efficacy, and side effects. An editorial in the *Journal of the American Medical Association* pointed out that the drug companies composed and paid for the package inserts, thus making them little more than "promotional items." Indeed, the FDA did not participate in the preparation of these pamphlets; the agency left decisions about their specific content to the manufacturers, so long as they met the basic requirements for drug labeling as outlined by the legislation.

The extended FDA regulations created a new category of drugs available by prescription only. While government regulation was designed to protect consumers from unscrupulous drug manufacturers, it also removed a significant amount of decision-making about medical treatment from the patient's, or consumer's, domain. After 1938, patients relied on physicians to instruct them on which drugs to purchase and to use. The doctor controlled not only the patient's treatment, but also the degree to which the patient understood the complexities of that treatment.

The day after the FDA Commissioner announced his intention to require the insert, the *New York Times* published the proposed text. Entitled "What You Should Know About the Birth Control Pill," the 600-word document described in lay language the health risks, side effects, and contraindications of oral contraceptives. Although Edwards indicated that the insert was necessary because doctors did not adequately inform patients, the leaflet assured women of the competence of their doctors: "Your doctor has taken your medical history and has given you a careful physical examination. He has discussed with you the risks of oral contraceptives and has decided that you can take this drug safely." Ten of the fifteen paragraphs in the proposed text referred to the doctor as the proper authority on oral contraceptives; the leaflet encouraged the woman to consult her physician in no fewer than six different situations.

In spite of this deference to the doctor, the medical profession strongly opposed the insert, claiming that the pamphlet would intrude upon the doctor-patient relationship. The pharmaceutical industry contended that the proposed leaflet overstated the potential risks and overlooked the benefits of oral contraception. Even the Department of Health, Education, and Welfare (HEW), which housed the Food and Drug Administration, argued that the leaflet needed to be revised to satisfy somewhat murky legal issues. (The *New York Times* reported that HEW was irked at having been left out of the loop on the development of the insert.)

In response, the FDA backed away from its initial proposal and substituted a much shorter, less detailed version. The revised text, 100 words in length, mentioned only one complication of oral contraception, blood-clotting disorders. Whereas the first draft had included statistics on increased risk and mortality rates from thromboembolism, the edited version omitted this information. It encouraged women to see their doctors if they experienced side effects, listing just five symptoms and conditions whereas the earlier draft had listed more than twenty-five.

Outraged, women from D.C. Women's Liberation staged a sit-in at the office of HEW Secretary Robert Finch to protest the watered-down version. They came with their children and they sang,

making up pill songs to the tunes of nursery rhymes, like "The doctors give the pill, the doctors give the pill, heigh ho the derey-o, the women take the pill, the women they get ill, the doctors send their bill." Alice Wolfson, organizer of the demonstration, said, "Those of us who had babies . . . we brought them everywhere, and when anyone would say, 'Take the kids out of the hearing room' or this or that, we would say, 'Well, that's fine, where's the day care center?' All of these issues were always linked."

Secretary Finch did not see the feminists that day, but agreed to meet with them a few days later. On March 30, 1970, Secretary Finch, FDA Commissioner Edwards, and Surgeon General Jesse Steinfeld met with six representatives of the feminist group, including Barbara Seaman and Alice Wolfson. Wolfson reported in the feminist newspaper *off our backs* that after an hour of discussion, "Finch stormed out of the room, tailed by Edwards and Steinfeld, claiming we were just wasting his time."

The feminist petition to reinstate the stronger version of the package insert did not sway the officials of HEW and FDA. On April 10, 1970, the FDA published the abridged draft in The *Federal Register* and invited all interested parties to respond with comments. Letters from more than eight hundred individuals and groups flooded in. About a third requested more information about the insert and about the oral contraceptives in general. Many had not read the actual notice in the *Federal Register*, but had heard or read about it in the news. More than half wrote to object to the abridgement of the text. Most of these were copies of form letters distributed by women's and consumers' groups which complained that the insert did not provide full disclosure on the adverse effects of the pill and called for public hearings on the matter. Over a hundred women and men wrote their own letters to protest the reduction in the length and scope of the insert. Some of them objected to the unequal distribution of power in the doctor-patient relationship:

I have inadvertently received the physician's copy of facts and cautions now included in each 3-pack of Ortho-Novum pills; the first time I told the people who had given it to me they said, "You're not supposed to see that. That's only for doctors." I was outraged and insulted at this; the only reason I can see for doctors or other parties [to] withhold medical information from patients is the desire to maintain their psychological and monetary power over us.

Others added their concern about the integrity of the pharmaceutical industry and its control over government agencies:

In the *Chicago Daily News*, March 24, 1970, I read that the FDA has called for toning down the wording of the precautionary literature on oral contraceptives which HEW has in the planning stage. It was clear from the article the HEW is bowing to pressure from the drug industry, the AMA, and many private physicians, all of whom feel that a precise report will harm the [p]ill's market and their own pocketbooks.

Still others expressed the opinion that women had the right to full disclosure on medical matter: "I DEMAND, that as a woman, having the option to take the pill or not, I have *all* the facts in front of me!"

Much of the public interest in the oral contraceptives can be attributed to the publicity generated by the Nelson hearings and the consistent coverage by the news media. It is less easy to explain why people moved beyond mere interest to direct action—in this case, writing letters of protest. Most likely the climate of the times spurred many individuals to act. In a society attuned to the issue of rights and conducive to political activism, people felt empowered to speak out against what they perceived as a denial of the right to informed consent. During this time, many Americans felt angered by the secret policies of the government in the Vietnam War; by 1970,

the demand for public information extended to a broad range of government activities. In addition, Congress had recently passed the Freedom of Information Act (in 1967), which both entitled and emboldened citizens to seek information previously withheld from them.

Doctors also wrote to the FDA. The majority opinion of the medical profession was represented in letters from the American Medical Association and other national and state organizations. With very few exceptions, doctors strongly opposed the patient package insert, which they claimed would interfere with the doctor-patient relationship. Excerpts from physicians' letters reveal their indignation at regulation from outside the medical profession:

I deeply resent the Government of the United States coming between me and my patients in the matter of a single class of prescription items . . .

This practice can serve no useful purpose except [sic] to frighten patients. Furthermore, it represents an undesirable entry of government into the practice of medicine.

I would sincerely hope that before such a proposal becomes an accomplished fact, strong consideration be given to the far-reaching [e]ffects such legislation [regulation] will have on the medical community of this country, which has been so frequently maligned. . . . The determination of appropriate use of medications must continue to rest in the hands of the physician . . . To remove this clinical relationship would be just another method of eroding the foundation of American medicine.

A few physicians expressed approval, agreeing with consumer advocates that the patient should be fully informed before making the decision to use birth control pills. One doctor argued that the insert would "serve as a protection for the doctor rather than as a cause for initiating lawsuits." One would think that this reasoning would appeal to the pharmaceutical industry as well; by 1970 more than a hundred lawsuits had been filed against birth control pill manufacturers.

However, drug companies vehemently opposed the inclusion of an FDA-mandated warning. The president of the Pharmaceutical Manufacturers Association (PMA), which represented 125 drug companies, articulated the industry's objections; four companies also wrote letters supporting the PMA position and offering additional comments on the proposed wording. The drug industry sided with the medical profession in preserving the sanctity of the doctor-patient relationship.

The content of the insert that became a requirement in June 1970 was significantly modified from the version proposed in April. The *New York Times* reported that the change resulted from pressure from physicians; clearly, the FDA bowed also to the interests of the powerful pharmaceutical industry. Although it did describe abnormal blood clotting as "the most serious known side effect," the insert did not list any symptoms; instead, it told the reader to "notify your doctor if you notice any physical discomfort." Four of the seven sentences in the insert described the availability of an information booklet, which the patient could request from the physician.

This 800-word booklet was written by the American Medical Association in conjunction with the FDA and the American College of Obstetricians and Gynecologists; it resembled in scope and content the original insert. The package insert merely informed the patient that further information was available; the onus fell on the patient to ask her doctor to give her the booklet.

In late June, a woman announced that she planned to sue the FDA and HEW under the 1967 Freedom of Information Act for disclosure of all clinical and toxicological records on eight different brands of oral contraceptives. According to HEW, release of the data from laboratory and clinical tests "would only confuse the average citizen." The plaintiff sought to challenge that assumption.

In another lawsuit, an associate of the consumer advocate Ralph Nader lost a battle to have the booklet included directly in packages of birth control pills in lieu of the shorter insert. Barbara Seaman was "very shocked when we learned that it was going to be distributed to doctors' offices, not by pharmacists, and that the prescribing physician would give out the booklet. . . . I spent a lot of time buttonholing women and asking them if they had received this, and I invariably found that if they'd been to a clinic, the chances were very good they had gotten it. Private physician, forget it! I don't know if I ever found one person whose private physician gave it to her."

The battle over the patient package insert demonstrated the influence and power of the medical profession and the pharmaceutical industry over the FDA. Yet, in spite of its watered-down wording, the insert still represented an important turning point in the doctor-patient relationship. Patients had demanded the right to know about the medications prescribed for them, and the package insert legitimized this claim.

Eight years later the FDA ordered the minimal package insert replaced by a lengthy information leaflet. In 1977, the FDA issued patient information requirements for estrogens used in hormone replacement therapy. In the wake of this mandate, the FDA revised the oral contraceptive requirements to be consistent with those of other estrogen products. This 1978 version of the patient package insert represented what consumer and feminist groups had wanted all along.

THE WOMEN'S HEALTH MOVEMENT

Oral contraception was not the first reproductive health issue to engage women activists in the decades after World War II. The La Leche League began to promote breast-feeding as a better alternative to infant formula in 1956, challenging the authority of "scientific motherhood" and advocating the return of mothering to the mother. At the same time, women dissatisfied with the anesthetized experience of hospital childbirth turned to the "natural childbirth" techniques of Grantly Dick-Read. Another early feminist health issue centered on the promotion of physical therapy for radical mastectomy patients to prevent the loss of mobility in their arms. All of these initiatives sought to redress problems created by the medicalization of women's health in the twentieth century.

By the late 1960s, women around the country gathered in informal "consciousness raising" groups to share their experiences as women in a sexist society. Many of these groups focused their discussions on medicine, health, and the body. In Boston, women frustrated with the existing system of medical care decided to do research on health-related topics; the resulting papers written by members of this Boston Women's Health Book Collective formed the basis for the best-selling *Our Bodies, Ourselves.*

A rallying point for the early health feminists was the legalization of abortion. Members of D.C. Women's Liberation became more interested in women's health issues as they fought for legalized abortion. Alice Wolfson recalled: "We found that one of the leading causes of maternal death in D.C. General Hospital, which is the only public hospital in Washington, DC, was botched abortions. So when we began to scratch that surface, we began to find out lots of other things about health care for women, and also began to develop a kind of analysis of the health care system and the relationship of women to power and the health care system as being kind of a microcosm of women's place in society in general at the time." It was only a short step from activism on abortion and sterilization abuse to activism on a broader range of health-related issues. In 1970, many abortion rights advocates were still working at the state level. The pill hearings, however, took place on Capitol Hill and attracted national attention.

At the Nelson hearings, Barbara Seaman met Alice Wolfson, thus bringing together the "uptown" and the "downtown" feminists on the issue of the safety of the pill. Seaman used the term "downtown" to describe the more radical feminists who belonged to militant groups such as the Redstockings, Bread and Roses, and D.C. Women's Liberation. "Uptown" referred to those feminists who belonged to more mainstream organizations such as Betty Friedan's National Organization for Women. Seaman described herself as an uptown feminist . . . until she met Wolfson: "I instantly struck up a friendship with Alice. I just thought everything she said was right, putting her political analysis on all of this. I thought, yes, yes, why didn't I see it this way, why didn't I understand it this way all along? But of course, if I had seen it that way, I wouldn't have been suitable to write for the *Ladies' Home Journal* or to write the kind of book I wrote. So in the scheme of things, it's just as well that I saw it from my particular lens up until that moment in January 1970, when I met Alice."

The two women remained in close contact after the hearing; Wolfson lived in Washington and could keep track of the developments at the FDA. Soon thereafter, she invited Seaman to testify at the women's hearings on the pill, to meet with HEW Secretary Finch, and to "sit in" at a closed meeting of the FDA's Advisory Committee on Obstetrics and Gynecology: "Alice and I went down there [to the FDA] and we walked in [to the room where the Advisory Committee met] and we sat down and everybody said to us, "What are you doing here?" And Alice said, "Well, why shouldn't we stay? It's our bodies you're discussing." They told us we had to go out, and they would discuss whether we would be allowed to stay. We sat on the floor in the hallway right outside for about a half an hour, and then somebody came out and said okay, we could stay. I think that was the first time that the advisory committees were made open to the public." For both women, full disclosure and informed consent remained at the heart of all of their battles.

Wolfson and Seaman were in the vanguard of what became the women's health movement. In 1975, they joined with other health activists to form the National Women's Health Network. The network acted as an information clearinghouse for women's collectives around the country. It represented women's health interests in hearings held by Congress and the FDA and published a newsletter on health policy and legislation. Twenty years later, the organization remains actively engaged in women's health issues.

The goals of health feminists in the 1970s differed dramatically from those of their predecessors. A generation earlier, Margaret Sanger and Katharine McCormick lobbied for women's right to reproductive control. To achieve their goal, they enlisted the help of scientists and physicians and encouraged these experts to develop a solution to the problem of birth control. Sanger and McCormick hailed the oral contraceptive as a scientific triumph for women and gladly entrusted contraception to the hands of physicians. In contrast, the women's health movement rejected the hegemony of the medical-pharmaceutical complex and instead advocated lay control over the delivery of health services. Health feminists objected to the birth control pill on several grounds: insufficient clinical trials, potentially fatal side effects, and a lack of informed consent among its millions of users worldwide. In 1970, feminists interpreted the pill as representative of patriarchal control over women's lives; it was this issue that catalyzed the rise of the women's health movement.

Although not as well organized nor as powerful as the established medical profession and the pharmaceutical industry, health feminists were determined to take on these male-dominated institutions and their traditional assumptions and practices. In the decades to follow, the interests of feminists, female patients, physicians, drug manufacturers, and government officials would clash many times over issues such as diethylstilbestrol (DES), intrauterine devices, Depo-Provera, Norplant, and abortion. All of these debates had their own unique set of concerns; however, in each one the matter of informed consent, as articulated in the controversy over the safety of oral contraceptives, remained central.

Julie Is Not a Statistic

BARBARA SEAMAN

Barbara Seaman, "Julie Is Not a Statistic," in *The Doctors' Case Against the Pill,* New York: Peter H. Wyden, 1969. Reprinted by permission.

To five blue-eyed little girls, she was "mommy." To her husband, she was "the heart of our home." To her older sister, she was a "born mother. That was the thing God meant her for."

Whatever she was meant to be in life, Julie Macauley was not a statistic. She became a statistic only when she died at the age of twenty-nine from a pulmonary embolism and left her beloved husband, Tom, a widower and her children motherless.

Julie had been on the pill for less than a year. Her husband is convinced that it killed her and he is bitter against the doctors and drug manufacturers who he feels let death come so unnecessarily to his Julie.

"They say, 'Oh, it's only one in a thousand that's going to have trouble,'" he scoffed. "But this one in a thousand is my wife. She was the mother of five children. She was a real person. She was not a statistic."

Dr. Wood, a gynecologist in the large Midwestern city where Julie lived, placed her on the pill to regulate a long-standing menstrual irregularity. He testified in court that he had read drug company pamphlets and medical literature reporting more than 400 cases of clotting and thirty-seven deaths among pill users through 1964. Nevertheless, he had placed Mrs. Macauley on the pill in 1965 without warning her of its possibly dangerous side effects.

The doctor said that he considered the statistical evidence of clotting to be "quite small. . . . I think the physician is supposed to exercise judgment. That's what I did. I felt I would be doing the lady a disservice to report it to her. You can scare a patient to death."

The fact is that Julie would not have been "scared to death" if the doctor had come straight out and told her the risks she was facing. She was not the type to be stampeded. Her sister Peggy described her to us as a "solid, steady sort of person—very quiet, very determined. She just went her own way."

She had been independent even when she was a baby, Peggy said. "She was tall for her age, but when she was three and four, she always walked around with a little chair so she could get things she couldn't reach without having to ask for help. She was very tall and gangly by the time she reached her teens. She was really awkward then. And those long, gangly legs! They were always bent over chairs and things like that."

When Julie outgrew the gangly stage, she turned out to be a real beauty. She was tall, slender, blond. Her friends told her she should be a model. "She was a good student," her sister said, "but she didn't really like school. She didn't date much at first, but when she started to blossom, she dated quite a bit. And then she met Tom the summer right after she graduated from high school."

RHYTHM DIDN'T WORK

Anybody who knew Julie at all knew what was going to happen to her. She was going to get married and have a big family and live as happily ever after as real people ever do in real life.

"I met Julie when I was a sophomore," Tom Macauley told us. "We went together for two years before we got married, but I knew from the first that we were going to get married. When we were courting, we used to talk about the children we were going to have. We decided we wanted a large family, perhaps seven or eight children."

Julie and Tom got married while Tom was still in college. Their first daughter, Anne Marie, arrived within the year. The Macauleys decided that they should wait until Tom was through college before having another child. They turned to the only form of birth control acceptable to them as Roman Catholics.

"We practiced rhythm," Tom explained, "but it was very difficult." Julie had had very irregular cycles all the way from the time when she started having her periods. "It would vary between, say, twenty-eight days up to fifty-five or sixty days," Tom recalled. "Well, we kept track of it. We took her temperature every morning and recorded it versus the day of the cycle. We tried to avoid relations during the period when she would have ovulated and been fertile."

Despite their meticulous recordkeeping and their careful study of the charts, the result had been four more blond, blue-eyed girls in seven years. With such a history, Julie should have acquired the right in her obstetrician's office to be regarded as a human being with a very human problem. Instead, she was just an anonymous white record card. Her doctors were a team of three specialists who shared a suite of offices and practice. Tom described it as "a big assembly line."

When Julie made an appointment to see one of the doctors, she pointed out to him that the rhythm method of birth control obviously wasn't working for them because her periods were so extremely irregular. The doctor suggested that she take the pill. "Julie told him right away that she was a Catholic," Tom said. "And he said, 'Well, I'm giving it to you for medical reasons. I won't prescribe it for you until you go first and tell your priest.' He said that the pill had a tendency to adjust the hormone system of the body in some way so that the cycle became more regular.

So Julie "went to Monsignor O'Hara," Tom said, "who was our pastor. He said that it was a strictly medical matter. Julie called the doctor back and he phoned the prescription to the drugstore so we could pick it up."

OH, WE HAD PLANS

Tom paused and recalled softly: "I remember, I think the most joyful look I ever saw on her face was when our first child, Anne Marie, was born. The nurse brought the baby into the room. It was the first time she saw the baby, you know, and fed it. I never saw such a look of joy on a person's face as I saw that time. I got a little of an understanding of what this means to a woman from the expression on her face."

Tom recalled: "Julie was always happiest when we were working together or doing something as a family. "One particular incident I remember. We went out and bought one of those outdoor swing sets that were so popular for the backyard. All the kids had to stand around, of course, and watch Daddy put the swing set together. Lots of giggles and laughs. Of course Mommy and Daddy had to do a little clowning around. I think kids get the greatest kick out of their parents clowning around.

"I got the camera out and took a few pictures. And Julie took one of me sliding down the sliding board. I was obviously too big for the sliding board. It's things like this that I remember as our happiest moments, that I keep remembering.

"She was always busy. She liked to knit. And she did all the mending. We were thinking about buying a sewing machine and had started looking at the different models . . ."

He paused and shook his head.

"In 1963, we moved into this house. It was September that we moved in and she died just two years later.

"We had so many plans. We used to sit back and plan and say, 'Well, some day we'll have a couch here and a new rug. We'll get a new dining room set.' Oh, we had plans."

Peggy knew the pride her sister took in the new house and spent many hours talking with her about how it should be furnished as soon as there was enough money. "The sad part of it," Peggy said, "she was just beginning to reap the benefits of all their struggles and sacrifices so that Tom could get his degree. Life was just beginning to be a little more easy. They had a nice home now, but she never lived to see it the way she wanted it."

For a time, it seemed that Julie and Tom were indeed destined to live happily ever after, but when Julie started taking the pill to control her menstrual

irregularities, their life began to change. Tom tried to recall exactly what had happened. "Julie would become very upset and cry. It seemed like it didn't take anything at all to set her off. She would kind of go into a mood and it would last for a day of two.

"And then her attitude toward things changed. She became pessimistic. For example, she would feel that we were in real bad financial shape and things were not going to improve. She used to talk about our financial condition before, but she wouldn't get depressed and pessimistic. Our finances were typical for someone in our position. Naturally we weren't putting a lot of money in the bank or anything like that. But we were paying our bills. There were a lot of time payments, but I think any young married couple with five children has a lot of time payments."

ALL OF A SUDDEN . . .

Julie was depressed, on and off, for several months. But neither of them connected this change in her normally cheerful disposition with the pill. Tom was accustomed to doing a fair amount of traveling in connection with his job. Sometimes he would be away just overnight; other times, it would be for as long as a week. On the Tuesday before Julie died, he had to go on a trip.

"I returned Friday afternoon and found my wife sick," he told us. "She had been trying to get hold of the doctor. She had called the three rotating physicians, but they couldn't come out to see her.

"She told me she had had several incidents where she would be going about her business and all of a sudden, she would get very dizzy and break out in this cold sweat, become pale, and feel very sick. This occurred once when she went shopping, and I think it happened another time when she went to get her hair fixed. When she went shopping, she had a whole cart full of groceries and she felt so bad, she couldn't even bother with the groceries. She just told the girl to put them back and she got in the car and came home.

"She had been taking bed rest and trying to get

hold of a doctor all day. I finally succeeded in getting one to come out Friday night." The doctor checked her over and recommended that she go down to the hospital in the morning so that he could run some tests. He mentioned a chest X-ray, blood tests, and a urinalysis.

"The next morning," Tom recalled, "Julie wasn't feeling real well. There were no episodes of this dizziness, though, during the night. When we got ready to go down to the hospital, she wanted me to help her walk. She felt a little unsteady. I was surprised at how weak she was. We got to the hospital about 8:30 AM."

The doctor came out to talk to Tom after the tests on Julie had been completed. He seemed cheerful and unconcerned. "He said that he didn't see any reason to admit her to the hospital," Tom said. "The X-ray didn't show anything particular. He said something about a broken blood vessel showing up on the X-ray, but later on he said, 'I was mistaken about that.'

"He told me there was some pus in the urine and there was some indication of infection. But it wasn't anything that couldn't be cured with bed rest and a little bit of medication."

"I thought there was something more serious," Tom said. "And so did my wife. The doctor saw that we were uneasy about it. I said something to the effect that I thought she ought to be admitted to the hospital anyway or something like that. He came back and said there is nothing in these tests that indicates any reason for having your wife admitted. And I felt a little bit relieved when he said, 'Just bed rest and take this medication. It's just a mild infection.'"

So Tom and Julie went home. He fixed up the sofa in the living room for her with pillows and a blanket and they watched a football game on television together.

"I fixed her a steak, a broiled steak," Tom said. "She ate well."

But she stayed close to the sofa all afternoon. They started watching Jackie Gleason and Julie suddenly became very sick.

Tom remembered every moment of it. "She became pale and she broke out in a sweat. She started to breathe real hard. She told me, 'Quick! Call an ambulance!' They arrived fifteen minutes later.

"She asked me to fan her," Tom went on. "She was having trouble getting her breath. And she was white as a sheet, kind of a bluish white, I guess you'd say. And then all of a sudden her chest heaved up and her eyes rolled back in her head and she passed out."

Julie's mother had come over that day to care for the children, and she pitched in trying to help. She joined Tom at the sofa, fanning Julie. Her daughter looked up at her, just before she passed out and said, "Oh, Mommy, I don't think I'm going to make it."

"The ambulance came," Tom said, "and I held the oxygen on her mouth and we got her to the hospital. She was put in the emergency room. I was in the waiting room. The doctor came out later. I don't know exactly how much later it was, about forty-five minutes or so. And he said it didn't look too good. And then the nurse came up to him and I could see from the look on her face that she was dead . . .

"The doctor said, 'I don't understand it. I don't understand it.'"

Tom was not the sort of man who was ready to leave without understanding. He signed the release for an autopsy. And then he made an appointment with a well-recommended internist.

HAD JULIE DIED IN VAIN?

The first thing the doctor asked was, "Was she taking birth control pills?"

Tom was surprised. "Yes, does that have anything to do with it?"

"I'll bet," said the doctor, "that the autopsy will show a pulmonary embolism, a thrombus in the ovarian vein."

And he was right. The attending doctor told Tom later that Julie had died from "a thrombus in the right ovarian vein, which caused an embolus which eventually caused the pulmonary embolism."

Tom was not only stunned by the suddenness of Julie's death. He was determined to find out what had really happened. He made a point of researching the effects of the pill. He read everything relevant that he could get his hands on. He pored over the medical journals and talked to whatever experts were available. He became increasingly convinced that his wife's death had been unnecessary, that just a little time and a little interest would have made the crucial difference as to whether or not the doctor would have prescribed the pill for medical reasons.

He particularly resented that his wife had not been warned of the dangerous side effects. Slowly, quietly, he became angry. And the more he learned, the angrier he became. Tom sued the drug company that had manufactured the particular pill. He lost the case.

The jury of four women and eight men sat for two weeks while pathologists, blood coagulation specialists, gynecologists, and other authorities testified whether or not, in their opinion, the blood clot that killed Julie was unquestionably caused by the pill. Some of the experts maintained that the clot was indeed pill-induced; others, testifying for the drug company, dismissed the idea and voiced their opinion that an upper respiratory infection was more likely to have caused Julie's death.

The jury decided in May 1969 that the manufacturer was not guilty. But this group of responsible men and women had obviously been moved to worry deeply about the medical testimony they had been hearing. Indeed, they had become so concerned that they accompanied their verdict with an unusual and urgent comment. They said that they felt that the manufacturers of this oral contraceptive should make it a regular practice to warn doctors and patients that these pills may be dangerous.

Tom had sought $750,000 in damages from the drug company, but to him the money was not principally at stake (although it can be very expensive to bring five children up without a mother). Tom's crusade had been a valiant attempt to ensure that Julie had not died in vain, that her death would become widely known and turn into a warning to other women.

And perhaps it will. The trial was covered by the major news services and many newspapers sent their own reporters. Reports of the testimony and proceedings appeared in newspapers from coast to coast.

Today Tom tries not to look back. His life and that of his daughters is in the future. But it is hard. He keeps remembering—how they all ate together at the big dining table, the baby in the high chair beside Julie, how they all piled in the car for a week's visit to his folks to show the girls off to the relatives.

He keeps telling people, "She was a real person, the mother of five, not a statistic. And she was an important part—she and a thousand other mothers—of what we call the human race."

Philip Corfman

INTERVIEW BY TANIA KETENJIAN

Philip Corfman, MD, OB-GYN, was a member of the National Institutes of Health, the World Health Organization, and the Food and Drug Administration. This interview was conducted in June 1999.

TK: In its Tenth Anniversary Issue in 1982, *Ms.* magazine voted you one of forty male heroes of the women's movement. You were nominated for your "sensitive response to feminist health activists." *Ms.* lauded your "efforts to change the direction of birth control research so that male methods were included and safe methods for women were emphasized." What made you take paths that diverged from those of your male peers? Why do you have an interest in women's issues?

PC: It's hard to be objective about the reasons for your own interests, but I'll try to respond. Perhaps it started early in my life with my grandmother, Minnie Corfman, who told me that she could drive a team of horses "like a man," or my mother—a housewife—who told me that she earned half of my father's income. My father was a good model for me in that he shared in the housework and enjoyed it, as I do. Going to Oberlin, the first coeducational college, helped, and my wife, Eunice, whom I met there, was a feminist but didn't know it. She played on Oberlin's women's basketball team, and really hated having to play by "women's rules"— only three dribbles, for instance. And I remember her telling me just a few months before she died how she stopped her car to watch some kids playing soccer, and when she saw that they were girls she was so happy that she burst into tears.

TK: So a feminist perspective was ingrained in you very early on?

PC: Yes, I'd say so. And it's certainly enhanced by my partner, Harriet Presser, the demographer, who is a true feminist in that she not only believes in women's rights, but works aggressively for them.

TK: Tell me a little bit about what your aspirations were when you first became an obstetrician and gynecologist.

PC: After Oberlin, I went to medical school at Harvard and took all my specialty training in Boston. I chose obstetrics and gynecology because of the interesting combination of medicine and surgery that the specialty provides, and because even then I was interested in the population problem and the attendant reproductive health issues, particularly the need for better contraceptives.

After our nine years in Boston—during which time we had four children, built a house ourselves, and Eunice published several short stories and had a TV drama produced—I entered a clinical practice in upstate New York. I loved it. My patients were ex-urbanites from New York and farmers. I particularly liked obstetrics. Childbirth is usually a happy time, and I was often able to involve the husband in the delivery.

TK: Why did you leave clinical practice?

PC: I left after four years—during which time we built another house—because I simply didn't want to be only a clinician the rest of my career. I was offered a Macy Fellowship in New York to do cancer research, and took it.

Then, after less than two years, I was asked to join NIH [National Institutes of Health] as a "consultant in obstetrics and gynecology." It was clear that I would work on reproductive health issues— including contraceptives—but at first the responsibility couldn't be alluded to in my title.

TK: How long were you at NIH?

PC: I was at NIH for twenty years, from 1964 to 1984. I became the first director of the Center for Population Research in 1968. The Center originated from growing concern and recognition of the "population problem" in the US and worldwide. It also originated out of concern for the safety of the pill. The Institute was given three million dollars to study this problem in 1965 and I was put in charge, so we started our research work on contraception even before the Center was established.

We originated and supported a large prospective study in California, called the "Walnut Creek Oral Contraceptive Drug Study, somewhat similar to studies underway at the time in the UK. Ours was a ten year study that monitored the health of women who elected to take the Pill and to see if anything bad happened to them. Fortunately, no unexpected adverse effects of note were discovered. Another major pill study was a retrospective study by the Centers for Disease Control which demonstrated that the pill protects women against ovarian and endometrial cancer.

TK: As I remember there were problems with the Walnut Creek Study at the end. I understand that Dr. [Savriti] Ramcharan—who was the principal investor near the end of the project—is thought to have accepted drug company money to promote the pill and later went to Canada. All this led the women's health movement to have some doubts about the study. Do you think their doubts are justified?

PC: Certainly not. Only the general practice study in the UK equaled the Walnut Creek Study for its design and scope, and Dr. Ramcharan didn't work with the project long enough to have an effect on the quality or significance of the published findings. I'd say that Dr. Diana Petitti, a world-class epidemiologist who's now research director at Kaiser of Southern California, and Dr. Susan Harlap, another world-class epidemiologist—both of whom worked on the project much longer that Ramcharan—had a far greater effect on the quality of the work.

TK: Could you mention some of the other work that was done at the Center?

PC: The Center's program covered four very broad areas: basic reproductive biology research in humans and experimental animals; the development of new contraceptives; ascertaining the safety of contraceptives in use; and social science research in the population sciences. Since this involves an incredibly wide range of subjects over a twenty year period it would take a book to describe the work and the findings in a meaningful way.

TK: What led up to your becoming involved in activities at the Food and Drug Administration in 1968, when you were the director of the Center, and working at the National Institutes of Health?

PC: In 1966, before becoming Director, I was appointed by the FDA to its Obstetrics and Gynecology Advisory Committee, first as a consultant then as a Member. This committee was the first formally constituted Advisory Committee at the Agency. It was formed initially to deal with the safety of the birth control pill, but then was asked to address many other OB-GYN issues, such as the IUD, drugs for obstetrics, and hormone replacement therapy.

The Committee was appointed at a very active time in reproductive health issues. It was at the time that I testified at the Nelson hearings on the safety of the pill about the work that NIH was doing on this problem. That's when I first met Barbara Seaman. I met her again soon after that when she and her colleagues, who were sitting in the corridor outside the Committee meeting, were invited into the meeting by the members so that they could express their views. The FDA staff didn't want them to attend because up to that time, at least, such meetings were closed. Now, of course, most meetings like this are open to the public, in part because of the activism of Barbara and her colleagues.

This was also at the time that Barbara Seaman and others established the National Women's Health Network. I recognized very early that it was essential that Network staff participate in the Committee's meetings and would call them as soon as I knew that a meeting was scheduled.

I continued to attend Committee meetings either as a member or as an NIH Consultant until I was sent by NIH to work at the World Health Organization in 1984. When I returned from Geneva in 1987, I was asked by the FDA to become a medical officer to review new drugs for obstetrics and gynecology, and to be the executive secretary of the very committee that I had been on for many years. Its name had been changed by then to the Fertility and Maternal Health Drugs Advisory Committee, and more recently it was changed again to the Reproductive Health Drugs Advisory Committee.

TK: Why were you recruited to these two quite different positions at the FDA?

PC: I was recruited to the medical officer job because of my training and experience, particularly in reproductive health. As for being the Committee's executive secretary, the original intention when the committee system was set up was to have physicians as executive secretaries, since they were expected to know both the science involved and the scientists who worked in the field. I believe that this applied to me.

I very much enjoyed being executive secretary,

because the Committee provided a forum to discuss issues such as the safety of the Pill, or the value of hormone replacement therapy before the public, and it often became possible to take action on such issues rather rapidly.

TK: On January 23, 1970, during Senator Gaylord Nelson's hearings on the birth control pill, Alice Wolfson and her associates from D.C. Women's Liberation interrupted your testimony. The Wolfson women were cleared from the room by guards, as usual. The many other expert witnesses who were interrupted during those weeks of hearings and demonstrations seemed indignant, impatient, neutral, sometimes amused, but, the record shows, even those who most deplored the pill didn't want to hear about it from mere patients. Only you, of all the scores of witnesses, took the occasion to speak up in the demonstrators' defense. When Senator Nelson said, "Doctor, go ahead, you may proceed," you veered off from your prepared testimony to exclaim, "Some of the questions placed by people who interrupted our hearings were quite important." What were you feeling and thinking when you said this?

PC: Well, the questions were and are important; no one can deny it. The activists were women worried about the safety of the pill, and had a right to be heard. They also had a right to be wary of the predominance of men on the Committee and the fact that almost all of those giving expert testimony were also men.

TK: What made you decide to let Alice and Barbara listen in on the advisory committee meetings?

PC: The committee was taking a break when we saw Alice and Barbara waiting in the corridor outside the room. When we asked them what they were doing there, they said they wanted to attend the meeting because we were talking about the safety of the pill. The committee caucused, and, against the wishes of FDA staff, asked Alice and Barbara to join us and tell us what they had in mind. As I remember, the most important thing they said was

that women should be better informed about pill safety. This led in time to the patient package insert [PPI] for the pill—a really big step for which Alice and Barbara deserve much credit.

TK: Why do you think PPIs on the pill and estrogen are so important?

PC: Simply because patients should know just as much as possible about the pills their doctors prescribe. This applies to all drugs, not just the pill and other drugs for women.

TK: So why aren't patient package inserts applied for all drugs?

PC: It's primarily a political problem. At the end of the Carter administration, the FDA had in the works a plan to provide inserts for most drugs, but one of the first thing the Reagan administration did was to stop it. Later, when I was at the FDA, we tried to resurrect this plan, but it's bogged down someplace. Advocates must apply political pressure if they want to see some action on this issue.

TK: Years later you took your work to a global scale at the World Health Organization.

PC: After twenty years at NIH, I thought I'd like a new challenge, so I requested a detail by NIH to WHO to help manage the "Human Reproduction Programme." This was an activity quite similar in some ways to what we were doing at the Center, except that it was international in scope, and directed to the interests of developing countries. I very much enjoyed this work, and believe that I made a meaningful contribution. Of particular note was the research then underway at WHO which led to the availability of RU-486 in three European countries.

TK: And then you returned to the FDA?

PC: My detail to WHO ended in 1987, and I was fortunate to be offered a medical officer position at the FDA, where I worked until I left the public health service in 1998.

I had ten super years at the FDA. In some ways

I enjoyed the FDA more than other assignments because what I did was so close to actual clinical practice. We did practical things when I was there, such as bringing the pill label up to date. Labels may seem unimportant, but I assure you that they are not: a label is the government's record of what a drug is for, what its safety has been determined to be, and how it is to be used. We updated all the scientific information in the label, and added a health benefit section which notes that the pill prevents anemia, promotes regular cycles, prevents endometrial and ovarian cancers, as well as prevents pregnancy. Some of these findings were based on work that was done when I was still at NIH.

At another time we changed the label to say that a physical exam doesn't have to be done before the woman goes on the pill. Indeed, I think that the pill should be available without prescription, but that's another issue. We also removed from the market the higher dose pills which had been shown to be no more effective and somewhat more hazardous than lower dose pills.

Other contraceptive issues that came up during my watch were the approval of Norplant and Depo-Provera. We also were faced with issues relating to drugs for obstetrics and hormone replacement therapy.

TK: Looking back on all these changes in the health and the drug industries, what do you see as the effect of there now being more women in medicine?

PC: It's been great for patients. Women patients, at least, really prefer female doctors, and some men do too. A recent article in the *New England Journal of Medicine* attests to this. Barbara Seaman said some time ago that my specialty, at least, should have predominantly female practitioners, and that's happening: more than half the residents of obstetrics and gynecology are now women. The old boys are fading away.

A Pill for Men

BARBARA SEAMAN

Barbara Seaman and Gideon Seaman, excerpt from *Women and the Crisis in Sex Hormones*, New York: Rawson, 1977. Reprinted by permission.

The human male is a prodigious maker of sperm. In a single ejaculation he releases, to whatever destiny, some 80 million of these tiny life-bearing sex cells. Sperm are manufactured from precursor cells, in a process that takes about seventy days. Spermatogenesis is stimulated by two hormones, follicle-stimulating hormone (FSH) and luteinizing-hormone (LH), which issue from the pituitary.

Once the female was also a prodigious bearer of eggs. She, or rather her fish and amphibian foremothers, deposited a milky "egg clutch" into sea water and tidal marshes. The male dropped off his sperm in the same neighborhood, and they merged.

Out of the primordial slime, the mammal, the primate, and humankind evolved. Evolution *depended on dramatic advances in female reproduction*. She reduced her cyclical egg release from an enormous quotient to a selected few or one. *She* retained the conceptus—the product of conception—within her own body, developed a placenta, and nourished her babies from her own blood and bones. The advances that make us humans rest, as modern embryology explains it, on adaptations that the female of the evolving species made.

Male reproduction—and this is not to minimize its importance—is still much like reproduction in the amphibian and fish. Sperm production is extravagant, not conservative, and the male role is biologically ended when sperm go on their way. The reproductive role of woman is longer, harder, and much more dangerous to her.

Revolution—often it is sounded to drama, drums, and discussion, but sometimes it just settles over us like mist. While some fortunate women always had access to vaginal spermicides (Cleopatra, for example, used a mixture of honey and dried crocodile dung) it was *male contraceptive methods,* first withdrawal, and later the condom, that drastically reduced the birth rate in modern times.

Carefully used, these are far more effective than modern people imagine, but each has obvious drawbacks. Although it requires skill and discipline, withdrawal was the sole method of contraception used by two-thirds of the couples in France and Hungary *until 1960!* The birth rate in these countries was admirably low. It shouldn't be overlooked as a method for emergencies.

Margaret Sanger, among other feminists, believed it was essential for birth control to be in women's hands, but, of the new devices, many have proved injurious to health. Senator Gaylord Nelson's hearings on the pill were forced to recess on January 23, 1970, after a raucous demonstration by Alice Wolfson and a group of young, articulate Washington DC, health feminists.

"Why are there no patients testifying?" the Wolfson women demanded. "Why is the press whitewashing all the adverse comments against the pill? *Why is there no pill for men?*"

EARLY WORK ON A MALE PILL

The fear that a pill for men might alter male libido or the sex organs has been a major deterrent to research. *Hormones can have this effect on some users of either sex.* Masters and Johnson have stated that when a woman who was previously orgasmic loses her ability, the first question they must ask is, "Has she been taking the pill?"

Scientists view diminished *male* sex drive more ominously than the female equivalent. After all, they argue, libido is needed to *put sperm into action* but *not* to position the ova in place. Species continuation rests on the libidinous male. One government population official recently put it like this:

Many women don't have those orgasms you read about, anyway. A lot of that Masters

and Johnson and women's lib stuff is about the extremes, almost the abnormal. I never heard any hesitation based on whether the pill would affect whether a woman would have an orgasm.

Among the early human subjects to be tested for male fertility control were eight psychotic mental patients in a Massachusetts state hospital. They received an early form of Enovid in the 1950s. Ten milligrams a day of Enovid had a definite sterilizing effect. However, one young man was found—at the end of the five and one-half months' trial—to have shrunken testicles; his scrotum had become "soft and babyish," according to his doctor's report.

The sex drive of these patients—they can hardly be called volunteers—was not, in general, altered by Enovid. Their psychiatrists kept an eye on them, and they masturbated as much or as little as before.

Therefore, although Enovid was early shown to work for men, the fellow with the shrunken testicles put a damper on follow-up experiments. His side effect was viewed more seriously, we are sorry to report, than the unexplained *deaths* of three Puerto Rican women, during some of the early experiments with the pill.

Sex hormones, whether taken by implant, injection, or mouth, turn off sperm production, just as they do ova production, because they "fool" the pituitary into diminishing its natural output of the pituitary hormones FSH and LH. Within about two months' time (seventy days), sperm will be gone from the semen. Any sex steroid may have this effect, but the pills used for women are too feminizing to be suitable for men. (In fact, it's a little startling to realize that experiments on human males, proving beyond any doubt that *various hormones produce infertility,* date all the way back to 1939.)

Why not use more malish hormones, the androgens? (Both sexes produce male *and* female hormones, actually, but in different proportions.) Testosterone-only contraceptives for men do not cause feminization but may pose other problems, such as heart attacks and an increase of red cells in the blood. (Pills for women also cause heart attacks and blood disturbances, but men fear the former more acutely since they are *normally* at greater risk.)

A logical solution is to find a combination of male and female hormones so balanced that they avoid feminization on the one hand, or immediate overstimulation of the heart, blood cells, and prostate on the other. Such products are being clinically tested by, among others, Dr. C. Alvin Paulsen of the University of Washington, and Dr. Julian Frick from Innsbruck, Austria. Paulsen and Frick are investigating different combinations of drugs, which, inconveniently, involve taking *both* oral pills and monthly injections.

Any contraceptive that works through pituitary suppression is bound to have some long-range effects on the total system. The pituitary mediates *many* body functions, and it is always chancy to tamper with it. Thus, at best, male contraceptives *based on hormones* are unlikely to be safer than the current female pills. They "pool" the risks, but do not eliminate them, and should provide a fine sincerity test for men who claim they would die for love.

A MALE PILL THAT'S ALREADY HERE

The Paulsen and Frick formulations will not reach the market for years—certainly not, it is estimated, until the 1980s. But there are already products on the shelves of every drugstore that promise to be just as suitable.

These are the previously mentioned androgen and estrogen combinations, currently marketed as a treatment for osteoporosis, or bone loss, in aging individuals of both sexes and for the syndrome some people call male menopause. Their effectiveness as a bone treatment is disputed, but *hundreds of thousands of men have taken them, usually for long periods.* Some of the preparations include vitamins and mood brighteners, in addition to their dual sex hormones. *One also contains speed,* and is understandably hard to give up. More than a dozen brands are available, including Ayerst's Mediatric and Formatrix, Leferle's Gevrine, Reid-Provident's Estratest, Schering's Gynetone, Upjohn's Halodrin, and many more.

Far from being feminizing, such products usually contain substantially more androgen than estrogen (up to 500 times as much!) and so—while they are promoted as suitable for men or women—their manufacturers usually issue warnings such as the following:

> Watch female patients closely for signs of virilization. Some effects, such as voice changes, may not be reversible even when the drug is stopped.

Recently, Drs. Michael and Maxine Briggs of the Alfred Hospital, Melbourne, Australia, discovered that elderly men who use these products develop evidence of severely reduced sperm production without any such side effects as developing breasts, shrunken testicles, or grossly abnormal libido changes. They called for younger volunteers and selected five, who were instructed to take the osteoporosis pills twice daily with their meals.

At the end of the projected seventy days, or sooner, four of the five had stopped manufacturing sperm. The fifth patient took twice as long, but finally he stopped also.

The Briggs volunteers stayed on the hormones for thirty-four weeks, during sixteen of which their wives gave up birth control. No pregnancies resulted. Sperm production returned to normal in all cases within five weeks after stopping the drug.

Three of the five men had occasional mild nausea, but there were no anatomical effects. Two complained of decreased libido in the first eight weeks, which then returned to normal for the remainder of the trial. Another man had an increased sex drive, which leveled off when he stopped the medication. A fourth reported no changes while he took the hormones, but a decrease in sex drive when he stopped. This outcome might puzzle readers who are unacquainted with the aftereffects of the female pill. Any powerful drug suppresses some of our natural functions, which may in turn have some trouble reasserting themselves. As many of us have learned the hard way, we may all be too susceptible to a new infection right after taking an antibiotic.

What are the ethics of giving *an approved drug,* like these osteoporosis or male menopause remedies, *for an unapproved use,* such as contraception? Such questions are hotly debated among doctors, many of whom *do* prescribe hormones for purposes never dreamed of by the FDA or their own manufacturers. Two recent examples are the use of DES and Premarin as a morning-after female contraceptive, and a group of anabolic or "body-building" hormones, frequently prescribed to put flesh on athletes. Anabolic hormones could, in addition to building muscle, cause cancer of the prostate, breast cancer, and blood clots in athletes. They are rumored to have done just that to members of a professional football team.

Should any untoward effects occur, the doctor is in a weak legal position. However, he may get around it by asking the patient to sign a release.

This much can be said for the "new" male pill from Australia, limited as its contraceptive testing has been: A lot more is known about its side effects on men than was known about Enovid when *it* went on the market for women.

HIS SAFETY OR HERS?

In return for the wonders it may perform, any hormone is bound to have side effects. To pass off such potent pharmaceuticals as "natural" is nothing but fraud. The honorable way to prescribe drugs is to admit the risks, and let the patient decide whether he or she wants to take them. The Rx pad belongs to the doctor—but the body is the patient's alone. To prescribe a drug without informed consent is a violation of the Bill of Rights, we think—a kind of chemical assault.

The female pill was approved after little testing.

The side effects of the pill are quite well known now, but 50 million women worldwide are willing to take it. The pill is still the preferred method of one in five fertile women in the United States. Its male "twin," however chancy, will find a market as well, for, contrary to predictions of drug manufacturers and some researchers, men are not unwilling to share the risks. When Dr. Paulsen of Seattle ran a small ad in a college newspaper asking for volunteers, he was overrun with responses. He and others who supervise male programs get letters today by the handful.

Why has the research only just started? Why was male contraception ignored for twenty years (the 1950s and 1960s) while fortunes were being poured into finding new female products? Only in 1974 did funds for male studies start making any dent in the federal health budget. Nonprofit research groups, like the Population Council, are also supporting male projects, but not as generously as they might. Some $20 million is now being spent annually, the *Wall Street Journal* estimates, which is but one-fifth the amount needed to develop a contraceptive rapidly.

Unfortunately, drug companies have sharply reduced their efforts to deveop new contraceptives. Many projects have been abandoned. Executives say they are disenchanted with stringent federal test requirements (making it take longer than formerly to get a new drug on the market) and with costly lawsuits over the pill and the IUD.

A spur to research has been the arrival of a new medical specialty called andrology, concerned with male fertility. Another spur was the feminist charge of discrimination—denied, at first, by scientists who then rallied rather quickly to correct their course. The effort to find a male pill is hardly of crash proportions, but it exists. It is taken seriously. It may bear fruit.

Must a male pill rely on hormones? We hope not. There may be better ways of interrupting male fertility, *without involving the pituitary and higher brain centers.* Theoretically, a *safer* pill for men than for women might be devisable, but no one knows yet for sure. Discussion centers on the greater complexity of the female system. Sheldon Segal estimates that *there are fourteen stages at which a woman's fertility might be interrupted, but only seven in men.*

These male-female differences are looked at two ways. It can be argued, and is in some quarters, that woman's greater complexity affords more chances for interruption. It can be, and is, conversely argued that man's greater simplicity yields more opportunity to intervene *locally*, without widespread bodily effects. In women, reproduction is intertwined with many other functions, more so than in men.

Another debate centers on the natural history of ova and sperm. Unlike woman, whose lifetime supply of eggs is intact at birth, man produces new sperm as he goes along for most or all of his adult time span. It is feared that an imperfect fertility drug might allow a few damaged sperm to escape, producing defective fetuses. An opposing view is that permanent damage or latent drug effects on the sperm cells are less to be feared in the male. When he stops the pill he is set to manufacture brand-new sperm, whereas a woman's future-ripening ova might be residually influenced by a drug she once took.

OTHER SPERM INHIBITORS

The hypothalamus, a walnut-sized collection of brain cells, might be called the conductor of our endocrine symphony. In breakthrough research, Andrew Schally of New Orleans has recently isolated the hypothalamic chemicals that trigger the release of LH and FSH from the pituitary. Scientists in many laboratories are seeking hypothalamic suppressants based on his discoveries.

We mention Schally's work for its profound importance, as it much advances our knowledge of reproduction in both female and male. But we think it unlikely that a safe contraceptive will emerge from it. These hormones would affect both the hypothalamus and pituitary, and it is inadvisable to mess with them just for birth control. Local action in the genitals would be safer.

In England, Belgium, and Australia, scientists are working on a protein substance that might be able to block pituitary FSH secretion without altering LH. If the dream materializes, the protein may halt sperm production without at the same time inhibiting natural testosterone, or requiring supplements of the same.

Many drugs inhibit sperm formation in the testes or, if you prefer, testicles (the words are synonymous) without interfering with natural hormones. Thus far, all have exhibited unacceptable side effects, but the search goes on. One group, the nitrofurans, has had wide use as inhibitors of bacterial growth, but dosages high enough to sterilize are extremely toxic. Other sperm suppressants are found among cancer drugs (at least in mice) in a sugar analogue.

In 1960 a drug to treat intestinal amoebae was tested on prisoners and completely suppressed their sperm. When tried on men enjoying more normal circumstances, it was noted that the drug had the effect of Antabuse, causing dizziness and vomiting when alcohol was consumed. It might still have been marketed for teetotalers, except that during the two-month recovery period, abnormal and bizarre sperm and heart irregularities were reported.

Drugless intervention, such as heat, X-ray, diathermy, and laser beams, may also inhibit sperm and are being investigated.

Heat experiments were initiated, years ago, by Dr. I. Tokuyama of Japan, whose volunteer medical students submerged their scrota in hot water baths for half hour daily. Elevation of scrotal temperature by just a few degrees proved highly effective in sterilizing some men.

Next, Dr. John Rock, co-developer of the pill, got seventy-five of his students to either sit in hot water or wear insulated scrotal supporters—Rock's Hot Jock, they were nicknamed around Harvard. Now in retirement, Rock insists that the method *works*, but of course he was also the scientist who declared the pill to be safe.

In any case, Rock says that of his seventy-five volunteers only one complained of a side effect—sweating—and one other failed to show the usual reduction in sperm count. Subsequently, the wives of a number of these students conceived and bore normal children.

There is little question today that heat, including fever, reduces fertility some of the time. Hippocrates was aware of this, and today the first thing specialists tell their *infertile* patients is to stop wearing tight jockey shorts and trousers which, by generating heat in the scrotum, inadvertently sterilize some stylish men.

The great promoter of TMS (shorthand for "the thermatic method of temporary male sterilization") was Martha Voegeli, an indomitable Swiss physician using TMS in India since 1912.

Here is how she described her method: For three weeks, a man takes a daily 45-minute bath in water of 116°F. He then remains sterile for six months, after which normal fertility returns. If desired, the treatment can be repeated. (We suggest that men who try this get a sperm count done afterward to make sure it worked.)

At the University of Missouri, Dr. Mostafa Fahim, chief of Reproductive Biology, has been studying ultrasound for many years and has already designed a chair apparatus to administer ultrasound birth control in doctors' offices. He dreams that an ultrasound machine could become a standard home bathroom fixture. His trials on humans are mired down by requirements that, for the time being, he try ultrasound only on men with prostatic cancer, who (should the ultrasound prove dangerous) are already in line to have their testicles removed. At last report he'd located only one such patient—and he must find ten before he can proceed with healthy humans. Fahim complained: "We inject hundreds of chemicals into the woman's uterus but we never touch the testes." Some of the most militant feminist supporters are men who are trying to do contraceptive research—on their own sex.

WHAT DES TAUGHT US ABOUT MALE FERTILITY

After leaving the testes, sperm move on to the epididymis, a compact 2-inch oblong tissue lying within the scrotum, against each testicle, and containing six or more yards of tubing. Here in the epididymis, where sperm remain for about two weeks, maturation and storage take place. The epididymis is highly sensitive to drugs, and in theory could be "selectively" treated without ill effects on other system. When epididymal function is altered, sperm may be produced in normal numbers, but won't be competent to fertilize eggs.

At Cornell University, Dr. C. Michael Bedford, a veterinarian and physiologist, is doing important research into these crucial but long-neglected components of male reproduction. We are still a long way from a safe epididymal suppressant, but if and when it arrives, it might be the ideal method we have all awaited.

Recently, the epididymis has been in the news for a most unfortunate reason. Sons of mothers who were given the hormone DES to strengthen their pregnancies have a 10 to 25 percent incidence of cysts of the epididymis, which impair fertility. The same effect has been observed in laboratory animals.

Most of these DES sons are perfectly normal in other respects, which reaffirms scientific belief that the epididymis is an especially susceptible target organ.

SPERM SWITCHES, SPERM BANKS

Sperm is found in the testes, matured in the epididymis, and transported in the vas deferens, the spaghetti-like site where male sterilization—vasectomy—is performed. *Reversible* vasectomies, or "sperm switches," involving clamps, plugs, and faucets, have been so discussed and prematurely publicized that many men ask for them, thinking they are available.

They are not. While research continues at ten

universities and private laboratories, many observers are doubtful of success—ever. A narrow living channel like the vas is all too apt to scar over any temporary blockage, making the blockage permanent. No man should agree to be a test subject for one of these devices unless he is prepared to accept final sterility.

If "sperm switching" does not seem imminent, "sperm banking"—that is, preserving live sperm by freezing—prior to vasectomy may have a better chance. Animal sperm banks, especially for cattle, have been highly successful, but, in humans, the resurrection of frozen sperm still remains unpredictable. It is no more than 70 percent successful, at the most. No one yet knows why some sperm can take freezing and others cannot.

Seminal fluid has an amazing composition, which includes trace materials such as iron, zinc, and magnesium, and carbohydrates that appear to be an important source of energy for sperm. An alcohol which may be oxidized into fructose, a sugar, is also present in the human variety.

Certain oral medication such as sulfonamides may be traced in seminal fluid. Thus it is possible that the right oral drug might so influence the fluid as to keep the sperm from "capacitating." Sperm are not fully competent (capacitated) until they traverse the cervical mucus and womb, on their way up the fallopian tubes to the ultimate egg. The apparent purpose of seminal fluid, the ejaculate, is to carry the sperm from male to female. Still, its chemical complexity, including so much nourishment, suggests that it also plays a part in the sperm's final development. Products that inhibit capacitation on the sperm's last journey might either be added to the seminal fluid, or given to the woman.

When a woman is fertile, the progress of sperm through her vagina, cervix, and womb has been likened to spinning along on a highway; at other times in her cycle, the sperm's journey is more like slogging through a swamp. Altering the chemical environment provided by *her vagina* as well as by *his seminal fluid* offer possibilities for relatively safe birth control. Foundations and government bodies say that they want to develop new contraceptives for men. Until the 1970s they merely chortled at the notion, so it appears that genuine progress is afoot.

But, as Dr. Philip Corfman of the National Institutes of Health explains, a lot of research that *sounds* male-ish could just result in more new products for women to use. Sperm capacitation is an excellent example; contraceptives ensuing from these studies could well be vaginal suppositories or further female pills.

In the meantime, men who truly want to "participate" could experiment with TMS, according to Martha Voegeli's instructions. They could ask their doctors for one of the male menopause treatments, employed by Michael and Maxine Briggs; or they could buy quality condoms, thin ones, in Japan. They could go to France or Hungary for tutoring in withdrawal, and, of course, they can get a vasectomy, too.

Norplant: The Contraception You're Stuck With

BARBARA SEAMAN

Barbara Seaman, excerpt from "Norplant: The Contraceptive You're Stuck With," in *The Doctors' Case Against the Pill*, New York: Hunter House, 1995. Reprinted by permission.

Gregory Pincus, a father of the pill, was wary of estrogen, uncomfortable with its possible role in the development of cancer. His dream was to create a progestin-only contraceptive, and that is what he intended to test in his historic 1956 Puerto Rican clinical trials. Those were the trials, remember, when hundreds of mostly poor and uneducated Puerto Rican women were given the newly developed pill experimentally. In August 1956, several months into the study, Pincus sent a curious letter to his colleagues in San Juan. He apologized that a recent shipment of experimental pills was "contaminated" with a small amount of estrogen, and he reassured them it would not recur.

There was a problem with progestin-only contraceptives: they produced irregular and unpredictable spotting, or conversely, a complete absence of menstruation. Cycles ranged from just a few days in length to many months, a condition aptly called *menstrual chaos*. Pincus, after wavering back and forth, eventually put estrogen back into the pill being tested.

How much Pincus wavered is evidenced in his papers, which are now available at the Library of Congress and comprise 213 containers, 85.2 feet of shelf space, and approximately 44,000 items. His records reveal an awesome scientific and entrepreneurial brinkmanship and make one wonder why he didn't burn the evidence.

Evidence of what?

Well, for example, evidence that late in the study, the FDA informed Pincus that he would need a control group, and when the recruiter at the Family Planning Association in Rio Pedras could get no volunteers, Pincus instructed her to relabel the drop-out folders as "controls."

This made the records especially confusing, since it wasn't until May 1959 that the then-final formula, with the final amount of estrogen officially added to the progestin, was fabricated and shipped to the trial participants. Thus, the so-called control group was not only a drop-out group, but it was a drop-out group from a different pill.

It is interesting to note that female medical students and nurses at the University of San Juan were fearful of the study and refused to participate. According to a doctor who corresponded with Pincus, the medical students were punished with lower grades. The letters don't say what happened to the nurses.

THE PROGESTIN-ONLY CONTRACEPTIVE YOU CAN'T QUIT ON YOUR OWN

Since the days of the very first pills, the fatal flaw in progestin-only contraceptives has never been overcome. These products may be safer than those containing estrogen. They may be less associated with cancer, blood clots, and other crippling side effects, though whether or not all progestins are truly less of a cancer risk than estrogens remains unknown. But no scientist has ever been able to make them mimic the normal menstrual cycle in a majority of users.

Despite the menstrual chaos so often precipitated by progestin-only pills, they arrived on the market in the late 1960s, about ten years after Pincus' first pill, Enovid. Today these brands include Micronor and Nor-Q-D (both of which contain norethindrone, the first orally effective progestin) and Ovrette (which contains norgestrel and which some doctors suggest women might wish to "test-drive" if they are contemplating Norplant).

Norplant is a system of six matchstick-size Silastic capsules, which are implanted in the fleshy underside of a woman's arm, above the elbow. They contain levonorgestrel, a synthetic progestin, which slowly leaks out of the capsules and enters the bloodstream, providing a high degree of protection against pregnancy for up to five years.

Research for the development of Norplant was begun in the 1960s by Drs. Sheldon Segal and Horacio Croxatto of the Population Council, a nonprofit organization dedicated to global population control. More than ten compounds were evaluated and discarded.

A troubling fact about Norplant is that although it was tested for decades prior to receiving FDA approval, some of its worst "bugs" have never been corrected, and vital questions about long-term safety remain unanswered.

Norplant has a threefold effect. About half the time, it suppresses ovulation. However, should ovulation occur, Norplant has thickened the cervical mucus, preventing migration of sperm through the cervical canal to the uterus. Finally, Norplant suppresses the endometrium, so a pregnancy cannot be supported.

THE SELLING OF NORPLANT

In 1983, Finland became the first country to license Norplant, and Leiras Pharmaceuticals became its manufacturer. Although the product is assembled in Finland, its constituent hormone—levonorgestrel—is owned by US manufacturer Wyeth-Ayerst, who is also the distributor in the United States.

While Leiras has kept the price to developing countries at $23 per set, the cost in the United States was set much higher. Wyeth-Ayerst obtains its capsules from Leiras, repackages them with a few inexpensive items such as a plastic inserter, and resells the kits for at least $350 wholesale. The health care provider or pharmacy may then add a retail markup, which averages $75. Norplant insertion runs $100 to $250, and removal runs as high as $400 to $500. Thus, the cost for a woman in the United States to try Norplant today can be over $1,000.

Price notwithstanding, Norplant's debut in the United States in 1991 was most auspicious, due in part to aggressive promotion by Wyeth-Ayerst and the Population Council.

HOW SAFE IS NORPLANT?

The answer to the question of Norplant's safety, in terms of immediate deaths and disabilities, would seem favorable. Cynthia Pearson of the National Women's Health Network has received reports of only one death, and that was from general anesthesia used during a difficult removal.

Is it all right to insert Norplant immediately after childbirth, or should implantation be deferred? The Population Council warns against giving Norplant to nursing mothers, but this advice is often breached. Traces of Norplant occur in breast milk; how might this hormone exposure effect the nursing baby when she or he grows up?

In addition to unanswered questions, the evidence we do have about Norplant is not entirely unbiased. In large-scale surveillance studies of Norplant, the comparison or control groups tend to be IUD users. IUDs also create a measure of menstrual chaos, as well as pelvic inflammatory disease, so studies cannot tell us how Norplant users fare compared to women with normal, healthy menstruation.

Some women on Norplant may bleed for two to three weeks, then spot for any number of days, then bleed again for another two to three weeks. Other women may go several months without a period, then bleed or spot irregularly.

OTHER SIDE EFFECTS

Besides menstrual chaos, other side effects of Norplant have been reported: gain or loss of more than five pounds (32 percent); headaches, nervousness, or depression (15 to 33 percent); androgenic effects, including acne, growth of facial hair, and loss of scalp hair (up to 15 percent). Less common but also notable side effects include dizziness, breast soreness and nipple discharge, nausea, rashes, and infection or chronic pain at the insertion site.

These side effects, however, don't normally kill. The Norplant manufacturer relays warnings of more crippling or lethal complications, most of which are associated with blood clots. These warnings are based on experience with estrogen-containing contraceptives and may or may not be applicable to Norplant, or, if applicable, may occur much less frequently than with combination estrogen-progestin pills. It is hard to understand why, after decades of development, scientists have not yet determined whether Norplant may be implicated in strokes, heart attacks, birth defects, blood clots, or cancer, and why no solid information about long-term side effects exists. In the blunt words of Native American health advocate Charon Asetoyer, "The manufacturers of Norplant are marketing their product based on an assumption that the drug is not dangerous. There is no proof of this. Such overt negligence is inexcusable on the part of the company."

Wyeth-Ayerst, the US distributor, lists the following as absolute contraindications for Norplant's use:

➤ Pregnancy
➤ Acute liver disease, noncancerous or cancerous liver tumors
➤ Unexplained vaginal bleeding
➤ Breast cancer
➤ Blood clots in the legs, lungs, or eyes

Patient information pamphlets place other conditions in a "gray zone"—meaning they do not preclude Norplant use, but require medical supervision. These include: breast nodules or other abnormalities; diabetes; elevated blood fats; high blood pressure; headaches; gallbladder, heart, or kidney disease; history of scanty or irregular menstruation; and smoking.

Norplant users are advised to expect tenderness and swelling in the upper inner arm for a couple of days, while the insertion site heals. The implication is that, thereafter, the discomfort disappears. For many women, perhaps a majority, this is simply not so: a low to moderate level of tenderness, and sometimes inflammation, persists.

THE IMPACT OF NORPLANT ON A WOMAN'S LIFE

The World Health Organization, the Population Council, and the Norplant manufacturer have all set standards and conditions to be met before Norplant use, including a pregnancy test to assure that the patient is not pregnant, and a complete medical history. In addition, Norplant should not be given to a nursing woman, and no woman should be pressured to use it.

These guidelines, however, are often disregarded. Nursing mothers have routinely been started on Norplant without being advised that hormone residue will appear in their breast milk. Since women cannot remove their capsules without medical intervention, they become captive to them, regardless of worries or side effects. Even satisfied women who keep their implants for five years must in the end have them removed but may not be able to afford the often hefty price for the removal. They have no choice but to leave them in and suffer the consequences.

Providers of Norplant make little or no effort to grasp what the menstrual chaos may mean in a woman's life. In Thailand, pharmacist Judith Richter observed that at one hospital, half of the women provided with Norplant were prostitutes. When bleeding, they were unable to work and were deprived of their livelihood. In Indonesia, social anthropologist Jannemieke Hanhart learned that many Norplant recipients couldn't work because they were devout followers of Islam and, under Islamic law, women cannot pray, cook, wash their hair, fetch rice from the rice barn, plant certain crops, have intercourse, or participate in social ceremonies while they are bleeding. The women in one village lived seven kilometers from a water source; their water was carried on horseback or motorcycle to the village, so the more frequent washing of themselves and their clothing during menstruation was onerous.

If there is a positive outcome from the menstrual chaos caused by Norplant, it is that the most popular argument for omitting barrier methods from population programs has finally been laid to rest. In *The Politics of Contraception,* Dr. Carl Djerassi, the father of modern progestins, took issue with this author and other health feminists for suggesting that women in developing countries should be offered barrier contraceptives: "On safety grounds the diaphragm is clearly the best female contraceptive, and . . . may be ideal . . . for the motivated American woman willing to use it, but it is totally unsuitable for the impoverished woman living in a hovel lacking running water, toilet and privacy. . . . How can an affluent American female recommend to her impoverished sister in some Asian country that she use a diaphragm when this woman has not even any storage place for it or the jelly?" Norplant, which requires the most washing up of any contraceptive, opens the door for promoting safer methods.

THE POTENTIAL ABUSE OF WOMEN'S RIGHTS

Norplant presents abundant opportunities for coercion and social control. In Indonesia, where the government is making efforts at population control, the army has been used to scare people into trying implants.

No sooner was Norplant approved in the United States than some judges, penal authorities, and state legislators moved to use it coercively. They recommended a two-pronged approach: rewards, such as paying welfare mothers to go on it, and punishments, such as sending abusive mothers to jail if they refused it.

A report by the Hastings Center suggests the following guidelines for policy makers and health care providers for "the safe and respectful use of Norplant."

➤*Fair pricing.* "The current pricing structure of Wyeth-Ayerst is questionable and should be changed. . . . [Norplant's] development and testing were supported by the federal government and private foundations," so the company can't claim it is only trying to recoup its development expenses.

➤*Insurance coverage.* When women have public or private insurance coverage for Norplant or IUDs at the time of insertion, they risk being uninsured when they wish its removal. "Financial guarantees of removal should be extended at the time of insertion. . . . Insurance coverage of removals should be unconditional."

➤*Service delivery systems.* If skillful insertion and removal and appropriate follow-up care are lacking, the method should not be offered.

➤*Availability to adolescents.* As with adults, appropriate access requires adherence to informed consent and confidentiality.

➤*No links to public assistance.* Making Norplant a requirement for receiving public assistance is inappropriate. "A woman's health may make it dangerous for her to use a hormonal method, or she may be unable to tolerate the side effects. . . .

Her local health care system may lack personnel with adequate training and expertise. . . . She may be celibate or perfectly happy with her current method and competent in its use."

WHAT DOES THE FUTURE HOLD?

The word is that Norplant is in trouble. Sales are down to the point that the Population Council—which counted on a certain royalty from the sale of the implant—has had to freeze salaries.

Three separate class-action lawsuits seeking damage for hundreds of users have been filed. The plaintiffs assert that they were sorely wounded by Norplant, suffering "severe pain and scarring" when their practitioners attempted to remove the contraceptive. Either large, impenetrable masses of scar tissue, called "fibrous envelopes," formed around the capsules, or the capsules were incorrectly implanted and proved difficult to find, or the capsules broke, or they dislodged from their original location and moved to areas deeper in the body, or the practitioners lacked training and expertise in removal. How much more responsible and productive the introduction of Norplant could have been if these concerns had been taken seriously and the following suggestions thoroughly addressed.

First, no coercion will be used. Second, no practitioner will be licensed to place Norplant until she or he has demonstrated skill at removal. Third, every practitioner inserting Norplant must sign a document agreeing to remove the capsule, free of charge, at the user's request. Fourth, no woman with any of the problems Charon Asetoyer mentions—overweight, diabetic, or a heavy drinker—will be given Norplant until the health concerns about these matters are clarified by the industry. Fifth, veterans of studies in remote places must be located and assisted with contraceptive removal. Sixth, women whose activities, religious or mundane, would be sabotaged by menstrual chaos will be offered Norplant only if they fully understand what might happen. Seventh, along with her $600 Norplant installation kit, a patient will receive a generous supply of condoms—in a variety of colors and textures—and be reminded that, with or without Norplant, sex can kill, and barrier methods must be used as well.

Today, we check the claims for new products. With Norplant, women's health advocates are performing and publishing their own studies, and pooling information at international conferences. In the United States, through such organizations as the National Women's Health Network, the Boston Women's Health Book Collective, the Black Women's Health Project, the Native American Women's Health Education Resource Center, and the Committee on Women, Population and the Environment, we are spreading awareness.

Cycles of Hot and Cold: Trying to Learn Fertility Awareness in North America

KATIE SINGER

Katie Singer, "Cycles of Hot and Cold: Trying to Learn Fertility Awareness in North America." © 1999. Original for this publication.

Several years ago, my boyfriend and I drove from Santa Fe toward a cabin north of town to celebrate my birthday. "I've got another yeast infection," I said quietly.

The traffic had thinned. Our views of northern New Mexico's mesas and spring wildflowers were now unobstructed. "Well, that's lousy," he said.

The lousiness wasn't that I was sick but that we wouldn't be able to make love. Already that year I'd had several yeast infections because of irritation from the spermicide I used with my cervical cap.

How do I get out of here? I wondered. Out of feeling like my birthday celebration is only about sex, out of birth control that makes me sick?

Sex, fertility, love. Like the burning in my groin, they made a tangle too hot to touch.

A few years later, I heard about fertility awareness (FA), also called the sympto-thermal method or natural family planning (NFP), and decided to learn it. By daily charting her basal (waking) temperature and the secretions from and changes in her cervix, a woman can tell when she's fertile. If they want to conceive, couples who chart know the best time to try. To avoid pregnancy, they postpone intercourse on fertile days.

Fertility awareness is not the same as the (ineffective) rhythm method, which determines fertility by past cycles' patterns. FA gauges fertility as the woman's daily chart evolves. According to the World Health Organization, when used properly for birth control, it's virtually as effective as the pill.

I began learning fertility awareness primarily by taking classes and reading literature put out by Catholic organizations. Many statements in the literature didn't suit me. Despite my discomfort, I started to observe and record my fertility signals. I began to experience explosions of awe: I had never conceived or tried to, but now I could see bona fide proof of my fertility. My cycles had often been erratic, but now (from knowing when I ovulated), I could predict when my period would come. I was with a new man while I learned the method, and his interest in my cycles helped both of us appreciate my femaleness. As awareness of my fertility patterns emerged, they gently took the lead in our relating.

I began to see that while the rhythm of masculine sexuality is often on all the time—men are fertile all the time—feminine cycles invite periodic rest from sexual intimacy. Women are fertile, on average, only one-third of each cycle. Despite my feminist perspective, I came of age expecting that I should be available for sex all the time. I remember one three- or four-month period when I was physically able and wanting to have sex every day. Surely, I thought, my boyfriend and I would stay together if I could keep this up. And how did my access to artificial birth control contribute to such thinking?

Indeed, sterilization, the pill, the IUD, the diaphragm, the cervical cap, and condoms give women the option of having fewer children than earlier generations. These methods allow choice about the course of our lives. Usually, however, these methods are distributed without substantial information about how our bodies or the methods work. Artificial birth control allows people to explore sex without awareness of their fertility.

I began to wonder what price we pay when we don't know this basic information about ourselves.

In the first part of her menstrual cycle, while she's maturing an egg, a woman's body is cooler. Men's testicles, where sperm are produced, hang outside their trunks for the same reason: human eggs prefer cooler temperatures during production. Women heat up after ovulation, during the cycle's second phase, to support an embryo's gestation; they cool down when a new cycle begins. These patterns can be seen when a woman charts her waking temperature.

Cervical fluid (CF) typically cycles through the following pattern: after the period (which some FA teachers assume to be fertile, since CF can't be discerned through blood), a woman will experience several "dry" days. The CF samples she takes with toilet tissue or a clean finger from just inside her vagina will not feel slippery or textured. Then the CF (which, when fertile, can keep sperm alive in the cervix for up to five days) will build up, beginning with a moist sensation and/or a sticky texture. Near ovulation, her CF tends to become slippery and clear—like raw egg white. After ovulation, it typically becomes dry again. A woman who charts can identify her days as infertile or fertile.

Women are like the earth, whose surface continues to develop through processes of heating and cooling and moistening and drying.

Charting began to feel like spiritual practice. I felt much more connected to myself and to other women who understood their own cycles. And as we learned and practiced fertility awareness, my partner began to realize, "I used to wake up and ask myself, 'When was the last time I masturbated? Have I had intercourse in the last twenty-four hours?'" With FA as our birth control, he wondered instead if I was fertile or infertile.

Why hadn't we learned this method before?

Because of my passion for the method, I began writing a story about its availability in northern New Mexico. I called Shirley Hoeffler, the director of a natural family planning clinic at St. Joseph's Hospital in Albuquerque. Her program teaches a cervical fluid–only method. Just from looking at a woman's charts, Hoeffler told me, she can tell if the woman is prone to miscarriage, ovarian cysts, and other gynecological problems.

When she said she would be offering a course to train people to teach the method, I asked for an application.

"I could send you one," Hoeffler said, "but I couldn't accept you."

I was stunned. "Why?" I asked.

"Because you have genital contact."

"Because I'm not married?" I asked, groping for clarity.

"No," she said. "Because you're single and you have genital contact." If I was celibate or married, then her program could accept me.

This was June 1997.

Hoeffler's policy propelled me onto a tour of conversations with nurse practitioners in women's clinics, the director of medical affairs for Planned Parenthood, the medical journalist Nona Aguilar, and finally Suzannah Doyle, who writes about the method for *Our Bodies, Ourselves.*

Laurie Holmes is a highly esteemed certified nurse-midwife in Santa Fe who dispenses birth control, primarily to low-income women. "I've seen too many unwanted pregnancies with fertility awareness to feel entirely comfortable endorsing it," she said. "I bring it up, but people need time to learn it and stay with the daily charting. I think you need to be open to failure if you use it. I also find that people don't want abstinence."

I told Laurie (who, like most health care practitioners, is not trained to use or teach FA) about the first woman I met who used it. She'd had two abortions by the time she was twenty-one, then vowed never again to have an unwanted pregnancy. After her second abortion, she chose FA for birth control, and 115 cycles later, she hasn't conceived again.

Laurie Holmes found it exceptional that a woman would have the discipline to take her temperature every morning all those years.

I began to wonder if fertility awareness is not taught as well in the women's community as it is among Catholics (certainly it's less available), and how this figures into practitioners' lack of faith in the method and people's capacity to commit to daily charting. Are the teaching methods, commitments, and self-control expressed in the Catholic community not available to others?

Kara Anderson, Planned Parenthood's director of medical affairs, explained that their practitioners rarely have more than twenty minutes with each client. "Most of the people who come to us have been sexually active for six months—without any birth control.". . . If a client asks to learn fertility awareness (which is unusual), she's usually referred elsewhere—often to a teacher affiliated with a Catholic organization. "To learn this method well," Anderson said, "a woman needs to be in close touch with a teacher for three or four months. In many areas, Catholic organizations seem to provide the method's only teachers."

But how to administer such time-intensive classes? Who would pay for them?

The Couple to Couple League is staffed primarily by volunteer, married couples who perceive teaching as "service," and it's therefore able to offer classes at a nominal fee. Indeed, the CCL admirably meets the needs of religious Catholics. Their classes last for four months, and couples new to the method are encouraged to stay in touch by phone with their teachers.

Currently, there are 525 volunteer couples who teach NFP through the CCL. These teachers are required to sign a principle statement advocating, for example, rejection of abortion and homosexual behavior, and marriage and breast-feeding as necessary ingredients in healthy families.

While I appreciate CCL's clear outlaying of their beliefs, their style discourages individual decision making around very personal issues. For me, this makes learning fertility awareness with them awkward at best.

Nona Aguilar's book *The New, No-Pill, No-Risk Birth Control* presents thorough, accurate information on how to chart fertility signals. It also includes inspiring testimony from couples who switched to this method and found it significantly enriched their intimacy. Her book was a treasure, one of only two books I found on the subject after a year of scouting Santa Fe stores, and it didn't come with a moral bias. Aguilar was my heroine.

I told her so when I reached her, then described my frustration that I was not acceptable to the Albuquerque training program.

"Well," she said respectfully, "I agree with that policy."

I leaned back in my chair. "Okay," I said. "I don't understand this. Please explain."

"Properly used, prayerfully used," she began, "sex is about emotional and psychological union. In our culture, artificial birth control—which feminists have strongly advocated—has made sex a recreational activity. But it's meant to be a transcendent one. Sex is the life-bearing force of humankind. When lovemaking is turned into something recreational, it's a little like being colorblind during sunset over the Grand Canyon. Union becomes harder to experience, and that's a loss."

Aguilar's thoughts stirred me deeply and encouraged me to revere fertility awareness more than before. Our conversations also clarified my desire for classes that teach people how our bodies work, how various kinds of birth control affect reproductive systems and risk the transfer of sexually transmitted diseases, and that offer opportunity for individuals to differentiate between their personal inhibitions around sexual issues and the prohibitions suggested by society. And still, I felt qualified to teach such classes despite my not being celibate, despite my never having felt moved to marry.

Finally, I called the Boston Women's Health Book Collective. I was given the number of Suzannah Doyle, who's written about the method for the last several issues of *Our Bodies, Ourselves.*

Like Shirley Hoeffler, Suzannah can read a woman's charts and tell if she's prone to miscarriages or ovarian cysts. "That's not hard to learn," she said.

Indeed, charting speaks to a tradition (before male doctors took over the delivering of babies, distributed the pill, and provided abortions) when women were in charge of their own health care.

Doyle explained that fertility awareness teachers usually tell their clients that they have choices during their fertile times: barrier methods to prevent pregnancy, sexual expression that doesn't include genital-genital contact, or postponing intercourse. "In either case," Doyle said, "since women are fertile only one-third of their cycle, using birth control for two-thirds of it is a waste."

Doyle also confirmed that most of the scientists who've done research in this field have been male, Catholic MDs. Until the 1980s, fertility awareness was only available from a Catholic perspective. Since then, nonreligious teachers (who usually learned the method through Catholic organizations) have offered classes.

Now, the fertility awareness community is often divided between those who are pro-choice and pro-life. "I like to call myself" *pre* -choice," Doyle said.

Currently, there is no national group that advocates fertility awareness and informed choice. There are several organizations—including the Ovulation Method Teachers Association, the LA Regional Family Planning Council, and the Fertility Awareness Network—which, however small, conduct classes in using the method and training for teachers. But usually, those who teach fertility awareness in their own communities are in touch with each other informally, without institutional support.

I'm dreaming now: of adolescents knowing how their reproductive systems work before they become sexually active and before they choose a birth control method; of women and men being as aware of our fertility as we are about our sexuality; of fertility awareness classes as available as the pill; of alliances between those who provide health care education in women's and Catholic communities; of alternative and allopathic medical students learning how to diagnose and treat women's imbalances based on charting of fertility signals;* of medical researchers making use of women's fertility awareness charts; of every person knowing, intimately, the sacredness of their procreative powers.

---

*In China, charts of women's basal body temperatures (BBTs) are routinely used to diagnose gynecological health, as the pulse and the tongue are used to gauge overall health. Like the approximately thirty acupuncturists in the United States who have special training in gynecology, mine uses the BBT as a diagnostic tool to treat gynecological imbalances.

CHAPTER 4

Menstruation

In the beginning, the menstrual process inspired fear and wonder in human beings. Both men and women saw at once that woman's blood set woman apart from man in a mysterious, magical way. This blood flowed but did not bring death or disability; it came and went with a regularity that no human act could change.

—Janice Delaney, Mary Jane Lupton, and Emily Toth

THERE ARE FEW EXPERIENCES that are as formative for women as getting your first period. One way or another, it forces you to examine and ask important questions about your biological and social identity. For some of us, periods are a difficult thing—they mean struggling monthly with pain, mood swings, and sometimes crippling cramps. For many others they are just a minor inconvenience made well worth it by their monthly message that pregnancy isn't happening.

Menstruation has historically been a point on which discrimination against women was initiated, and while the subject is no longer "in the closet"—women speak openly about it, and joke about it in ways that range from the helpful to the hurtful—it is still a process on which sexism runs rampant. Recent debates about the role of women in the military reveal that long-held stereotypes about bleeding are still alive and well: but what if she gets her period?

Perhaps more insidiously, anxiety about menstruation is used by pharmaceutical companies to sell a variety of drugs. Irregular periods are used to push birth control pills on young girls. When Eli Lilly's blockbuster antidepressant Prozac was set to go off patent in 2000, Lilly made a new market for the drug by re-branding it Sarafem and prescribing it in a patronizingly pink fashion for the treatment of premenstrual dysphoric disorder. What, exactly, is PMDD? It turns out that most people aren't sure—the American Psychiatric Association has been unable to agree that it exists. Generally it is defined as depression or severe mood disruption that has a relationship to the menstrual cycle. The problem is, it is hard to distinguish this new "disease" from either regular clinical depression or from the normal mood fluctuation associated with premenstrual syndrome.

Most respectable health professionals called the "discovery" of the disease what it was—an effort to protect a profitable pill at the expense of women.

In the past several years a new myth of menstruation is gaining steam—the myth that periods are obsolete. Not coincidentally, theories suggesting that it would be healthier for women to bleed less (like our ancestors who were in near constant gestation) have come just as new birth control pills that cut down or cut out periods are being pushed on the market. First there was Seasonale, a pill that cut the yearly twelve periods to three. Now there are others—Seasonique and the period-stopping Lybrel. While certainly a percentage of women suffer monthly from debilitating pain, most don't. Makers of these new pills, in addition to spreading fear about the body's natural processes, don't widely publicize the fact that their new wonder drugs are associated with a huge incidence of intermenstrual spotting and also carry the recommendation that users take a monthly pregnancy test. That marketers missed this crucial function of the period—telling a woman that she isn't pregnant—shows the disconnect between the pill pushers and potential consumers. For women who unwittingly become pregnant, the outlook may not be good. We know from the tragedy of DES that extended exposure to estrogen in utero causes sexual and reproductive problems, and even cancer. Another possible danger of the drugs, says Dr. Richard Crout, is that they prevent the shedding of the endometrial lining, which may eventually lead to greater incidences of endometrial cancer.

The larger point, perhaps, is that women are still fighting cultural and social attitudes that would tell them that their bodies, as they exist naturally, are diseased. Much like menopause, which has been medicalized for decades, it seems that periods are being increasingly made the province of the doctor and the pharmacist. Such an outlook can only come from holding a male body to be normative and seeking to "cure" the processes that make our bodies distinctively female.

If Men Could Menstruate

GLORIA STEINEM

Gloria Steinem, "If Men Could Menstruate: A Political Fantasy," *Ms.*, October, 1978. Reprinted by permission.

A white minority of the world has spent centuries conning us into thinking that a white skin makes people superior—even though the only thing it really does is make them more subject to ultraviolet rays and to wrinkles. Male human beings have built whole cultures around the idea that penis envy is "natural" to women—though having such an unprotected organ might be said to make men vulnerable, and the power to give birth makes womb envy at least as logical.

In short, the characteristics of the powerful, whatever they may be, are thought to be better than the characteristics of the powerless—and logic has nothing to do with it.

What would happen, for instance, if suddenly, magically, men could menstruate and women could not?

The answer is clear—menstruation would become an enviable, boast-worthy, masculine event:

Men would brag about how long and how much.

Boys would mark the onset of menses, that longed-for proof of manhood, with religious ritual and stag parties.

Congress would fund a National Institute of Dysmenorrhea to help stamp out monthly discomforts.

Sanitary supplies would be federally funded and free. (Of course, some men would still pay for the prestige of commercial brands such as John Wayne Tampons, Muhammad Ali's Rope-a-Dope Pads, Joe Namath Jock Shields—"For Those Light Bachelor Days," and Robert "Baretta" Blake Maxi Pads.)

Military men, right-wing politicians, and religious fundamentalists would cite menstruation ("men-struation") as proof that only men could serve in the army ("you have to give blood to take blood"), occupy political office ("can women be aggressive without that steadfast cycle governed by the planet Mars?"), be priests and ministers ("how could a woman give her blood for our sins?"), or rabbis ("without the monthly loss of impurities, women remain unclean").

Male radicals, left-wing politicians, and mystics, however, would insist that women are equal, just different, and that any woman could enter their ranks if only she were willing to self-inflict a major wound every month ("you must give blood for the revolution"), recognize the preeminence of menstrual issues, or subordinate her selfness to all men in their Cycle of Enlightenment.

Street guys would brag ("I'm a three-pad man") or answer praise from a buddy ("Man, you lookin' good!") by giving fives and saying, "Yeah, man, I'm on the rag!"

TV shows would treat the subject at length. ("Happy Days": Richie and Potsie try to convince Fonzie that he is still "the Fonz," though he has missed two periods in a row.) So would newspapers. (Shark Scare Threatens Menstruating Men. Judge Cites Monthly Stress in Pardoning Rapist.) And movies. (Newman and Redford in *Blood Brothers*!)

Men would convince women that intercourse was more pleasurable at "that time of the month." Lesbians would be said to fear blood and therefore life itself—though probably only because they needed a good menstruating man.

Of course, male intellectuals would offer the most moral and logical arguments. How could a woman master any discipline that demanded a sense of time, space, mathematics, or measurement, for instance, without that built-in gift for measuring anything at all? In the rarefied fields of philosophy and religion, could women compensate for missing the rhythm of the universe? Or for their lack of symbolic death and resurrection every month?

Liberal males in every field would try to be kind: the fact that "these people" have no gift for measuring life or connecting to the universe, the liberals would explain, should be punishment enough.

And how would women be trained to react? One can imagine traditional women agreeing to all these arguments with a staunch and smiling masochism. ("The ERA would force housewives to wound themselves every month": Phyllis Schlafly. "Your husband's blood is as sacred as that of Jesus—and so sexy, too!": Marabel Morgan.) Reformers and Queen Bees would try to imitate men and pretend to have a monthly cycle. All feminists would explain endlessly that men, too, needed to be liberated from the false idea of Martian aggressiveness, just as women needed to escape the bonds of menses envy. Radical feminists would add that the oppression of the nonmenstrual was the pattern for all other oppressions. ("Vampires were our first freedom fighters!") Cultural feminists would develop a bloodless imagery in art and literature. Socialist feminists would insist that only under capitalism would men be able to monopolize menstrual blood. . . .

In fact, if men could menstruate, the power justifications could probably go on forever.

If we let them.

The Selling of Premenstrual Syndrome

ANDREA EAGAN

Andrea Eagan, "The Selling of Premenstrual Syndrome: Who Profits from Making PMS 'The Disease of the '80s'?" *Ms.*, October 1983. Reprinted by permission.

In the summer of 1961, I was working as a laboratory assistant at a major pharmaceutical firm. Seminars were regularly given on recent scientific developments, and that summer there was one on oral contraceptives. As a rule, only the scientists went to the seminars. But for this one, every woman in the place showed up. Oral contraception sounded like a miracle, a dream come true.

During the discussion, someone asked whether the drug was safe. Yes, we were assured, it was perfectly safe. It had been thoroughly tested, and besides, you were only adjusting the proportions of naturally occurring substances in the body, putting in a little estrogen and progesterone to fool the body into thinking that it was "just a little bit pregnant." The dream, we now know, was much too good to be true. But we learned that only after years of using the pill, after we had already become a generation of guinea pigs.

Since then, we have presumably learned something: we have become cautious about medical miracles and scientific breakthroughs. To suddenly discover, then, that thousands of women are rushing to get an untested drug to cure a suspected but entirely unproved hormone deficiency which manifests itself as a condition with a startling variety of symptoms—known by the catchall name "premenstrual syndrome" (PMS)—is a little shocking.

When I began seeing articles about PMS and progesterone treatment, I immediately had some questions. Why was PMS suddenly "news"? What did we really know about progesterone? And who were the advocates of this treatment?

PMS itself was not news. It was first mentioned in the medical literature in the 1930s, and women presumably had it before then. Estimates on the numbers of women affected by PMS vary wildly. Some claim that as many as 80 percent are affected, while others place estimates at 20 percent. Similarly, the doctors' opinions vary on the number and type of symptoms that may indicate PMS. They cite from twenty up to 150 physical and psychological symptoms, ranging from bloating to rage. The key to recognizing PMS and differentiating it from anything else that might cause some or all of a woman's symptoms is timing. The symptoms appear at some point after ovulation (midcycle) and disappear at the beginning of the menstrual period. (It should not be confused with dysmenorrhea or menstrual discomfort, about which much is known, and for which several effective, safe treatments have been developed.)

While PMS is generally acknowledged to be a physical, as well as a psychological, disorder, there is little agreement on what causes it or how it should be treated. There are at least half a dozen theories as to its cause ranging from an alteration in the way that the body uses glucose to excessive estrogen levels—none of which have been convincingly demonstrated.

One of the most vocal proponents of PMS treatment is Katharina Dalton, a British physician who has been treating the condition for more than thirty years. Dalton believes that PMS results from a deficiency of progesterone, a hormone that is normally present at high levels during the second half of the menstrual cycle and during pregnancy. Her treatment, and that of her followers, relies on the administration of progesterone during the premenstrual phase of the cycle.

Although she promotes the progesterone treatment, Dalton has no direct evidence of a hormone deficiency in PMS sufferers. Because progesterone is secreted cyclically in irregular bursts, and testing of blood levels of progesterone is complicated and expensive; studies have been unable to show conclusively that women with PMS symptoms have lower levels of progesterone than other women. Dalton's evidence is indirect: the symptoms of PMS are relieved by the administration of progesterone.

Upon learning about Dalton's diagnosis and cure, many women concluded that they had the symptoms she was talking about. But when they asked their doctors for progesterone treatment, they generally got nowhere. Progesterone is not approved by the FDA for treatment of PMS, there is nothing in the medical literature showing clearly what causes PMS, and there has never been a well-designed, controlled study here or in England on the effect of progesterone on PMS.

Despite some doctors' reluctance to prescribe progesterone, self-help groups began springing up, and special clinics were established to treat PMS. Women who had any of the reported symptoms (cyclical or not) headed en masse for the clinics or flew thousands of miles to doctors whose willingness to prescribe progesterone had become known through the PMS network. And a few pharmacists began putting progesterone powder in suppository form and doing a thriving business.

How did PMS suddenly become the rage? At least part of the publicity can be traced to an enterprising young man named James Hovey. He met Katharina Dalton in Holland several years ago at a conference on the biological basis of violent behavior. Returning to the United States, he started the National Center for Premenstrual Syndrome and Menstrual Distress in New York City, Boston, Memphis, and Los Angeles—each with a local doctor as medical director.

For $265 (paid in advance), you got three visits. The initial visit consisted of a physical exam and interview and a lengthy questionnaire on symptoms. During the second visit, the clinic dispensed advice on diet and vitamins and reviewed a monthly record the patient was asked to keep. On the third visit, if symptoms still persisted, most patients received a prescription for progesterone.

Last year, James Hovey's wife, Donna, a nurse who was working in his New York clinic, told me that they were participating in an FDA-approved study of progesterone, in conjunction with a doctor from the University of Tennessee. In fact, to date the FDA has approved only one study in progesterone treatment of PMS, which is conducted at the National Institute of Child Health and Human Development, an organization unrelated to James Hovey.

Similar contradictions and misrepresentations, as well as Hovey's lack of qualifications to be conducting research or running a medical facility, were exposed by two journalists last year. Hovey left New York and gave up his interest in the New York and Boston clinics. He is currently running a nationwide PMS referral service out of New Hampshire.

In a recent interview, Hovey said that the clinic business is too time-consuming, and that he is getting out. His "only interest is research," he says. At last report, Hovey still headed H and K Pharmaceuticals, a company founded in 1981 for the manufacture of progesterone suppositories.

Hovey's involvement in PMS treatment seems to have centered on the commercial opportunities. Others, such as Virginia Cassara, became interested for more personal reasons.

Cassara, a social worker from Wisconsin, went to England in 1979 to be treated by Dalton for severe PMS. The treatment was successful and Cassara returned to spread the good news. Cassara began counseling and speaking, selling Dalton's books and other literature. Her national group, PMS Action, now has a budget of $650,000, seventeen paid staff members, and forty volunteers. Cassara spends most of her time traveling and speaking.

Cassara's argument is compelling, at least initially. She describes the misery of PMS sufferers, and the variety of ineffective medical treatments they have been subjected to for relief. For anyone who is sensitive to women's health issues, it is a familiar tale: a condition that afflicts perhaps millions of women has never been studied; a treatment that gives relief is ignored. Women, says Cassara, are pushed into diet and exercise regimens that are difficult to maintain and don't always work. One valid solution, she feels, is progesterone.

According to FDA spokesperson Roger Eastep, initial studies have yet to be done for progesterone. But in the meantime, more and more doctors are prescribing the hormone for PMS.

Dr. Michelle Harrison, a gynecologist practicing in Cambridge, Massachusetts, is one physician who does prescribe progesterone to some women, with mixed feelings. "I've seen it dramatically temper women's reactions," she says. "For those women whose lives are shattered by PMS, who've made repeated suicide attempts or who are unable to keep a job, you have to do something. But I have a very frightening consent form that they have to sign before I'll give progesterone to them." Harrison also stresses that a lot of PMS is iatrogenic; that is, it is caused by medical treatment. It often appears for the first time after a woman has stopped taking birth control pills, after tubal ligation, or even after a hysterectomy, in which the ovaries have been removed.

When doctors do prescribe progesterone, their ideas of the appropriate dosage can vary from 50 to 2,400 mg per day. Some women are symptom-free as long as they are taking the drug, but the symptoms reappear as soon as they stop, regardless of where they are in their menstrual cycle.

For all these reasons, some women are taking much higher doses than their doctors prescribe. Michelle Harrison had heard of women taking 2,400 mg per day; Dalton had heard about 3,000; Cassara knows women who take 4,000. Because PMS symptoms tend to occur when progesterone is not being taken, some women take it every day, instead of only during the premenstrual phase. Some bleed all the time; others don't menstruate at all. Vaginal and rectal swelling are common. Animal studies have shown increased rates of breast tumors and cervical cancer.

Reminding her of the history of the pill, DES, and ERT, I asked Virginia Cassara whether she was concerned about the long-term effects of progesterone on women. "I guess I don't think there could be anything worse than serious PMS," she responded. "Even cancer?" I asked. "Absolutely. Even cancer." Later, she said, "I think it's very pa-ternalistic of the FDA to make those choices for us, to tell us what we can and cannot put into our bodies. Women with PMS are competent beings, capable of making their own choices."

I don't have severe PMS, and I don't think I fully understand the desperation of women who do and who see help at last within reach. But given our limited knowledge of how progesterone works, I do not understand why women like Cassara are echoing drug company complaints of overregulation by the FDA. I'm alarmed to see women flocking to use an untested substance about which there is substantial suspicion, whose mode of action is not known, to treat a condition whose very cause is a mystery. And I fear that, somewhere down the line, we will finally learn all about progesterone treatment, and it won't be what we want to know.

One doctor, who refused to be quoted by name, cheerfully assured me that progesterone was safe. "Even if a woman is taking 1,600 mg per day, the amount of circulating progesterone is still only a quarter of what is normally circulating during preg-nancy." And I couldn't help but think of the doctor at the seminar more than twenty years ago: "Of course it's safe. It's just like being a little pregnant."

No More T.O.M.

SARA GERMAIN

Sara Germain, "No More T.O.M.," 2008. Original for this publication.

Brace yourselves ladies, it is time to celebrate. Those medical experts have finally landed on the one thing that will make our lives, as women, blissful and carefree. That is right. No. More. Periods. At long last we no longer have to fear Aunt Flo's visit, the curse will be lifted, the crimson tide will cease flowing and we can all finally con-tribute fully towards society without the monthly debilitation of our periods that leaves us all in such a state of helplessness. Our savior, the new birth control pill Lybrel is here. Praise the Food and Drug Administration (FDA).

Lybrel was approved by the FDA in May of 2007. This blessed little pill is so far considered to protect against pregnancy as effectively as many other mainstream birth control pills with one dif-ference: Lybrel does not include a week of placebo pills, thus women who are taking it receive a con-tinuous supply of hormones that will cease the monthly shedding of the lining of their uteruses. Or so they say.

The FDA approved Lybrel based on two clinical trials, each lasting for one year, of more than 2,400 women aged eighteen to forty-nine. These clinical trials held by Wyeth indicated that the elimination of these monthly periods comes at a cost. Indeed, unanticipated "breakthrough bleeding" occurred in half to most of the women involved in the trials. Breakthrough bleeding is bleeding that occurs while taking the active pills of oral contraceptives, in other words, the pills that are not placebos. Wyeth states on their website that "Unscheduled bleeding or spotting is likely to occur while you are taking Lybrel. The convenience of having no regular menstrual periods should be weighed against the inconvenience of unscheduled or unplanned breakthrough bleeding or spotting." Thus, while Lybrel will theoretically eliminate our monthlies from plaguing us, it will come at the cost of never knowing when breakthrough bleeding might occur. Is this worth it?

If you listen to advertisements for Lybrel, then it certainly is. Headlines and ads all over are proclaiming Lybrel as the new pill for the *modern* woman who, for the first time, will have control over her own body. In this way, she will be able to rise above her bodily functions. She will be in control, rather than nature.

The entire basis of this pill lies on the assumption that menstruation is an undesired burden that a sensible woman would want to avoid. While it is very true that there are some women who experience very severe symptoms with their monthly periods, they are in the minority. Most women, believe it or not, can function quite normally while in the process of shedding their uterus linings, although many of us have been conditioned to think otherwise.

This trend of shame over one's periods can be observed through looking at the line of "feminine products," or pads and tampons. Pads, more politely referred to as "sanitary napkins," have become both smaller and more tightly packaged as time has gone on, so as to allow the menstruating women to walk to the bathroom with the pad properly concealed in a pocket or purse, and to shield her from the embarrassment of letting others know that she is experiencing feminine problems. Tampons, too, have aimed to become smaller while still absorbing the same amount of fluid, so as to be slipped skillfully inside a woman's purse. Menstruation is not considered a topic decent for every day conversation, and thus, is it

any wonder most women feel such shame around their periods?

Karen Houppert, author of *The Curse: Confronting the Last Unmentionable Taboo, Menstruation*, states that "every time women start demanding access to this or that, there is a rash of studies 'proving' that menstrual cycles render them unsuitable."[1] In the late 1800s there was a belief that women should not be educated, lest the blood move from their uteruses to their brains, causing their uteruses to shrivel up and leave these women barren and unable to perform their function of bearing children. After all, we all know that a woman is only as good as her uterus.

Of course, no one was concerned about women's shriveling uteruses during WWII when women were needed to fill the jobs that men left behind. Menstruation was not considered so debilitating during this time.

There seems to be a contradictory struggle in the advertising techniques over how to go about pushing this pill on women and convincing them that Lybrel is really what they need. While one technique includes displaying the modern woman who just has no time for such base things as her period, another technique takes the complete opposite route, and flat out states that monthly periods are unnatural. A headline stating this appeared in *Glamour* magazine in July 2000 next to other cover headlines that read "Does This Make Me Look Fat?" "What Makes a Woman an Unforgettable Lover," and "The New Sex Accelerator." This leads to another unavoidable aspect of this pill: no monthlies means sex is available all the time.

Just like the good old days before birth control was invented! In this same *Glamour* article, period-suppressing pills are explained by stating that the *natural* state of woman is that of the cavewoman, who was always either pregnant or breastfeeding, and thus menstruated less. In this way, Lybrel is being pitched as either the newest and most modern pill in the most advanced scientific research, or the pill that puts women in their more natural place, back to the days of the cavewomen. I ask you what is more natural, letting your body perform its monthly cleansing cycle or interrupting it with a period-suppressing pill?

Some are going so far as to force the idea that having your monthly period can make you sick or even cause cancer! It is cited that women who never go through pregnancy or breast-feeding have higher risks of endometrial and ovarian cancer, since their bodies never get a "break" from their monthly cycles. In other words, if you are not a good woman who performs her duties as defined by her body's abilities then you will suffer the consequences and will inevitably get cancer. Perhaps this is the same line of reasoning over why the new vaccine that protects against cervical cancer, Gardasil, is not offered to women over the age of twenty-six—at that point a good woman would be in a monogamous marriage where HPV will no longer be an issue.

In regards to cancer, many women are rightfully demanding to know whether period-suppressing pills will lead to greater health problems down the road. Looking at the history of birth control pills, and women's health in general, this is a very valid concern. When the birth control pill was first introduced in the 1950s it contained estrogen levels ten times the amount that are present in most birth control pills on the market today. In just looking at Barbara Seaman's 1969 book *The Doctors' Case Against the Pill*, I think most people would be alarmed. Chapter titles read: "Blood-Clotting: No. 1 Danger," "Strokes and the Pill," "How the Pill Can Spoil Sex," "Sterility and the Pill," "Cancer and the Pill," "Heart Disease and the Pill," "Diabetes and the Pill," and "The Pill and Jaundice, Thyroid Function, Weight Gain, Urinary Infections, Arthritis, Skin and Gum Problems, etc." Needless to say, birth control pills have always affected women's health, and in most cases, as seen above, the effect has been negative.

At this point, the long-term side effects of constantly exposing your body to the hormones in Lybrel are conveniently not yet determined. Con-

sequently it would appear that the only negative side effect of Lybrel is the spotting and break-through bleeding. I have to wonder, however, how allowing the lining of the uterus to continually sit inside and never shed itself will affect women's health. It has also been determined that the hormones produced naturally inside a woman throughout the cycle that includes her period affect other aspects of her body besides that of reproduction. Similar to the discovery that a woman's ovaries continue to produce hormones that are needed by her body after menopause, so too does a woman's period and her cycle affect the overall health of her body. Functions as broad as metabolic rate, temperature regulations, pain, gastrointestinal function, reaction to insulin in diabetes, and immune function are all affected by the delicate production of hormones that a woman's cycle goes through. The age range that is being targeted by advertisements of Lybrel also poses some serious health questions, as young women who are just beginning to menstruate have very different health needs than women who have been menstruating for a longer period of time. The consequences of starting young girls on this pill when they are just beginning to menstruate could be disastrous. For example, there has been a discovery that such pills prevent young girls' pelvic bones from widening, and thus cause a much increased chance of having to undergo a Cesarean section later in life. How the continuous exposure to these hormones will affect young girls is something to cause much worry.

Perhaps it should also be considered that taking hormones that will determine one's monthly cycle is hardly exercising personal control; rather, your body will become dependent on these pills, learning to take its cue from them rather than running its own cyclical course. This pill promotes hatred of one's own body, teaching women that there is something wrong and dirty about themselves, and that they need science to intervene and protect them from their own selves. Personally, I have never felt more in control of my body than when I went off of the birth control pill that I was taking. In order for the pill to work properly, it has to be taken every day at about the same time. It appears to me that these pills hold more influence over us than we do over them.

And let us not forget the not-so-little fact that our periods are necessary in order to tell us if we are pregnant. Because of this, Wyeth has issued a recommendation that women who are taking Lybrel receive a monthly pregnancy test, since taking these pills while unknowingly pregnant can cause real harm to the fetus. Add this to the breakthrough bleeding and we have ourselves a real convenience here!

Several gynecologists have predicted that these pills will not make it on the market. What with the breakthrough bleeding and the constant stress over never knowing if you are pregnant, perhaps women are not ready for Lybrel. Seasonale, the less extreme version of Lybrel, which causes women to have a period every eighty-four days, has significant breakthrough bleeding as well. Perhaps pills such as Yaz and 24-4, which contain twenty-four active pills and four placebo pills, and thus cut down the amount of days women are menstruating per month, will be more accepted. Some gynecologists even predict that the body has a way of "righting" itself, and that a woman's periods cannot be suppressed forever.

It has been reported that after Lybrel is no longer taken, menstruation and the ability to become pregnant return within three months. Many women have stated that they consider their periods a significant part of what makes them female, and that, believe it or not, they do not dread their monthly bleedings. Perhaps rather than hiding behind a pill, we women should try to rid ourselves of the shame and embarrassment that comes along with our periods. Or, as a good friend of mine told me, we should walk down the hall with our "sanitary napkins" out in the open for all the world to know that we are menstruating.

It would be better for women if we embraced and celebrated menstruation rather than treated it as a cause of shame. Perhaps it should also be considered that before we attempt to turn a birth control pill into a period-managing tyrant, we should enter an almost unknown realm of, dare I say it, creating a birth control pill for men. Much can be learned about society's standards just by looking at the drugs on the market for women and for men. If women's health were given as much support and concern as Viagra is given, then women would have much less to worry about.

NOTE

1. Karen Houppert, "Final Period," *New York Times*, July 17, 2007.

CHAPTER 5

Pregnancy and Birthing

IT WAS DURING THE BIRTH of my first child—my son Noah—that I first became radicalized on the subject of women's health. While I was carrying him, I discussed my intention to breast-feed with my doctor. It seemed like a given to me: my mother had breast-fed me and I wanted the same experience. My doctor's response surprised me: "You wouldn't make a good cow," he said with the patronizing confidence of the male physician in the 1950s. At that time, doctors had been convinced by infant formula companies that their product was more nutritious than mothers' milk. I argued with him and eventually thought he understood my position.

Flash forward several months and I had a new baby who had been healthy at birth, and quickly became sick and started losing weight. I couldn't imagine what was going wrong with my perfect son, but it was terrifying me and potentially threatening his life. What I discovered enraged me and put me on the road to a career as a health activist. My doctor had ignored my stated intention to breast-feed and had prescribed a laxative that had entered my breast milk. My baby wasn't wasting away because of some nasty virus or birth defect—rather, it was because my doctor didn't respect me enough to listen to what I was saying. I began writing about the experience and other women's health topics, which eventually led to my first book about the dangers of the birth control pill.

In certain ways, the experience of giving birth in America is almost unrecognizable from the one I knew in the 1950s. Women continue to work during their pregnancy and after their baby is born. A far cry from the over-medicalized experience that almost always involved drugs, fear, and didn't involve fathers, women now can choose to work with midwives and birthing centers, experience home births, or even deliver in the water. As Naomi Woolf has pointed out, many of the old problems still linger—she writes with passion about the pressure she received from obstetricians who thought she would be crazy not to have an episiotomy and an epidural—but over the past half-century, women have fought to create options and choices when they decide to become mothers.

Today there are new issues and controversies facing would-be parents.

Treating infertility has become a multi-billion dollar industry, yet the safety of various drugs and strategies employed by clinics has yet to be demonstrated. Instead, people struggling to conceive have too often become easy prey for irresponsible doctors who are all too ready to push potentially carcinogenic drugs on women's bodies. Egg donation and other reproductive technologies have created conversations about how one becomes a parent, and what different models of motherhood might look like. Same-sex parents continue to push these boundaries as well, helping to create new ways of imagining families.

Many of the conversations we were having in the 1970s are still being echoed in the voices of young activists. How a woman decides to balance work and family life is still a huge issue, as well as the extent to which medicine should play a role in the natural process of giving birth. Choosing when and how to become a parent is different in many ways, but fundamental issues remain the same. In the 1970s, we were very concerned with reproductive choice—that a woman should be able to decide for herself at what age and in what circumstances to become a parent. Amy Richards wrote with honesty in 2004 about her decision to reduce her three conceived fetuses to one baby, which she carried to term. Richard's candor angered pro-life activists and she received death threats following the publication of her article in the *New York Times*.

Childbirth in America

EDITED BY VICTORIA ENG AND SONIA LANDER

Richard W. Wertz and Dorothy C. Wertz, excerpt from *Lying In: A History of Childbirth in America*, New York: Free Press, 1977; Margaret Charles Smith and Linda Janet Holmes, *Listen to Me Good: The Life Story of an Alabama Midwife*,

Columbus: Ohio State University Press, 1996. Reprinted by permission.

Margaret Charles Smith, the subject of Listen to Me Good: The Story of an Alabama Midwife, *attended over 3,000 births, had nearly perfect results, and adapted to the mother's choice of birth position, however awkward it might be for Smith herself. In contrast, the experimental maternity techniques of nineteenth-century male physicians, as described here by Richard and Dorothy Wertz, seem needlessly bloody and barbaric. How these doctors lured some (by no means all) women to forgo midwives for the new "technology" remains a puzzle.*

Richard and Dorothy Wertz's book *Lying In: A History of Childbirth in America* vividly illustrates the takeover of midwifery, and ultimately of women's bodies and health, by male physicians. Women in childbirth often suffered greatly because of the ignorant practices of male physicians. These barber-surgeons often resorted to the use of horrific surgical tools. The following passage begins with an excerpt from Dr. Samuel Bard's *Compendium on the Theory and Practice of Midwifery* published in New York in 1815.

[The young doctor] will probably fail at first, for want of judgment, to discriminate accurately between one case and another, as well as for want of skill and dexterity in the application of his instruments; and finding himself foiled in the use of safer lever and forceps, he will become alarmed, confused, and apprehensive for his patient's safety, as well as for his own reputation. And now, deeming a speedy delivery essential to both, and that, having taken the case into his own hands, and began his work, he thinks he must not desist before he has accomplished it, he flies to the crotchet [an instrument for killing, cutting, and extracting a fetus lodged in the birth canal] as more easy in its application, and more certain in its effect—with this he probably succeeds; and although the poor infant is sacrificed, yet he persuades himself, perhaps honestly believes, this was necessary.

After 1750 American men began to return from medical education abroad to practice in colonial towns and cities. Perhaps the most notable medical attainment they brought, in terms of potentially widespread and concrete medical benefit, was new knowledge and skills to aid women in birth in ways that uneducated American midwives could not match. The doctors called their science and arts relative to birth by the traditional term "midwifery," but they realized that it constituted medical science's first major practical advance. . . .

French doctors had come to regard the birth process as a natural process and defined midwifery as a science. . . .

By defining birth as a natural process that followed its own laws, as a machine with shapes and movements of its own, the French reduced its potentially awesome aspects and removed its emotional and spiritual associations from their consideration. They could then look intently at what determined the success or failure of birth, and that would be their arena for further scientific and medical art.

They could have done this and have been wrong. It was common practice at that time to sever the sacred and the natural and to posit mechanical models for natural processes. But the mechanical model of birth was fortuitously accurate and adequate to describe many of the normal and abnormal events of birth.

The French achievement consisted primarily in finding a better understanding of birth rather than in discovering new techniques to aid it. Even their mechanistic view did not explain many of the pathologies of birth. It led some surgeons to make deep cuts to expand the birth canal or to open the abdomen, but, since the women usually died, they had to abandon such attempts to reshape or circumvent the birth medicine. . . . Often knowing that the canal was misshapen or inadequate only enabled them to announce that a woman would die. . . .

The new midwifery had a different beginning in England. There it was not associated with medical institutions in which generations of birth attendants accumulated experience and formulated a new view of birth's processes. Rather, it began in the often desperate struggles of poorly educated medical empirics, the barber-surgeons, to save the life of the mother by extracting the child with whatever tools they could devise. . . .

These empirical operators had a wide range of instruments—in fact, a real armamentarium—to extract the fetus, living or dead. They had blunt hooks to bring down the thighs in a breech delivery, sharp hooks (crotchets) and knives and perforators to puncture the fetus's head when it was completely impacted or dead, and the ancient device of the *speculum matricis* to dilate the vagina and make it easier to cut out obstructions or reach the fetus. Often they used the fillet, a strip of flexible but firm material, to slip into the uterus and loop around the child to pull it out. Most often the surgeons had to kill the impacted child in order to save the mother's life. Their efforts were not those of scientific observers but of desperate practical technicians, experimenting with various tools to aid delivery, rushing to save life often by killing life.[1]

In the mid-nineteenth century, after Queen Victoria elected to use chloroform during her own deliveries, it became acceptable to use anesthetics to relieve labor pain; from then on, the comfort of the patient was considered more important than the safe delivery of the baby. Class prejudice and Victorian notions of modesty played key roles in the development of clinical training in obstetrics.

Male midwives, as they called themselves, went to great pains to protect the chastity and purity of their middle-class and upper-middle-class patients, often at the expense of good clinical practice.

The medical profession claimed that a doctor who could not practice "by the sense of touch alone" was incompetent in midwifery, and American textbooks on midwifery, drawing from French originals, obligingly illustrated that point by showing the doctor on one knee before his standing patient, feeling under her long skirts, with his eyes averted and staring abstractly into the distance.

The problem for modesty became not touch but sight, whether the male doctor could see the genitalia and whether the patient could see the doctor seeing her body. Exposure during physical examination and during delivery were the matters of most extreme delicacy in nineteenth-century America, for both doctors and patients. Exposure had been a problem in the previous century also, and British instructors in midwifery, such as [William] Smellie, had to resort to using a "mock-woman" to demonstrate the processes of birth to most students, although occasionally Smellie, [William] Shippen, and other instructors found poor women who were willing to allow male students to observe their deliveries. . . .

A committee of the American Medical Association deprecated the exposure of a patient during delivery as unnecessary since a physician had to learn to conduct labor by touch alone or he was unfit to practice. Other national responses were more varied, some pointing out that clinical training in obstetrics had long been common in foreign countries and had contributed to new knowledge and better skills for complications of birth and other female conditions. Other doctors feared, however,

that, if men could not perform obstetrical operations (including catheterization, forceps, and even embryotomy) "as well without the eye as with it," obstetrical practice would so offend women that they would choose female attendants and thus ruin many male doctors' practice.

The fit doctor was to be essentially a blind man. . . .

Most doctors went forth to attend birth with no clinical experience; those from better medical schools associated with clinics or hospitals may have had experience of the touch alone. A desire to overcome the restriction on clinical training, which often created ignorance and mishap, prompted Dr. James White of Buffalo to demonstrate a delivery upon a living patient before a group of medical students in 1850. The woman was from the country poorhouse, was having her second illegitimate child, and was one of the recent Irish immigrants in Buffalo, a group of second-class citizens who had only shortly before won the right to enter the state legally. The presence of such a low-status female population may have been essential for clinical midwifery to proceed, for doctors could classify such women as not needing or deserving the same symptomatic treatment given to respectable women. . . .

In the early decades of the nineteenth century in many cities doctors and philanthropic patrons did establish separate maternity hospitals as charitable asylums for poor or unmarried women who the doctors and patrons believed deserved a clean, comfortable, and moral environment in which to deliver and to rehabilitate themselves. . . .

After the Civil War doctors realized that maternity hospitals provided occasions for clinical obstetrics; students might learn and professors teach and research. Doctors therefore struck a bargain with the charity patients in such hospitals; in exchange for medical treatment, the women would allow themselves to be exposed to the eye of medicine. Doctors could do this because respectable women patrons supported such institutions for the deserving poor, who were valuable to the patrons as object lessons about the redeemability of the poor and the value of charity.

The maternity hospital was an interesting example of the exchange of benefits between social classes, for what the doctors learned in treating the poor they could use in treating respectable women in their home. Doctors could study birth more intently . . . for they could disregard the scruples and feelings of poor charity patients more readily than those of respectable women. Since doctors acquired little status from treating the poor, the maternity hospital allowed obstetrics to transcend the barrier of modesty and to begin to transform itself into a science that looked primarily at the physical processes of birth rather than at patients.[2]

Despite these atrocities, professional, male-dominated, scientific procedures were considered safer and more socially acceptable than those of women's midwifery. Male doctors were largely ignorant of the midwives' methods, and perhaps because they felt competitive with these women, they set about to discredit and ultimately destroy the longstanding tradition of lay midwifery.

But the patients of barber-surgeons—the recognized pioneers in the practice of obstetric medicine—had much higher mortality rates than those of lay midwives. One such woman, Margaret Charles Smith, the subject of *Listen to Me Good: The Life Story of an Alabama Midwife* is notable for her sterling record: Smith attended over 3,000 births during her long career, and lost not a single mother and very few babies.

Lay midwives had no formal education and delivered babies for poor women (both white and black); sometimes (probably because the care was considered so good) they delivered the babies of middle- and upper-middle-class white women as well. Over the course of time, laws were passed that strictly regulated the role of midwives. However, enforcement of these regulations did not extend into poor black America—and that is why Smith was able to keep most of her methods intact.

The following passage, told in Margaret Charles Smith's own words, discusses many traditional birth techniques that midwives used.

When I first get to the mother's home, I'd see if I can find stuff to make a pad for them to deliver on. If they have some newspaper, I'd sit down and twirl that newspaper together and tack it so it won't slip and slide. If you put twenty sheets together, you won't have no trouble. See, you twirl them and fold them in a certain way, and then you tack it in each corner. I put that in the bed. That would catch the waste, so it won't get on the mattress, and it won't get on the sheet. I learned how to make the basket to catch the afterbirth out of newspaper. I learned that in Tuskegee.

Then sometimes, I'd tell the mother to go take a hot bath, and that hot water helps a lot. I sit their feet in hot water or let them sit in that tub, if they got it, a number three tub. I was willing to let them have their way until push comes to shove. Some of them would say, "I don't want to take a bath."

I'd say, "Just get in the tub, and I'll bathe you." I was right there to get them out, but some of them just wouldn't do it.

You are sitting there to do what you can for her, rub her or put something under her back, trying to rest her back some. That's what you are there for, talk to her. If you like tea, you can make them some hot tea, and that will pick them pains up. Then you can rub the stomach and make the pains start back. I'd put some grease in my hand or whatever the lady happened to have and rub it in. Sometimes I'd rub their back. That's where the misery was—in their back and stomach, but you know, if I go rub their stomach that would make some pains rise, and they'd want me to stop rubbing their stomach, so I'd rub their back, and some of them had all their pain in their back.

Sometime they want to get up, and I'd help them up. Walk around the room. Walk a pain off then get back in the bed. A lot of people get a kick out of walking. Go into different rooms and sit in different chairs, or get down on their knees—anywhere they think they can get ease. But there's no ease for birth till it's over with. It's good to walk, but you'll have to stop sometime. You can pretty much do what you want till you get down to the real nitty-gritty.

Now, some of the mothers be talking all this slack talk. But you're the midwife. So you, well, you got to take that. You could get up and tell them, "It doesn't make a difference. I don't care. It ain't no skin off my teeth."

I don't think that would be the words to speak. You are there. You just as well make the best of it you can, talking kind, giving kind words, and rubbing her hands. That means a lot. That means all of it. Kindness whipped the devil. Kind words, that's right, and belief. If somebody is sick, and you start talking rash to them, that hurts their feelings, but if you talk kind to them, why, that makes a lot of difference.

I'd just tell them, "Well honey child, you're going to have to hurt before your baby's born. It ain't no way around that. You can expect that. Now the pains ain't hard now, but they're going to be hard. I want you to be aware of what's coming, and you'll have to learn to take it as it comes, and it will soon be over. If you are going to buck and ram and holler, you ain't going to help you none. You might as well settle yourself down and do the best you can."

See, a midwife just can't say, "You got to do so-and-so."

You know what you got to do, and you got to do it, but you can go around in a better way and make it more pleasant, the way I see it. You keep a-talking to them until they realize they got to bear to it.[3]

Women had more control over the process of their labor under the traditional practice of midwifery. This is in stark contrast to the procedures of clinical deliveries, which required women to be passive.

When it comes time to deliver, most of them want you to fold a quilt and put it down on the floor and turn down a straight-back chair like that one yonder with the cane-seat bottom. You put the pillows on back of it. Turn it down where they can be halfway kind of sitting up like, and their bottom part be scooted out. Somebody holds their bottom part, and somebody holds their knees. You take this chair and turn it down where she could feel the heat from the fireplace. The mother can't get cold, 'cause if she gets too cold, that's going to cut the pains down.

And then some of them get on their knees. If they're on their knees, they got some pillows on the back of the chair. They just open their knees out. Some people won't have a baby no other but that way. Mostly there be two or three women around. They use the back of the chair to support their back, and the people help them get down.[4]

Smith, however, was forced to submit to some of the regulations. Here, she recounts her decision to abandon the use of herbal remedies that were considered threatening by the medical establishment.

Now, the nurses didn't know what was good and what was bad. You can take too much of anything. You just need enough to warm you up inside and get those pains a-moving, if you done done everything you can do on the outside.

I had to stop fooling with teas and things in labor because my name was getting out.

"Miss Margaret, how come you are not using some of that stuff you used on Emma or Lucille. She was telling me about what good stuff you had. Why don't you give me some? Fix some for me so I can get through with this baby."

See, my name was getting where I could hear it. I stopped right then. I had been practicing a good while. I was going by what Miss Ella Anderson taught, but I stopped. I already knew about the teas 'cause I was going with this other midwife. They used to make teas for the mothers to pick the pains up.

The woman told us in the clinic, I think we had a meeting of all the midwives, the woman was from Selma.

She said, "No more pepper tea, no dirt dauber, no kind of root or nothing unless you give them some hot tea, regular. But not no roots and things like that."

They said, "They better not catch nobody giving nobody no tea of no kind. If they do, she was going to jail and from there to the pen."

You know, they're quick to think teas and things are going to kill somebody. One midwife told the nurse when we had the meeting, she just told her, "I think I'll bring my bag in and give it to you all because you all are not there when this labor is going on. You don't know how it goes. Rubbing helps and teas help. If I can't give them some hot teas which I know will help, I just well ought to give it up." . . .

So I quit. I quit trying to do anything

but what they gave me to work with. I had been working a good while when I threw that root out my bag.[5]

Smith's account of her life and work paints a picture of the commitment and investment made by the midwife, qualities that were phased out of the medical profession with the invention of such tools of convenience as the early models discussed by Wertz and Wertz. There seem to be four main reasons why midwives had more success than medical doctors. Doctors, restricted by Victorian rules of modesty, practiced medicine blindly, whereas midwives were able to actually look at their patients as they treated them. Doctors practiced various types of medicine, but midwives were specialized in treating women. Doctors tended to rely on tools, while midwives relied on hands-on experience. Finally, and perhaps most importantly, doctors—ignorant of germ theory and basic aseptic techniques—were more likely to carry infection from one patient to the next.

NOTES

1. Samuel Bard, *Compendium of the Theory and Practice of Midwifery* (New York: Collins and Perkins, 1815), 29–35.
2. Ibid., 84–100.
3. Margaret Charles Smith and Linda Janet Holmes, *Listen to Me Good: The Life Story of an Alabama Midwife* (Columbus, OH: Ohio State University Press, 1996), 88–90.
4. Ibid., 92–93.
5. Ibid., 99–100.

The Cultural Warping of Childbirth

DORIS HAIRE

Doris Haire, excerpt from *The Cultural Warping of Childbirth: A Special Report to the International Childbirth Education Association*. Originally published in *ICEA News*, Spring 1972. Reprinted by permission.

While Sweden, Finland, and the Netherlands compete for the honor of having the lowest incidence of infant deaths per 1,000 live births, the

United States continues to find itself outranked by fourteen other developed countries.

Several explanations for our poor national infant outcome have been advanced. Some try to explain our poor standing on the grounds that our statistics are more reliable, but according to the Statistical Office of the United Nations our statistics are no more accurate than those of other countries listed in all of which use the same UN standard for "live birth" without regard for gestational age or birthweight, and most of which collect their statistics on a uniform basis through their national health services. Analyses by Chase of the United States Public Health Service and more recently by Wegman, writing in *Pediatrics*, acknowledge slight variations in the collection of this data but report that, when cross-checked by other statistical data, the variations do not significantly alter the statistics.

In light of the fact that in most of the other listed countries there is no strong feeling of obligation to use extraordinary measures to preserve life when a live birth results in extreme prematurity, severe congenital malformation, or impairment, their incident of infant mortality should be greater than ours, not less.

No one will dispute the fact that socioeconomic factors play a significant role in any infant mortality statistics. However, research has demonstrated that among mothers of the lower socioeconomic groups infant outcome can be substantially improved by changing the pattern of obstetrical care offered these mothers during labor and birth.

There is no question that the welfare of their patients has always been the deep concern of American physicians, nurse-midwives, and nurses. The unphysiological practices which have become so much a part of American obstetric care—to the point where such practices have been generally accepted as normal accompaniments of birth—appear to have gradually built up as a result of social customs and cultural patterning. But cultural patterning can be changed if mothers can be helped to recognize the importance of their accepting some inconvenience and discomfort (and at times pain) in order to achieve the best possible birth and good health for their babies.

Educating mothers for the childbearing experience and improving the quality of emotional support given to mothers during labor and birth have been clearly demonstrated to lessen or eliminate the mother's need for obstetrical medication and obstetrical intervention during labor and birth. The benefit of individualized emotional support and care during this time of stress was made evident in a report by Levy, who notes that during a two-year medically directed, nurse-midwifery program carried out in California, in which nurse-midwives were employed to provide complete care for normal maternity patients, the incident of infant deaths decreased significantly. In order to avoid the inference that it was the additional access to prenatal care alone which made the difference in infant mortality, Levy compared the incidence of infant deaths among women who had had *no prenatal care at all* before, during, and following the pilot program. He found that the incidence of infant deaths among mothers who had had no prenatal care at all, but who were attended during labor and birth by a nurse-midwife, dropped significantly during the nurse-midwifery program and then almost doubled when the nurse-midwifery program ended. Across the continent the success of the California nurse-midwifery program has been essentially duplicated by the Frontier Nursing Service in remote Leslie County, Kentucky, one of the poorest counties in Appalachia.

Obviously we cannot produce enough nurse-midwives overnight to fill the demand, but we can do much to improve our incidence of infant mortality and morbidity by maximizing the emotional support offered the childbearing woman in order that she may cope with the discomfort of labor and birth with a minimum of medication and its attendant hazards.

A spokesman for the National Foundation March of Dimes recently stated that according to the most recent data, the United States leads all developed countries in the rate of infant death due to birth injury and respiratory distress such as postnatal asphyxia and atelectasis.

According to the National Association for Retarded Children, there are now 6 million retarded children and adults in the United States, with a predicted annual increase of over 100,000 a year. The number of children and adults with behavioral difficulties or perceptual dysfunction resulting from minimal brain damage is an ever growing challenge to society and to the economy. While it may be easier on the conscience to blame such numbing facts solely on socioeconomic factors and birth defects, recent research makes it evident that obstetrical medication can play a role in our staggering incidence of neurological impairment. It may be convenient to blame our relatively poor infant outcome on a lack of facilities or inadequate government funding, but it is obvious from the research being carried out that we would effect an immediate improvement in infant outcome by changing the pattern of obstetrical care in the United States. It is time that we take a good look at the overall experience of childbirth in this country and begin to recognize how our culture has warped this experience for the majority of American mothers and their newborn infants.

As an officer of the International Childbirth Education Association (ICEA) I have visited hundreds of maternity hospitals throughout the world—in Great Britain, western Europe, Russia, Asia, Australia, New Zealand, the South Pacific, the Americas, and Africa. During my visits I was privileged to observe obstetric techniques and procedures and to interview physicians, professional midwives, and parents in the various countries. My companion on many of my visits was Dorothea Lang, CNM (certified nurse-midwife), director of Nurse-Midwifery for New York City. Miss Lang's experience as both a nurse-midwife and a former head nurse of the labor and delivery unit of the New York Cornell Medical Center made her a particularly well-qualified observer and companion. As we traveled from country to country certain patterns of care soon became evident. For one, in those countries which enjoy an incidence of infant mortality and birth trauma significantly lower than that of the United States, highly trained professional midwives are an important source of obstetrical care and family planning services for normal women, whether the births take place in the hospital or in the home. In these countries the expertise of the physician is called upon only when the expectant mother is ill during pregnancy or when labor or birth is anticipated to be, or is found to be abnormal. Under this system the high-risk mother—the one who is most likely to bear an impaired or stillborn child—has a better opportunity to obtain in-depth medical attention than is possible under our existing American system of obstetrical care where the obstetrician is also called upon to play the role of midwife.

Deprivation, birth defects, prematurity, and low birthweight are not unique to the United States. While it is tempting to blame our comparatively high incidence of infant mortality solely on a lack of available prenatal care and on socioeconomic factors, our observations indicate that, comparatively, the prenatal care we offer most clinic patients in the United States is not grossly inferior to that available in other developed countries. Furthermore, the diet and standard of living in many countries which have a lower incidence of infant mortality than ours would be considered inadequate by American standards.

As an example, when one compares the availability of prenatal care, the incidence of premature births, the average diet of various economic groups, and the equipment available to aid in newborn infant survival in two such diverse countries as the United States and Japan, there are no major differences between the two countries. The differences lie in (1) our frequent use of prenatal and obstetrical medication, (2) our pathologically oriented management of pregnancy, labor, birth, and postpartum, and (3) the predominance of artificial feeding in the United States, as opposed to Japan.

If present statistics follow the trend of recent years, an infant born in the United States is more than four times more likely to die in the first day of life than an infant born in Japan. But survival of the birth process should not be our singular goal. For every American newborn infant who dies, there are likely to be several who are neurologically damaged, because the major differences in infant mortality between the United States and Japan are represented by our comparatively high incidence of infant deaths due to birth injury and respiratory distress, such as postnatal asphyxia and atelectasis, conditions which are more likely to occur if the mother has received obstetrical medication. The better records of infant outcome in Japan is even more dramatic when one considers that, according to a recent report by the Japanese Ministry of Health, the maternal death rate due to toxemia is five times greater in Japan than in the United States. Whether this is due to diet or lifestyle is not yet scientifically established.

Most American mothers do not, as yet, realize that the management of labor is even more important than the management of birth in determining how an infant will fare, not only during the first critical hours but perhaps throughout life. A poorly managed labor can result in an infant who shows no signs of respiratory distress and who scores well on the Apgar scale, while, in fact, a more scientific evaluation of the infant's condition may indicate lingering signs of oxygen deprivation in utero resulting from obstetrical medication administered to the mother.

Hellman and Pritchard state that the respiratory center of the infant is highly vulnerable to sedative and anesthetic drugs administered to the mother and that such medication may jeopardize the initiation of respiration of the infant at birth. They point out that sluggish respiration is observed to some extent in the majority of infants whose mothers received sedation during labor. The added burden on the newly born infant of having to detoxify indirectly acquired obstetrical medication as he adjusts to extrauterine life is the subject of abundant scientific literature in the past and present.

An outstanding monograph entitled "Effects of Obstetrical Medication on Fetus and Newborn,"

published by the Society for Research in Child Development in June 1970, makes it evident that we can no longer assume that the apparent recovery of an asphyxiated infant after successful resuscitation is a guarantee that the infant has come through unharmed. (This monograph should be required reading for all obstetrical personnel.) A baby with a heartbeat after cardiac massage may appear to be recovered but, in fact, may be irreversibly brain damaged. Virtually all obstetrical medications—nausea remedies, diuretics, sedatives, muscle relaxants, analgesics, regional anesthesia, and general anesthetics—tend to rapidly cross the placenta and alter the fetal environment as they enter the circulatory system of the unborn infant within seconds or minutes of administration to the mother. As Dr. Virginia Apgar bluntly puts it, the placenta is not a barrier but a "bloody sieve."

If prolapse of the umbilical cord or premature separation of the placenta occurs during labor, the fetus is compromised. If obstetrical medication is administered to the mother during labor and either of these conditions occurs, this compounds the danger to the unborn infant. No one can guarantee the mother that such conditions will not occur.

While respiratory distress is one of the more obvious hazards of obstetrical medication, the more subtle effects of such medications are now being noted. Sedatives containing barbiturates administered to the mother during labor have been shown to adversely affect the infant's suckling reflexes for four or five days after birth. The prolonged effects of some commonly used obstetrical medications, such as meperidine (Demerol), have been detected in the infant several weeks after birth.

Regional anesthesias appears to be an improvement over general anesthesia, but research indicates that even in the most dedicated hands regional anesthesias can compromise the mother and her infant. All regional anesthesias, including pudendal block, tend to alter the fetal environment and to inhibit the mother's ability to push her baby down the birth canal, which in turn, tends to increase the need for fundal pressure, uterine stimulants, and forceps extraction—conditions which should be avoided if possible in the best interests of the child. L. Stanley James, chairman of the Committee on Fetus and Newborn of the American Academy of Pediatrics, cautions, "Regional techniques are gaining popularity but they are not without problems." He points out that it is difficult to give spinal anesthesia—caudal, epidural, or saddle block—without any change in maternal blood pressure, and that even if pressure is restored by the use of vasopressors, there is no assurance that regional circulation through the uterus remains normal.

Because he must fill the role of both obstetrician and midwife, the overburdened American obstetrician frequently manages his maternity patient's labor by telephone and arrives at the hospital shortly before a birth is anticipated. This type of management must depend on reports from the mother's labor attendant, who may or may not have had specialized training in evaluating the effects of labor and obstetrical medication on both the mother and her unborn infant. But in countries which enjoy a lower incidence of infant mortality than ours it is the hospital-assigned, professional midwife who manages the prenatal care, labor, birth, and postpartum care of the normal mother and the care of the normal newborn infant. The professional midwife receives special training in maintaining the delicate physiological balance between mother and child during labor and birth, and is trained to recognize conditions which require the medical expertise of the physician.

Because the professional midwife also is involved in the postpartum care of the infant, and not just labor and delivery, she is fully aware of the importance of providing individualized and skillful emotional support for the laboring mother as a means of reducing or eliminating the mother's need for obstetrical medication, with its possible narcotizing effect on the fetus and newborn infant.

The active encouragement of breast-feeding by the professional midwife also appears to affect the incidence of infant mortality in the various countries, for in those countries such as Sweden, the Netherlands, and Japan, where breast-feeding is still the predominant pattern of initial infant feeding, the incidence of infant mortality is significantly lower than in those countries where artificial feeding is the predominant initial form of infant feeding. It is interesting to note that in those older age categories, when the customary times for weaning occur, such countries as Sweden, the Netherlands, and Japan begin to lose their statistical advantages.

Unfortunately, the American tendency to warp the birth experience, distorting it into a pathological event, rather than a physiological one, for the normal childbearing woman is no longer peculiar to just the United States. In my visits to hospitals in various countries I was distressed to find that some physicians, anxious to impress their colleagues with their "Americanized" techniques, have unfortunately adopted many of our obstetrical practices without stopping to question their scientific or social merit.

Few American babies are born today as nature intended them to be. Among the 55,000 children included in the American Collaborative Prenatal Study carried out by the National Institute of Neurological Diseases and Stroke, there was no apparent effort made to include a control group of normal mothers who were educated to cope with the discomfort of childbirth without the use of medication. With rare exceptions, those mothers in the Collaborative Study who did not receive obstetrical medication were those who had a precipitous labor or those whose unborn child showed signs of fetal distress which precluded the use of obstetrical medication.

Although there is a tendency to think of paracervical and pudendal block anesthesia as relatively harmless, research indicates that they too can compromise the fetus and newborn infant. Rosefsky and Petersiel noted a drop in fetal heart rate in almost half of a group of ninety mothers who were observed after receiving paracervical block anesthesia. In another series the incidence of infant depression and Apgar scores (see Table 1) of six or less was almost three times greater among those infants whose mothers had received paracervical block than among the controls. The fetal hazards of depression with occasional death associated with paracervical block have been clearly demonstrated. Transient fetal bradycardia may appear to be relatively harmless, but an abnormal drop in fetal heart rate usually indicates a decrease in the oxygen saturation for the fetus. How much depletion of oxygen can be sustained by a given fetus or newborn infant before neurological damage occurs may not be recognized for several years, for the effect of even a relatively small decrease in oxygen saturation of the fetus and newborn has yet to be assessed. It is ironic that transient fetal bradycardia is taken so lightly, for no one would purposely inject medication or apply a device to a newborn infant which would possibly decrease his oxygen supply for even a few minutes without grave cause.

The relaxed attitude in the past toward the use of obstetrical medication was not due to a lack of concern for the fetus and newborn infant but to an unawareness of the problem. However, newer scientific methods of evaluating the immediate and prolonged effects on the fetus and newborn infant of obstetrical medications and many of our common obstetrical practices now make it evident that they do, in fact, tend to alter the normal fetal and infant environment. The effect of minimal brain damage on the child's personality and his ability to learn and to cope with our complex society is only now beginning to be fully understood. Research by Lewis indicates that infants who were rated between seven and nine on the Apgar scale at birth were significantly less attentive than were those infants rated ten, and that the difference, in general, held true over the first year of life. It is not unlikely that unnecessary alterations in the normal fetal environment may play a role

TABLE 1:
METHOD OF SCORING FOR APGAR SCORE

Sixty seconds and again at five minutes after the complete birth of the infant (disregarding the cord and placenta) the following five objective signs are evaluated and each given a score of zero, one, or two. A score of ten indicates an infant is in the best possible condition. Infants with scores of five to ten usually need no immediate treatment. A score of four or below indicates the need for prompt diagnosis and treatment.

SIGN	0	1	2
Heart rate	Absent	Slow (below 100)	Over 100
Respiratory effort	Absent	Slow, irregular	Good crying
Muscle tone	Limp	Some flexion of extremities	Active motion
Reflex irritability: response to catheter in nostril	No response	Grimace	Cough or sneeze
Color	Blue, pale	Body pink, extremities blue	Completely pink*

*American professionals are frequently amazed to see the consistency with which Scandinavian and Dutch newborn infants "pink up" to the very tips of their fingers and toes a few seconds after being born.

in the incidence of neurological impairment and infant mortality in the United States. Infant resuscitation, other than routine suctioning, is rarely needed in countries such as Sweden, the Netherlands, and Japan, where the skillful psychological management of labor usually precludes the need for obstetrical medication. In contrast, in those European countries, such as Belgium, where the overall pattern of obstetrical care is similar to our own the incidence of infant mortality also approaches our own.

Obviously there will always be medical indications which dictate the use of various obstetrical procedures, but to apply the following American practices and procedures routinely to the vast majority of mothers who are capable of giving birth without complication is to create added stress which is not in the best interests of either the mother or her newborn infant.

Let us take a close look at our infant mortality statistics and then at some of our common obstetrical practices from early pregnancy to postpartum which have served to warp and distort the childbearing experience in the United States. While not all of the practices below affect infant mortality, it is equally apparent that they do not contribute to the reduction of infant morbidity or mortality and therefore should be re-evaluated.

After you have read each section below, check the appropriate box if the obstetrical care in your community includes the practice discussed. The total number of check marks that you record will provide some idea as to how far obstetric practices in your community have digressed from normal physiological childbirth.

WITHHOLDING INFORMATION ON THE DISADVANTAGES OF OBSTETRICAL MEDICATION

Ignorance of the possible hazards of obstetrical medication appears to encourage the misuse and abuse of obstetrical medication, for in those countries where mothers are not told routinely of the possible disadvantages of obstetrical medication to themselves or to their babies the use of such medication is on the increase.

There is no research or evidence which indicates that mothers will be emotionally damaged if they are advised, prior to birth, that obstetrical medication may be to the disadvantage of their newborn infants. Offering the mother accurate, printed information (adapted from that which appears in the package insert of every obstetrical medication) on the relative safety and hazards of commonly used obstetrical medications and practices, prior to her confinement, may seem a nuisance, but such a precaution helps to protect the hospital, physician, or professional midwife from legal liability resulting from the mother's uninformed consent and allows the mother to share in the responsibility for her own well-being and that of her child in utero. To withhold information as to the possible complications of obstetrical medication is to delude the mother into assuming that there are no risks involved.

We must keep in mind that it is the mother who must ultimately bear the major emotional burden of a damaged or impaired child, even if that child is institutionalized. Under normal conditions no one should usurp the mother's prerogative by placing her unborn or newborn infant at a possible disadvantage without her informed consent. As the public becomes more aware of the possible effects of obstetrical practices on infant outcome, failure to disclose or inform the mother of the possible adverse consequences of some of the obstetrical practices discussed herein may become the basis of legal liability if or when those adverse consequences occur.

AMBIVALENT PRENATAL COUNSELING ON BREAST-FEEDING

In most of the countries of the world breast-feeding is actively encouraged during the prenatal counseling and during the mother's hospital confinement. Breast-feeding is particularly encouraged if birth is premature. If an infant is too premature or ill to suckle his mother's breasts, the mother is frequently asked to return to the hospital in order to express her milk in the presence of her baby, since the closeness tends to increase the mother's production of milk. In contrast, most American mothers are merely asked prenatally to state their preference for breast-feeding or bottle feeding, without being offered any information as to the relative benefits of breast-feeding for their babies. Once the mother has stated her preference to bottle-feed, little or no effort is made to suggest to her the advantages of breast-feeding. Yet the incidence of allergy among formula-fed infants is steadily on the rise in the United States.

While not all of the protective mechanisms of breast milk are understood, many scientists have demonstrated that there is significantly less incidence of illness among children who are breast-fed. A survey of over 3,000 children living in a housing project in England (postpenicillin) showed that the death rate was nine times greater among children who were artificially fed from birth. All of the children in the project received their health care from the same doctors and nurses. Yet among those children who were breast-fed there was significantly less incidence of common colds, bronchitis, pneumonia, eczema, asthma, hay fever, colic, gastroenteritis, otitis media, mastoid, whooping cough, measles, German measles, and scarlet fever. Colostrum and breast milk contain antibodies against three strains of polio, Coxsackie B virus, two types of colon bacilli which can cause fetal infant diarrhea, pathogenic strains of *E. coli*, and gram-negative infections.

Diseases resulting from malabsorption, such as delicate syndrome, and sudden infant death syndrome (SIDS) rarely occur among completely breast-fed babies. Unfortunately, there are too few breast-fed infants in the high-incidence SIDS study areas to make up an adequate number of breast-fed controls.

Newborn infants who are breast-fed excrete more strontium than is ingested in breast milk whereas bottle-fed infants accumulate strontium.

There are now indications that the protective effects of breast milk may go far beyond the weaning period. Various researchers suggest that there is less incidence of dental caries, orthodontic disproportion and orofacial dental deformities, premature atherosclerosis, and ulcerative colitis among young people and adults who were initially breast-fed. One can only wonder about the future incidence of ulcerative colitis among adults whose initial food was foreign protein, fed at a temperature 25° below the temperature of breast milk, an infant's normal, species-specific food.

Research is strongly supportive of the use of breast milk for the premature infant. Mothers who breast-feed were noted by Paffenberger to show a decreased susceptibility to delayed postpartum hemorrhage. In light of the abundant research showing the medical value of breast-feeding it would seem that a statement such as "One is just as good as mother" can hardly be applied to the initial form of feeding of a newborn infant.

For additional information and references on this subject read, "The Nurse's Contribution to Successful Breast-Feeding," prepared by the author and available from ICEA's Education Committee or Supplies Center.

PERMITTING THE MOTHER TO FACE CHILDBIRTH UNINFORMED OF WAYS IN WHICH SHE CAN HELP HERSELF TO COPE WITH THE DISCOMFORT OF LABOR AND BIRTH

All mothers should be offered the opportunity to be physically and emotionally prepared to cope with the discomfort of childbirth because circumstances frequently preclude the use of obstetrical medication, even if the mother requests it. Dr. Charles Flowers, former Chairman of the Committee on Obstetric Analgesic and Anesthesia of the American College of Obstetricians and Gynecologists, states, "Gymnastics are not necessary in the preparation of the patient for childbirth but the ability of a person to know what to do and how to relax and how to breathe during labor is of fundamental importance."

A well-controlled research program by Enkin of Canada demonstrated that mothers who were prepared for the possibility of effectively participating in the birth process tended to experience significantly shorter labors, to require less medication and less obstetrical intervention, and to remember the experience of birth more favorably than did those mothers who were motivated to ask to be prepared to cope with childbirth but could not be accommodated in classes.

According to Dr. Pierre Vellay, a pioneer in childbirth education, the ability to relax is the key to pain relief during labor and birth and the breathing patterns act as a distraction from painful stimuli. Experience in several countries indicates that the type of controlled breathing patterns, either chest or abdominal, taught in class or in the labor room is relatively unimportant since it is the mother's intense concentration on the controlled breathing patterns, and not the breathing patterns in themselves, which makes her less aware of the discomfort or pain of her contractions.

The psychoprophylactic method of childbirth training, developed and still used successfully in Russia, involves no controlled breathing patterns. While controlled breathing patterns may be unnecessary in the future, such patterns serve a useful purpose at this point in our culture. The recent de-emphasis on breathing patterns will help to avoid hyperventilation (according to McCance, hyperventilation rarely occurs in animals) and will help to bring childbirth educators into greater agreement.

REQUIRING ALL NORMAL WOMEN TO GIVE BIRTH IN THE HOSPITAL

While ICEA does not encourage home births, there is ample evidence in the Netherlands and in Chicago (Chicago Maternity Center) to demonstrate that normal women who have received adequate prenatal care can safely give birth at home if a proper system is developed for home deliveries. Over half of the mothers in the Netherlands give birth at home with the assistance of a professional midwife and a maternity aide. The comparatively low incidence of infant deaths and birth trauma in the Netherlands, a country of diverse ethnic composition and intermarriage, is evidence of the comparative safety of a properly developed home delivery service.

Dutch obstetricians point out that when the labor of a normal woman is unhurried and allowed to progress normally, unexpected emergencies rarely occur. They also point out that the small risk involved in a Dutch home delivery is more than offset by the increased hazards resulting from the use of obstetrical medication and obstetrical tampering which are more likely to occur in a hospital environment, especially in countries where professionals have had little or no exposure to normal labor and birth in a home environment during their training. We cannot justify deprecating a system of care which rarely produces a newborn infant with an Apgar score less than nine when we in the US have a predicted yearly increase of more than 100,000 retarded infants. If the increasing American trend toward home deliveries is to be contained, it is imperative that an effort be made to make birth in the hospital as normal, as homelike, and as inexpensive as possible.

ELECTIVE INDUCTION OF LABOR

The elective induction of labor (where there is no clear medical indication) appears to be an American idiosyncrasy which is frowned upon in other developed countries. In discussing electric induction of labor in *Williams Obstetrics*, 14th ed., Hellman and Pritchard caution that the conveniences of elective induction are not without the attendant hazards of prematurity, prolonged latent period with intrapartum infection, and prolapse of the umbilical cord. They report that studies involving almost 10,000 elective inductions indicate that perinatal deaths due to premature elective inductions occur despite efforts to comply with specific criteria.

In reviewing the results of 3,324 elective inductions of labor at the University of Pennsylvania Hospital, Fields stresses the importance of caution in the selection of candidates for elective induction. He states, "Amniotomy carries with it the risk of injury to the mother or fetus and displacement of the presenting part, resulting in malposition, prolapsed cord, prolonged latent period and infection. The hazards of the use of oxytocin in labor are related directly to the dose for a given individual. Overdosage results in uterine spasm with possible separation of the placenta, tumultuous labor, amniotic fluid embolus, afibrinogenemia, lacerations of the cervix and birth canal, postpartum hemorrhage and uterine rupture. There may be water intoxication due to the antidiuretic effect of oxytocin. There may be fetal distress due to anoxia and intracranial hemorrhage, and trauma may result from tumultuous uterine contractions. Fetal and/or maternal mortality are, of course, ever present dangers."

The elective induction of labor has been found to almost double the incidence of fetomaternal transfusion and its attendant hazards. But perhaps the least appreciated problem of elective induction is the fact that the abrupt onset of artificially induced labor tends to make it extremely difficult for even the well-prepared mother to tolerate the discomfort of the intensified contractions without the aid of obstetrical medication. When the onset of labor occurs spontaneously, the normal, gradual increase in contraction length and intensity appears to provoke in the mother an accompanying tolerance for discomfort or pain.

Since the British Perinatal Hazards Study found no increase in perinatal mortality or impairment of learning ability at age seven among full-term infants, unless gestation had extended beyond forty-one weeks, there would be no medical justification for subjecting a mother or her baby to the possible hazards of elective induction in order to terminate the pregnancy prior to forty-one weeks gestation. The elective induction of labor, when there is no specific medical indication, could be considered obstetrical interference in the normal physiology of childbirth and may leave the participating accoucheur legally vulnerable unless the mother is offered accurate information as to the possible hazards of elective induction of labor.

SEPARATING THE MOTHER FROM FAMILIAL SUPPORT DURING LABOR AND BIRTH

Research indicates that fear adversely affects uterine motility and blood flow, and yet many American mothers are routinely separated from a family member or close friend at this time of emotional crisis. Mice whose labors were environmentally disturbed experienced significantly longer labors, as much as 72 percent longer under some conditions, and gave birth to 54 percent more dead pups than did the mice in the control group. Newton cautions that the human mammal, which has a more highly developed nervous system than the mouse, may be equally sensitive to environmental disturbances in labor.

In most developed countries, other than the United States and the eastern European countries, mothers are encouraged to walk about or to sit and chat with a family member or supportive person in what is called an "early labor lounge." This lounge is usually located near but outside the labor-delivery area in order to provide a more relaxed atmosphere during much of labor. The mother is taken to the labor-delivery area to be checked periodically, then allowed to return to the labor lounge for as long as she likes or until her membranes have ruptured.

The rapid acceptance by professionals of permitting the mother to be emotionally supported by a family member during birth is perhaps the most dramatic change in obstetrical care throughout the developed countries. However, in some countries where multiple-bed delivery rooms are prevalent, such as in the eastern European countries and Asia, husbands are usually excluded.

CONFINING THE NORMAL LABORING WOMAN TO BED

In virtually all countries except the United States, a woman in labor is routinely encouraged to walk about during labor for a long as she wishes or until her membranes have ruptured. Such activity is considered to facilitate labor by distracting the mother's attention from the discomfort or pain of her contractions and to encourage a more rapid engagement of the fetal head. In America, where drugs are frequently administered either orally or prenatally to laboring mothers, such ambulation is discouraged—not only for the patient's safety but also to avoid possible legal complications in the event of an accident.

The disadvantages to the fetus resulting from the mother's lying in a recumbent position during labor have been recognized for several years. It is not unlikely that research will eventually find that the peasant woman who labored in the fields up until the moment of birth may have been well served by this physical activity.

SHAVING THE BIRTH AREA

Research involving 7,600 mothers has demonstrated that the practice of shaving the perineum and pubis does not reduce the incidence of infection. In fact, the incidence of infection was slightly higher among those mothers who were shaved. Yet this procedure, which tends to create apprehension in laboring women, is still carried out routinely in most American hospitals. Clipping the perineal or pudendal hair closely with surgical scissors is far less disturbing to the mother and is less likely to result in infection caused by razor abrasions.

WITHHOLDING FOOD AND DRINK FROM THE NORMAL UNMEDICATED WOMAN IN LABOR

The effect on the fetus of depriving a mother of food and drink for many hours, as is the custom in the United States, has not been sufficiently investigated. Intravenous feeding, as a substitute for light eating, only adds to the pathologic environment of an American hospital birth. In most developed countries one of the incentives for an expectant mother to take advantage of prenatal care is the fact that she will be allowed to eat and drink lightly during labor only if her prenatal examinations show her to be normal. Since anesthesia is not routinely administered during childbirth, light eating and drinking has not been found to increase the incidence of maternal morbidity or mortality in these countries.

The inhalation of gastric fluid by itself can be hazardous to the anesthetized mother. Therefore, to avoid this hazard obstetricians in most countries require that the mother's stomach be emptied or special precautions be taken if for any reason she must be anesthetized for delivery.

PROFESSIONAL DEPENDENCE ON TECHNOLOGY AND PHARMACOLOGICAL METHODS OF PAIN RELIEF

Most of the world's mothers receive little or no drugs during pregnancy, labor, or birth. The constant emotional support provided the laboring woman in other countries by the nurse-midwife, and often by her husband, appears to greatly improve the mother's tolerance for discomfort. In contrast, the American labor room nurse is frequently assigned to look after several women in labor, all or most of whom have had no preparation to cope with the discomfort or pain of childbearing. Under the circumstances drugs, rather than skillful emotional support, are employed to relieve the mother's apprehension and discomfort (and perhaps to assuage the harried labor attendant's feeling of inadequacy).

The fallacy of depending on the stethoscope to accurately monitor the effects of obstetrical medication on the well-being of the fetus has been demonstrated by Hon. While electronic fetal monitoring is more accurate, the fact that some monitoring devices require that a mother's membranes be ruptured and that the electrode penetrate the skin of the fetal scalp creates possible hazards of its own. Therefore, obstetrical management which reduces the need for such monitoring is advisable.

Many professionals contend that a "good experience" for the mother is of paramount importance in childbearing. They tend to forget that, for the vast majority of mothers, a healthy undamaged baby is the far more important objective of childbirth. The two objectives are not always compatible. Human maternal response has not been demonstrated to be adversely altered by a stressful, unmedicated labor if the mother has been prepared for the experience of birth. To expose a mother to the possibility of a lifetime of heartache or anguish in order to insure her a few hours of comfort is misguided kindness, for while analgesia and anesthesia for the laboring woman may be the easier route for the nurse, midwife, or physician, the price of a narcotized mother may be a narcotized or damaged newborn infant whose ultimate potential for learning is forever diminished.

CHEMICAL STIMULATION OF LABOR

Oxytocic agents are frequently administered to intensify artificially the frequency and/or the strength of the mother's contractions, as a means of shortening the mother's labor. While chemical stimulation is sometimes medically indicated, often it is undertaken to satisfy the American propensity for efficiency and speed. Hon suggests that the overenthusiastic use of oxytocic stimulants sometimes results in alterations in the normal fetal heart rate. Fields points out that the possible hazards inherent in elective induction are also possible in artificially stimulated labor unless the mother and fetus are carefully monitored.

The British Perinatal Study appears to consider twenty-four hours as an outside limit for the first stage of labor, with a second stage of two or three hours or more. The average labor is about thirteen hours for a primipara and about seven and a half hours for a multipara. Shortening the phases of normal labor when there is no sign of fetal distress has not been shown to improve infant outcome. Little is known of the long-term effects of artificially stimulating labor contractions. During a contraction the unborn child normally receives less oxygen. The gradual buildup of intensity, which occurs when the onset of labor is allowed to occur spontaneously and to proceed without chemical stimulation, appears likely to be a protective mechanism that is best left unaltered unless there is a clear medical indication for the artificial stimulation of labor.

MOVING THE NORMAL MOTHER TO A DELIVERY ROOM FOR BIRTH

Most of the world's mothers, in both developed and developing countries, give birth in the same bed in the same hospital room in which they have labored. Since most European labor-delivery beds do not have adjustable backrests, mothers are supported into a semisitting position for birth by their husbands or a midwife. The midwife assists the mother, and if necessary, performs an episiotomy from the side of the bed, rather from the end of the bed. The suturing of an episiotomy is done by the side of the bed, or the bed may be "broken."

American nurse-midwives, especially those who have been trained abroad, are now beginning to permit American mothers the same privilege. This may seem innovative to many Americans until we realize that there is no research or evidence which indicates that a normal, essentially unmedicated mother should be required to give birth in a delivery room, rather than in a labor room which is equipped with portable or permanent sources of oxygen, suction, and high-intensity lighting. The pathological environment of the modern American delivery room is not conducive to a relaxed, normal childbirth experience.

The low temperature of the average delivery room has in the past been more suitable for the staff than for the infant. The American Academy of Pediatrics, acting as the infant's advocate, now recommends that the temperature of the delivery room should be maintained between 71.6 and 75.2°F.

DELAYING BIRTH UNTIL THE PHYSICIAN ARRIVES

Because of the increased likelihood of resultant brain damage to the infant the practice of delaying birth by anesthesia or physician restraint until the physician arrives to deliver the infant is frowned upon in most countries. Yet the practice still occurs occasionally in the United States and in countries where hospital-assigned midwives do not routinely manage the labor and delivery of normal mothers. One of the benefits of husband-attended deliveries noted by many chiefs of American obstetrical departments is the tendency for obstetrical coverage by attending physicians to immediately improve.

REQUIRING THE MOTHER TO ASSUME THE LITHOTOMY POSITION FOR BIRTH

Some contend that the low incidence of spontaneous birth among American mothers is due to the disparity in the size between the parents, resulting from the differences in their ethnic background. However, there is gathering scientific evidence that the unphysiological lithotomy position (back flat, with knees drawn up and spread wide apart by "stirrups") which is preferred by most American physicians because it is more convenient for the accoucheur, tends to alter the normal fetal environment and obstruct the normal process of childbearing, making spontaneous birth more difficult or impossible.

The lithotomy and dorsal positions tend to:

1. Adversely affect the mother's blood pressure, cardiac return, and pulmonary ventilation.

2. Decrease the normal intensity of the contractions.

3. Inhibit the mother's voluntary efforts to push her baby out spontaneously, which, in turn, increases the need for fundal pressure or forceps and increases the traction necessary for extraction.

4. Inhibit the spontaneous expulsion of the placenta, which in turn, increases the need for cord traction, forced expression, or manual removal of the placenta—procedures which significantly increase the incidence of fetomaternal hemorrhage.

5. Increase the need for episiotomy because of the increased tension on the pelvic floor and the stretching of perineal tissue. The normal separation of the feet for natural expulsion is about fifteen to sixteen inches, or thirty-eight to forty-one centimeters, which is far less separation than is allowed by the average American delivery table stirrups.

Australian, Russian, and American research bears out the clinical experience of European physicians and midwives—that when mothers are supported to be a semisitting position for birth, with their feet supported by the lower section of the labor-delivery bed, mothers tend to purchase more effectively, appear to need less pain relief, are more likely to want to be conscious for birth, and are less likely to need an episiotomy.

The fact that the extended delivery table or bed spares the mother the common but often unspoken fear of involuntarily expelling her baby onto the floor before the doctor or midwife is ready to receive the infant, or the fear that the accoucheur might accidentally drop her baby may inhibit the mother's ability to relax her perineum during the second stage of labor.

The increased efficiency of the semisitting position, combined with a minimum use of medication for birth, is evidenced by the fact that the combined use of both forceps and the vacuum extractor rarely exceeds 4 to 5 percent of all births in the Netherlands, as compared to an incidence of 65 percent in many American hospitals. (Cesarean section occurs in approximately 1.5 percent of all Dutch births.) These differences are even more striking when one considers that in modern Holland, which has a population almost as heterogeneous as our own, the average pelvic measurements of the Dutch mother and the average circumference of her baby's head are the same as those of their American counterparts.

Manual removal for the placenta occurs in approximately 0.6 percent of all Dutch births despite the fact that oxytocin is not administered to mothers routinely.

Although the author knows of no specific research which verifies the incidence, clinical experience in the United States suggests that mothers who give birth in the semisitting position, with their legs resting on the bed, are less likely to sustain postpartum backache and fracture of the coccyx. A scientific investigation is long overdue.

THE ROUTINE USE OF REGIONAL OR GENERAL ANESTHESIA FOR DELIVERY

In light of the current shortage of qualified anesthetists and anesthesiologists and the frequent scientific papers now being published on the possible hazards resulting from the use of regional and general anesthesia, it would seem prudent to make every effort to prepare the mother physically and mentally to cope with the sensations and discomfort of birth in order to avoid the use of such medicaments. Regional and general anesthesia not only tend to adversely affect fetal environment pharmacologically, which has been discussed previously herein, but their use also increases the need for obstetrical intervention in the normal process of birth since both types of anesthesia tend to prolong labor. Johnson points out that peridural and spinal anesthesia significantly increase the incidence of midforceps delivery and its attendant hazards. Pudendal block anesthesia not only tends to interfere with the mother's ability to effectively push her baby down the birth canal due to the blocking of the afferent path of the pushing reflex, but also appears to interfere with the mother's normal protective reflexes, thus making "an explosive" birth and perineal damage more likely to occur.

While there are exceptions, the use of regional and general anesthesia usually dictates that:

1. The mother must be restricted from eating or drinking from the onset of labor.

2. The mother's uterine contractions must frequently be pharmacologically stimulated.

3. The mother must be moved to a delivery room which is equipped for obstetrical emergencies (obstetrical medication tends to increase the need for resuscitative measures for the infant).

4. The mother must be placed in the lithotomy position for delivery since she will not be in control of her legs.

5. Fundal pressure and/or the use of forceps and an episiotomy will be needed to facilitate the delivery of the infant.

6. The infant's umbilical cord will be clamped early to facilitate immediate resuscitative measures for the infant and to shorten the infant's accumulation of obstetrical medication.

7. Fundal pressure or manipulation, cord traction, pharmacological stimulation of contractions, or manual removal of the placenta be employed in order to facilitate the prompt delivery of the placenta to prevent maternal hemorrhage.

FUNDAL PRESSURE TO FACILITATE DELIVERY

Cooperman cites the past work of Pennoyer as he points out that the application of pressure on the fundus during delivery has been shown to depress oxygen saturation in the newborn infant. The use of obstetrical medications which tend to precipitate the use of fundal pressure should be avoided in the best interests of the mother and her infant.

THE ROUTINE USE OF FORCEPS
FOR DELIVERY

There is no scientific justification for the routine application of forceps for delivery. The incidence of delivery by forceps and vacuum extractor, combined, rarely rises about 5 percent in countries where mothers actively participate in the births of their babies. In contrast, as mentioned previously, the incidence of forceps extraction frequently rises to as high as 65 percent in some American hospitals. Research in Europe, where there are more natural births to serve as controls, has demonstrated that, when forceps are used for delivery in order to relieve maternal distress, those infants so delivered are more likely to sustain intracranial hemorrhage and damage to the facial nerve or the brachial plexus. There are obviously times when indications of fetal distress dictate the use of forceps to facilitate the safe delivery of an infant, but there is no scientific support for the routine application of forceps during birth.

ROUTINE EPISIOTOMY

There is no research or evidence to indicate that routine episiotomy (a surgical incision to enlarge the vaginal orifice) reduces the incidence of pelvic relaxation (structural damage to the pelvic floor musculature) in the mother. Nor is there any research or evidence that routine episiotomy reduces neurological impairment in the child who has shown no signs of fetal distress or that the procedure helps to maintain subsequent male or female sexual response.

Pelvic Relaxation: The incidence of pelvic floor relaxation appears to be on the decline throughout the world, even in those countries where episiotomy is still comparatively rare. The contention that the modern washing machine has been more effective in reducing pelvic relaxation among American mothers than has routine episiotomy is given some credence by the fact that in areas of the United States where life is still hard for the woman,

pelvic relaxation appears in white women who have never borne children. Interviews with gynecologists in many countries suggest that the incidence of pelvic relaxation is strongly influenced by genetics. The condition, although comparatively rare in both Fiji and Kenya, occurs more frequently among Indian women in those countries than among black women, although the living habits and fertility rate of both groups of women are much the same. Whether a resistance to pelvic relaxation is due to diet, physical activity, practices or position used during birth, or any other factor is not clear. The fact remains, however, that susceptibility to pelvic relaxation appears to be a genetic weakness which has not been shown to be eliminated or reduced by routine episiotomy.

Neurological Impairment: Shortening the second stage of labor by performing an episiotomy when there is no sign of fetal distress has not been shown to be beneficial to the infant. The scientific evaluation of 17,000 children, born in one week's time and followed for seven years in Great Britain, indicates that a second stage of labor lasting as long as two and a half hours does not increase the incidence of neurological impairment of the full-term, average-for-gestational-age infant who shows no signs of fetal distress.

Sexual Response: In developed countries where episiotomy is comparatively rare the physiotherapist is considered an important member of the obstetrical team—before as well as after birth. The physiotherapist is responsible for seeing that each mother begins exercises the day following birth which will help to restore the normal elasticity and tone of the mother's perineal and abdominal muscles. In countries where every effort is made to avoid the need for an episiotomy, interviews with both parents and professionals indicate that an intact perineum which is strengthened by postpartum exercises is more apt to result in both male and female sexual satisfaction than is a perineum that has been incised and reconstructed.

Why, then, is there such an emotional attachment among professionals to routine episiotomy? A prominent European professor of obstetrics and gynecology recently made the following comment on the American penchant for routine episiotomy, "Since all the physician can really do to affect the course of childbirth for the 95 percent of mothers who are capable of giving birth without complication is to offer the mother pharmacological relief from discomfort or pain and to perform an episiotomy, there is probably an unconscious tendency for many professionals to see these practices as indispensable."

Interviews with obstetrician-gynecologists in many countries indicate that they tend to agree that a superficial, first-degree tear is less traumatic to the perineal tissue than an incision which requires several sutures for reconstruction. There is no research which would indicate otherwise. It would appear callous indeed for a physician or nurse-midwife to perform an episiotomy without first making an effort to avoid the need for an episiotomy by removing the mother's legs from the stirrups and bringing her up into a semisitting position in order to relieve tension on her perineum and enable her to push more effectively.

EARLY CLAMPING OR "MILKING" OF THE UMBILICAL CORD

Several years ago De Marsh stated that the placental blood normally belongs to the infant and his failure to get this blood is equivalent to submitting him to a rather severe hemorrhage. Despite the fact that placental transfusion normally occurs in every corner of the world without adverse consequences there is still a great effort in the United States and Canada to deprecate the practice. One must read the literature carefully to find that placental transfusion has not been demonstrated to increase the incidence of morbidity or mortality in the placentally transfused infant.

Routine early clamping or milking of the umbilical cord may appear to save the professional a few minutes time in the delivery room, but neither practice has been demonstrated to be in the best interest of either the essentially unmedicated mother or her infant. Placental transfusion resulting from late clamping, whereby the infant receives approximately an additional 25 percent of his total blood supply, is part of the physiological sequence of childbirth for most of the world's newborn infants in both developed and developing countries where the dorsal, squatting, or semisitting position is preferred for birth. The lithotomy position for birth, preferred by the American obstetrician because it is more convenient for him, makes placental transfusion inconvenient since there is no end of the bed on which the obstetrician can place the wriggling infant. The practice of "milking" the cord in order to save three minutes time does not appear to be in the best interests of the newborn infant.

Early clamping has been demonstrated by research to lengthen the third stage of labor and increase the likelihood of maternal hemorrhage, retained placenta, or the retention of placental fragments. The latter condition frequently necessitates the mother's return to the hospital in order to stop inordinate bleeding and to prevent infection. Because early clamping tends to interfere with the spontaneous separation of the placenta, making the need for obstetrical intervention more likely . . . , such a practice also tends to increase the incidence of fetomaternal hemorrhage or transfusion. Fetomaternal transfusion, which occurs when fetal blood cells pass into the maternal circulatory system, increases the likelihood that an Rh negative mother of an Rh positive baby will develop antibodies. If a mother has already developed such antibodies, fetomaternal transfusion should be avoided in order to lessen any complications for any future Rh positive fetus the mother might carry.

Whether early clamping increases the incidence of anemia in the rapidly growing child has not been sufficiently investigated, but research has demonstrated that the red cell volume of late clamped full-term infants increases by 47 percent.

ROUTINE SUCTIONING WITH A NASOGASTRIC TUBE

Although the use of a nasogastric tube attached to a deLee trap is now a widely used method for removing mucus from the newborn infant's nasopharynx, Cordero and Hon suggest that blind suctioning with a nasogastric tube is a hazardous procedure. They point out that the procedure can cause severe cardiac arrhythmias and apnea—conditions which do not tend to develop when the suctioning is accomplished by the use of a bulk syringe.

APGAR SCORING BY THE ACCOUCHEUR

No one can be completely impartial in judging his own skills, no matter how objective he or she may try to be. As one pediatrician put it, "Asking the person who delivers the infant to determine that infant's score on the Apgar scale is like asking a student to fill out his own report card." In countries where obstetrical medication is the exception rather than the rule the Apgar score of the majority of newborn infants seldom falls below nine. Therefore, it would appear that an infant's Apgar score is possibly more influenced by the management of labor and delivery than the physical condition of the mother.

Although there is a "maximum dosage" level and time interval recommended by the manufacturer of most obstetrical medications, there are no recommendations, guidelines, or restrictions on the use of several medications administered to the mother at the same time. Nor is there any recommendation or guideline for determining safe time intervals between administration of multiple medication. A review by the hospital joint obstetric-pediatric committee of any Apgar score of seven or below would very likely tend to improve infant outcome.

Treatment of a slow learner or retarded child may be facilitated by knowing the Apgar score of the child under observation. Since the Apgar score of an individual is now always accessible several years after birth (many hospitals discard birth records after seven to ten years) parents should be given a copy of their baby's Apgar score for retention, even if the score is coded.

OBSTETRICAL INTERVENTION IN PLACENTAL EXPULSION

The most common mismanagement of the third stage of labor involves an attempt to hasten it. Cord traction, the use of uterine stimulants such as oxytocin, ergonovene, etc., manipulation of the fundus, and manual removal as a means of accelerating the expulsion of a reluctant placenta are pathological procedures which tend to increase the incidence of fetomaternal transfusion, maternal blood loss, and the incidence of retained afterbirth or placental fragments. Such obstetrical intervention is rarely found necessary when (1) the mother has received little or no medication, (2) she has been supported to a semisitting position for birth, and (3) placental transfusion has reduced the volume of the placenta.

SEPARATING THE MOTHER FROM HER NEWBORN INFANT

There is no evidence that the full-term infant of a relatively unmedicated mother will suffer an abnormal drop in temperature if he is dried off quickly, wrapped in a prewarmed blanket, and placed in his mother's arms during the recovery period. Experience at Yale–New Haven Hospital in Connecticut indicates that when the above procedure is followed and the mother is allowed to hold her baby for two hours or so, the infant's body temperature remains stable. In light of the present concern over the possible hazard of infant warming devices in the delivery room, perhaps we should recommend one of the most logical of warming devices—the mother's arms.

A mother-baby recovery room, staffed with skilled nursing personnel, makes it possible for even the high-risk or postoperative mother to be with her baby during the first hours of life.

Recent research by Klaus and Salk has demonstrated that the conventional hospital postpartum routine tends to inhibit rather than engender maternal response and nurturing. The first twenty-four hours following birth appear to be a critical period for the establishment of the normal mother-infant bonds. Separating the mother from her infant during this time tends to interfere with the mother's normal responses to her baby. Salk suggests that the mother's increased sensitivity to her newborn infant during the first twenty-four hours following birth may be a biochemical mechanism which is not yet understood. Both Salk and Klaus have demonstrated that maternal responses and nurturing are adversely affected a full one month after birth when the mother and her baby have been restricted to the usual hospital postpartum schedule (a glimpse of the baby shortly after birth, brief contact and identification at six to twelve hours, and then twenty to thirty minutes every four hours for feeding). How long this initial restrictive pattern of contact adversely affects maternal behavior is yet to be assessed.

As I visit hospitals throughout the world I am always impressed by the effort made in most countries to keep mothers and their babies together from the very moment of birth. Even when there are abnormal conditions which require adjustments to be made, there is still great emphasis placed on the importance of mother-baby contact during the immediate postpartum period.

DELAYING THE FIRST BREASTFEEDING

The common American practice of routinely delaying the time of the first breast-feeding has not been shown to be in the best interest of either the conscious mother or her newborn infant. Clinical experience with the early feeding of newborn infants has shown this practice to be safe. If the mother feels well enough and the infant is capable of suckling while they are still in the delivery room, then it would seem more cautious, in the event of tracheoe-sophageal abnormality, to permit the infant to suckle for the first time under the watchful eye of the physician or nurse-midwife rather than delay the feeding for several hours when the expertise of the professional may not be immediately available.

In light of the many protective antibodies contained in colostrum it would seem likely that the earlier the infant's intake of species-specific colostrum, the sooner the antibodies can be accrued by the infant.

Research on several species of animals suggests that the earlier the newborn's intake of colostrum and maternal milk the earlier gut closure will occur. Gut closure, whereby the colostrum acts as a sealant to the intestinal lining, appears to prevent or lessen the passage of harmful bacteria or foreign protein through the intestinal lining. Although similar research has not been carried out on the human infant, it is not unlikely that such a similar protective mechanism exists.

OFFERING WATER AND FORMULA TO THE BREAST-FED NEWBORN INFANT

The common American practice of giving water or formula to a newborn infant prior to the first breast-feeding or as a supplement during the first days of life has not been shown to be in the best interests of the infant. There are now indications that these practices may, in fact, be harmful. Glucose water, once the standby in every American hospital, has now been designated a potential hazard if aspirated by the newborn infant, yet it is still used in many American hospitals.

It is a comment on the American penchant for the artificial that there has never been any research carried out in the United States which attempts to evaluate the safety of colostrum as the infant's first intake of fluid, yet nature obviously intended the initial fluid intake of the newborn infant to be of the same consistency as the relatively thick, viscous colostrum.

Whether the human infant experiences a gut

closure, as is seen in animals, and whether the administering of water or formula initially to the infant who is to be breast-fed will interfere with normal gut closure has not been scientifically investigated. Experts in the raising of cows make great effort to see that species-specific bovine colostrum, not milk or water, is the first fluid received by the newborn calf. It is ironic that we do not give the same consideration to human newborns.

Unless the physician or the nurse can be absolutely sure that an infant has no familial history of allergy, it would be cautious to obtain the mother's permission before offering her infant formula in the nursery. Offering the infant formula in the nursery interferes with the normal progress of lactation in so many ways that the subject cannot be adequately discussed herein.

RESTRICTING NEWBORN INFANTS TO A FOUR-HOUR FEEDING SCHEDULE AND WITHHOLDING NIGHTTIME FEEDINGS

Although widely spaced infant feedings may be more convenient for hospital personnel, the practice of feeding a newborn infant only every four hours and not permitting the infant to breast-feed at all during the night cannot be justified on any scientific grounds. Such a regimen restricts the suckling stimulation necessary to bring about the normally rapid onset and adequate production of the mother's milk. In countries where custom permits the infant to suckle immediately after birth and on demand from that time, first-time mothers frequently begin to produce breast milk for their babies within twenty-four hours after birth. In contrast, in countries where hospital routines prevent normal, demand feeding from birth, mothers frequently do not produce breast milk for their babies until the third day following birth.

Widely spaced feedings, which limit the normal suckling stimulation of the breast:

1. Restrict the infant's normal intake of colostrum at a time when he is most in need of the protective antibodies in colostrum.

2. Increase the likelihood of dehydration in the infant by suppressing both the onset and production of breast milk.

3. Interfere with the maintaining of the normal, relatively constant level of glucose in the infant's blood which occurs when an infant is fed on demand.

4. Increase the likelihood of overdistention of the breast by interfering with the normal clearing of colostrum from the lactiferous ducts before the onset of milk.

5. Increase the likelihood of poor "let-down" of breast milk due to the mother's discomfort or pain resulting when the overly hungry infant tugs anxiously at his mother's engorged, unyielding breast which is overdistended with accumulated milk.

Physiological jaundice, which, if it does occur, usually appears about the third day of life, appears to be quite common among infants in those cultures where breast-feeding predominates. The switching of an infant from his mother's milk to foreign protein because he shows evidence of physiological jaundice is a practice which has not been justified by scientific research.

A scientific evaluation of the relationship of prenatal diuretics and other pharmacologic agents to the incidence of postnatal jaundice should be carried out.

PREVENTING EARLY FATHER-CHILD CONTACT

Permitting fathers to hold their newborn infants immediately following birth and during the postpartum hospital stay has not been shown by research or clinical experience to increase the incidence of infection among newborns, even when those infants are returned to a regular or central nursery. Yet, only in the eastern European countries is the father permitted less involvement in the immediate postpartum period than in the United States (eastern European fathers are usually not permitted to enter beyond the foyer of the maternity hospital and are not allowed to see their wives or babies for the entire seven- to nine-day stay). Research has consistently confirmed the fact that the greatest sources of infection to the newborn infant are the nursery and nursery personnel. One has only to observe a mother holding her newborn infant against her bathrobe, which has probably been exposed to abundant hospital-borne bacteria, to realize the fallacy of preventing a father from holding his baby during the hospital stay.

ASSIGNING NURSING PERSONNEL TO MOTHERS OR TO BABIES (RATHER THAN TO MOTHER-BABY COUPLES)

The traditional American system of assigning postpartum nurses to mothers and nursery nurses to babies has done much to distort the normal pattern of initial mother-baby interaction. The European concept of assigning nursing personnel to care for mother-baby couples, then letting them care for their assigned babies in the mothers' rooms or in the nursery, has not been shown to increase the incidence of infection. The latter pattern of assignment has been approved by the Committee on Fetus and Newborn of the American Academy of Pediatrics.

RESTRICTING INTERMITTENT ROOMING-IN TO SPECIFIC ROOM REQUIREMENTS

Throughout the world great effort is made to keep mothers and babies together in the hospital, no matter how inconvenient the accommodations. There is no research or evidence which indicates that intermittent rooming-in should be restricted to private rooms or to rooms which have a sink, or which provide at least 80 square feet for mother and baby. Such requirements are based on conjecture and not controlled evaluation. Nor is there any scientific support for requiring that each room used for intermittent rooming-in be supplied with a covered diaper receptacle. A simple system, whereby soiled diapers and baby linen are placed

in plastic bags which are tied to the crib (for the mother's convenience) and then changed at the end of each shift, has been found to be safe. This system would appear less likely to be a source of infection than using communal diaper receptacles and is far less expensive for the hospital.

RESTRICTING SIBLING VISITATION

The common American practice of prohibiting toddlers and children from visiting their mothers during the hospital stay is an emotional hardship on both the mothers and their children and is unsupported by scientific research or evidence. Experience in other countries and in several hospitals here in the United States suggests that where sibling visitation is permitted a short explanation as to the importance of not bringing suspect illnesses into the hospital seems to be effective in controlling infection.

SUMMARY

As mentioned previously, most of the practices discussed above have developed not from a lack of concern for the well-being of the mother and baby but from a lack of awareness as to the problems which can arise from each progressive digression from the normal childbearing experience. Like a snowball rolling downhill, as one unphysiological practice is employed, for one reason or another, another frequently becomes necessary to counteract some of the disadvantages, large or small, inherent in the previous procedure.

The higher incidence of fetal, neonatal, and maternal deaths occurring in our large urban hospitals, as opposed to our smaller community hospitals, is undoubtedly due, in part, to the greater proportion of high-risk mothers in the urban areas. But we in the United States must stop looking for scapegoats and face up to the fact that, by individualizing the care offered to maternity patients, much can be done immediately to improve infant outcome without the slightest outlay of capital.

There is currently an increasing emphasis on consolidating maternity facilities. However, we in ICEA do not see the consolidation of community obstetrical facilities as being always in the best interest of the vast majority of mothers who are capable of giving birth without complications. There should, of course, be centers where those mothers who have had no prenatal care or who are anticipated to be obstetrical risks can be properly cared for. But to insist that every healthy mother must go to a major maternity facility which is unnecessary for her needs and inconvenient for her family, and where she is very apt to be "lost in the crowd," will only spur the growing trend in the United States toward professionally unattended home births.

Throughout the United States the current inclination of many expectant parents is to seek out, to "shop around" for the type of physician and hospital they feel they need in order to have the type of childbearing experience they want. They not only want a doctor who will support them in their efforts to have a prepared, natural birth, with a minimum of or no medication, they also want a hospital which offers education for childbearing and a supportive family-centered atmosphere. These expectant mothers appreciate the availability of such facilities as an early labor lounge, a dual-purpose labor-delivery room, a mother-baby recovery room, and a children's visiting room if they have older children. But most of all they want a supportive atmosphere in which they can share the childbearing experience to the extent that they desire and one which makes an effort to meet the individual needs of the mother, the father, and their newborn baby as they form their family bonds during the hospital stay.

By working together in an interdisciplinary effort, the professional and lay members of the International Childbirth Education Association of the USA and Canada, the National Childbirth Trust of Great Britain, and the Parents' Centers of both New Zealand and Australia have served as catalysts to the improvement of maternity care throughout much of the world. We stand united in the belief that parents should be educated and prepared for childbearing and then be given the freedom to participate effectively in the birth of their children in order to insure the quality of life's beginning.

Motherhood

LETTY COTTIN POGREBIN

Letty Cottin Pogrebin, "Motherhood," *Ms.*, May 1973. Reprinted by permission.

I'd like to interview everybody," I announce at a recent meeting of our women's group. "I'm writing an article on motherhood."

"Oh God," my friends respond. "How boring! How old hat! How *could* you!"

One evening at the dinner table I question my children about their thoughts on motherhood.

"Is that like Robin Hood?" asks my five-year-old son.

One 3-year-old daughter assumes an angelic expression and recites: "Motherhood is a great thing because a mother is a person's very best relative."

"A mother is someone who looks good in hoods," offers her twin sister, overjoyed at her own wit.

My husband shifts the conversation to a more pressing problem: "Now let's see if we can't all agree," he begins patiently, "that a family in midtown Manhattan has no business buying a hunting dog."

During the next several weeks I declare to every woman I meet that I need some input on motherhood. A couple of young unmarried friends admit that they're afraid to have children. It seems too difficult, too demanding.

A mother of teenagers confirms that kids are not easy but, for her, life would be incomplete without them.

"I don't think motherhood is for me," says a married woman who is childless at age thirty-one. "At least not until I feel that fatherhood will really mean something to my husband."

"I want to have children whether I have a husband or not," declares a single woman who has given the subject much thought.

A mother who is also a lesbian states flatly: "I wouldn't have missed having and living with my child for anything in the world."

"I believe you can mother problems and projects if you're not the type who can mother kids," explains a busy activist. "But I admire someone who enjoys motherhood and does it well."

As I listen I think about how these statements would surprise the many people who seem to believe (with the aid of media distortion) that the women's movement is rabidly antimotherhood. In some minds, the all-purpose "women's libber" is either a self-serving single career girl who has an abortion every spring, or a Marxist lesbian who hates men, motherhood, and the flag.

Sure, there are a small number of radical women who argue that total biological equality between the sexes could be brought about by the development of test-tube pregnancies and the elimination of marriage, the nuclear family, and even "childhood" itself. However repellent this may seem to some, many people are intellectually engaged by the political ramifications of such visionary social changes. But the bottom line is that these few of our revolutionary sisters usually deliver themselves of opinions, not babies.

The rest of us, scores of feminists of every age, race, marital status, and sexual persuasion are talking seriously, thoughtfully, and candidly about motherhood.

We either have children already or wish to retain that option in our life spans. We care deeply about children whether we have our own or not. We work to improve educational curricula, child care facilities, health services, and the childbirth experience. We are saying that men are parents, too; that fatherhood need be no less important or time-consuming than motherhood. We are examining the guilt feelings that force us into involuntary servitude in the home. Fears about the loss of our freedom; skepticism about our readiness for sharing that responsibility equally—all these serpentine doubts are writhing out in the open where we can get a grip on them.

We are trying, too, to make peace with the fecund wombs that have been used by sexist society to prove our weakness—sometimes a prideful peace and sometimes a peace of resignation. Most of us choose to see the female's "inner space" as a physiological reality, not an internal psychic or spiritual void. We refuse to believe that women are hollow shells unless and until we have brought forth issue.

Truly, feminists are talking about choice: about *making* the decision to become pregnant and *choosing* a motherly role that is right for ourselves and our children.

It sounds simple. And logical. Yet, in this area, the notion of choice is a new one for our generation. In the minds of so many women, motherhood is prescribed; nonmotherhood is deviate. Childless women are to be pitied. Motherhood is synonymous with womanhood (in a way that fatherhood has never been considered sufficient to fulfill a man or to prove manhood). Caring for a child is, in the old view, a shortcut to self-respect, maturity, and even martyrdom. For women who grew up believing in the inevitability of motherhood, the notion of choice is in itself disturbing and heretical. And so, when these women try to relate to the movement—no matter how much they may agree with its pragmatic goals—there is a point of alienation.

"Women's liberation makes me feel defensive about being a mother," my neighbor tells me. "I think feminists are looking at me and thinking: Is that all she can do?"

A woman at our local playground solemnly questions the loss of distinctions: "Once the nurturant role was woman's manifest destiny. Now psychologists are disproving the maternal instinct, and new fathers are demanding paternity leaves. Will there be anything special left for women?"

"I've come full circle right back to where my Victorian grandmother was," says a pregnant friend with a toddler on each hand. "Granny had to hide her condition out of modesty. My belly is embarrassing in 1973 because it labels me a population exploder or an exploited baby machine."

I am troubled by this new lament. It seems to proclaim that women are divided on the point that should most unite us. Right now, a discussion of motherhood can shake sisterhood to its roots. There is intransigence and enmity. The extremists' requiem for motherhood is premature; the traditionalists' Hallelujah Chorus is anachronistic. Yet no one seems able to orchestrate an ideology about motherhood that plays right for both audiences.

At this point in my investigations I become convinced that if anything can be said at this time about being a mother and a committed feminist, it must be no more ambitious and no less honest than a personal commentary—even if it comes out disconnected, vulnerable, and frankly sentimental.

I have found myself, now and then, in fierce arguments with people who can see no merit whatsoever in having children. These are not the proponents of zero population growth; they are arguing as if they believe in zero population. And no matter how I resolve never to proselytize parenthood, I find myself extolling the joys of a small child's smile in answer to their accusations that I produce offspring to guarantee my own immortality. (Since I have a profession, I am spared the aspersions about substituting procreative for creative energy. But those guns are at the ready for women not presently gainfully employed.)

The plot thickens. While the militant childless may have no ideological sympathy with the women's movement, they freely borrow and distort whatever feminist rhetoric is serviceable.

Under attack I begin to understand how, without its nuances explained, any monolithic party line can make women defensive and hostile. Because I am a mother of three, I make a clear target for the militant childless. And I realize that everything I say about the meaning of children in my life becomes a platitude echoing Sophie Portnoy or Rose Kennedy. It gives one pause.

Can we verbalize some of the components of motherhood or does analysis of the parts tend to trivialize the whole? If one has never known thunderous fear when a child is lost in a crowd, or shared the sweet intensity of a small boy's secret, or felt the blissful vertigo of a little girl's first bicycle solo, then explaining mother love—or father love, for that matter (though here I must speak only for myself)—will be rather like explaining the sea to a landlocked people. One puts sand in their palms and conchs to their ears and trusts the rest to human imagination.

I cry in natural childbirth movies. When the baby's head emerges, I want to cheer. The appearance of shoulders and arms makes me laugh, and finally the sight of the entire tiny creature bathed in primal slime moves me to awe, and more tears and whispered sobs about God and miracles. My emotional upheaval always peaks at that excruciatingly tender moment when the mother first sees her baby—still anchored to her by a twisted cord, but real, alive, and bawling triumphantly. It is a moment I profoundly missed when my first child was born.

Of necessity, cesarean sections are somewhat impersonal and antiseptic. So it was only after the total anesthesia wore off that my twins were brought to my hospital room in wheeled carts, and I saw my babies for the first time just as any visitor could have seen them: placid dolls sponged clean and swathed in neat bunting wraps. I remember nothing of their grand entrance into life; it could have been the stork that brought them after all.

Women who adopt their babies report that the life-cycle shock of motherhood can happen the instant your child is placed in your arms. In my case, missing the actual birth made the advent of motherhood seem remote and unreal. All I know is I badly needed a mother during thirteen hours of labor. Next thing I knew I was a mother myself. Perhaps the problem was that I was drugged during the drama of transition. Or maybe the fault lay with my preconceptions of what it would feel like to be a mother. Like many women, I had shaped a transcendent ideal out of my childhood image of my own mother. And I truly believed that ripeness, solidity, and wisdom would gestate within me along with the fetus, and that I would give birth to my own adult persona at the same time as I delivered my first child.

Well, it didn't happen that way. My first child was children, plural—which may have crowded out the gestating persona—and the fully mature mother I intended to be never quite materialized.

Next time around I refused to undergo childbirth *in absentia*. Although my third child also had to be delivered surgically, this cesarean was by appointment, and I insisted upon an anesthetic that would allow me to remain numb but conscious. My view was obscured by a tent of green sheets until the doctor yanked out the baby and hoisted him up in the air like a victory banner. True to form, I cried and laughed, clapped and whooped until the doctor warned that my display was making it impossible to suture the incision. He ordered a mask of gas to put me out of my ecstasy.

This time, because I had witnessed the birth I expected to wake up feeling transformed at last. But watching my son taken from my body like a vital organ did not change my perception of myself as unalterably unmotherly; motherhood as a state of mind was no more palpable than before.

Since then the years have passed cheerfully. I'm having a terrific time with my children and they claim I'm a good mother. I gladly answer when someone calls, "Mom." But I can't help feeling still that a mother is someone you *have*, not someone you *are*. Knowing myself since childhood, I simply cannot fit myself into my own abstraction of a Mother. I suppose the only one who ever could was my own mother. And perhaps that is as it should be after all.

If the truth were known, all parents have their favorite child-development state. Infancy was my least favorite period. I find that the more expressive and independent my kids become, the more I enjoy being with them.

Of course I know that nonverbal communication can be full of feeling and that caring and ministering to a baby is a kind of interchange. But personally, I have never been particularly gratified by dependency. I get no satisfaction out of being needed by someone who is totally powerless. (By contrast, one of my friends says she never thought of herself as independent until she had someone she knew was dependent on her. She views her babies as living proof that she is important and competent.) In my opinion, however, once a child can say "I think" or "I won't," the mother-child axis becomes more balanced, complex, and interesting.

Naturally, infancy is a period of justifiable dependency, and during my children's earliest months, I responded to their needs without resentment. But feeding, bathing, burping, or diapering aren't acts of love. They are functions one performs lovingly for a child (and I believe mothers, fathers, or surrogates can perform them); they are not the best that motherhood has to offer. To call them rewarding, or to romanticize them in Pampers, Gerber's, or Ivory soap commercials is to mislead women (and men) and to risk starting parenthood with disillusionment.

The mother who glorifies and prolongs infancy may be clinging to her one opportunity to exercise control. In a world that disapproves of women in positions of authority, she is allowed and encouraged to be "in charge" of the children. Her helpless children are "her job." When they leave infancy, their growth toward self-sufficiency is a rebuke to the mother's indispensability and an erosion of her "job." Because the dependency mechanism can be habit-forming, it seems to me we must learn to love our children enough to let them grow away from us. And value ourselves enough so there is something left over when they leave.

Living with children has humanized me. Though I cannot claim an undifferentiated appreciation of all kids, the existence of my own children gives me a personalized empathy with the children of others.

The sterilized news of Vietnam couldn't disguise the fact that "defoliation" meant crops were being destroyed, and children were starving; "pacification" meant homes were leveled, families displaced; "accidental civilian casualties" meant babies had been maimed and slaughtered.

Everywhere—in the bizarre and the commonplace—I am sensitive to the discomforts of the children. In restaurants I see them hushed up and scowled upon. On public streets I see them slapped or dragged along disdainfully. In friends' homes I see them roughly scolded in the name of the parents' standards but without regard for the children's dignity. All too often, in the presence of the young, adults smile "Partridge Family" smiles and talk in condescending clichés. I don't remember noticing any of this eight years ago, before the children came.

Having children has also revitalized my sense of the future. I feel a greater responsibility for my own survival—not because "my children *need* me" but because I am deeply curious about the unseen scenario for all five of us. There is a difference, though, between my concept of future for the children and the one I attempt to contemplate for my husband and myself.

For example, since I am still in my early thirties, becoming forty is an abstraction. I can only try to imagine how it will feel and what I will want to do and be. I have never been forty before. But when my children turn twelve or seventeen years old, I shall have a million points of reference. I have been there before. And no matter how the children choose to design those years for themselves, I will always have a sense of my own participation in an observed future that is more familiar than my own. I enjoy being a witness to the possibilities.

Which is not to say that I want to mold their lives in my image or to make my children, at twelve or seventeen, all the things I couldn't be. It seems to me one can share and enhance a child's life without dominating it. As one mother puts it: "I am not a sculptor who molds a child from clay. I'm the gardener who tends a seed that will grow to become itself." Another metaphor maker compares the process to apprenticeship: the protégé (child) lives with the sponsor (parent) in order to benefit from experience, minimize stress, and become professional at living in this world.

Childhood, I believe, is something one can experience twice. The first time directly, with growing pains and discovery, frustration and endless wonder. Living through childhood as a child is the universal purgatory, for our first real childhood is not ours to control. But our children's childhood is our second chance. And if we have kept our memories sharp and sensitive, we can help support a more endurable purgatory for our daughters and sons than the one we remember distilled in nightmares and dreams.

"Let's have a private talk, Mom."

It's an invitation I cherish. One child and I, without distractions; we banish other family members, close the door, lounge upon the big bed, and prop ourselves against the pillows. We are close. Trusting. A time for emotional refueling. Or for venting anger. Occasionally, one child simply wants to boast to me about something the others might call bragging or teasing. But most often we meet behind closed doors to discuss disappointment, confusion, and fear.

"When they said we had eight and a half players on our side, I knew I was the half, Mom, 'cause I was the only girl on the team."

I remember how it feels to be "just a girl" when boys are choosing up sides. (It still happens to me now, as a woman among men.) I remember once playing hide-and-seek. Secluded behind a wooden fence, I waited endless minutes for the boys to find me. Finally I understood that I had been tricked; they had run away to play without me.

After our talk I ask you to read aloud to me because it is your certain skill and I know no other child your age who can read with the exuberance that you give to a story you love. And a few days from now we will go to Central Park and we will throw baseballs and run and bat the ball into the trees until you feel strong and whole again.

"Mommy, I feel like sleeping with the lamp on tonight."

You were upset today when we saw war protestors lying in the street. And you were troubled when I explained that this was a symbolic reminder of real people dying in a faraway land. I know it is on your mind and you are frightened. Long ago, my father had an air-raid helmet, and my mother doused the lights, and we practiced being bombed in New York City. That was 1944, but I have not forgotten that a child doesn't always know how to tell what is real from what is make-believe.

"Did you get undressed in the bathroom when you and Daddy first had sexible intercourse?"

I tell you there are times when we display our bodies proudly, like poems that we have written to read aloud to someone we love. You confide your confusion: What about privacy? Why do women cover their breasts? Why do boys laugh when they see a girl's underwear? You ask why you sometimes feel ashamed. There's so much you want me to explain but, I suspect, in my way I'm as muddled as you. I teach you to feel good about your body, and yet I say you cannot lie naked in the sun. I explain that some people are perverted, and others are easily offended. Can I possibly make sense of it? In this second chance at childhood, I hack through a forest of sexual memories to clear a path for you that is not as tangled as my own was. I try not to fumble, although it's very difficult and I am not sure of myself. But for you, perhaps there should be less modesty so that there will be less shame.

I have often asked my mother-in-law for her secret.

"How did you raise him? What did you do that was different?"

I'm looking for a clue to explain why my husband is so easy to live with. It would be immensely helpful to me in raising my own son if I could know how my husband's mother produced a male with such a generous spirit, so innate a respect for women, such an absence of *macho* tensions, so much humor and love to give to me and the children. My mother-in-law shrugs. She claims the only secret she can pass along to me concerns the making of perfect stuffed cabbage.

When I ask my husband about his childhood, he tells me that he and his father always did the vacuuming.

I find both answers a trifle too glib. What I need is a signal that I'm on the right track with my son. While his father is a direct model, I also seek a special kind of relationship with our little boy. I'd like to avoid the classic conflicts and all the small-scale sex-role charades that I've seen mothers and sons act out over the years. So for the time being I have decided not to differentiate between my daughters and my son in the way I love and counsel them. With each of the three I have an organic mothering relationship that defines itself in new ways all the time.

Still, I wonder. How do you help a boy to be confident but not arrogant? How do you teach reason and compassion in a world where masculinity is equated with violence? As a woman, a feminist, and a mother, I have a certain mandate: what I transmit via example—and what my husband transmits via attitude—will affect my son's experience with women and men for the rest of his life. Together, his father and I will establish for him what we believe manhood is all about.

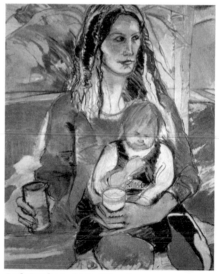

Lady Madonna by Jeri Drucker.

When my son bullies his two older sisters, I sometimes question whether aggression may be inborn after all. When he points a carrot at me and shouts, "Pow! You're dead!," I feel I'm not getting through. And when he announces to our role-free household "Daddy's the boss," I'm totally baffled.

But there are times when he loses himself in painting or requests *The Nutcracker Suite* for his bedtime record or spends long periods playing gently with his infant cousin, and then I decide he is a well-balanced short person indeed. The other day I even had a glimpse of a brave new world in which children will choose freely what they like to do and want to be; a world where competence and interest are not sex-typed quantities but are uncensored expressions of the self.

I had brought home several new things that the girls needed for school: paraffin, notepads, some colored yarn. My son looked up from his caravan of toy trucks, saw the haul of packages, and whined: "That's not fair! There's nothing for me." I told him we might get him something one day soon and asked what he'd like to have.

"A sewing kit," he said.

Time and again when I lecture, I am introduced as a "wife and mother of three." That credential precedes me to the podium like a disclaimer on the label of a dangerous drug—as though the audience could not tolerate a dose of feminist opinion without marriage and motherhood to make it palatable.

Isn't it obvious that by categorizing one another in opposing terms such as "career gal" or "working mother," we perpetuate the straitjacketing roles that limit women's lives? When was the last time we heard a serious male speaker introduced to an audience as "husband and father of three"? Who calls a businessman a "career guy" or "working father"? Sexist semantics is the verbal shorthand for sexist institutions. It's time we all kicked the habit.

I find it remarkable that traditional women's groups only ask to know that I am a mother—not whether I am a good mother or a happy mother. Once assured that I am one of them, however, an extraordinary thing happens: they then insist that I be *better* than they. If they can believe that I am superwoman and supermother, then they can exempt themselves from what I may say about self-actualization, expanded options, and women's participation in social change. They would like some proof that I am special—more educated, organized, energetic, younger, older, calmer—so that they can deny our commonality. It is a crafty device to protect themselves from identifying with what I have to say.

But I refuse to play that game. When they ask me how I "manage," instead of how I feel or think, I point out that their question betrays something like my own tendency to make motherhood fit an abstraction. I tell them that there is no right answer; I am not special; I don't have the formula for perfect motherhood. I am only trying to work it all out for myself and my children.

We all carry the secret fear that every other woman is doing a better job of it and only we are failures at "managing." It is one of our many common obsessions.

Pity. If only we could talk together about guilt and resentment, frenzy and frustration, devotion and love, then perhaps we could begin to arrive at the truth about our children and our lives. Unless we demythologize motherhood for all women, there will always be suffering for those who fear to be Gorgons, and despair for those who expect to be goddesses.

I came to terms with motherhood when one of my plainspoken daughters asked me the ultimate question. It was an average Saturday. Chaos was loose in the house. My husband was grumbling about a troublesome legal issue while trying to dress our son for a birthday party. I was alternately wrapping the birthday gift, working at the typewriter, and helping one daughter to make papier-mâché.

Then the other daughter began complaining. She was bored. *No one* was paying attention to her. When would *somebody* have time to play with her. Totally frazzled, I explained that after her father took her brother to the party, he was going to the library to do some research. I had an article deadline to meet and would be at my desk all afternoon with the door closed. It was up to each girl to find activities for herself. No loud noise please. No interruptions. No fussing!

That was when she asked, "Did you ever wish you never had us in the first place?"

I think I became partially paralyzed. Guilt flooded my cheeks with blood. The glands in my neck seemed suddenly swollen. I've scarred her, I thought: I've made her feel like a burden—unwanted, unloved, rejected. Then I realized she was waiting for an answer. We both deserved to know the truth. I sorted my ragged thoughts and took her onto my lap. Gentleness wrapped around us like a fog. When I finally spoke, I believe I was answering an unasked question in my soul.

"Sometimes my life is a little too full because I have you children," I said, "but, for me, it would be much too empty if I didn't."

In Which a Sensible Woman Persuades Her Doctor, Her Family, and Her Friends to Help Her Give Birth at Home

BARBARA KATZ ROTHMAN

Barbara Katz Rothman, excerpt from "In Which a Sensible Woman . . . ," *Ms.*, December 1976. Reprinted by permission.

December 17

Dear Linda,

I need you to be fairly impartial, to act as a "sounding board." Hesch is as supportive and helpful as a husband can be, but he's just too involved. And I think everyone else thinks I'm crazy. So as sister (and aunt), you're elected.

I do not want to have the baby in the hospital. I've started to do some reading, and it does seem to me that the hospitals create as many problems as they solve—with too many drugs, and delivery tables that force you to give birth against gravity, and just too much interference.

I really don't feel ready to be thinking about all this so soon—I won't even look pregnant for another four months—but I know that if I don't start now, I'll surely end up in a hospital.

So—I made about 60 phone calls to obstetricians today, and I just may have found a doctor. She's never done it, but at least she'll talk to me about it.

My breasts are hurting. That's certainly planning ahead, isn't it?

Love, Barbara

December 29

Dear Linda,

It's been quite a day. We got into a strange kind of bargaining situation. She promised a "relaxed hospital environment," no prep (enema and shave), and I can go home as soon after the delivery as I want to—measured in hours, not days. All I have to do is go to the hospital. It took the wind out of my sails.

I don't know what to do. Maybe I ought to just be a good girl and go to the hospital like everybody else.

Love, Barbara

January 17

Dear Linda,

You're right. I don't know what a "relaxed hospital environment" is supposed to mean either. It's like that George Carlin routine on inherent contradictions: jumbo shrimp, military intelligence, etc.

I don't want my consciousness raised on the delivery table. I'm a feminist and I'm pregnant. That shouldn't be contradictory. There has to be a way of having a baby with dignity and joy—as a feminist, not in spite of being a feminist.

I've been reading about "natural childbirth." First off, they prefer to call it "prepared" rather than natural, there being nothing particularly natural about breathing and relaxation exercises you have to learn. I gather that if you're a very good girl and you show how cooperative you're being, then probably the nurses won't strap your hands down. If you're very polite and rational with your doctor, then maybe you won't be anesthetized when you don't want it. Terrific. It seems to me you should be able to make these decisions when you're at your best and be able to expect that nobody will double-cross you when you're defenseless.

Does that sound paranoid? We've been raised with the idea that hospitals are not just the best, they are the *only* place to give birth—and we lose sight of the fact that hospitals are a fairly recent invention, and like all institutions, they are run more for the comfort of the staff than for those they ostensibly service. And so when I remind people of that, they tell me: "We all have our hangups." It's an interesting, and frightening, way to dismiss my ideas.

Love, Barbara

March 12

Dear Linda,

I am now recognizably pregnant, and people are starting to respond to me differently. My belly is public property.

I'm getting basically two kinds of response to the idea of having the baby at home, now that people are beginning to believe I mean it. First, an astonishing number of women say they were talked out of it. I had no idea that so many women wanted it. It makes it all the harder for me to understand why nobody's doing anything about it.

The second response is for people to tell me that it's not safe. Some people tell me how they, or their mother or aunt or friend, would have died if they hadn't been in a hospital. And when I ask why, it so far has always turned out to be not as it first sounds. Some were in labor for frighteningly long times and needed medical assistance, even a cesarean. Long labors, by definition, are not sudden medical emergencies. Some were breech births, or RH problems—but those things you know about weeks ahead of time. When you have good reason to expect a problem, then you *do* go to a hospital.

But the best story was the friend who told me that her mother would have died without emergency care. Why? The hospital had given her the wrong drug and if she hadn't been in a hospital, they couldn't have corrected the error!

I started wearing maternity clothes. Did you ever look in a maternity department? One of my friends says that if a man from Mars arrived, he'd think that in pregnancy the breasts swell, the belly grows, and little puffs appear on your shoulders.

Maternally yours, Barbara

May 15

Dear Linda,

I'm getting bigger and bigger, and the time is getting closer. And I can't seem to get a real commitment from the doctor. I wrote her a letter, and I'm sending you a copy.

Barbara

Dear Marcia:

This has something very basic to do with questions of control, power, and authority. At home, I have it; in the hospital, it's handed over to the institution. I don't want this to come across in such a way that it is offensive to you, but the way I see it is that I am hiring you to do a service for me. In your office, I can hold on to that idea. Not so in other offices I have been to. The asymmetry of forms of address sets the tone for an entirely different relationship ("The Doctor will see you now, Barbara." "Hello, Dr. Stevens." "Hello, Barbara.").

I have read arguments for home rather than hospital delivery that spoke about privacy. I think it's less a question of privacy and more a question of authority. At home, nobody's coming in the door that I did not choose to have come in. I chose you and I am therefore delegating my control over my body to you, or pretty much anyway. I'll do what you tell me to do, and see you as the "expert." But that's because I expect you to be making decisions on the basis of your medical expertise, and not on the basis of "them's the rules" or what's most convenient in an institution that is simultaneously processing umpty-seven baby-making women.

Besides the authority/control issue, there are other reasons. As Hesch pointed out the other day, I am having a baby after all and not an appendectomy. It is a condition of health, not of illness. You do not put someone in hospital gowns on hospital tables under hospital lights with little bracelets on, and not create the image of patient.

At home I will go into labor and I'll call you and the nurse and eventually someone will show up and eventually the baby will be born and eventually you'll all leave. There is a continuum. The hospital alternative means, first I go into labor and then we have to decide when it's serious enough for me to be driven to the hospital. From there on I am processed through, in clearly demarcated states—labor room, delivery room, wherever one goes after, and then back home. It is partly a question of how the situation is defined and again partly a question of control over self and situation.

I think I first got the idea seriously about six or seven years ago. I saw two childbirth films. One was the Lamaze film with everybody running around and carrying on in French at this woman all draped in white on a table. The other was a film of a down-south black midwife at work. The black woman giving birth did not know from beans about panting in rhythm or any other fun and games. And she was definitely feeling pain sometimes. But she was in her bedroom with this one nice woman she knew, and sometimes they chatted and sometimes not, and the midwife dealt with her as an entire person; helping her get out of her nightgown when she was hot, and wiping her face and delivering her baby. Her husband came in sometimes, but it was definitely woman's territory only. And you could see the sun going down through the windows, and hear kids playing outside, and it was all of a piece.

Now, about safety. You asked how I am going to feel if something goes wrong. And that points up something very interesting I have to deal with. Anything that goes wrong is going to be my fault if we do it at home—is going to be perceived as my fault. I have to take on that responsibility personally—can't even really share it with Hesch. It's my problem. If this kid is born without arms or

something, somehow it's going to be seen as my fault for having it at home.

It's a tricky question, maybe best dealt with through the sociology of knowledge, as to what we define as risk-taking behavior and what as normal, acceptable behavior. There are some risks I could take that are totally socially acceptable. I am not held accountable, for example, for how I choose a doctor. If I just chose the local doctor because I hate subways, that would be considered legitimate. And if he/she screws up, that's not my fault. Or, for another example, I could be asked to be drugged out of it completely, and I would not be held socially accountable for whatever risks that entailed. A friend's mother took diet pills all through her pregnancy because the doctor prescribed them. The pills have since been taken off the market for everybody, let alone pregnant people. A friend of my mother's was given that drug, diethylstilbestrol (DES), to prevent miscarriages, and they're still waiting around to see if the daughter by that pregnancy gets cancer. But none of these women are responsible, because they followed the doctor's orders. The moral is that the more control I give up, the more responsibility I give up for the consequences, and the more socially acceptable my behavior is.

That pretty much covers my ideological, philosophical, sociological arguments. And now, last of all: I don't want to act sentimental, but I am having a baby, and I do want it to be as positive and beautiful an experience for Hesch and me as we can make it.

See you on Thursday.

Barbara

June 1

Dear Linda,

She's going to do it. She read the letter, she understands, and she's going to do it. Hesch and I sat in her office and talked it all over. Even the baby picked up the vibes and jumped around!

We're going to do it without any drugs, without trying to deal with emergencies in the home that should be dealt with in the hospital. If anything is even questionable, we'll head for the hospital.

So, Linda, it looks like you get to do the whole staying-downstairs-and-boiling-water number. Try and come in soon—you won't want to miss this!

Love, Barbara

Around 3:30 AM on a Tuesday morning, the week before my due date, I woke to find myself in labor. It must be awkward and make a person feel silly to go rushing off to the hospital on a "false alarm," but to bring the doctor to me if I wasn't really in labor was unthinkable.

By 8:30 I decided it was time to get mobilized. I woke up Hesch, handed him the watch and the lists (things like make sure we had ice cubes, and clean the bathroom, make the bed, sweep—baby or no baby, we had company coming!). I left a message with Marcia's answering service that I was almost certainly in labor, and called my mother and asked her to drop off the cushions she was re-covering for my big platform rocker.

I sat in my rocking chair while Hesch cleaned up. He found pretty music on the radio, and chatted and timed contractions. On Hesch's list (we are crackerjack list makers) he noted that at 11:00 AM I was looking happy and self-satisfied, beginning to feel an outward, downward thrust to the contractions. But by 11:30 AM he noted that I was looking decidedly uncomfortable.

Marcia had returned our call and told Hesch to remind me that it really was going to hurt. It helps us understand what is going on when we speak of "contractions" rather than "pains," but the contractions of labor are painful, and I guess it's easier to deal with if your expectations are realistic. If I had been going to the hospital, that is probably the point at which we'd have gone. Contractions were strong and every three minutes. I was still sitting in my rocking chair, with Hesch sitting opposite me and very gently rubbing my belly, when Marcia arrived, at around two o'clock. By then we

had given up timing, no longer able to sort the pain out into separate contractions. Marcia timed the contractions at two and a half minutes, with 10-second rests, and told me I could expect a "horrendous but short" labor.

All afternoon our family had been arriving, one by one. My mother sat tensed at the bottom of the stairs while Hesch's mother compulsively cooked chickens. Fathers and siblings sat around. When I cried out during a particularly painful examination, Marcia went out afterward to explain to them that I was okay—and came back with the message that they were all bearing up well.

Sometime after 4:00 PM, I entered the phase of labor called transition, in which the last few centimeters of dilation takes place, the cervix opening up completely to let the baby come through. The contractions may have been more painful, I really don't know, but they started sorting themselves out into separate entities—maybe ninety seconds and sixty off. Again, I'm not sure. But they did have peaks and, blessed be, valleys. Hesch (who never moved from his seat opposite me) suggested I deal with the contractions by using two pants and a blow. That was the smartest thing I'd ever heard in my life. I was impressed by how clever and insightful he was—it sounds silly, but that's just the way I felt; how clever an idea. That, I gather, is what they mean when they say you need strong direction during labor.

I'd read that women get a "second wind" once they're fully dilated and ready to begin pushing the baby out, and it was certainly true for me. Pushing was the strangest, and in some ways the nicest, sensation I've ever had. I could actually feel the shape of the baby, feel myself sitting on the head as it moved down. Marcia said I looked comfortable enough on the chair, and I didn't have to get to the bed if I didn't want to. So there I was, on my rocking chair, with my feet up on two little kitchen chairs, with Hesch on one side and Marcia on the other, and pushing like crazy. It was like moving a grand piano across a room: so hard, but so satisfying to feel it move along.

Eventually, Marcia said I could have the baby in two pushes with an episiotomy (the small incision to widen the birth outlet), or maybe ten pushes without. I said no thanks. I thought, hell, I still wasn't sure it was happening, maybe I could accept the reality of it given the few extra minutes. I really needed the time to prepare myself, like the last-second cramming before the exam booklets are passed out.

So there I was, on my rocking chair with my feet up, pushing like crazy.

Hesch said my mother wanted to come in. My mother-in-law came in shortly after. It didn't take me ten pushes, just five. I heard noises coming out of my throat that I couldn't believe—like the soundtrack of a horror movie, but I had no time to laugh. And then I felt myself sitting on the head, felt myself opening, felt the head push through. A beautiful, total sense of opening and roundness. The shoulders seemed big and the shape was less comfortable than the symmetry of the head. And then slurp, wriggling, warmth, wetness, and there was a baby. He was up in the air, upside down, Marcia holding him over me. The longest few seconds in the world passed and then this gray-blue thing became alive and pink and breathing. Marcia handed him to my mother. I kept reaching out for him, but my mother was too dazed to move. I watched the cord being clamped and cut, and my baby, my son, Danny, was suckling by the time the placenta was out.

After maybe five minutes I stood, spilled blood all over the floor, and my mother walked me to the shower. As much as I had needed Hesch's support before, I felt the need for mothering then. I got the shakes—part physical, part emotional reaction, I guess. She bundled me up so I was warm and helped me put on a sanitary napkin—it was like the first time I got my period and was initiated into all the mysteries. Once I was changed and back into the rocker and Hesch and his mother had cleaned up the blood that had spurted from the cord, the whole world was in my room. Brothers and sisters and parents, suddenly aunts

and uncles and grandparents. They brought with them champagne and flowers and a teddy bear and a silver spoon, and looks of wonderment and love. It was the best birthday party I had ever been to.

As much as I had wanted it, I don't think even I understood how good it can be to have a baby at home. I gave birth, freely and consciously—I was not *delivered*. And my baby and I were surrounded by love, not efficiency. Images pass through my mind—my mother-in-law helping me get my breast out of the nightgown and to Danny; my brother carrying a big plastic garbage bag down from the bedroom singing "afterbirth" to the tune of "Over There"; my mother and Hesch trying to clean up the meconium (the baby's first bowel movement) in the middle of the night without waking me. I am sure there are more efficient ways to do these things—but who needs them?

The pediatrician came the next day to examine the baby. She kept telling us we were crazy. The baby looked so big and healthy (he was eight pounds, five ounces, and had been a nine-plus on the Apgar newborn scale of ten) and I looked so good, dressed and walking around, up and down stairs, but still we were crazy.

How Late Can You Wait to Have a Baby?

BARBARA SEAMAN

Barbara Seaman, excerpt from "How Late Can You Wait to Have a Baby?" *Ms.*, January, 1976. Reprinted by permission.

Men like to think they can all go on reproducing as long as Chaplin, and apparently some do. But where fertility is concerned, women fear that we must use it or lose it, that it's risky to delay having children. We worry about time running out on our bodies. We lose the luxury of postponing "the baby decision."

The reproductive capacity of women—and

men—deteriorates with advancing age. But physically, there is no ideal time to have a baby, for mother and baby do not operate on the same trajectory of risk. Maternal risk is lowest in the late teens and twenties, rises slowly but steadily through the thirties, and after forty may be as much as ten times higher than for women in their twenties.

Infant mortality, on the other hand, is lowest when mothers are in their late twenties and only rises again very slowly thereafter. The infant mortality rates for mothers aged thirty-five to thirty-nine are the same as the rates for mothers aged twenty to twenty-four, while the rates for mothers over forty are comparable to those aged fifteen to nineteen.

A most dangerous time to have a baby, in terms of risk to *both mother and child,* is in the early teens, the years just after menarche. It's as if the female reproductive system were warming up, but is not yet ready to go the distance. Impoverished countries where very early marriage prevails have strikingly higher infant and maternal mortality figures than comparable countries where marriage occurs later.

Thus, for your child's sake there is much to be said for delaying motherhood until your mid-twenties at least. The children of young mothers also have more health problems and accidents, and a higher mortality rate at ages 1 to 4. Mothers under twenty, or even under twenty-five, produce more babies of precariously low birthweight. Might the junk foods and crash diets in which adolescent girls indulge leave a deficit that takes some years to correct? If the female sexual response does not reach peak efficiency until the late twenties, or beyond, are our reproductive organs still, in some hidden aspects, short of their optimum maturity in the early twenties?

We have been oversold on the health advantages of starting our families early. This may sound coutrary to everything you've heard about Down's syndrome and malformed infants being born to older women, but here are the surprising facts.

The statistics on birth defects are exceedingly difficult to sort out, because they are recorded in so many diverse ways. Consider, for example, a handicap such as deafness, which is not usually diagnosed until the second year of life, or dyslexia (reading disability), which is not diagnosed until school age. These disorders, among many others, are not and cannot be reported on ordinary birth records. The figures, then, on the frequency of birth defects in *any population* range from about 1.5 to about 8 percent, depending on who's counting what—and how.

Birth defects are associated with a variety of causes, some of which are better understood than others. Of particular concern to older women is one group of defects called "chromosomal abnormalities," of which the best known is Down's syndrome. *It is only this special group of birth defects—the chromosomal abnormalities—which have been proved to occur with greater frequency to older mothers.* Malformations and birth defects that are *not chromosomal in origin* are rarely, if ever, associated with maternal age. A number of defects do appear to be associated with low birth-weight (under five pounds), which in turn occurs most commonly in very young mothers, poorly nourished mothers, mothers whose pregnancies were spaced at less-than-two-year intervals, and white, but not black, mothers who have a history of mental illness. In recent years we have also become aware that some birth defects are *iatrogenic* (doctor-caused) are associated with the injudicious administration of drugs to pregnant women, excessive limitations on weight gain during pregnancy, misuse of anesthesia, the confined birth position, and other kinds of mismanagement of labor and delivery.

In 1959 it was discovered that children with Down's syndrome have forty-seven chromosomes in most cells of their body, instead of the normal forty-six. It is thought that the egg cells which give rise to babies with Down's syndrome have become overaged, so that their cell division does not function properly. The risks of Down's syndrome may be especially high in women who have already started menopause.

Another birth defect which is chromosomal in origin is Klinefelter's syndrome, afflicting one in 400 males. It is marked by small testes, which will not produce sperm, and is sometimes associated with mental retardation. Klinefelter's syndrome is associated with parental age, and some rarer chromosomal defects may be also, although the evidence is not conclusive.

All told, it is estimated that serious chromosomal defects, including Down's and Klinefelter's syndrome, occur once in every 200 births, regardless of maternal age. The number of *conceptions* involving such defects is considerably larger, but since many are incompatible with life, an estimated 88 percent abort spontaneously.

Chromosomal defects can now be detected during pregnancy, by means of a procedure called amniocentesis. The older mother who has "passed" her amniocentesis test may have no more reason to fear birth defects than a comparable woman many years her junior. At the centers which specialize in it, amniocentesis is better than 99 percent accurate.

At Columbia University, sociologist Amitai Etzioni and his former research associate, Nancy Castleman, have also been puzzled by the failure of many physicians to notify "high-risk" patients that amniocentesis is available. In their random sampling of 500 board-certified gynecologists, only two-thirds of the 40 percent who responded stated that they inform their older patients about the procedure. In 1973, a forty-two-year-old Brooklyn woman appealed to Dr. Etzioni for support in her malpractice case against her obstetrician. Having already had a defective child, she inquired about amniocentesis, but her doctor dismissed her as "a worrier," and her child was born with Down's syndrome. The woman received a settlement.

At thirty-six, Marlene Sanders, the television producer, became pregnant a second time. Sanders now explains, "I put off having children because I was getting established in my work. Then Jeff, my first son [born when she was twenty-nine], turned out to be a great kid."

In the third month of her second pregnancy, Sanders started bleeding. She was treated with hormones. "It didn't occur to me that it would be better to abort."

Her second son had Down's syndrome.

"Anyone who's had a baby with Down's syndrome in the family, who's seen these children, knows how essential it is for women to be informed. My son doesn't even know that I'm his mother. They say there are compensations in having a child with Down's syndrome, but I can't think of any—not one—except that I learned that life is unpredictable, and random bad luck can strike at any time."

Several years later, Sanders's thirty-eight-year-old sister-in-law took the test and was reassured that her unborn *daughter* had no chromosomal defects.

Amniocentesis does reveal the sex of the child, and this troubles some physicians who fear that parents may use the knowledge casually to preselect daughters or sons. Others are reluctant to suggest any procedure that could result in a midpregnancy abortion. Still others hesitate to send their patients to a colleague for amniocentesis, for fear that doctor switching may result.

Some geneticists have cautioned against amniocentesis on the grounds that it will "weaken our biological heritage," by encouraging parents who have already had one defective child to keep trying for a normal child. These normal siblings of Down's syndrome children, it is feared, may turn out to be carriers of the defect.

While the politicians and futurists slug it out (should the procedure be imposed on all women . . . or completely withdrawn?) only Etzioni and Castleman have thought to propose that medical specialists might simply be required to *inform* women and allow us to each make a personal choice.

Of equal importance is the question of what risks are faced by *mothers* over forty. In the United States there were twenty-four maternal deaths per 100,000 live births in 1972—good compared to the early 1950s figures of 83.3 deaths, but bad compared to the 1972 figures from countries such as Denmark and Sweden, whose rates were under fifteen maternal deaths per 100,000 live births. Preliminary reports from the National Center for Health Statistics indicate that 1973 may have brought marked improvement in the United States, our figure finally declining to 15.2, which puts us in the same ballpark with other technologically advanced nations. Only 477 maternal deaths were recorded in the United States in 1973.

In one sense time is on a woman's side, for as she grows older and wiser, obstetrics does too. In 1940, the US maternal death rate for women of *all* ages was 376 per 100,000 live births. By 1950, it had dropped to 83.3.

Physicians who feel comfortable delivering older women—and many do not—claim that the after-forty mortality figures are somewhat misleading. They point out that many more deaths from all causes occur in the forties than in the twenties, regardless of pregnancy, and that most maternal fatalities occur in women whose general health is poor.

Says Dr. Arthur Davids of Manhattan: "A lot of nonsense is published on this subject. The American woman is not old at forty. Physically she can pass for thirty if she's well-nourished and has good medical care . . . Kidney disease, hypertension, diabetes, cardiac disease, these have to be ruled out, but younger women can get them too. I can't remember ever telling a patient never to get pregnant *unless she had a chronic disease.* We're getting more women in their thirties having a first child, and more unmarried women deliberately getting pregnant."

Is the delivery process itself more complicated for an older woman? Statistically, the answer is yes. Her cervix may not dilate well, labor may be prolonged, and her chances of requiring a cesarean section are greater. A 1967 story by Dr. Sidney H. Kane entitled "Advancing Age and the Primagravida" indicated that abnormal fetal presentation (any position other than headfirst) was 18 percent among women aged twenty-five to twenty-nine,

but 31 percent among women aged forty to forty-four. Postpartum hemorrhage due to uterine inertia (weak contractions) rose from 2.7 to 6.2 percent for the same two age groups. Still, at an advanced medical center with conscientious attendants standing by, the absolute risks arising from such complications are not very high. I, who have long been a critic of (some) obstetricians for intervening when things are going normally, am happy that we have the good physicians—and, yes, even their fetal monitors and Brave-New-World-ish intensive care delivery rooms—when complications arise. I do not think that a woman in her forties should try a home delivery.

To mother *and* child, the order of risks is somewhat higher for a first pregnancy (whatever the mother's age) than for a second and third. However, after the fourth, the risks rise again.

First labors tend to be somewhat longer than subsequent labors, presumably because the uterus (up to a point) gets more efficient with practice. However, these statistics don't tell the stories of the women who, having had a grueling first experience, decline to repeat it.

Regardless of the mother's age, spacing children closely, at less than two- to three-year intervals, somewhat increases the risks. But spacing them far apart, at more than five-year intervals, somewhat diminishes the benefits derived from an "experienced" uterus. Generally, a woman's best labor is apt to be her second or third—if it follows more than two but less than five years after the one before. A woman who has deferred childbearing until thirty-five or after, may not have done so by choice. Many such women have had fertility problems, repeated miscarriages, or gynecological conditions such as fibroids, endometriosis, or cystic ovaries. Still others have systemic diseases which they were waiting to get under control. The risks to women who *had* to postpone a first birth for medical reasons are obviously higher than the risks to women who *chose* to wait. Actually, some of the complications associated with older pregnancy occur *more* frequently with later than with first births. Women past thirty-five are, for example, about three and a half times more likely to have placenta previa (a condition producing hemorrhage during labor) than those under twenty-five. But, the chances of placenta previa in older mothers are lower if it's a first birth than if it's a later one.

No woman can be positively assured that she will remain as fertile at forty as she was at twenty. Besides aging, which does lower fertility in an absolute sense, infections such as venereal disease may intervene. So may drug effects, systemic diseases, and possibly radiation and other environmental influences. Age also lowers fertility in men, and while there are many exceptions, most women continue to select sexual partners who are their own age or older. (A biological imperative may be at work. Several studies reveal that, mysteriously, birth defects occur much more frequently when the age between mother and father is substantial.)

The woman who appears to have marginal fertility in her youth—as suggested, for example, in scanty and irregular menstruation—may find it especially hard to conceive in her thirties and forties. Frequent, repeated abortions may reduce fertility, as may use of the pill and perhaps the IUD. But one advantage of waiting to have a child is that some women discover they were not so keen on becoming mothers after all.

Finally, let's stop being so susceptible to what psychiatrist Anne Seiden calls "Old Doc's Tales," whether they be alarming, or falsely reassuring. Having a baby is never, strictly speaking, safe.

In a social sense, we who are at risk should determine the laws and practices surrounding birth control, abortion, and emerging reproductive issues such as amniocentesis. In a personal sense, we must inform and preserve ourselves.

For a healthy, affluent woman in 1976, the comparative risks of childbirth after 35 have been exaggerated—especially if she lives near a fine medical center. You can't expect objectivity from the sort of people whose textbooks, in this day and age, refer to women having their first child after thirty as *elderly primaparas*.

But the insults and patronizing suffered by affluent women are as nothing compared to the neglect suffered by the poor. The risks faced by poor mothers and their babies at the two extremes of the reproductive life span are inexcusable.

Given our current technology, and social trends, we would serve women and children better if we worried less about advancing age per se, and worried more about delivering medical and social services to mothers who are too poor or too young.

The optimum time for starting a family can be anywhere from twenty-five to thirty-five. However, as Dorothy Nortman points out in her authoritative 1974 study entitled *Parental Age as a Factor in Pregnancy Outcome and Child Development*, "It cannot be stressed too often that, if other factors are favorable, age alone should not deter a woman who wants a child from bearing one."

How Science Is Redefining Parenthood

BARBARA KATZ ROTHMAN

Barbara Katz Rothman, "How Science is Redefining Parenthood," *Ms.*, July–August 1982. Reprinted by permission.

The United States has produced its first "test-tube" baby. I read about it in the newspaper. Some woman bore it, of course, but the child, I am told, is a product of medical technology. Doctors put it in, and interestingly, doctors took it out—this baby, like Louise Brown, the first of the test-tube babies, was also removed surgically, born by cesarean section.

All the fanfare that has greeted the birth of these babies, the marvel at their "production," is itself an interesting thing to observe. In vitro fertilization—sperm joining ovum in a test tube (actually on a glass dish, but let's not quibble)—is not just one more treatment for infertility. It is that, certainly, and no small thing—"New Hope for the Childless," the headline read. But it is also a challenge to traditional definitions of parenthood, the latest in a long line of such challenges, and that's where we'd best pay attention.

What does it mean to be a parent in this society? The first thing we do is to separate social from biological parenthood. The modern, anonymous adoption taught us that distinction: a woman who adopts a baby is its social mother. She is not simply a woman raising a child, she is the child's *mother*, with the rights and obligations of motherhood. Women have always done a certain amount of raising one another's kids—taking in a dying sister's child or taking on one twin. In some societies that makes you a mother, and in some it doesn't. Making it formal, legal, and especially *anonymous* clarified the social-biological distinction.

Being a social parent now clearly means being a child-rearer, and is usually but by no means always associated with biological parenthood. But what is biological parenthood? We can now think in terms of "genetic" parents, those who provide half of the genetic material for a child; "physiologic" or biological parents, those who nurture an embryo/fetus in their bodies; and "social" parents, those who rear a child.

Women never before were able to think about genetic motherhood without pregnancy, or pregnancy without genetic motherhood: if we were biological mothers (carrying babies) then we were genetic mothers. But making the inseparable separate is what the technology of reproduction is all about. And it is this issue that we are now facing: women, for the first time, have the potential for genetic parenthood without physiologic motherhood. At all. No pregnancy. No birth. No suckling. Women are about to become fathers.

THE TECHNOLOGY OF BIOLOGICAL FATHERHOOD

Biological fatherhood has meant genetic parenthood: a biological father contributes half of the genetic basis for the child-to-be. Men can make their genetic contribution to conception without mating with the mother, substituting an "artificial" form of insemination. The continued secrecy surrounding artificial insemination is telling. Adoption is discussed openly, and the parents of babies fertilized in vitro are holding press conferences, but very few people who have used artificial insemination with donor sperm (AID) seem ready to come out of the closet. Maybe that is because biological fatherhood still means genetic parenthood, and social fatherhood is so ambiguous. It's not really being a child-rearer—so many fathers do so little child-rearing. What makes a man "really" the father of a child in this society, if not genetics? And a child without a father in a patriarchal society is called illegitimate. Men as social fathers "claim" or name children, legitimate them.

Like in vitro fertilization, "artificial" insemination is a treatment for infertility. An important difference is that AID is a treatment for male infertility. Women do not really need men to have children—we need only their semen. Men, on the other hand, do need women, if they are to have children. Much as we have been taught to think mechanistically about our body "parts," a womb does not live without a woman. When we are pregnant, we are pregnant with our whole bodies—to have children, men need living whole women. Our wombs really cannot themselves alone be rented or sold. But once women have the semen, we do not need the man's body to have our babies. And in a capitalist society, semen, along with blood and with milk, the essential fluids of life, is for sale.

While women without mates have used AID as a route to the socially fatherless child, the most common, and surely the most socially sanctioned, use of AID, is for the fertile woman married to the infertile man. In most of the literature on AID the reader is asked to sympathize with her plight, and to view artificial insemination as the solution.

Historically, when infertility was assumed always to be the "fault" of the wife, husbands were given the recourse of divorce. Now, given the technological sophistication available that can prove beyond all doubt that the male is responsible for the "barren" state of the couple, in this situation maternity is a privilege rather than an obligation of the wife.

Defining artificial insemination as a "gift" for the woman, something a husband "allows," means two things. One is that we gloss over the range of choices the woman in the situation has: she after all can be a mother by taking on a new husband, or simply taking a lover. The second consequence is that in the emphasis on genetic ties as defining fatherhood, the sharing of a pregnancy and birth by the woman's husband is dismissed as meaningless. In some states in the United States, the husband of a woman who has had artificial insemination (even at his written request) must formally adopt the child. He adopts a sperm. Thus the potential of biological fathering is reduced to a single-cell genetic contribution, and trivialized, purchased cheaply.

THE TECHNOLOGY OF BIOLOGICAL MOTHERHOOD

Biological motherhood encompasses both aspects of biological fatherhood, the genetic and the sexual, and a great deal more. Biological motherhood also involves pregnancy, the birth process, and suckling the baby. As the technology has become and continues to become available to make substitutes for one or another of these aspects of motherhood, the problem of defining biological motherhood, defining female infertility, gets more complicated.

Before the advent of the rubber nipple, the pasteurizing process for cow's milk, and the development of formulas to substitute for breast milk, if a woman could not produce milk, she could not be a mother: her babies would die. Her only alternative was to find a substitute, or surrogate mother, a wet nurse. Often that meant the sacrifice of the wet nurse's baby for the purchaser's baby. In modern America we no longer think of the breasts as necessary for fertility.

A woman with a very small pelvis, perhaps deformed from an accident or from rickets in childhood, cannot "give birth"—her baby must be removed surgically. Before the advent of the techniques necessary to do cesarean sections, women with small pelvises were perforce infertile; they could not produce a live baby and survive.

Pregnancy may in fact end quite early, and still produce a live baby. With the advent of the technology for caring for premature babies, it became the rule rather than the exception for premature babies to survive. This particular technology got even more media attention than did the current "test-tube" babies: incubators with preemies were a world's fair exhibit, and an exhibition at Coney Island. A baby in an incubator, fed on formula by a tube, was a "manmade" or "artificial" product. But that too got incorporated into our definitions of motherhood, and an inability to carry a pregnancy to term does not now mean infertility.

So far the test-tube babies like Louise Brown, like all of the previous "artificially created" babies, the artificially incubated, artificially fed, artificially (surgically) born babies, have all been the genetic offspring of their social/biological parents. There is no reason why they should have to be so any longer. Extrauterine or in vitro fertilization might in fact be a lot easier from the technological standpoint if the source of the ova were not a woman who was to host it. Yet the "ethical" guidelines established by the Ethics Advisory Board to the Secretary of the Department of Health, Education, and Welfare, and the current convention, are that in vitro fertilization is to be used only with married couples as the genetic parents.

Closely related to in vitro fertilization is the technology of embryo transplants. Embryo transplants are being done routinely with several species. When embryos, or just ova, can be transplanted from one woman to another, then who is the biological mother: the "donor" or the "host"? How different is the "donor" using this kind of technology from the woman who, in an earlier technology, used a wet nurse? Both are using the reproductive capacities of another woman. But looking at it another way, the donor is not a mother at all. She is a father: she contributes half of the genetic material, her "seed."

Now let us consider it from the perspective of the "host," the woman who carried the pregnancy. For women who cannot conceive, who are currently therefore infertile, a new option opens up: they can enter biological motherhood at the point after conception, carrying and birthing what will be their social children. Such a woman might not be a genetic parent, but social motherhood would begin with a biological tie, with pregnancy. With the new technology, an inability to conceive, or even to ovulate, will not mean infertility, any more than an inability to lactate or to labor now means infertility.

MODELS FOR THE NEW MOTHERHOOD

We used to talk about futuristic, science fiction–sounding things like embryo transplants as 1984 visions. Well, that may be right on target. There is no technological reason why human embryo transplants should not be available by 1984.

In *The Dialectic of Sex,* Shulamith Firestone says that new reproductive technology could free women from motherhood, and that would indeed free women. Not all of us shared that view of the relation between motherhood and feminism then, and even fewer of us share it now. This new technology is not being used to free women from motherhood. Quite the contrary, it is being used to make biological motherhood available to more women.

One of the standard objections made to proceeding with the new technology of reproduction is that it is an unwise and ultimately exploitative use of resources. With all the unwanted babies in the world, with overpopulation and world hunger, why should we invest so much energy in getting a few elite women pregnant? Indeed. Why not adopt? we say. Biology shouldn't matter. People can have the full experience of parenting by adopting. Well, yes. And no. Women do sometimes want simply to be pregnant, to give birth. These too are expe-

riences, like the parenting experience, which a woman, or a woman and her mate, may want to have. But there is an even more serious objection to the why-not-adopt argument.

Adoption has been based on another set of exploitations: the exploitation of biological mothers. Where exactly do people think adoptable babies come from? They used to be available because the demands of a patriarchal system created them. Pregnant women had so few choices.

Because women are no longer so tightly bound by the rules of the patriarchal family in America, we have lost the supply of domestic babies. So we turn to third-world women, and cash in on their "surplus" babies, the babies they would have aborted or would have kept, had life offered them choices. Loving, eager parents take these babies home from airports and raise them, accepting the genetic and biological donations of anonymous parents.

Does adoption provide us with a model we can use for managing embryo transplants? Will we come to think of some embryos as "adoptable"? Will a market for embryos develop, like the market for adoptable babies, with those of the whitest, healthiest, best-fed, best-educated women the most prized?

Because elective abortions for nonmedical reasons will be the most readily available source of healthy embryos for transplantation, once the technology is perfected, this may change the very meaning of abortion. When one woman's abortion becomes another woman's pregnancy, and ultimately another woman's child, then just what is an abortion? Can it be some kind of an adoption procedure?

Another meaning of pregnancy, a definition for which feminists have fought, is that it is a condition of women, a state of our bodies, like menstruation, ovulation, or menopause. If pregnancy is an undesired state, abortion is a remedy. That meaning of pregnancy essentially denies the presence of a future or potential child. The argument goes that just as there is a potential for a child with an early pregnancy, so too is there that potential with each ovulation. We will no more mourn the loss of a child with an early abortion than we would a few weeks earlier at the time of menstruation. With this set of meanings, donating an embryo is much like donating an ovum. That should be much like donating semen.

But is it? And do we want it to be? Will women accept this kind of nonresponsible, irresponsible parenthood? If we are going to become fathers, is that the kind of father we want to be?

Neither adoption nor sperm donation provides the model we should be seeking, a way of dealing with biological motherhood that is ethical, feminist, moral, fair. The history of surrogate mothers too has been largely a history of exploitation, in which rich mothers used poor mothers, in which slave mammies and peasant wet nurses sacrificed their own motherhood.

But the potential for nonexploitative surrogates, like the potential for women being good fathers to their genetic children, is really there. The new technology offers us another opportunity to work on the definitions of parenthood, of motherhood, fatherhood, and children. Earlier technologies *could* have revolutionized the family, but were incorporated instead into the existing family. Think of how formula might have changed women's and men's roles in child-rearing.

With this new technology the opportunity once again exists to evolve new relations between parents and children, to ask new questions and rethink old answers. We can now ask, should genetics matter at all for mothers? If we say no, then what are we saying about the meaning of biological fatherhood? Should the biology of motherhood, the carrying and birthing of babies, matter at all for mothers? And again, what does our answer tell us about fatherhood?

Reproductive technology will not make social change; as long as our social definitions remain the same, the technology will be used to support those definitions.

But not if we say no. Not if women want to be good fathers to their genetic children. As fathers we can perhaps be like aunts—aunts too share a genetic tie to their nieces and nephews. Not if we reject being or using "surrogates," reject the idea of one human being substituting for another. Not if we join together to form new families—a reproductive communism, with each giving according to his or her ability. We do not have to be "donors" and "hosts" and "surrogates"—we can be mothers and fathers and aunts and uncles. We can take away the gender assignments and leave the relationships. We are coming to understand this with social parenting, that several people, including fathers and other men, can "mother" a child. Perhaps we will learn the lesson for physical parenthood too.

Having Anne

LAURA YEAGER

Laura Yeager, "Having Anne," *The Missouri Review* 21(3), December 1998. Reprinted by permission.

I have stopped taking lithium so that I can have a child. It's that or heart birth defects. My psychiatrist says that I may not get high if I stay on the drug, but we're not taking any chances. We've hired a "sitter," someone to stay with me for nine months during the day. Her name is Penelope, and she wants to be an actress, but she fully understands that she must stay here with me from 9:00 AM to 5:30 PM until Richard gets home. I've informed her that until I start having symptoms, she can take an occasional audition if it is all that important. And if she gets a show, we'll just have to find someone else.

This baby-sitting idea is Richard's. He's seen how I speak in half sentences, how I can't sleep for days, how I have direct communications with God. I'm not sure he would have married me if I'd had manic depression when we met.

I was twenty-four, a perfect innocent who designed children's activities for the art museum. Once, he wandered into my finger-painting exercise, looking for the john. People often did that. The bathrooms were next to the children's room in the basement.

"It's the next door on your right," I said, my fingers smeared in yellow, blue, and red. I was teaching the joys of color combinations. I pointed.

He stood there in a beige raincoat that was a little wet and said, "Thank you."

That was the first time I saw him. I remember he walked directly over to the table and looked at the children's paintings. Over one child's purples and greens, he said, "Beautiful."

"We're learning how to mix color."

He was neither tall, nor short, nor fat, nor thin, nor blond, nor brown.

What stood out about him was his face, which seemed to burst into the world.

"Color," he said. He had a paper under his arm, and the museum booklet for the visiting exhibit upstairs.

I remember he looked at me, and I know I must have looked small to him, in a turtleneck and—oh, God—I think, a tartan skirt, my hair in a ponytail, my face covered by the huge, round black glasses I was wearing in those days. Over my clothes, I had on a white lab coat, which was covered in paint smudges.

"What do blue and yellow make?" he asked one child. At the time, he was thirty-two—eight years older than I. "Do they make green?" he said when the child refused to answer. The child ignored him. Another kid, a boy, spoke up. "Yes, green. They make green."

"What is this?" he asked, looking around.

"This is the children's room."

I began to wonder when he was going to go to the bathroom. He was making me nervous. I admired Stacey's ability to not speak to the handsome stranger. She, at four, knew how to behave around men. As he walked away, I thought of my grandmother's fear at meeting my grandfather. They'd met under an awning in a rainstorm in Akron, Ohio. He had offered her a ride in the taxi. She had not spoken to him, simply followed, petrified.

As the color ran off our fingers into the tiny sinks on the far wall of the room, I wondered who he was and if I'd see him again.

Five years ago, I was perfect. I had a small apartment near the museum, with white furniture and sheets on the windows bunched up into knots to let the sun in. I drank the right teas with honey, served scones on the right-textured dishes, watered my plants, fed my cat. I listened to the right classical station and had friends in. Oh yes, I bought fresh flowers and sat them in blood-red vases on my glass coffee table. I dated occasionally. One guy, Rex, was a part-time museum guard, full-time graduate student in American History. We did things like see movies at the museum, visit my family or his, go for walks, and cook things out of our mutual gourmet cookbooks. Rex's only problem was that he worshiped me. I began to feel unreal around him.

I'd also go to restaurants occasionally with a guitar player who repaired watches. My boyfriends at the time were, compared to Richard, marginal, and they were also young. Richard, whom I did see again—this time when I was eating grapes in the cafeteria—had arrived. He cleaned up hazardous-waste dumps.

The cafeteria, like all of the museum, is white. Richard stood out because that day he was wearing a black jacket and pants. Still carrying a paper, he filled a cup with coffee and proceeded to pay for it.

Eating the grapes was more of a pastime than anything. I had twenty minutes of lunch hour to kill. That was one of the rare days I had forgotten a book. I had, by this time, grapes on all five fingers.

Richard sat down at a table where he could watch me. Recognizing him, I took the grapes off my fingers and ate each one with a fork.

Richard emptied three creams into his coffee and stirred. He smiled at me.

He waved.

I waved back, a twenty-four-year-old woman who'd never been to the hospital before for anything.

Six months after our wedding, I broke. Richard, who was used to disasters, handled it logically.

At 8:00 AM, I wake up when Richard grabs my toe. "She'll be here in an hour," he says. This is Penelope's first day. I have spent the last two days cleaning the house so that Penelope will be reassured that this is a nice place to work. She has asked Richard about health insurance, but he's declined to pay for it. He's upped her salary to $275 a week—not bad for simply being my companion. Although, if I get bad, she may have to come looking for me in the car, or God knows what.

I lie here for a few minutes, remembering the weight of Richard on me, his even, reasoned thrusts, his patter of kisses.

As Richard ties his tie, I force myself out of bed and into the bathroom that smells like cleanser—into a tub which Richard has politely left as spotless as it was yesterday. I wait while the water warms, looking at him, with his one-day-old haircut. I like him best like this—trim and neat. He looks, in this hairstyle, capable of making and sticking to an earth-shattering, possibly billion-dollar (if money enters into it) decision.

Standing naked in my first trimester, I can see that my nipples have darkened. My breasts are tender, and I'm craving apple juice and cream cheese with scallions. I look around the porcelain bathroom and see that I have gotten everything I wanted. I do not feel guilty that my husband provided it for me. But I do feel a twinge at trying to carry this baby with this disease. I know that I'm putting myself and the baby in danger. I know that at three months, my psychiatrist will demand (because it's procedural in cases of manic depression) that I go back on lithium. I know that I won't. I know that I may go months without sleep. I comfort myself with the fact that we've done some digging and have discovered that ocean-wave music helps manics sleep.

I'm in the shower when Richard says, "Bye. I'll defrost your muffin. It'll be in the microwave."

"Thanks."

In the hot steam, I allow myself, amidst all my worries, to remember the night of our first date.

He must have been taken with me because he came back to the children's room when we were making prints with apples. This was an older group who could use butter knives to carve designs into their apple halves.

"Don't you work?" I asked. I know I must have been fearless then, and I'm sure this attracted him to me.

"Would you like to go roller skating with me?" he said, half smiling, not waiting for a private moment.

Boys went, "Wooooo."

The girls giggled.

"I get off at five."

He was sly in the activities he chose for us to do—they all reeked of adolescence—innocence. He must have thought I was a virgin. I wasn't. I'm sure all along the courtship titillated him because he saw me as a small, young woman in a plaid skirt, yet he did not worship me. This I was grateful for.

His palm sweated as we spun around with seventh graders.

"This is corny." I closed my eyes and imagined what it would be like to be blind and doing this. Men terrified me for that reason. I was afraid they wanted to lead me. His first kiss was cool and airy. A guy in junior high said, "Look at that."

Penelope comes when I'm just about to eat my muffin. Wanting to make a good impression, I've dressed in a pink lamb's-wool sweater and skirt. As I open the door, I realize we're peers. I can see lines around her eyes. She has to be twenty-seven or twenty-eight, maybe even twenty-nine, the same age as I.

"God, I couldn't find it," she says. "Am I late?"

"No."

Penelope takes off her long red coat. She has a bag with her, full of scripts, books, and knitting. "Good. I brought some stuff with me."

"That's fine. I'll be working in the upstairs office. Come on in."

She follows me into the kitchen.

"This is a great place," she says. I don't tell her that *Better Homes and Gardens* has approached us for a story. We're considering it. A magazine pictorial of my home almost frightens me—it's too public. Richard agrees.

"Would you like a muffin?"

"That would be great. I didn't have time to eat."

Penelope, I can tell already, is very dramatic. She opens her eyes wide and smiles as if for a camera. She looks good—trim and supple from all kinds of dance classes.

"How old are you?" I ask.

"Twenty-eight."

"I'm twenty-nine."

"I'm trying to make a go of theater," she says. "I'm giving myself till thirty. Then it's time for a real job."

"I had a real job."

"What did you do?"

"Children's activities coordinator for the museum."

"Neat," she says, showing her teeth again. She has beautiful blond hair, which she swings to one side like Julia Roberts.

"Now I do newsletters on a computer upstairs. Freelance—churches, plumbers. It's not too exciting."

I hand Penelope a warm muffin and a cup of coffee.

"Thank you."

"You can do whatever you want," I say. "Watch TV, use the StairMaster, read, talk on the phone. If you're going out, tell me."

"Okay."

"Maybe we can do something together every day."

"Sure."

"Take a walk or go shopping, go to a matinee. This is going to be a long eight months."

Penelope wipes her nose. She seems appreciative. I suddenly become worried that she might be a kleptomaniac.

Switching on the computer upstairs, I look at our wedding picture we've framed in gold. I remember our wedding day. Penelope is downstairs reading lines from some show.

We got married at St. Anthony's (the patron saint of lost items) with a Baptist minister cocelebrating the ceremony. The two men on the altar seemed to like each other and practically made small talk during the service. Father Nick, who'd confirmed me, swung his arms wildly when he talked. The minister kept saying, "I agree with you. I agree with you," during Father's sermon. For some reason, everyone cried, even the men. The minister, Richard's father's friend, kept saying, "Marriage is a lot of cleaning up after meals."

Father Nick said, "Yes, and a whole lot more."

We held our reception in the art museum—hors d'oeuvres and drinks. We had enough chairs for everyone, but most people stood, gazing up occasionally at an 8-foot by 8-foot Madonna and child or at a portrait or two of a nobleman. It was a cool summer night, and we had both doors of the gallery open so that a wind blew through the place. The wind kept blowing out the Sterno underneath the hors d'oeuvres, and Richard kept pausing to light the cans. Eventually, we let all of them go out, and people still ate every single one of the tidbits. Richard had one beer, and water with lemon all night because he said he wanted to be awake when we got to the hotel. I'd guzzled down 7Up and grenadine—Shirley Temples with cherries in them. By this time, our priest and minister had decided to run some joint seminars on God. We promised to attend. I felt married, even more married than the first time I saw him.

When we were finally alone, he unzipped my gown, which had cloth-covered buttons sewn on top of the zipper. I was down to one of those white bustiers and a slip. We had, I don't know how, managed to wait. After five minutes in bed with him, I said, "Something has got to happen. Something has got to happen." It did.

Placing our wedding picture back in its place on the desk, I bring up the masthead of the newsletter

I'm working on. *Notary News,* for notary publics in the area. With the title comes preset margins. This is a template—something I find very reassuring. For all I know, Penelope could be downstairs robbing us blind. She is unpredictable still; yet no matter how well we get to know each other, she'll never be fully predictable, not like this template before me.

I type in the first article about a new notary in the area—Rod Owens, on 24th Street. Rod has full power to witness any kind of signature, to process titles and registrations.

"Penelope," I yell.

"Yes." She hears me.

"Are you all right down there?"

"Yes. Are you?"

"I'm fine." With the article typed in, I press a button, and it filters into its proper place on the page. "Fine." I get up to take a pee, something I do all the time these days.

I watch Penelope make herself lunch—wheat crackers, slices of cheese, and strawberries. She has brought this food and asks if she can leave it in the refrigerator.

"Of course."

She's dieting. I have six newsletters before me, and I'm trying to edit them. I always edit on the kitchen table. It goes back to college days, when all I had was a kitchen table to edit on.

Penelope doesn't eat. She nibbles. "How are you doing?" she asks in a tone that suggests she sees this question is part of her duty. I suddenly feel like a small child.

"No flights of fancy yet."

"What's it like?" She bites into half a strawberry. "If you don't mind talking about it."

"Pregnancy or mania?"

"Mania."

I circle a spelling error in a mortuary science newsletter. "You feel as if you're communicating with everyone. I feel sometimes that I can read minds."

"Do you think the baby will have it?"

Penelope, I can see, does not mince words. "How should I know?"

Penelope smiles, appearing to be happy in my confession that we are controlled by larger forces.

"Anything else?" she asks.

"About the illness?"

"Yes."

"I travel a lot, spend a lot of money. And everything is so colorful. I hear messages on the radio."

"Am I supposed to restrain you if you get like this?"

"There's a straitjacket in the closet."

Penelope drops a piece of cheese.

"I'm only kidding. You're supposed to take me into a dark, quiet room, turn on the ocean-wave music, rub my back, and tell me things are normal, but we might not even have to resort to that."

"I'm an alcoholic," Penelope says.

She seems too proper to be an alcoholic.

"I've been sober for two years."

"Congratulations."

"I have admitted that I'm powerless over my life. I could break down and have a drink any minute. Sometimes I feel like something is following me, or worse yet, like I'm inside of something, and I can't get out. At those times I have to make the bed, take the garbage out, and scrub the toilet."

"I know what that feels like. I feel like my head isn't attached to my body. Like people I love are trying to harm me. Richard isn't like this at all." I look down at page five of *Mortuary News,* the page that publicizes new morticians. "Richard doesn't seem to have anything big hanging over him except heaven. Maybe that's why I married him."

"How long have you been married?"

"Three years."

"How did you meet?"

"He was looking for the bathroom at the art museum. He took me roller-skating."

"That's cute." Penelope eats a strawberry. She seems to be eating now with more vigor.

"Are you seeing anyone?"

"I see a few men occasionally, nothing serious. I'm working on my career. My AA group doesn't recommend dating anyone at the meetings. It's hard to find men who want a commitment."

"Do you?"

"Part of me would love to get married and have a man support me, but then I realize it's completely unrealistic of me. I'm perfectly capable of supporting myself. The work isn't steady, but I can't have a full-time job and act, too. Plus, I can't find anyone. I go to these happy hours, and I can't drink, so I drink this lime soda water and sometimes I talk to men. I recognize some of them because I've temped a lot. Do you know what it's like to answer the phone for eight hours a day?"

"I've done it."

"When?"

"In college. I temped."

"Sometimes I crave alcohol. I was drinking eight drinks a day. I quit the day my kitty got lost, and I was trying to find him in the rain. It was pouring outside, and there I was staggering around yelling, 'Tony, Tony.' The police picked me up, asked me who I was looking for. I said, "My husband. I'm looking for my fucking husband." They didn't arrest me. They got me to confess that I was searching for my cat. I never found him. When I woke up, I had bruised kneecaps from falling down so much. The whole thing was pathetic."

While Penelope talks, I remember how what my psychiatrist calls "the break" happened. We were on vacation at Jekyll Island in Georgia. We'd been married two years. I can see myself jumping off the pier, feeling the fall, not knowing if I'd live or die.

"Excuse me, Penelope," I say, picking up my newsletters.

"Are you all right?"

"Fine. I'll be upstairs."

In the bathroom I splash water on my face and decide to get in the tub.

The jump off the pier terrified Richard. He leaped in after me, off a 20-foot pier, all the way to the bottom.

"What the hell is wrong with you?" he asked as we dog-paddled.

Little did we know, I was breaking.

"We never do anything fun," I said. "Want to do it again?" I knew I wouldn't die. I had no fear.

Later that evening, we joined two couples we had never seen in our lives.

"Hello," I said. "We made it. We're here."

"Who are you?" asked one of the wives.

"Excuse us," Richard said. "We thought you were someone else."

"Let's sit with them," I said. I thought we were famous, that everyone would want to sit with us.

This craziness hadn't just appeared out of nowhere. A month prior, I hadn't slept well. I thought two pigeons at the park were God. They were perfectly white.

In the tub, remembering, I take a bar of lemon soap and soap my neck. And then, when I was in the hospital, Richard visited me every night. Every day it was a different flower delivered to the locked doors.

"Hello." Penelope knocks on the door. "Taking a bath?"

"Yes."

"Did I upset you?"

"No."

"Come down when you get out."

"Okay."

"Where are you going?" asks Penelope.

I have been reclining in Richard's chair for the past two hours, playing off and on with an Easter toy, an egg that opens up to reveal a yellow chick when I press a silver button. I can't watch TV. I feel as if they're talking to me, and Penelope gets embarrassed when I talk back. She feels like she's not doing her job. We haven't told my psychiatrist. For all he knows, I'm lucid. She's knitting up a storm out of sheer nervousness. She's frightened of me, but she's sticking this out because she thinks it will inform her acting.

"I need to be near water," I say, patting my five-month-old baby, who is, at the moment, quiet. I felt the first kick last week.

My mind, now, is always on. The only way I can get to sleep is if Richard rubs my feet in time to the ocean-wave music, but this keeps him up.

We're averaging five hours apiece. This isn't good, and I don't imagine Richard is a joy at work. We've stopped having sex.

"I'll come up with you," says Penelope, following me up the stairs.

One thing I so want is privacy. I never get any of it with Penelope and Richard watching me all the time. But Penelope does wash my back, and this does clear my mind. My heart slows down. She washes me in a circular motion, with a washcloth and soap, which seems to center me. When I rinse, I lie on my back and gaze at my stomach. The warm water feels good on my legs and back. My obstetrician has prescribed exercise to relieve the cramps and aches. I like the tub. At this point, Penelope picks up a novel she keeps on the john for this purpose.

I think about our day. We managed to go to the pet store to watch fish. Staring at swimming fish is one of my favorite pastimes now. They seem so orderly and calm.

"Do you have any razors?" I ask Penelope.

She burps. "Razors?"

"Yes, razors."

"What for?"

"I want to shave."

"Richard said you can't have them."

"Look at me, Penelope. I'm covered with hair. I feel gross."

Penelope cranes her neck to see my legs. I raise my arms; a small bush is growing in each armpit.

"What do you need to shave for?" she asks. "Who's going to see you?"

"I'll feel better, Penelope. God, I'm not suicidal."

"Richard thinks you might accidentally cut yourself."

"Oh, shit." I recline in the tub, submerging my head, wondering why I had to be born with this disease. God, what I wouldn't give for some lithium. I don't know how much more of this I can take.

"Penelope, my dear," I say, sitting up.

"Yes."

"Would you shave me?"

She puts her novel down, looking scared.

"I'm not homicidal either."

"This isn't in the job description."

"Neither is breakfast, lunch, and dinner and all that perfume I gave you."

"All right," says Penelope. "What if I cut you?"

"Go slowly. I won't move."

I place my leg on the rim of the tub while Penelope brings the shaving cream and a new razor. With precision, she sprays a long white stripe of cream on my leg. I pat it all over, and she shaves me from ankle to knee. Making slow, smooth strokes, she takes off the first layer of hair. I rinse off, and she repeats until my left leg is smooth. We do the right. This reminds me of when I was hospitalized, except Richard is stricter than the nurses. We were allowed to shave ourselves. They sat themselves next to the tub and listened, picking their fingernails, bored. Their glasses would fog up from the hot water, and their clothes would become damp.

I raise each arm one at a time. Penelope has the poise of a painter gliding a brush along a surface. She does not look at my breasts. When she's finished, I say, "You did it without a nick."

"Beginner's luck." She helps me out of the tub and leaves me to dry off.

With a wet finger, I flick on the radio to station 99.3, a station I believe is in touch with the president of the United States. I feel that these songs reveal what kind of mood the president is in. I feel as if he's set up this system to inform me of his moods because he values my input on world events.

I report back to him by going through station 101.5. I haven't told anyone about this little cataclysmic information-gathering and -relaying device. They'd think I was crazy.

Then, with my clean-shaven limbs, I throw up—morning sickness at 4:35 PM.

"Hi," says Penelope to the owner of the pet shop.

He's taking people's change with a huge snake around his shoulders. "Hi."

"A sign," I say.

"From whom?" says Penelope.

"From God. This man is Adam, only he's getting along with the devil."

"Shhh." Penelope tries to quiet me.

"This is no devil. This is Bob," the owner of the shop says. "He's my pet boa."

"Bless you. You are a chosen one," I say. At this point, I believe slightly that I am Jesus Christ.

"Let's look at the fish," says Penelope. "That always helps you."

We watch the silvery creatures swim in the green water. It's their order that quiets me. They never run into each other, have the ability to glide and turn—like thoughts. I manage to sit down in front of the tank.

The owner wanders back to the fish area, still holding Bob.

"That's a very beautiful snake," I say. "Come out of there."

"Who's she talking to?" the owner says.

"The devil. She's having a bad day."

"That's some bad day."

"She likes to look at the fish."

"I've noticed."

I look very pregnant and funny sitting on the floor, and a total stranger comments on my condition.

"First one?" she asks.

Her attention adds to my other delusion that I am famous.

"Yes," I say.

"Who's your obstetrician?"

"Lucas." Penelope speaks for me.

"She's good."

"My dentist is Jones," I say. "My psychiatrist, Donovan. My podiatrist is Mills. My psychologist is Smith."

The lady backs away when I say this.

"You too will be saved," I tell her.

"What's she talking about?"

"The end of the world," Penelope says. "It's here, by the way. Should be closing up tomorrow."

"Boy, if you could only feel my stomach. My baby knows Morse code."

"Is this lady for real?" the owner asks.

"My baby's kicks have become a full language."

"She has manic depression. We won't come anymore if you don't want us to," Penelope says.

"She likes the fish?" the owner asks.

"They calm her down."

"She can come anytime." He rearranges the snake on his shoulders, as if it were a stole.

I'm getting a glass of water when the exterminator comes in. At seven months without drugs, I believe he's trying to kill me. I'm psychotic. I need some Mellaril too. I freeze and drop the glass.

Penelope comes running in. "We had the service canceled," she says.

"What's wrong with Mrs. Darrow?" the exterminator asks. He has a particularly breezy voice from the chemicals he inhales.

"She's a little tense these days."

I start crying and run out of the room.

"He's the enemy. It's 3:00. He was due here at 2:30." Penelope has me by the shoulders. "He's the exterminator. We canceled him, and he came anyway."

"We did? No, he's tapped our phone."

She hugs me. "It's okay."

"I'm so tired, and I can't sleep. Whenever I lie down, the baby starts kicking, and my mind won't stop racing."

"You poor thing. Let's see if you'll go to sleep. Come on." She talks to me as if I'm a child. We lie down on the bed, and she rubs my back. "Everything is going to be all right."

"For you, but not for the rest of us."

"What?"

"You're going up the mountain soon."

Later in the day, I hear Penelope talking on the phone. "She thinks people are trying to kill her. What if she thinks I'm trying to kill her? Why am I doing this?" She's talking to her sister who has a 1-800 work number. "I don't want to be Dad's secretary. I don't want to sit in that damn garage and talk to truck drivers all day, but this is getting dangerous."

"Penelope," I interrupt. She jumps.

"Yes?"

"I don't love you."

"That's nice."

As usual, she disregards what I say.

"I like being in bed with you better than I do Richard."

"What?" She puts her hand over the receiver.

"You can calm me down better than Richard can."

"Have you told Richard this?"

"No."

"I should start spending the night?"

I can tell Penelope wants the extra money.

"I think you should. I'll ask Richard. Does this mean I'm gay?"

"No. It doesn't mean I'm gay either."

"What's it mean?"

"It means I can bring you down."

Richard and I sit in the waiting room of Dr. Lucas, my obstetrician. He has a wave machine I like to watch. It's a box full of liquid that sloshes back and forth, creating waves. They're never the same twice. "Can Penelope start sleeping with us?" I ask.

People in the waiting room raise their eyebrows. Someone chuckles.

"Why?" Richard asks.

"She gives a good back rub." I know I should save this for later, but I need to know.

"I stay awake for six months to rub your back, and you don't like it?"

"I love it, but Penelope puts me to sleep faster."

"And where would she sleep?"

"With us."

"The three of us in bed?"

"We have a king-size bed."

"Do you feel it's necessary?"

"Yes."

A lady gets up and moves across the room.

It takes extreme concentration to act sane when Dr. Lucas examines me, but I have managed up to eight months to keep her in the dark as to my psychiatric condition. I just don't say anything. I lie on my back and look at the colors in the fluorescent lighting. I can see blue and yellow. I can see a rainbow in the plastic covering the bulbs.

"The baby has turned," she says. "This is good. The baby's head is now in a downward position. How are you feeling?"

"My stomach is itchy."

"That's completely normal."

"I have varicose veins."

"Also completely normal. Everything looks normal."

Before all this happened, Richard and I could go shopping and have fun. Richard would take me to fancy lingerie stores. He'd sit outside the dressing-room door while I'd try on G-strings and push-up brassieres. Richard was usually businesslike at these occasions. "Try the peach on again," he'd say. Sometimes he'd come into the dressing room and fondle my nipples so they were hard. He loved navy blue. I must have six navy blue bras.

The colored lingerie has become a sign of my lucidity. When I'm high, I wear nothing but white. The fancy stuff makes me feel unclean, like a hooker.

But then, before all this happened, it was always Christmas.

Richard agrees to Penelope spending the night. This will allow us both to get more sleep. We'll pay her $50 to sleep with us.

"What will she do for $50?" Richard asks.

I'm not too manic to know this is a joke. "Blow us both."

"You're terrible."

"Just think of her as a big child smack dab in the middle of the bed. We're going to have to worry about that soon, anyway."

"What?"

"A baby in the bed."

Richard wears his clothes, his top button buttoned; Penelope, a cotton nightgown. I wear a large T-shirt that says "Baby."

Penelope seems the most attractive she's ever

been. I can see she's hot-rollered her hair. She's wearing lipstick. I know she likes Richard, and I'm afraid she'll steal him. "I changed my mind. I can sleep. We don't need you tonight."

"Hush, come on, get in bed. We'll all just sleep," Penelope says.

The way she says "just" makes me wonder what else she wants to do. Richard is snoring in 15 minutes. With one of Penelope's back rubs, I'm down in an hour.

I wake Richard up in the middle of the night. "Do you want her?"

"Who?"

"Penelope. I know you want her."

"I don't want her."

"I'm afraid she'll never leave our house."

"I'll leave," Penelope says sleepily.

Blowing up this orange balloon relaxes me. I take deep breaths and blow, exhaling into the orange rubber. This baby shower was Penelope's idea. I'm afraid it will expose to my family and friends how sick I am. Penelope just says, "Everyone needs a baby shower." We have a few guests—my three sisters, my mother, Richard's mother, two of my girlfriends, and Richard's sister. They've all been briefed as to my condition.

"Why didn't she let the doctor wean her off of the lithium?" my sister Denise asks.

"She thought she'd been on it long enough. She thought she wouldn't have any problems," Penelope says. "Now, we're going to keep this simple. No games, just ice cream and cake and open presents."

"Where's my address book?" I ask.

"It's in your room. Do you want it?" asks Penelope.

"Yes, I do."

"What do you need your address book for?" my mother asks.

"I need to check something."

"Okay, here's the first present," my mother says, with tears in her eyes.

"Why are you crying, Mom?" I ask.

"I hate seeing you like this."

"Like what?"

"Out of your head."

"I'm not out of my head."

"What do you want your address book for?"

"You know."

"It's time to read the names of the chosen," my mother says.

This is what I did when I broke the second time. She was driving me to the hospital, and I was reading the names and the addresses of friends—the chosen ones.

"Here, open this. It's from me. I hope this baby is worth it," my mother says.

"Mom!" my sister Donna says. "How could you say that?"

"I think we should play a game," says my sister Abby.

"No games," says my mother.

"What about that one where you have to remember items on a tray?"

"That's no fun," I say. I hate shower games.

"Okay, here's your address book," Penelope says.

My mom is motioning not to give it to me. "Take that back from her," she says.

"Why?" asks Penelope.

But it's too late. I've begun to read the names. "Henry Dugan, 291 Merdle Avenue, Cuyahoga Falls, Ohio 44221."

"Why is she doing that?" Donna asks.

"These are the chosen. I must read them. Paula Harrington, 6279 Park Road, Stow, Ohio 44224."

"Well, we might as well open the presents," Penelope says. "Who would like to open the presents?"

My friend Dolores volunteers.

"Karen Johnson, 1901 Pullen Drive, Tampa, Florida 33609." She opens a package of receiving blankets.

"Jan Wynn, 54 Riverside Drive, New York, New York 10024."

She opens a baby hamper, a box of diapers, baby T-shirts, footed sleepers, a lamp.

"Michael Gill, 110 West End Avenue, New York, New York 10023."

I need to read loudly, delivering my message. If

I can read their names to the universe, they will be saved.

"Oh, look, a rocking horse," my friend Joan says.

They've begun to ignore me. It's their shower now.

"Are you with her all day, dear?" Richard's mother asks Penelope.

"Yes."

"God bless you."

Days later, I'm swimming in cool water. My water has broken.

"We can't go to the hospital," I say.

"Why not?"

"They'll keep the baby." I double over from a contraction.

"They won't keep the baby. The baby is ours."

"They'll get our baby mixed up with someone else's, and we'll raise it for ten years, and then discover it's not ours. Where's Penelope going?"

"She's going with us."

"Why is she packing?"

"She's packing your clothes."

"She's going to Vegas."

"Penelope is going to the hospital with us. How do you want to do this?" he asks Penelope.

"I think she'd climb out of a car at this point."

"I'll call an ambulance. Lord, why did we do this?"

A contraction grips my back and lower abdomen. "Both of you are going to Vegas, aren't you? You're deserting me."

"God. I've never called 911," Richard says.

"There's a first time for everything."

"Christ, I can't take this. I have to have this baby."

And then I do it. I grab the phone from Richard and say, "249 Pierce Place. Hurry." I start pacing, terrified. I think that God is punishing me for something, for not taking my medicine, for trying to have a baby, for attempting to be normal. Manics should not try to live normal lives. They need their medicine. Their babies will be crazy. I fight back the pain. And then the ambulance comes.

At the birth, I believe not that I'm Christ, but that I'm delivering Christ. I am convinced that the birth is being televised worldwide, a far cry from a stable with farm animals standing around. Each doctor and nurse is an instant saint. The viewing of the miracle cures everyone of anything.

I lift myself off the cart and onto the delivery table. I'm surrounded by stainless steel. I suck on ice chips and hold Richard's hand. My feet are cold, so Richard gives me his socks. I don't want footies from the hospital. Because my mother had an enema and because they shaved her, I ask for these two procedures.

"Times have changed," a nurse says.

"But I want to be as clean as possible."

"We'll get you clean. Don't worry."

I say a Hail Mary and an Our Father. My contractions are two minutes apart. All I want to do is push.

The doctor catches God with both hands, and Richard cuts the cord. I remember now that she is a girl.

Little Christ has a weird-looking pointed head from squeezing through my cervix. Her eyes are blue, and her hair is light brown. She's eight pounds, five ounces. I love to hear her cry. She's crying for the world.

The baby is fine. My psychiatrist meets us here—calm but furious. Twenty-four hours later, I'm on 1,200 milligrams of lithium and 100 milligrams of Mellaril. I can barely speak.

Richard brings flowers and climbs in bed with me. "Are you hearing messages in the TV?"

"No."

"What about from people in the hallway?"

"I thought she was Christ."

"You know she's not, don't you?"

"Yes."

"Well, no harm done."

"Richard, I love you."

"She's the most beautiful baby I've ever seen."

"What should we call her?"

"Penelope?" Richard says.

"I don't like that name."

"Joan?"

"What about Anne?"

Saying good-bye to Penelope is hard. We take her to lunch and attempt to give her the recommendations we promised her, yet she doesn't take them, telling us she's landed the part of a waitress in a show. It's a shame because they're good recommendations.

And now, I rely on cool, pink lithium tablets—three a day—to save, preserve, and keep me. After what happened, I love the sound of the pills rattling when I open the bottle. I used to hate this sound. I used to avoid it by sticking my pointer finger inside and pulling out one pill at a time.

Preface to *With Child*

ARIEL CHESLER

Ariel Chesler, preface to Phyllis Chesler, ed., *With Child: A Diary of Motherhood*, New York: Four Walls Eight Windows, 1997. Reprinted by permission.

With Child is more than just a book to me. It is a very personal account of the beginning of my life. It carries me to pasts that I could never have seen on my own and allows me to understand my mother in a much deeper way. I am able to see her not just in relation to me, but as her own person. A book written for me and about me is the most welcoming gift that I could have received from my mother upon entering this world.

With Child is not fiction but a fierce reality. It charts the time of my mother's pregnancy, my own birth, and our relationship, which began long before I was conceived and will last until forever. I am the fetus, the growing clump of cells, the newborn baby in every line of this book, and have been given insight into the reality of my creation, and all mothers' histories.

This book is not only important for women, or young mothers, to read. I think that children can learn from this book. It can help them to see the importance of a strong bond with their own mother. It has shown me the beauty of that bond and the real reasons that we all should deeply respect our mothers.

I think that men should be aware of what the pregnancy process is really about. This will help all men to think about their own roles in the process. We should neither be terrified by nor ambivalent toward pregnant women. We should see the beauty in pregnancy, in that earth-round belly that holds a child.

My mother has given me life and love. I am flesh of her flesh, bone of her bone. I was born of her body, linked to her by nature. Thus, is she not my Adam, am I not her Eve? Must Adam really be male? Or is she my Eve since she has nourished me with forbidden fruit? Yes! She gave me knowledge of good and evil. The only difference is that she valued and praised the "forbidden" knowledge that she gave me. If we have sinned, by her sharing of knowledge, then at least we are exiled together.

My mother writes poetically and beautifully. She writes with passion, bravery, and strength. At certain moments, in the book, I can envision her singing the book. It is her warrior's tale and she is an ancient bard. She sings a prayer that is her *Sh'ma*, her motherly prayer. She writes: "Hear, O Israel, I am one. Mother and Child. Male and Female. Past and Future. My belly warms the sunglown stones." The *Sh'ma* is the most important prayer in Judaism. I can also hear a fairy tale–like sound to her story when she writes: "In colors of blood and air I spin without stopping: colon, foot, eye. By day, by night, for nine months. I weave you: precisely. Faithfully." This is so witchlike, her spinning me into gold, into body. She recites her thoughts throughout this book in song, with a pulsing rhythm and a graceful melody.

My mother does not begin with the beauty of children or family, or even her ideals of motherhood. She begins with the fact of her vomiting. This is her truth, the pure physical reality of pregnancy. Her voice is an honest, helpful, and questioning voice, which she maintains throughout the book.

When I read this book, I feel my mother talking to me. I see her eyes, smell her cappuccino, and hear her voice. I can always pick this book up if I want to converse with my mother. Her questions force me to ask her questions too. I want to ask about her childhood, about her past. I want to learn more about my childhood, and how she dealt with bringing up a male child. I wonder too how she brought me up in a feminist manner and why our relationship is so unique.

I always thought of my mother as "macho" when it came to work. She never took breaks, never relaxed her mind, but I guess she just couldn't (and still can't) allow herself to. This of course is due to the importance of her work as well as the time she devotes to it. However, when she had the additional responsibility of caring for a child, she realized that she could not handle all of her jobs on her own.

In some ways this book can be seen as quite comical. Here was a PhD, an intelligent woman, who was naïve when it came to being a mother. She only knew how to ask questions of other mothers, and the more she asked the less she comprehended.

With Child is not only a personal account of motherhood. It is of the utmost political importance for everyone. It signifies a radical revisioning of motherhood for the coming generations.

This book clarifies that, contrary to myth, women do not exist only to give birth to children. They all have their own lives, desires, and needs. In my mother's case, motherhood really hit her hard and shocked her. I brought her back to earth from wherever she was.

The book you are holding is as precious as a newborn child. In fact, imagine that you are actually holding an infant when you pick this book up. Imagine that this infant is still as small as I was when this book was first published. Imagine how difficult it would be for you to carry this book around with you everywhere you go. Then add about 6 pounds. Think about the time it would take to feed the book, clothe it, put it to sleep,

change it, entertain it, and still have your own life and career remain intact.

Now, imagine that the book is alive and cannot survive without you. If every time you left the room, the book looked at you, would you leave as quickly? If you loved the book would you be able to leave at all? If you helped to create the book and loved every bit of it could you let anyone else take responsibility for it? Could you even handle the responsibility yourself? Would your nerves shake every time you held the book, since dropping it could mean death?

My mother's office door is shut, but that means nothing to me, I am her one and only son. A mother can always be taken for granted, a mother can always be counted on. I knock calmly on her door and enter before she can reply. Her books surround her as usual and she sits with a pen in hand. "I'm off duty!" she informs me. I do not comprehend that phrase and reply, "You are not a taxi, Mom, I need to talk to you."

This scene was quite common throughout my childhood. I would upset my mother daily, by trying to interrupt her. Although I found her work interesting and was proud, I was jealous of the time and attention it took away from me. In a sense, despite being an only child technically, feminism was my baby sister, the one who got all the attention, it seemed to me, because she was cuter and more important.

However, feminism has had a profound and positive effect on my life. I was thrust into a world of feminism by birth. Ironically, I never became truly involved with feminism throughout most of my youth, despite my exposure to thousands of books, articles, and events. I was surrounded by feminist leaders, including my own mother; so I took the movement for granted. It was only when I ventured out on my own to college, that, without my mother's encouragement, I began to take women's studies courses. I loved them instantly, and discovered my affinity for my mother's work.

It is often quite frightening for me when I compare my political views to those of my peers. Although my friends are intelligent, liberal, and even progressive, that doesn't always mean they are feminist. I have come to realize that like my mother, I, too, am a radical feminist. It's not as easy as I assumed. I am constantly forced to defend all of my views, to enemies as well as my best friends. It becomes quite taxing and I only pray for the strength to voice my opinion in public, especially to other men.

Over the years, many of my friends have asked me what it's like to have a book written about my birth. "Is it weird?" they asked. "Does it cover your conception?" I guess the answer to both questions is yes, but I don't usually think of it that way. Who else has a gift like this? What better birthday gift could I have received? That is exactly what this book is—my birthday present. It is a tangible, never-ending gift to celebrate my life. I feel so blessed, so lucky to have this book. I can't believe that I didn't even read it until I was about fourteen. Perhaps I wasn't ready for it until then.

In fact, I was quite embarrassed by this book when I was younger. I hated the attention I often got because of it. I remember being ashamed when my mother read to my fourth-grade class, and described my strong bond with her as a marriage. "Because of you, I'll return to Earth, transformed: no longer a virgin, but a mother, married to a child." I was so embarrassed by this book that I wrote a parody of it. Oh, if I only knew! My piece was entitled "With Mother" and it was hilarious, at least to a fourth-grade sense of humor. Apparently even then I was attempting to come to terms with this book in my life.

I wonder what I would be like if I didn't have this book or if my mother was a traditional mother. I wasn't aware that my childhood was that different from many of my friends. To me, the way I grew up was normal, although my household was quite different from the people I knew. For example, in my house one would be more likely to see me cooking eggs for my mother, rather than her cooking anything for me. I had sophisticated concepts and "adult" issues thrown at me daily from a very young age. I learned how to travel around New York City on my own. I took care of myself quite often. I spent time alone in our house, when my mother had business. I learned to rely on friends and others for help that my mother could not always give me. I had to learn not to rely on my father. I had to redefine "family" for myself. I was in contact with brilliant, even revolutionary people whom I regarded as simply my mother's friends. I also had to deal with attempts to exclude me from feminist events specifically because I was male. I was forced into becoming responsible, independent, and free of the usual stereotypes. That's why I've become who I am today. I think that the freedom I had growing up was the most important and helpful part of my maturation.

I received respect as an individual from the time that I was born. Although this respect quickly brought responsibility (mental, spiritual, and physical) and maturity to me, it was worth it. In fact, my mother seemed to consider my wishes even before I was born. Like most parents, she and my father discussed my name at length. I could have been named Daniel at one point. Not that Daniel isn't a fine name. I even know some very nice people named Daniel. But it's just not for me.

When my mother was about six months pregnant, I visited her in a dream. I told her, from the womb, what I wanted, what I felt, and she listened. I requested a name that began with the letter A. A name that belonged to me, not just given to me, one that I chose. My mother writes, "I dream a wonderful dream. I give birth to a little blond boy. . . . Have you really visited me in a dream? Are you requesting a name that begins with A?"

I love my name, what it means, how it sounds. This seems extremely important because my name is a big part of who I am. I am glad to be a Shakespearian spirit, a lion of God, a secret nickname for the city of Jerusalem, a small city in Israel, and even a little mermaid if people must insist on it. My name is Israeli, and it means "Lion of God." At times my name is my only path to my roots, my origins, a past that I yearn to know. It is at times my only connection to my father, who is Israeli. It is only when I say my name properly that I feel truly visible. When I say "Arriael," using that rolling *R* that I love, in that sweet, rolling Israeli way, I feel like me.

So ever since my mother's dream that mind-melding night, we shared the truth in great detail, until we understood one another.

Jan. 4, 1978. My mother writes: "Tonight I descend, tonight I rise. Tonight I am halved, tonight I am doubled. Tonight I lose you forever, tonight I meet you for the first time. Tonight I cheat death. Tonight I die."

Jan. 6, 1997. It is 5:17 AM. I am tired but my body wakes me up. I look outside to see cold winter waiting for me. Even my windows shivered with the wind. I do not want to leave the warmth of my bed to be born again, not even on my birthday. That comfortable, healing, mother-warmth that one's bed has for them keeps me under the covers. I roll over and go back to sleep.

Jan. 6, 1985. It is 5:17 AM and I crawl out of bed to be with my mommy. I stumble into her bed to cuddle with her on my birthday. I am here next to you, Mother, just like I was that first day. Your bed is special and it relaxes me more than anywhere else in the world. It is my earth-womb, the re-placement for my first sleeping quarters, your stomach. You also awoke at this time in the morning and we smile at one another, knowing that this is a rare and wonderful occurrence. Soon we fall asleep, with my head resting on your belly, at-tempting to return to my first world.

Jan. 6, 1978. It is 5:17 AM. Today I am born, today I am ended. I am wide awake. I am completely exhausted. I am freed from my mother's body, but enslaved by mine. I see everything around me, I am blind. I feel alone, I am surrounded by too many bodies. Everything is new to me, but I've seen it all before. I am cold, I am warmed by my mother's body. I have my entire life ahead of me, and my last one behind me.

My mother's last line of the book asks, "And who could be closer than we two?" To which I reply to her, No one, Mother. No one.

Misconceptions

GENA COREA

Gena Corea, adapted from "Preface," in Gwynne Basen, Margrit Eichler, and Abby Lippman, eds., *Misconceptions: The Social Construction of Choice and the New Reproductive and Genetic Technologies,* Hull, Quebec: Voyageur, 1994. Reprinted by permission.

An elderly couple walk among the physicians and scientists in the lobby of the Hilton Hotel Convention Center in Jerusalem in 1989 silently handing to each "technodoc" a photocopy of a letter they have written. The couple are afraid. Would these participants of the VI World Congress on In Vitro Fertilization and Alternate Assisted Reproduction call the police? Throw them out? That prospect was terrifying, yet, as the old man, Alexander Werba, sixty-seven, told me, that was actually—when he later thought about it—what he wanted: He wanted the police to scream in with sirens, and reporters to rush in with them, notebooks open, cameras rolling, and then he could tell them why he and his wife had come, how these doctors—no, they were not doctors, he said angrily, they were child-production engineers—how they had killed his daughter.

The letter the Werbas distribute states that their daughter, Aliza Eisenberg, died as a result of an egg capture procedure in the in vitro fertilization (IVF) program at Haddasah Hospital. It protests the fact that the physician who performed that egg capture had been named secretary of the congress.

I had spoken with the couple for hours the night before about the death of their daughter and they had shown me the letter they planned to pass out this morning at the congress.

They speak no English. If a technodoc reading the letter addresses them, they fear, they will be unable to understand or reply.

Prima approaches the huge lecture hall to which the technodocs will soon return. She tries to enter but a woman in the red uniform of the congress employees stops her. Prima is not registered for the congress. She has no badge.

Fearing the uniformed woman, Prima waits until she leaves. Then she enters the empty hall and places a letter on each of the seats, always looking to each side to see that no one is coming.

As she is leaving, she looks up, spots a young man, catches a glimpse of the name on his badge: It's him! The man who took her daughter's eggs. The man who left her daughter bleeding to death.

Prima quickly exits. She and Alexander are too upset, too frightened, to continue distributing the letter. Trembling, they leave the convention center.

The Werbas' fear went deeper than a concern that they would not be able to understand the techno-docs' English. They explained it to me later when I visited them in their home in Haifa.

Poles, they both survived the Nazi time in Europe. Alexander's parents had been transported in a train in Treblinka. After running away from a work camp and obtaining false identity papers, he lived on the Aryan side of Warsaw, working in the dark room of a photography shop, thankful that he did not have to be out in the dangerous streets. He was afraid all the time. The fear he had felt during that year and a half in Warsaw, before he joined the Resistance, was exactly the fear he felt at the IVF congress, he told me.

Prima "dreams that the Germans are running and shooting," Alexander tells me. "Soldiers and SS men. She sees that in her dreams very often. Now, after this case with our daughter, she dreams more about doctors. Every night."

She told me of her reaction to seeing for the first time the man who had attempted IVF on her daughter. "I was afraid like when I was with the Germans, when they led me to the crematorium in a cargo train."

"There were many people from the conference center to make sure that everything was in order and was going 100 percent smoothly," Alexander explains, "and she saw the Nazis in every such official in the red uniform. All these associations. Maybe they would throw us out. Or arrest us. You understand me? I didn't want it to come to that.

"But now I am sorry I didn't make a big scene where they called the police and arrested me or tried to throw me out. Then someone would have come from the press or television. I could have said in the press everything that was written in the letter. But at that time I was so—that was dumb. They were no Germans. Why was I so afraid? I wanted to go sit in a corner where no one could see me."

The association Prima and Alexander Werba made between life under the Nazis and their daughter's ordeal from reproductive technology experimentation is an association consciously made by a number of feminists. They recognize in these technologies the totalitarian project of controlling who will be allowed to be born into this world; the eugenic attempt to eradicate, even before birth, the lives of those judged "unworthy of life."

The Nazis' "Final Solution" originated within mainstream medicine. More than 70,000 people—patients all—were killed in gas chambers installed in psychiatric hospitals. The doctors and gas chambers were then moved to Poland to kill ("heal," in the Nazi metaphor) on a grander scale. The Nazis called this "the great therapy of Auschwitz."

Many Germans today feel a special responsibility to speak out against and stop the proliferation of new reproductive technologies (NRTs) because, unlike Americans, they well understand what is going on here and where it leads. In fact, it was German women who organized the first international feminist conference in resistance to the new reproductive technologies. I remember that 1985 conference in Bonn, Germany, well since I was invited to address it.

One of my memories from that conference is of Theresia Degener. A young woman in jeans, she delivers a paper to a speaker on stage. She holds the paper in her teeth. She has no arms. She had not been disarmed by her genes. (Genes are responsible for but a small portion—3 to 5 percent—of disabilities.) No. She had been injured by medical treatment, in the form of thalidomide, administered by well-educated, mainstream physicians.

The first time I met Theresia, in Frankfurt, Germany, she interviewed me for a magazine article. With her toe, she turned on her tape recorder. When the recorder malfunctioned, she impatiently pushed it aside with one foot, and pulled a pen and notebook out from her tote bag with her toes. As I spoke, she scribbled notes with the pen between two toes.

In the following years, we often worked together at conferences of the Feminist International Network of Resistance to Reproductive and Genetic Engineering (FINRRAGE). At one such conference in Spain, she told me at breakfast that she'd toiled much of the night on the paper she was to give that afternoon. She hadn't wanted to disturb her roommate's sleep, so she brought her typewriter to the hall outside her hotel room and typed there, with her feet. Several people had staggered drunk down the hall at 3:00 AM. She could just imagine them now at breakfast, she told me, her eyes sparkling in delight, saying they were so drunk last night they thought they saw an armless woman in the hall typing with her feet! We roared laughing.

Imagine Theresia, with her joy, empathy for others, courage, deep intelligence—all qualities she took to law school with her, all qualities that infuse her work in the feminist and the disability rights movement—imagine Theresia, on some prenatal test, judged "life unworthy of life"!

The fascist project of eliminating "unworthy" life through use of reproductive technologies leads feminists like Abby Lippman to pose this question: "Why have efforts to find every fetus with Down's syndrome become so important to us that universal triple screening is entering recommended medical practice, while ensuring early prenatal care for all women [the lack of which is a major cause of disability] is still an unachieved goal?"

It is not only reproduction that is now being engineered. The public discussion of the NRTs and of genetic engineering is also engineered. The forces behind medicine and industry have been largely successful in controlling the kind of information and the kind of interpretation ("stories," in Lippman's phrasing) we receive on the technologies.

The public discussion is framed in a way that excludes any consideration of the risks to women or the community, filmmaker Gwynne Basen points out. What's left out is just what feminists insist on including in the alternative framework we provide: the extraordinarily high failure rate of IVF; the experimental nature of the techniques; the damage of the techniques to women physically, emotionally, and spiritually; the preventable and ignored causes of infertility—including environmental factors and sexually transmitted diseases—some of those diseases, transmitted to the women when they were sexually abused as children; increasing medical and technological control over procreation; the violations of women's integrity, dignity, and freedom involved in the techniques; the unimaginable stress placed on women who suddenly become the mothers of three or four infants following the implantation of multiple embryos; the increasing industrialization of reproduction; the connections between the use and promotion of experimental contraceptives in dominated (third world) countries and the promotion of proceptives, like IVF, in dominating countries; woman's status in a sexual caste system; the increasing use of women as experimental models for other species.

When ethics are publicly discussed, women's experiences are largely absent from consideration. At the IVF congress in Jerusalem where the Werbas passed out their letter, the panel on ethics was entirely composed of men. The men did not notice the omission of women. It occurred to none of them that experimentation on women might be an ethical issue related to IVF. No one spoke of the Nuremberg and Helsinki codes on protection of human experimental subjects, let alone pointed out the many ways IVF violates those codes. (And IVF is experimentation, as feminist analysts have been documenting for years and as the World Health Organization has acknowledged.) Though the moderator of the ethics panel was on the IVF team at Haddaseh Hospital, Aliza Eisenberg's name never passed his lips.

Determination

BARBARA KATZ ROTHMAN

Barbara Katz Rothman, excerpt from "Determination," *Genetic Maps*, New York: W. W. Norton & Co., 1998. Reprinted by permission.

What are the characteristics that we think we can control when we plan our children? As the genetic map is unfolded and read, we expect finer and finer resolution. But we're looking at a map, not a crystal ball, and we're not dealing with three wishes from the blessing fairy. Our choices are limited to those things we believe are genetically determined.

The logic of genetic thinking as Evelyn Fox Keller summed it up is that genes are primary agents of life; to read genes is to predict traits; and to order traits you have to select or construct the genes. Want a blue-eyed kid? Select for the gene that causes blue eyes.

But are genes causes? Ruth Hubbard would have me never use the word "cause" for the action of a gene. A gene does not cause or do something, and it certainly is not "for" something. A gene is associated with, involved in, active in. And while I know she is right, somehow I think that the language of a gene that causes something, like blue eyes or sickle-cell anemia, is a reasonable way to speak. What, after all, ever causes anything in this world?

I fell down the stairs and broke my ankle. But it is perhaps a bit more complicated. How did I come to be on the stairs? My Aunt Joan lent us the down payment for this house with its big staircase. I was carrying the Chanukah presents at the time and couldn't see where I was going—Judah Maccabee fought the battle that Chanukah commemorates. American Jews only make such a fuss over Chanukah to compete with the commercialization of Christmas. And besides, some little child who shall remain nameless lest godforbid she get a complex, left a plastic bag on the third-from-bottom step. And how can you break both bones in your ankle by falling three steps? Look at a skeleton some time—the whole weight of the body tapers down to this absurdly thin point right above where the foot twists.

So what was the cause of my broken ankle? Aunt Joan, Judah Maccabee, Jesus Christ, American capitalism, a nameless child and an orthopedic design flaw.

"Causality" in science is basically only a hypothesis you can't disprove (yet). So with the hedging of my bets and all, I'm still ready to use the word "cause" sometimes in connection with a gene. I know that genes only code for the production of proteins. They don't do anything, they don't even produce the protein, but still, in the more-or-less approximate way I use to talk about cause, I feel comfortable saying that a gene causes, say, blue eyes. Sickle-cell anemia. What else?

We make a list of characteristics, qualities, traits, states of being, and then see if we can find a "gene for" the characteristic. Is intelligence, sexual orientation, schizophrenia, the tendency to divorce, depression, the inability to spell, genetic or not? The discussion too often seems to degenerate into "Is too!" and "Is not!"

Probably the most public, vociferous, and politically important of the discussions has been the long-standing one focused on genetic components in intelligence, and the more recent one focused on the "gay gene." The intelligence discussion has been hopelessly mired in the racism that surrounds it. So let's take a look at the "gay gene" discussion: Is there a "gene for" being gay? If an identical twin is gay, the chances of his twin being gay are 50 percent. That is considerably higher than chance, but an awful lot lower than the odds on eye color.

Chandler Burr has helpfully compared male sexual orientation with handedness. For both we have a dominant and a minority orientation. About 92 percent of the population is right-handed. Left-handedness has at various times in history been treated as evil, sick, sinful, or an ordinary variation. Handedness is experienced as a very powerful given: it is not changeable by an act of will, though one can hide or pass if necessary. And so it seems to be with male homosexuality.

But is handedness "genetic"? If an identical twin is left-handed, the chances of his twin being left-handed are 12 percent, or one and a half times chance. That is, the identical twin of a left-handed person is only one and a half times more likely to be left-handed than is the person sitting next to him on the bus. It is not a powerful argument for genetic causality. But it doesn't make handedness a "lifestyle choice."

It seems as if what we are really talking about when we invoke genes is predestination versus free will. Genes seem to function in our language and our thinking as equivalent to inevitability, determination, predestination, fate. Yet what we hear from the geneticists is that genes work as probability factors in a causal equation. They play their part.

If you keep leaving things on the steps (and if I've said this once I've said it a thousand times), someone's going to get hurt. And if people march up and down stairs day after day, year after year, it's no surprise when eventually someone falls. And if you carry packages and can't see where you are going, well, what do you expect? To each of these things, and probably a dozen more, maybe even one or two that are "genetic," having to do with bone structure, clumsiness and distractibility, we can assign a probability rating. What are the odds of falling under each set of circumstances?

Now we're approaching some basic philosophical questions about determinism and inevitability. Was it inevitable that I break my leg? Given everything that happened in the world to that exact second—including the history of architecture, my relationship with Aunt Joan, the world history that brought that nameless little child who shouldn't have a complex about this into my life, the invention of plastic, the evolution of the ankle—given all of it, was it inevitable? Did I have to put my foot there? Was it fate?

That is a fascinating philosophical question, but it is not terribly useful practically. For practical purposes, we focus on one or two of the factors that we think we can control. Don't leave things on the stairs. Watch where you are going. And we act as if—we have to act as if—we have control.

When genes become more and more important in our thinking, we start assigning them greater and greater causal power, moving them to more central positions. Sometimes that has meant giving up, that metaphorical throwing your hands up in the air and saying "It's genetic," meaning "And that's that." The "gay gene" might be useful as a political tool if involving that gene becomes another way of saying, give it up, you have to accept that some people are inevitably, determinedly, gay. But if the question we are looking at is not "Why are some men gay?" but "Why are more black men in prisons than in colleges?" then saying "It's genetic" is quite dangerous.

What complicates it these days is that the way things are going, "It's genetic" might very quickly not be a throwing-up-of-your hands kind of problem, but a rolling-up-of-your-sleeves kind of problem. "It's genetic" might be coming to mean, so let's fix it, let's engineer it, let's construct it to order. Let us make the determination and let us predetermine.

Take that highly publicized "gay gene," XQ28, now officially recorded as GAY1. The idea that there is a genetic component to being gay leads pretty quickly to either selecting against that gene or engineering to change it.

Gay is a highly politicized trait. But every day seems to bring some other "gene for" some other quality, characteristic, trait. Can we control all of it? Can we test and select, read and decode and splice our way to what we really want in our children, for our children?

And have we any right to do that? I'm not talking about our legal rights, our rights as citizens. Rather, I am thinking about our rights as parents in our relationships with our children. Do we even want to order them, to have them custom-made? Would we have wanted our parents to have ordered us, chosen our traits, predetermined whatever they could or wanted to about us? Whether it is what you like best or least about yourself, you probably won't like thinking about that as something your parents put on an order form.

Parenthood does not come with guarantees. Motherhood, I've often said, is one more chance for a speeding truck to ruin your life. The world has plans for your children, and your children have plans for themselves: you will not be able to control this.

Motherhood is not about consumer choice, and it's not about guarantees. The Dutch word for midwife, *vroedvrouw,* translates—as it does in many languages—to "wise woman." For wisdom on motherhood, I turn to midwives. The Dutch midwives worry about all of the new testing, and the implicit but false guarantee it seems to offer. Women say they want testing because they could "never raise a retarded child," or "couldn't bear" to have a disabled child. As if these things could be predetermined, as if they were all written in code ahead of time. Test, select, do what you think you can, but remember, as one midwife said,

> You are eager to have a healthy child, but after a chorionic villus sampling, amnio, an ultrasound and birth, your worries are not over yet. When the child is there you still have your concerns. Can he walk along the street on his own, and near the water, I hope he gets no accident, and I hope he doesn't get some wrong friends. It is a process, all life long, isn't it? Somehow or somewhere you have to let it go, you cannot control everything, and maybe you have to start to let it go at the beginning. You should dare to leave some questions without an answer.

Patenting Life: Are Genes Objects of Commerce?

BARBARA KATZ ROTHMAN AND RUTH HUBBARD

Barbara Katz Rothman and Ruth Hubbard, "Patenting Life: Are Genes Objects of Commerce?" *MAMM,* May 1999. Reprinted by permission.

When people think of patents, they think of patenting inventions—gadgets, tools—a self-wringing mop, the proverbial better mousetrap. They don't think of patenting the better mouse. But in this brave new world, the more profitable patent is likely to be on the mouse rather than on the mousetrap. OncoMouse was, appropriately enough, the first patented animal in the world. OncoMouse can develop all kinds of cancer, but it is for breast cancer that she was primarily designed and patented, and is best known. A mouse produced to order, like the mousetrap designed to specifications, has come to seem like a reasonable thing to patent.

And yet, there is something absurd about the idea of patenting animals or their—or our—genes. You can hold a mouse in your hands and make eye contact with it—can you imagine patenting a living being? And genes: Genes, we're being told, are the essential building blocks of life. So how can you patent life? How can you patent parts not only of mice, but of people? It just doesn't make sense.

Tell that to John Moore. Cancerous cells from his spleen were turned into the "Mo cell line," and used to develop a series of proteins for fighting cancer and bacteria. The cell line was making a lot of money—Moore sued for his share. But Patent No. 4,438,032 stands, and Moore is not getting a cut of the profits. The California Supreme Court ruled that while Moore could sue his doctors for not informing him of what they intended to do with his cells, the cells, once the doctors had them, were no longer Moore's.

HISTORY

Patenting in the United States dates back to the founding of the nation. Thomas Jefferson, himself an inventor, was one of the first patent commissioners. Patenting was designed to give individuals ownership of the fruits of their labors.

Governments issue patents when they recognize an invention as having three qualifications: novelty, nonobviousness, and utility, as they are termed. In other words, first it must be something new under the sun, something that didn't exist before. Second, it must not be an obvious variation on something already existing (Once the black Model T Ford was patented, you couldn't get a patent for a red one). Third, it must have a practical use—you can't patent a painting or sculpture.

The issuing of a patent gives its inventor, or the "holder" of the patent, exclusive rights to that invention for a limited time, during which anyone in that country who wants to use or sell the invention has to buy the rights from the owner, the patent holder. In the United States, most patents last seventeen to twenty years. During those years, the inventor can manufacture the object herself, sell the patent to a manufacturer, or license it for a fee or for a royalty, pay-per-use, or per-sale agreement. DuPont collects royalties on OncoMouse in the United States, and may soon in Europe.

How did we get from patenting gadgets and tools to patenting genes and mice? Thomas Jefferson, who patented his own inventions, such as the automatically closing French door, did not consider patenting plants even though he was a farmer and a plant breeder. (And if he could have seen where DNA testing was eventually going to land him—in the most famous and drawn-out paternity suit of all time—he might not have been in favor of DNA patenting at all!) Plant patents did not occur until 1930, when the first Plant Patent Act allowed for the patenting of nonsexually reproducing plants. This marked the beginning of agribusiness and its threats to biodiversity. Seed companies could buy the patent to a strain of crops, or develop and patent their own, setting us on the path to the patented fruits and vegetables that have appeared on our dining tables ever since.

But it was in 1980 that the brave new world of patenting living beings began to take shape. Ranajit Chakraborty, a researcher at the General Electric Co., used the new technology of gene-splicing to create a microorganism, a bacterium that would "eat" oil. The genetically modified bacteria, Chakraborty and GE claimed, thus met the qualifications for patenting: They were new, nonobvious, and useful.

And yet, bacteria are not machines, not things or a process—they are living beings, and so, many argued, patently unpatentable. Chakraborty and GE took the case all the way up to the US Supreme Court. In June 1980, by a five-to-four majority, the court upheld the validity of the patent. Living beings, albeit very small ones, had been patented, and that opened the floodgates. In 1985, the US Patent and Trademark Office declared that plants and seeds were themselves patentable, and in 1987 the patent commissioner announced that the license to patent also encompassed animals.

Europe was slower to go along, but in 1992, five years after the US patent, the European Patent Office granted Harvard a patent for OncoMouse. It opened the door to patenting of animals in all the European member countries. The patent, which will now affect all of the European member countries, hinges on whether there is sufficient medical benefit to justify the animal's suffering. OncoMouse, Donna Haraway says, is a Christ figure, promising us the salvation of a cure for cancer through her suffering.

But whether you think of her as a metaphorical Christ or just another product for better living brought to us by DuPont, OncoMouse is the world's first patented animal: We have gone from patenting the mousetrap to patenting the mouse.

PATENTING HUMAN GENES

What genes do is specify the compositions of proteins. We often talk as if there were a "gene for" something—a gene for being tall, or a gene for breast cancer, but genes are not order forms. By affecting the production of proteins they play a part in a sequence of events that may eventually lead, for example, to a girl growing up tall or a woman developing breast cancer. What is important to remember is that genes are only a part of the sequence of events, and that the genes themselves are not simple packages. Genes vary in their details from one person to another. Think of it as something like a nose: Everyone has one, and they all perform essentially the same functions, but they vary quite a bit. You can't really talk about patenting "the gene for . . ." any more than you can talk about patenting "the human nose." To patent a functioning gene sequence would mean patenting a whole set of sequences, the details of which may differ, and cannot even be fully predicted.

No one is suggesting that genes are patentable while they function in the body, any more than anyone would try to patent someone's nose. What some scientists are arguing, however—and the courts are finding reasonable—is that once a specific gene sequence has been taken out of a person, then either the scientists who isolated it or the institutions they work for should be able to patent it. It is the separation from the body that turns genes into "inventions."

Scientists have long maintained that they don't "invent" things, don't make things up: They just discover truths, facts, reality. It is ironic now to hear scientists forced by the system of patenting to describe their "discoveries" as "inventions." This is not just an academic distinction. Remember the purpose of patenting: to enable inventors to profit from the fruits of their labors. Patenting human gene sequences means enabling someone to "own" and thereby profit from that sequence.

And it is no longer really some "one." Very few patents of any sort in biotechnology are held by individual scientists, or "inventors," alone. It is corporations and universities—what is called the life science industry—that control patents. That industry includes chemical, pharmaceutical, and agribusiness companies. *Science* magazine identifies them as three interlocking circles—with corporations like DuPont and Monsanto at the center, working in all three spheres.

Patents are about profit: Biotechnology companies are not likely to fund research unless they can profit from it, and scientists rarely work unless they can get funded to do it—there are no lone scientists working weekends in their garages hoping to invent the cure for cancer. Though clothed in statements about intellectual property rights and how to extract the greatest benefits for suffering humanity, a struggle over competing rights to profits is at the heart of the debate about patenting.

PAYING THE COSTS OF PATENTING

And where does profit come from? Consumers. Us. While the United States permitted patents on gene sequences, the United Kingdom fought it. A British briefing paper called "No Patents on Life" was prepared in opposition to legislation making human gene sequences patentable in the European Union. The paper argued that medical costs would rise with patenting. After a ten-year battle, gene patenting legislation did indeed pass in the European Union; since May 1998, human gene sequences have been patentable throughout the member countries.

Most gene sequences have been found with the help of publicly funded research. Furthermore, many of the gene sequences being patented were found only with the voluntary cooperation of affected families. It is wrong that, at the point when the knowledge might produce useful results, its applications should be exploited for private profits. Genes should not be turned into objects of commerce.

Nor is patenting necessary to spur research. Proponents of patenting argue that unless scientists, universities, and private entrepreneurs can patent genes, they will not invest the necessary work and funding to create useful products such as diagnostic tests and therapies. But patents aren't just a way of encouraging research: They are also a way of hampering it. They introduce economic and proprietary barriers into what should be a free exchange of ideas and information. Scientists can no longer freely present their ideas at conferences or publish them in journals. They now must hold them in silence until patents have been applied for. The effort to establish patent rights is more likely to slow down scientific exploration than it is to further it.

Gene patenting is an ethical problem. No one, and no multinational corporation, should hold patents on our genes. As Jonas Salk said in a far-different era when someone suggested he patent his polio vaccine: "It would be like patenting the sun." Our genes are not commercial resources.

Geriatric Obstetrics: Oh, Baby!

CARRIE CARMICHAEL

Carrie Carmichael, "Geriatric Obstetrics: Oh, Baby!" *East Hampton Star,* July 17, 1997. Reprinted by permission.

In the new medical specialty of geriatric obstetrics (GO for short), you can accurately say the wrinkled newborn looks just like his old mom or old dad. That's some of the good news coming after the birth of a daughter to that sixty-three-year-old Californian who is for now the oldest new mother in the world.

Times have changed and so must the geriatric obstetricians. They must ask a new set of questions, like: "How many decades ago was your last period?"

"Will Medicare reimburse for deliveries?"

"During labor and delivery will the fetal monitor disable the mother's pacemaker?"

"Can I require a lie detector test about a prospective mother's age?"

"HMOs have already cut my income, now I must give a senior citizen discount?"

AARP TWOFERS?

It's not just the doctors who will have to change. The American Association of Retired Persons will have to revamp, too. It will have to add discounts if members are buying a twofer, such as a stroller and a wheelchair in the same week, dentures and teething rings, human eggs and chicken eggs, Ensure and baby formula.

Of course, discounts for diapers—both kinds. Depends and Huggies. The AARP should recommend that members make sure their new kids are out of diapers before they need them.

Can new old parents take their tots on Elderhostel trips?

START-OVER DADS

Not long ago the *New York Times* enshrined men it called Start-Over Dads (SODs). Guys in their sixties, seventies, and eighties. George Plimpton among them, who had no children until they were elderly or who hadn't bothered to take time out of busy career years to raise their first batches of kids.

Male geezers have long fathered babies, to the delight of the tabloids. Wink, wink, nudge, nudge. He can still do it! Tony Randall, a first-time dad at seventy-seven, is the most recent example. And he wants another baby right away. Quick, before he can no longer schlep the stroller and the baby bag.

The *New York Times* did not address the COKs (Cast-Off Kids) or COWs (Cast-Off Wives).

GEEZELLES

Techno-obstetrics evens the reproductive score for postmenopausal women. Now geezelles have equal opportunities to become SAMs (Scientifically Assisted Moms).

The conditions that attract young women to old, wrinkled, wealthy men now exist for old, wrinkled, wealthy women. A rich older woman no longer has to give up a younger man as a mate because he wants a child of his own. With enough money to pay for fertility treatments, she can have her baby boy and boy toy, too. As Oprah says, GO girl!

In fact, retired women can offer something younger women may not. No longer busy with careers, like rich older SODs, rich older moms can either hire young help to run after their kids, or marry it.

CERTAIN BLESSINGS

Being an older parent may be an asset. An elderly parent who needs less sleep now may already be up for the 4:00 AM feeding. Being an extremely old parent of a teenager may bring the blessing of not being able to remember at dinner the insults hurled at breakfast.

It seemed fitting when the news broke about the sixty-three-year-old mother that she lives in California, where looking young is coin of the realm and lying about your age common. Movie stars aren't the only ones to shave years. Anyway, sixty-three isn't as old as it used to be and plastic surgery can keep you from facing your years.

This latest GO mom had to lie about her age to get the fertility treatments. I wonder if GO dads face an age cutoff, too.

MIND-BOGGLING

With GO marching on, an older woman who wants a baby cannot count on breaking the record and becoming the oldest mother on record. She can't trust some tabloid will come along and cover the fertility treatments, finance her child's education, and enhance her retirement portfolio.

That is a long shot. Her older sister might beat her.

Let's not forget that the all-time geriatric motherhood award goes to Sarah in the Bible.

Margaret Mead wrote about PMZ, post-menopausal zest, the focused energy that women get after childbearing years. GO moms are going to need it.

Now that science has extended the possibility of giving birth almost to the point of death, what other mind-boggling possibilities are on the horizon?

NEVER SAY NEVER

I had my children premenopausally. One is in high school, the other in law school. I assumed my childbearing years were over. Science is now telling me, "Never say never."

Who knows? I may want to have more children when my future grandchildren are old enough to babysit.

I am single now. Maybe a young, offspring-hungry guy will cross my path. GO lets me say to him,"Baby, I want to have your baby."

Come to think of it, GO takes the pressure off the younger generation to produce grandchildren for us. My daughter can say, "Mom, do it yourself."

But not right now. My first batch of children is launched. My complexion is clear.

Bold Type: Childbirth Is Powerful

BARBARA FINDLEN

Barbara Findlen, "Childbirth Is Powerful," *Ms.*, January/February 1995. Reprinted by permission.

Outspoken, frank, and decidedly feminist, pregnancy and childbirth expert Sheila Kitzinger makes no bones about her mission: the empowerment of women in the birth process.

"Information is power," says the British author of eighteen books and mother of five grown daughters. "It's extremely difficult to act as your own advocate—unless you have the information to challenge doctors who often treat women as if they were irresponsible, selfish, and concerned only with their own emotions."

Thirty years after her first book, *The Experience of Childbirth,* hit the shelves, Kitzinger, a social anthropoligist, has released two new, very different books.

The Year after Childbirth: Surviving and Enjoying the First Year of Motherhood arose out of Kitzinger's realization that of the hundreds of books available about childbirth, baby care, and child development, "there was nothing that was woman-centered about the year after childbirth. All the books were about the baby, and the woman was marginalized."

By contrast, *The Year after Childbirth* focuses on the experiences and feelings of new mothers—with nods of inclusion to women with disabilities, lesbians, adoptive parents, HIV-positive women, survivors of sexual abuse, and single women. The book is full of practical information—tips on breast-feeding, advice on getting help and support from friends and family, realistic execise guidelines—combined with reassurance about what to expect emotionally.

All of this comes in the context of Kitzinger's lively, unadulterated feminism. For example, she calls episiotomy—an incision to enlarge the birth opening that is performed routinely in industrialized countries— "our Western way of female genital mutilation." She lambastes medical professionals who chalk up postpartum depression to women's hormones: "With all its joys—and these can be vivid and exultant—motherhood is intensely stressful. Research might be more productive and realistic if it examined why some mothers are not depressed."

In *Ourselves As Mothers: The Universal Experience of Motherhood*, Kitzinger compares childbirth and mothering in many different cultures. What emerges is a powerful critique of childbirth practices in industrialized countries, where doctors often induce labor or perform cesarean births for their own convenience, and where the whole process is depersonalized and taken out of women's hands. "Our society sets us up to feel socially isolated, guilty, and as if we are failures as mothers," she says. "In many traditional societies there is much more woman-to-woman support in pregnancy, during the birth, and afterward."

Kitzinger's family lives out a version of this supportive model. She and her husband, Uwe, live outside Oxford, England, with two of their daughters, their son-in-law, and their two young grandchildren. The extended family shares meals, laundry, and child care.

The author also practices what she preaches by running the Birth Crisis Network, a telephone counseling resource for women who have had invasive or humiliating birth experiences. "It's like a rape crisis line," says Kitzinger. "The emotional trauma after a violent childbirth is not unlike the trauma after rape. The woman's body has been forcibly invaded."

Kitzinger has been inspired by her mother—a pacifist and feminist who in the 1930s founded one of the first birth control clinics in southwest England—and her daughters, three of whom are radical lesbian feminists. "They call me a wishy-washy liberal feminist," she says.

"My work is all about women finding a voice, women growing in confidence, women sharing with each other," Kitzinger says. "All my writing has come out of my joy in birth."

Arlene Eisenberg

INTERVIEW BY TANIA KETENJIAN

Arlene Eisenberg is the author of several bestselling books including What to Expect When You're Expecting. *This interview was conducted in June 1999.*

TK: Dr. Spock's *Baby and Child Care* was the leading book of that genre before your *What to Expect in the First Year.* What do you feel is different in your book, and how does it replace Spock's?

AE: Actually, I used Dr. Spock's book when I was a young mother. But I think one of the big differences is that *What to Expect in the First Year* was written by three mothers. I think that we have more insight into what's going on.

TK: In *Memoirs of an Ex-Prom Queen,* Alix Kates Shulman discusses the contradictory feelings of a young mother when she brings her first child home. She attributes her confusion to Spock's suggestions, which went against her own instincts. So what is it that women as mothers (even first-time mothers) can grasp that male doctors simply cannot?

AE: When you've gone through breast-feeding, for example, you really know what it's like and what the problems are. And that goes for so many other aspects of parenting. I remember listening to a doctor talk about giving a child a healthy diet, and that that's all you have to do. Of course, you can give it to them, but they're not necessarily going to eat it; so therefore, it's a good idea to supplement with vitamins. So there are a lot of things doctors who aren't taking care of children just don't have any idea about. I think that was true about pregnancy.

TK: How did you arrive at that conclusion? What was the impetus that pushed you to write this book?

AE: The first book we wrote was *What to Expect When You're Expecting*; that was when my coauthor Heidi Murkoff was pregnant. She went out and bought a whole lot of books that were either very scary or very inaccurate, or both. Books tended to be written either from the point of view of the woman without full understanding of the medical aspects, or they were written by doctors who didn't understand the families' needs. So I think we were able to combine them both. One of my coauthors, Sandy Hathaway, has been an ob-gyn nurse, and I have a good medical background as well. So we combine medical backgrounds with being mothers, stay-at-home mothers at that. There are doctors who are mothers who go out to work and have somebody else take care of their kids; but we all took care of our kids; we all stayed home with them. So I think we had a big advantage.

TK: Did you find major contradictions when you were following Spock's book?

AE: I didn't have a lot of trouble with that. Actually, I first read Dr. Spock when I was about twelve years old for a Girl Scout badge. I think some of his ideas probably stayed with me. But it wasn't a complete guide. His book is a small book that deals with kids from birth through their teen years. Our books are big, fat books that deal with one or

two years at a time; they're just much more thorough; we deal with much more.

TK: Your book gained popularity by word of mouth. At that time, it was difficult for women to challenge their doctors. How did your book allow them to do that with confidence?

AE: Most doctors recommend our books; I think that is why women feel confident to use them from a medical point of view; and the doctors themselves use them. Over and over we hear from both pediatricians and obstetricians that they probably couldn't have gotten through their pregnancy or the first year of their child's life without our books. So they use them and they recommend them; that really has made a big difference.

TK: What do you think are the most potent messages in the book? How does it solve the problem of the contradictions that existed with Spock's book?

AE: Our point of view is that there isn't one answer that will work for every mother and every baby. It just isn't possible. Everybody is different, every baby is different, every mom is different. You have to use your own instincts and feelings and see what works for you and for your baby. There are four things that are invaluable. One is that you have to take care of your baby's health; there are certain things you must do: immunizations, regular checkups. Safety is the second thing. You have to make your house safe for your baby; you always have to use the car seat, that kind of thing. Then you have to love your baby; it's very important. And the other thing is that, along with loving your baby, you have to set limits. Limits are also very important, and different people have different ways of setting them, and different rules. In some households, you can't walk or put your shoes on the sofa; in others, they don't care about that, but there are other rules, like you can't eat sugar. It doesn't matter what they are, but there have to be consistent rules that your kids know they have to follow. Those are the four things that everyone has to be concerned with. Beyond that, there are no rules. You have to do what works for you, and what you're comfortable with, and that's different for each family.

TK: When you wrote *What to Expect When You're Expecting*, what made you so intuitively aware of the questions that mothers had?

AE: It helped that there were three of us because we all had different points of view in certain areas. We had different experiences with our pregnancies and with our doctors, so that started us off with a wide range. But we also did a lot of research and handed out a lot of questionnaires; that was extremely helpful in finding out what people were concerned about.

TK: You were already a writer before you wrote these books. Was it part of your vision to write a book and was *What to Expect When You're Expecting* the ideal one?

AE: I'd written books before that one. In 1975, I did a college textbook on health, which gave me a very good background in medicine. It took me four and a half years and I consider it to be my medical education. My coauthor, Sandy, is a nurse and has a DSN, and Heidi was also a writer. So we had expertise, which I think was valuable, because without knowing how to communicate as writers, we probably could not have done as good a job. We had the advantage of medical backgrounds, of being mothers, and also of being writers.

TK: You say expertise; how would you distinguish between professionalism and expertise? What would you say the differences are?

AE: We're not professionals because we don't get paid as medical personnel, but we do have expertise. Somebody told me she went in to ask a question of her doctor and the doctor said, "Excuse me a minute," and they looked up the answer in our book. So we do have a certain amount of expertise from our experience as well as from our research.

TK: What is the focus of the What to Expect Foundation?

AE: The What to Expect Foundation provides materials and programs for low-income and low-literacy moms, and dads as well, of course. We think that's important because the middle class has been able to use our books very successfully, but unfortunately, a lot of people in the lower income brackets either can't afford the books, or really find them overwhelming. We're going to provide books that are easier to read, and that deal with a lot of the ethnic and cultural issues that aren't in our other books.

TK: Until the nineteenth century, it was mothers who were writing books about how to care for children; but then, in the 1830s, it started being doctors, and that lasted until you wrote your ground-breaking book. What allowed that change?

AE: There was a feeling that doctors weren't always meeting the needs of patients because they didn't always understand. Our books have helped because they help doctors to better understand what mothers are going through during pregnancy, or as new parents. When we proposed the book to our publisher, his response was, "A doctor has to write this," and we said, "No, no, no." He was willing to listen to us and to go along with us. A writer knows how to research, how to gather material and make sure it's accurate; I've been doing that for over forty years.

TK: How much do you think has changed since the 1970s in regards to when a woman decides to have a child and what to do when she has a child? How have those views changed?

AE: A lot has changed. When we first wrote the book, there was an attitude that if you accepted any kind of pain relief during labor, you somehow failed in your job of natural childbirth. We took the position, which was different from that in many books, that if you needed pain medication, then you should have it and be willing to take it. I remember a young woman who cried after she delivered, saying, "I had medication; I failed"; she was really upset. The only thing that's really important is that you and your baby come through that delivery well and healthy; that's what really counts. Anything else is not important. There are women who deliver "naturally" around the world and yet one woman dies every minute in childbirth. "Natural" is not synonymous with healthy or right. I think we changed that attitude and that women now feel that if they need to take medication, it's OK. I think that we've tried to be non-judgmental about what people do. We think breast-feeding is by far the best way to feed a baby, but there are some women who just either can't breast-feed or don't feel comfortable doing it. If you're not comfortable breast-feeding, your baby's going to get that message anyway; so we tried not to be either judgmental or authoritarian, and we tried to say, "These are your choices; this is what is good about each thing, and you have to decide what's going to work for you." These are some of the things we had some impact on.

TK: Looking back at when you first wrote the book, would you do anything different now?

AE: We have been changing it. When we first wrote *What to Expect*, we actually did not include material about problem pregnancies and complications because we wanted to write a very reassuring book. Then we got letters from people saying, "But you didn't talk about this and you didn't talk about that." So in the revised edition, which came out in 1992, we added all that.

TK: Are there other books that you think are also pretty good?

AE: There are some books that we recommend in our book. One of them is Richard Ferber's book, *Solving Your Child's Sleep Problems.*

TK: The use of midwives seems more popular than it used to be and several people suggest that midwives are the way to go, what do you think of that?

AE: It's a matter of choice, of what you're comfortable with. Midwives are terrific in many cases,

but they should be either practicing in a hospital setting or in a setting where you can immediately get emergency care from a physician if it's necessary, for example, if an emergency c-section is needed. In England, they use midwives primarily, but they always have an ambulance standing outside ready to take you to the hospital. Midwives are wonderful because a lot of women are more comfortable with them, and they tell you more and give you more comfort and information, but you also have to be sure you get the best technical medical care as well. That combination is terrific.

TK: Are there any books that you would suggest for men when their wives are expecting?

AE: There are a few out, but I haven't really read them. There's a new one called *Business Dads,* which looks very good, that helps a father who has been working day and night to change his lifestyle in order to be home more with his family.

TK: Would you suggest to a man that he read *What to Expect?*

AE: We do have a section for men in it, and we do recommend that they read the whole thing, and a lot of men do.

TK: So that they understand where their wife is coming from.

AE: Absolutely, it's really valuable, otherwise you don't know. I think it's really important for them to read it.

TK: How quickly did the book become famous?

AE: It was slow. In fact, when it first came out, I think there were 5,600 books ordered, and I think either Barnes and Noble or one of the other big chains didn't even order it because they said they had too many pregnancy books already. It really took a little time for mothers to tell each other about it and then for doctors to start recommending it. It was a gradual, uphill thing. It was a couple of years before it really started to hit the best-seller list.

TK: That isn't too long.

AE: With most publishers, if you don't hit it right away, they stop pushing it. We were very lucky to be with Workman Publishing, which really tries to sell all the books they publish; they made a really good effort. The most important things in our books are not the answers to the questions, but the questions themselves. Because when you find out that everybody has the same questions and worries that you have, you start to think, "Ah-ha, I'm not crazy." A lot of the questions women have they don't want to ask their doctors because they think they're dumb. Our point is that there isn't such a thing as a dumb question. If you're worried about something, then it makes a good question, and when you see that everybody else has the same worries, you're comforted, and I think that is really important.

Lives: When One Is Enough

AMY RICHARDS, AS TOLD TO AMY BARRETT

Amy Richards, "When One is Enough," *New York Times*, July 18, 2004. Reprinted by permission.

I grew up in a working-class family in Pennsylvania not knowing my father. I have never missed not having him. I firmly believe that, but for much of my life I felt that what I probably would have gained was economic security and with that societal security. Growing up with a single mother, I was always buying into the myth that I was going to be seduced in the back of a pickup truck and become pregnant when I was sixteen. I had friends when I was in school who were helping to rear nieces and nephews because their siblings, who were not much older, were having babies. I had friends from all over the class spectrum: I saw the nieces and nephews on the one hand and country club memberships and station wagons on the other. I felt I was in the middle. I had this fear: What would it take for me to just slip?

Now I'm thirty-four. My boyfriend, Peter, and I have been together three years. I'm old enough to presume that I wasn't going to have an easy time becoming pregnant. I was tired of being on the pill, because it made me moody. Before I went off it, Peter and I talked about what would happen if I became pregnant, and we both agreed that we would have the child.

I found out I was having triplets when I went to my obstetrician. The doctor had just finished telling me I was going to have a low-risk pregnancy. She turned on the sonogram machine. There was a long pause, then she said, "Are you sure you didn't take fertility drugs?" I said, "I'm positive." Peter and I were very shocked when she said there were three. "You know, this changes everything," she said. "You'll have to see a specialist."

My immediate response was, I cannot have triplets. I was not married; I lived in a five-story walk-up in the East Village; I worked freelance; and I would have to go on bed rest in March. I lecture at colleges, and my biggest months are March and April. I would have to give up my main income for the rest of the year. There was a part of me that was sure I could work around that. But it was a matter of, Do I want to?

I looked at Peter and asked the doctor: "Is it possible to get rid of one of them? Or two of them?" The obstetrician wasn't an expert in selective reduction, but she knew that with a shot of potassium chloride you could eliminate one or more.

Having felt physically fine up to this point, I got on the subway afterward, and all of a sudden, I felt ill. I didn't want to eat anything. What I was going through seemed like a very unnatural experience. On the subway, Peter asked, "Shouldn't we consider having triplets?" And I had this adverse reaction: "This is why they say it's the woman's choice, because you think I could just carry triplets. That's easy for you to say, but I'd have to give up my life." Not only would I have to be on bed rest at twenty weeks, I wouldn't be able to fly after fifteen. I was already at eight weeks. When I found out about the triplets, I felt like: It's not the back of a pickup at sixteen, but now I'm going to have to move to Staten Island. I'll never leave my house because I'll have to care for these children. I'll have to start shopping only at Costco and buying big jars of mayonnaise. Even in my moments of thinking about having three, I don't think that deep down I was ever considering it.

The specialist called me back at 10:00 PM. I had just finished watching a Boston Pops concert at Symphony Hall. As everybody burst into applause, I watched my cell phone vibrating, grabbed it and ran into the lobby. He told me that he does a detailed sonogram before doing a selective reduction to see if one fetus appears to be struggling. The procedure involves a shot of potassium chloride to the heart of the fetus. There are a lot more complications when a woman carries multiples. And so, from the doctor's perspective, it's a matter of trying to save the woman this trauma. After I talked to the specialist, I told Peter, "That's what I'm going to do." He replied, "What we're going to do." He respected what I was going through, but at a certain point, he felt that this was a decision we were making. I agreed.

When we saw the specialist, we found out that I was carrying identical twins and a stand alone. My doctors thought the stand alone was three days older. There was something psychologically comforting about that, since I wanted to have just one. Before the procedure, I was focused on relaxing. But Peter was staring at the sonogram screen thinking: Oh, my gosh, there are three heartbeats. I can't believe we're about to make two disappear. The doctor came in, and then Peter was asked to leave. I said, "Can Peter stay?" The doctor said no. I know Peter was offended by that.

Two days after the procedure, smells no longer set me off and I no longer wanted to eat only sour-apple gum. I went on to have a pretty seamless pregnancy. But I had a recurring feeling that this was going to come back and haunt me. Was I going to have a stillbirth or miscarry late in my pregnancy?

I had a boy, and everything is fine. But thinking about becoming pregnant again is terrifying. Am

I going to have quintuplets? I would do the same thing if I had triplets again, but if I had twins, I would probably have twins. Then again, I don't know.

Following the publication of this piece in the New York Times *on July 18, 2004, Richards received an enormous amount of mail, some positive, much negative. Today she responds to those letters and reflects on what she learned through the experience of going public with this very personal experience.*

Hate Mail

AMY RICHARDS

Amy Richards, response to the *New York Times* article "When One Is Enough," 2008. Original for this publication.

When I initially approached the *New York Times* about doing an essay on selective reductions, I did so because I had two goals. First, I wanted to dispense information about this increasingly common procedure. I didn't want others to feel as in the dark as I did. What was it? What was the aftermath? What was the threat to the surviving fetus(es)? Second, I wanted to explore the political ramifications of this procedure within the broader context of the future of reproductive rights. Was a selective reduction an abortion? And was it really a rare procedure or just rare that people talked about it? In the future, could this procedure be used to eliminate one fetus and thus potentially be free of the stigma otherwise associated with abortions? After all, these were done in hospitals with doctors, specialists even, rather than in beleaguered clinics.

Not surprising the *New York Times* received hundreds of responses and, expecting as much, they were kind enough to call me days before the article's publication to confirm that my number was unlisted. Most surprising to me wasn't the hate mail, which is to be expected anytime someone talks about abortion, but those who wrote saying how brave I was. I didn't think being honest and public about what is more likely to be a reality in people's lives than not was doing anything out of the ordinary. This isn't to say that receiving hate mail is easy—nor is being called a baby-killer, especially when you have two small children—however, it is possible to persevere when you know that you made the best decision.

Equally surprising was how many people thought I was "tricked" or manipulated by the *New York Times*. Many in the pro-choice community were as uncomfortable with my level of honesty as those staunch abortion foes. Though the pro-choice community spends a disproportionate amount of time trying to break free from the stereotypes of those who have abortions—poor women who lack good judgment—when I came forward as a middle-class woman who chose an abortion, I was accused of not being sympathetic enough. They wanted me to be sad, express remorse; essentially they wanted me to be mourning this decision, just as the pro-life side wanted me to be mourning this loss of life.

The reactions I received to this piece illuminated for me the limitations the pro-choice side still has on its own perspective. The pro-life side is winning the moral debate partially because we are uncomfortable with simultaneously expressing our political belief, that abortion should be fully accessible to any woman who chooses it, and our personal perspectives, we consider some women's choices to be lame, reckless, and selfish. Yes, we have been beaten down by the pro-life side and become vulnerable to their sanctity of life argument, but also we haven't fully embraced our own moral superiority—we trust the women, even when we don't agree with them.

Love, Mom: A Mother's Journey from Loss to Hope

CYNTHIA BASEMAN

Cynthia Baseman, excerpt from *Love, Mom: A Mother's*

Journey from Loss to Hope, AuthorHouse, 2006. Reprinted by permission.

The night wore on and on and I continued to feel lousy. I sipped 7Up and tried to keep still under my sheets. A leaf rustling three blocks away can awake Neal from slumber to total wakefulness. He's been a tosser and turner since I've known him. But on that night, my numerous trips to and from the bathroom, the whirr of the bathroom pocket door, even my retching did not disturb his sleep. It was as if someone had cast a spell on him. Finally, I fell into an uneasy sleep.

A moment later, it seemed, Neal roused me from my bed. "Eight-thirty, my love. Bobby's looking for you. I gave him his breakfast."

I sat up. "What a night. You're lucky you could sleep through it all."

"Sleep through what?"

"My getting in and out of bed all night."

"Oh, honey. Why didn't you wake me up?"

"Doesn't one of us need to be conscious when this baby's born?"

In the kitchen, I poured a glass of Martinelli's apple juice. I had no food in my stomach and was feeling light-headed. Outside, I heard Neal start up his old blue Porsche and back out of the driveway. As he accelerated up the block, the engine grew fainter and fainter. The house was too quiet. I felt like even I wasn't supposed to be there.

The soft murmur of a *Sesame Street* video played in the den and I smiled when I heard Bobby giggle. I nibbled a piece of toast off Bobby's plate, expecting the baby to move any minute. The phone rang, startling me.

"I thought for sure you'd be in labor this morning," my sister-in-law Hayley said.

"Me, too! Last night I thought I was coming down with something and I couldn't feel the baby, so I saw Dr. Starre. He said everything was okay."

"Jesus, Cindy! You're feeling her now, though, right?"

"Well, not exactly. But I haven't had any food . . ."

"I don't like the sound of this."

"Give it a couple of minutes."

"Call Starre right away. And call me right back!"

Why did Hayley have to be such a drama queen? We hung up and I called Dr. Starre's office.

"Doctor says you ought to come in. Now."

Come on, baby. I ran my hand down my belly. *Let's get this show on the road.*

I called Neal, and though I tried to dissuade him, he insisted on coming home. He must have run every red light because when he showed up, I was just reaching over my abdomen to tie my tennis shoes.

At Dr. Starre's office, one of the nurses ushered me into the same examining room at the end of the hall where I'd been the previous night. The wallpaper didn't do much by way of calming me down. Women were in the other rooms with scheduled appointments, and here I was, cutting to the head of the line. It didn't sit well with me. The nurse was strapping the monitor to my belly and moved it this way and that, looking for the heartbeat. She cast her eyes down and fled the cramped room like a spooked horse. Neal and I exchanged worried glances.

I was here last night and everything was okay. The nurse doesn't know what the hell she's doing. Everything will be fine once Starre gets in here.

On cue, Dr. Starre swooped back in, gave a brief nod to Neal and me and took the monitor in hand. He slowly edged it to the left, then to the right like a safecracker searching for the right combination. Nothing clicked. Fear throbbed in my ears. Dr. Starre settled the monitor in one place and turned the unit's volume up. Way up. Finally we heard it. A heartbeat.

"Oh, thank God," I said.

I blew out the breath I didn't realize I'd been holding in and my heart swelled with gratitude for Dr. Starre. Like he'd been a witness to a near-miss car crash, Neal kept shaking his head back and forth. Hey, I wasn't even pissed at the inept nurse who flubbed it earlier.

"Let's go in the other room. I want to do an ultrasound," Dr. Starre said. I straightened out my shorts and pulled my shirt back down over my belly. Neal held his hand against my lower back, guiding me down the hall. The examining room where the ultrasound machine was kept was only two doors away. I lay down on the table and lifted my T-shirt and slid my shorts low across my hips.

Dr. Starre didn't say anything. He was all business and I figured he was under pressure, having squeezed me in between his regularly scheduled patients. He squirted the warm, clear conductor jelly on my belly and traced the ultrasonic probe along it, searching for the clearest view. Squinting, I tried unsuccessfully to find the baby amidst all the black and white clutter on the monitoring screen. After a moment, Dr. Starre held the probe still. The nauseating pink and green walls inched together, practically squashing Neal, Dr. Starre, and me into one being.

And there was my baby. I could make out her hands and her face, her image eerily still. Hello? Why wasn't Dr. Starre saying anything? There was no air in the stifling room. For fear of disturbing the image of the baby Dr. Starre held still on the ultrasound, I didn't move a muscle. The hum of the ultrasound machine was all I could hear. Dr. Starre lifted his hand, removing the ultrasound camera from my abdomen. His eyes were still on the monitor, where he had recorded a freeze frame of our girl.

"This baby is dead."

No, I thought. *That can't be right.*

Neal stepped closer to the monitor. "The heartbeat. We heard a . . ."

Dr. Starre cut him off. "That was Cynthia's."

Like an ox, I stared at Dr. Starre for my next cue. Go forward. Stop. Go right. Stop. For the first time in my life, I was at an absolute loss for what to do or say.

"Last night I should've done an ultrasound."

"I don't understand," I stammered.

"We'll know more in time. But for right now, we need to deliver this baby. Meet me at Westside."

While we lingered in the hallway, Dr. Starre arrived. Neal and I were holding hands like lost children.

"The delivery is not going to be painful. I promise." I floated along in a stupor of confusion and dread. Dr. Starre said the baby had to be delivered. My mind set a course on delivering the baby. I gave no thought to anything else. Who else could I trust? Trust him.

In about half the stillborn cases in the United States, many mothers don't even realize they've lost a child for days or even weeks. When a fetus dies, it's often without any warning, in a pregnancy that had seemed totally normal up to that point. Unfortunately, a woman's body has no automatic response, no built-in mechanism for delivering the baby.

To this day, I have no idea what caused me to become violently ill for twelve hours nor if there was a connection between my baby's distress and my illness. All I know is, over the course of nine months, I had become in tune with Samantha's cycles. The roundness of her face and the shape of her body became more familiar through each ultrasound viewing. I sang songs to her and she was my girl. If I sensed something ominous, it was quelled by Dr. Starre's assessment. Like Shakespeare's Macbeth, who was convinced by his trusted advisors, the witches, that he was safe as long as the forest never moved, I was lulled into thinking all was well and my child would never cease to move.

The nurses showed me to my private room, which was dim, somber, and windowless. They gave me a cotton gown and I changed out of my maternity clothes and slipped it on. Neal took my clothes from me and stashed them in a blue hospital-issue plastic bag. The nurses poked my forearm with a needle and I didn't blink. They hooked me up to an intravenous pitocin drip to jump-start labor into full speed.

During the series of events, I completely lost track of time. Dr. Starre came in and stood at the foot of the bed. "Breaking the bag of waters ought to speed labor along." He put a hand on each calf and spread my legs. The nurse, Maria, was a friendly face who had assisted in Bobby's delivery.

"I am terribly sorry for what has happened," she said.

"Thank you."

She handed Dr. Starre a long, thin tool resembling a knitting needle. Numb from shock, I didn't feel a thing when Dr. Starre inserted the tool inside me and punctured the bag of waters. A warm liquid poured out of me.

"Meconium was released," Dr. Starre said. His voice was grave. His manner reminded me of the kid who is sent to the principal's office and doesn't question it. Meconium is a black, tarry substance made of mucus and bile—a waste product only expelled in utero when a fetus is in distress. My mind went to work: How long had she been in trouble? When did she actually die? Did she suffer? Oh, God. Did she?

My mind turned to the immediate: labor. I didn't cry. I wasn't in hysterics. When the anesthesiologist came in, Dr. Starre instructed me to get on my side. Two and a half years earlier, I'd done all this during labor with Bobby. Back then, having a needle inserted into my spine scared the dickens out of me. This time around, it was about as intimidating as a manicure.

Dr. Starre's left hand steadied my head, while the other braced my back. I felt his strong fingers tremble. Instinctively, I raised my arm and held his hand. Why did I want to reach out to him? Why did his shaking hands stir me so? In some sense, this was his baby, too.

Maria helped the anesthesiologist gather his equipment and they both left the room. Neal said, "Are you okay for a couple of minutes? I want to talk to your mom and dad."

"Go ahead. It's alright." Neal kissed my forehead and stepped out. Alone in the darkened room with Dr. Starre, I lay still while he sat on the edge of my bed. How long had I been here? When I'd first arrived, Neal had taken my watch from me as the nurses suggested. The under-counter fluorescent lights cast a weird greenish glow in the room. Dr. Starre shifted on the bed.

"This was my fault. I should've delivered this baby last night."

He couldn't possibly mean that. Did he think I blamed him?

"You took a good look at me, right? If that was the call, you'd have made it."

He took a deep breath, almost talking to himself. "I should've done an ultrasound."

Given that Los Angeles is the sue-happiest town in the nation, I saw his confession as tantamount to a fireman entering a burning building; I admired the heroism and feared for his self-destruction. It had all the makings of an explanation but I wasn't convinced he was to blame. He had been my gynecologist for years prior to my getting pregnant with Bobby and I had always found him to be attentive and caring. How could I suddenly buy into him making a mistake as horrendous as this one?

My cervix was ripe, and where it had previously taken me eighteen hours to deliver Bobby, this labor and delivery took only three. And it didn't hurt in any conventional way. When Dr. Starre told me I could push, a tremor of fear pulsed through me. What if my baby was deformed? After all, something had gone wrong. I didn't know how wrong.

The panic flared up in my eyes as I started to push the baby out. Neal took one look at me and saw the fear. "It's okay."

I stared back at him, frozen with alarm. He fixed me with a stern look. "It's *okay.*"

Astonished, I peered down between my thighs and saw her, all curvy, white, and feminine in the palms of Dr. Starre's hands. She had plump little thighs with a couple rolls of fat. Her abdomen was long and rather slim. Her hands were pudgy and the nails needed a trim. Her hair stood out, dark brown against her fair face. Her eyes were still closed. Dr. Starre startled me as he swiftly cut the umbilical cord. My mouth started to open to object—wasn't that Neal's job?

When he handed her to me I was struck by how light she felt. A sleeping baby has weight and the reassuring motion of its chest rising and falling with each delicate breath. She was lighter than a shadow, an astonishingly beautiful, empty shell. It was unbearable to hold her because it was such a cheat; it wasn't her anymore. The baby I'd loved

and held inside of me was gone. The spark that was my baby's life, the rhythms of her sleep and her play, all that I'd learned to love, all the dreams I had for her and for us, had simply vanished overnight. Her face looked a lot like Bobby's; it was heart-shaped and full-cheeked. I stared at her lips. They weren't pink like a newborn's; they were a deep plum color like one of my lipsticks. In a moment's time, I handed her body back to Neal. It felt unsettling to hold this featherweight body in my arms as if it were my baby.

"She's not here," I whispered.

Dr. Starre's voice brought me back to the present. "We need to deliver the afterbirth. A couple more pushes . . ." My feeble attempts didn't get the job done.

"You've run out of steam," Dr. Starre said. His left hand firmly massaged my belly while his right hand coaxed out the afterbirth. Passive as a pigeon, I was stitched up, cleaned up, and fussed over.

"See this little kink?" Dr. Starre shows us the umbilical cord. "I think this may be where the cord twisted and cut off her oxygen." My eyes scanned the cord but I could not detect any such kink in its smooth, shiny surface. Unsure, Neal squinted and thought maybe he could see something. "So the cord wasn't wrapped around her neck or anything?" Neal said.

"But it could have twisted like a garden hose, and cut off her circulation. We should have an autopsy performed to rule out anything else for future pregnancies." Dr. Starre looked at me for a moment then turned his attention to Maria, gave her some instructions and left.

Out of nowhere, the fatigue slammed me. I hadn't slept the night before and the physical exertion of delivering a dead child finally knocked me down. My body began to shake and my teeth were clattering. It was all I could do to say one sentence: "I'm cold." Neal approached one of the nurses and asked her for an extra blanket. She quickly brought me one; it had been heated, I noticed. It wasn't enough, though. No matter how many warm blankets the nurses put over me, I still shook like I was standing naked in the sheet.

The hub of activity had no effect on me until one of the nurses I did not recognize wheeled a plastic bassinet into the room and parked it at the foot of my bed. I raised myself up on my elbows and saw through the clear plastic to a little lump covered with blankets. Neal and I exchanged an unsettled look.

"Excuse me?" I called softly to the nurse.

"Yes?"

"Can you please move her?"

She froze in her tracks.

"Some families want to spend time with their babies."

"Take her out of here," I said. My voice was as menacing as a growl.

"Wouldn't you like a few minutes alone with—" she persisted.

"No. I wouldn't!"

My eyes tracked her like a rifle sight as she backed up and wheeled the baby out like she was maneuvering a grocery cart through a tight space.

I sighed, glad she and the bassinet were out of sight. Unfortunately, when the door to my dim room swung open it was the nurse again.

"We're taking some pictures of her. Hospital policy."

Nurses took photos of dead babies? Good God.

"It's totally your decision as to whether you want to see them or not. If you do, they'll be ready in about a week. We'll call you."

Neal looked as surprised as I was.

"Why in the world are you taking pictures of . . . I mean, really, isn't this a little morbid?" I said. Sick, not morbid, is what I had on the tip of my tongue.

"A lot of parents want them."

If hanging on to that were your only memory, I'd rather forget.

Is This Any Way to Have a Baby?

BARBARA SEAMAN

Barbara Seaman, "Is This Any Way to Have a Baby?," *O, The Oprah Magazine*, February 2004. © 2004 by Barbara Seaman.

When Louise Brown, the world's first test-tube baby, was born, in 1978, no one followed the news reports with more excitement than Liz Tilberis, then a thirty-year-old fashion editor at British *Vogue*. After several years of trying to get pregnant, she and her husband, Andrew, had not been able to conceive. Although Tilberis had been told repeatedly that she was simply working too hard, she consulted a London gynecologist who prescribed three cycles of Clomid, a workhorse of a drug that stimulates the ovaries (the doctor referred to it only as a 'fertility booster'). Clomid gave Tilberis stomach pain, bloating, breast tenderness, occasional vomiting, and hot flashes (she was spared the more serious side effects like severe dizziness and blurred vision); when it didn't get her pregnant, the doctor sent her to famed fertility surgeon Ian Craft, MD. Craft performed an exploratory operation and discovered that both of Tilberis's fallopian tubes were blocked as the result of a sexually transmitted disease in her youth that had never been diagnosed. When he came to her hospital bed to tell her there was no way she was going to have children in her current condition, she later recalled in her memoir, *No Time to Die*, "I might have jumped out of the hospital windows if they hadn't been hermetically sealed. . . . That may sound shocking, but the psychology of infertility is pernicious and crushing."

Not long after, Tilberis underwent surgery to remove one ovary and fallopian tube and to clear the other temporarily, after which Craft invited her to become one of the original "test-tube tries" in his research clinic. She signed up instantly and began treatments while still sore from her operation. "In vitro fertilization [IVF] was truly the stuff of science fiction, something akin to cloning today," she would say, looking back.

"Augmenting a woman's chance to produce a viable egg with fertility drugs, then harvesting that egg and uniting it with sperm in a petri dish? I certainly shared the public thrill that such a thing was possible."

Each month on the eleventh day of her cycle, already swollen with Clomid and a second drug, Pergonal, and teary from their pharmacological effects on her emotions, Tilberis entered the hospital for her egg extraction. In rapt fascination, she watched the eggs "ready to burst out of their follicles" on an ultrasound screen, then was hurried into the operating room and given general anesthesia. The doctor made two incisions, one just below her belly button for the laparoscope to enter and locate the eggs, the other above her pelvic bone to accommodate the syringe that would aspirate them (these days egg extraction can be done with a local anesthetic). Only once did these efforts result in a petri dish fertilization. Tilberis was rushed to the hospital, where the embryo was inserted into her uterus. But it turned out to be a "chemical pregnancy"; hormones surged but the egg didn't implant, and it quickly ended in a heavy bleed. That fleeting embryo was the closest she came to the experience of giving birth, and she deeply mourned the loss.

After nine debilitating cycles, Tilberis adopted two dearly beloved sons, Robbie and Chris, and fast-tracked her career to become a distinguished editor in chief. Life was good. She and Andrew still adored each other. And she was doing so well at British *Vogue* that in January 1992, American *Harper's Bazaar* stole her away and brought her to New York. But less than two years later, in December 1993, she was diagnosed with advanced ovarian cancer. Her doctors suggested that her history of fertility treatments might have put her at a higher risk. She learned that Gilda Radner, the comedian who died of ovarian cancer at forty-two, had also taken fertility drugs. Radner's husband, Gene Wilder, had given her the shots of Pergonal himself after practicing on oranges and grapefruits.

"Being told I had cancer was not as hard as being told I was infertile," Tilberis said, but she demanded to know if there was a connection. "The unanticipated question that most affected my life was, what might this pushing of the reproductive envelope be doing to my ovaries?"

Louise Brown, now a postal worker in Bristol, celebrated her twenty-fifth birthday this past July. And today fertility treatments are taken lightly, so much a part of our landscape that they're constant fodder for sitcoms like *Frasier* and *Friends*. But as the industry thrives at $2 billion a year, reproductive medicine is in many ways a Wild Wild West where doctors can practice like cowboys, using drugs that haven't been approved for fertility, and where no one is regulating the clinics, which often boast inflated success rates. "A fertility doctor can literally set up a lab in his garage and hire his son or daughter to run it, and it would be perfectly legal," says Brooks A. Keel, PhD, professor of biomedical sciences and associate vice president of research at Florida State University. "A woman gets more regulatory oversight when she gets a tattoo than when she gets IVF." Surprisingly, although the Clinical Laboratory Improvement Amendments of 1988 set strict quality control standards for medical laboratories, facilities that deal with women's eggs are exempt. Senator Ron Wyden of Oregon, who has steadily pushed for regulation of the fertility field, managed to get a bill passed in 1992 requiring that clinics at least report accurate success rates. But today some facilities notoriously cook their books to show the kind of success rates that will attract new patients. And Wyden himself acknowledges, "There is no question people still get around the law." By many accounts, government agencies like the Food and Drug Administration (FDA) and National Institutes of Health (NIH) are looking the other way. Fallout, perhaps, from politicized controversies over stem cell research and frozen embryos.

As almost any woman who has gone the fertility route knows, these treatments are often painful and always costly, and only one in four who attempt a test-tube pregnancy will take home a live baby, according to the best data available, odds that plunge to 5 percent at age forty-three and only 2 percent after that. The grueling nature of even a single cycle is hard to grasp. "When I was on Gonal-F and Repronex, my abdomen got so swollen from the egg follicle production that I had difficulty breathing," says a woman named Mona P. who eventually did get pregnant with twins. "I gave myself subcutaneous injections in the stomach, and my husband gave the intramuscular injections in the hip. I hate needles. The night of egg retrieval, you take progesterone shots, which are extremely painful and create lumps under your skin. After retrieval my ovaries filled up with fluid, so I kept the uncomfortable bloated feeling for another three or four weeks. A horrible pain in my left shoulder lingered on and on. In all we paid $20,000 to the clinic, including about $4,000 for the drugs." Beyond discomfort, assisted reproductive techniques pose serious health threats like ectopic pregnancy (embryos may migrate or be inadvertently misplaced), and more than one out of three IVF deliveries are multiple births (which often result in childbirth complications and severe infant health problems). And it isn't just the physical trauma that lays women low, says Harvard professor Alice Domar, PhD, director of the Mind/Body Center for Women's Health at Boston IVF. It's also the rising disappointment with each treated cycle where hopes are raised, and then dashed. Without oversight of fertility clinics, many patients go through harrowing ordeals for nothing. I talked to some women who got the full monty of ovulation hormones only to later find out their husband's sperm was solely the problem, and others who were pumped with drugs before doctors realized their misshapen uteruses could never carry a fetus. In the absence of regulation, too, a rogue doctor is more likely to have free reign.

Famously, in 1995, Ricardo Asch, MD, at the University of California at Irvine, was accused of filching his patients' fertilized eggs to place in other women's wombs. And he was considered one of the best in the field, the man who invented GIFT, a technique in which the egg and the sperm are placed in the fallopian tubes and fertilized within the woman's body (the license plate on his Ferrari read "dr. gift"). Asch was indicted but fled to Mexico. Another hallowed specialist, Cecil Jacobson, MD, who ran a clinic in Tysons Corner, Virginia, was convicted in 1992 on fifty-two counts of fraud and perjury and sentenced to five years for performing "anonymous donor" fertilization, using his own sperm, in as many as seventy-five patients.

But even with the best doctors and most sterling clinics, there are still glaring gaps in our knowledge about the danger fertility drugs may pose and whether the benefits outweigh the risks. A leading scholar who prefers to remain anonymous minces no words: "This is a field that thrives in the absence of factual information. There is little work on animals to show safety, or randomized clinical trials to compare results. We make the same mistakes, but with increasing confidence."

Liz Tilberis died of her cancer at fifty-one, in April 1999, having revitalized *Harper's Bazaar* and presided over the Ovarian Cancer Research Fund. But her question about the connection between ovarian cancer and fertility treatments remains unanswered, the necessary clinical trials yet to materialize. In truth, it would take a brilliant scientist to devise a study capable of teasing out the individual drugs from the pharmaceutical stew many patients now end up taking. (Mona's list included "eleven vials of Repronex, thirty-three powders of Gonal-F, one order of Profasi, a month's supply of Lupron, nine days of Doxycycline, and two Valium.") But the major drugs of concern in terms of ovarian cancer are those that induce ovulation, like Clomid, the typical first step for most infertile women, and Pergonal, which increases the number of eggs produced, is often the second. Both were discovered in the 1950s and for some infertile women, they're wonder drugs. Pergonal (human menopausal gonadotropin) is extracted from the urine of postmenopausal women and must be given by daily injection into the muscles of the buttocks or thighs. Clomid (clomiphene citrate, also sold as Serophene) can be taken orally. It is derived from DES (diethylstilbestrol), the infamous synthetic estrogen given to pregnant women for thirty years before it was found, in the 1970s, to cause a rare form of cancer in their daughters, as well as birth defects like T-shaped uteruses and other anatomical distortions that make it difficult, if not impossible, to carry a baby.

Scientists theorize that the more often the ovaries are stressed by going through a monthly cycle ending in the rupture of an egg, the more prone they are to damage and to the development of abnormal cells that could become cancerous. Pregnancy and breast-feeding give your ovaries time off, and as a result, each child you have lowers your risk of ovarian cancer by 10 to 15 percent. Birth control pills, which suppress ovulation, are also known to decrease the cancer's frequency. Using this logic, hyperovulation caused by fertility drugs like Clomid and Pergonal would mean a higher risk.

In the early 1990s, two major studies linked such drugs to the occurrence of ovarian tumors, although in both cases the lead authors felt they had only shown enough evidence to warrant further investigation. Other studies failed to find a connection. In 2000, however, the well-respected Cochrane Collaboration, an independent organization that conducts reviews of medical studies, concluded that adverse effects of Clomid "include a possible ovarian cancer risk." Serono agrees that the relationship between its drug Serophene and ovarian cancer is "controversial" (the company also states that no causal link has been established for Pergonal). Dennis Marshall, PhD, executive director of medical affairs at Ferring, another fertility drug maker, notes that while there's no final answer on ovarian cancer, doctors are now using lower doses to stimulate patients' ovaries.

Whatever the risk is, shamefully, we do not yet have a handle on it. Last spring I received a letter from John Collins, MD, professor emeritus of obstetrics and gynecology at McMaster University in Ontario, who was an author of the Cochrane review and is considered an experienced evaluator of ovarian cancer studies. "The risk is not one that would be considered proven," he wrote, "and the subject does not seem to have had a high priority for further research in the last few years." Some new research, however, may be emerging, aimed at identifying particular women with genetic susceptibilities to ovarian cancer for whom drugs like Clomid would be dangerous. Two case reports published in the *New England Journal of Medicine* last August do "point to a potential subgroup of patients who could be at risk of harm due to ovulation-stimulant therapies," says Ursula Kaiser, MD, at Brigham and Women's Hospital in Boston, author of an accompanying editorial.

Whether Diane Leatherman was in this group or not is unclear. But the sixty-six-year-old nonprofit consultant and author (*Crossing Kansas*, a fictionalized memoir, and *Rebecca: A Maryland Farm Girl*, a children's book) was diagnosed with ovarian cancer about eighteen years after she took Clomid and Pergonal. (This was basically Tilberis's time frame, too.) Leatherman already had four children when, at age forty, she fell in love with her third husband. They decided to try for another child. After several rounds of the drugs, she got pregnant the natural way and one month short of her forty-eighth birthday delivered a baby girl. When Leatherman was diagnosed with cancer, the oncologist asked about her history of fertility drugs. "Anytime you go splitting cells, you can run into trouble," she recalls him saying. Today her ovarian cancer has spread to her brain. Her doctor has suggested she get her affairs in order.

Leatherman urges all women who have had ovulation treatments to watch out for signs of the cancer (thickening of the waist, feeling full after eating only a little, changes in bowel movements, pain during sex). Despite the haunting questions about its dangers, Clomid remains one of the most commonly prescribed fertility drugs in the country. As a couplet scribbled on the bathroom wall of a California fertility clinic puts it, Clomid: widely used, much abused.

The journal *Fertility and Sterility* published an NIH study last year showing that women who took human menopausal gonadotropin (Pergonal-type drugs) for at least six cycles had a risk of breast cancer two to three times greater than women who had never used fertility medication. The findings are very tentative, but a few experts believe that breast—more than ovarian—cancer may emerge as the real concern. Cancer, however, is not the only cloud hanging over high-tech baby-making drugs. Any potential patient would think twice if she had sat next to Suzanne Parisian, MD, when this former FDA official who wrote *FDA Inside and Out* studied the file of agency records on Lupron. A synthetic hormone that suppresses the pituitary gland, Lupron is often prescribed to both infertile women and egg donors to control the timing of ovulation. The drug, however, was never approved for this purpose. After writing a hundred-page report, Parisian sent me a note: "Lupron is approved for only two short-term applications in women, (a) preoperative treatment of fibroids in patients with anemia and (b) management of endometriosis for a limit of six months. The FDA never approved Lupron for more than six months because there is significant risk of irreversible bone loss." Prescribing drugs for an unapproved, or "off-label," use is legal and quite common in medicine. But patients should be informed when it happens. And some women—especially "frequent fliers," who go through many cycles hoping for a baby—get more than the FDA's limit.

Parisian goes on to say that Lupron produces a postmenopausal state in women ("it literally drops the floor right out from beneath them without any time for the body to acclimate to the hormonal change"). Perhaps most alarmingly, she writes, far from being approved for fertility, Lupron "is 'pregnancy category X,' which means it is labeled not to be given to women intending to become pregnant or already pregnant. The entire IVF field uses Lupron for physician convenience. It lets them plan when to do [egg] harvests at a comfortable hour for them. They bully women into using it, telling them that there will be an increased risk of failure without Lupron. There is absolutely no real science to using Lupron for IVF."

Another concerned physician, Susan C. Vaughan, MD, a psychiatrist and pharmacology expert, has had two successful IVF babies financed by the best-selling book she wrote, *Viagra: A Guide to the Phenomenal Potency-Promoting Drug*. Acknowledging that ovarian cancer may turn out to be more of a worry than she originally thought, Vaughan has taken a special interest in treating patients who suffer from anxiety and depression after going on fertility drugs. She charges that too many fertility doctors "underestimate how rotten people feel on Lupron. They'll advise, 'At your age, you should have such and such a dose,' but they don't consider the emotional effects. A woman who did well on two and a half vials of Pergonal cried hopelessly when she was given six of these injectables." Vaughan adds that the doctor and the patient may both push the envelope too hard, desperate to have the treatments work before the money—as much as $20,000 per cycle, with some patients spending $150,000 for six cycles—runs out.

Complaints about Lupron go well beyond mood swings. A small percentage of women, it seems, never recover from what was supposed to be a temporary pituitary shutdown. At least one lawsuit filed on behalf of five Florida patients who took Lupron—for endometriosis and infertility—alleges that the drug causes chronic physical distress. TAP Pharmaceuticals denies liability for all the charges. More than a dozen women interviewed for this story, however, went on record to report a litany of medical complaints they believed to be the result of Lupron. Among the more common: autoimmune diseases, neurological problems, stomach disorders, and severe unexplained pain. Marriages fell apart. Careers languished. "We've gone to what seems like 5,000 doctors," laments the husband of one woman who at twenty-five was put on Lupron to help get her pregnant (she's since been hospitalized for chest pains and extreme hives, and suffers from a battery of other ailments). "They say, 'Think of something that might have caused all these things to suddenly come about.' And I tell them, 'Yeah! She took Lupron, and she's been sick ever since.' But they say Lupron doesn't have anything to do with it. I'm watching my wife fall apart in front of my eyes, and no one wants to do a thing about it."

One woman trying to do something is Lynne Millican, forty-six. A registered nurse, she has also become a paralegal and a knowledgeable activist on the dangers of Lupron. Last year, as part of her ongoing efforts to get the government to investigate, she testified before Congress on behalf of thousands of women who have reportedly been harmed by the drug. Millican's own story began at age thirty-two, when she started the first of three IVF cycles. She was already taking Lupron for endometriosis, and her doctor continued giving her the drug. He neglected to mention that it wasn't approved for fertility treatment. In the fourteen years since taking Lupron, Millican has had twenty-two hospitalizations, and her problems have included a large, benign tumor in her gallbladder, which appeared a few months after the IVF; severe fatigue; and gastroparesis (paralysis of the stomach and intestines). Her medical history—typed out, single-spaced on a continuous ream of paper—stands seven and a half feet tall. One condition that never made it onto the list is pregnancy.

"I think every physician who uses Lupron has seen some scary things, and they're not sure if it's due to the Lupron," says Michael Zinaman, MD, who readily prescribes the drug for endometriosis and infertility, warning patients of possible negative effects. "I get calls saying, 'Have you ever heard of women taking Lupron and having this, this, and this?'" Zinaman, a professor of reproductive endocrinology and the head of Loyola University's fertility program in Chicago, believes 2 or 3 percent

of women using the drug have "really bad things happen to them." David Redwine, MD, a gynecologist at the St. Charles Medical Center in Bend, Oregon, has treated hundreds of endometriosis patients, many suffering from adverse reactions to Lupron, but says that, unfortunately, there are no studies tracking the long-term effects.

The push for effective fertility drugs has been fierce, fueled by the promise of pharmaceutical profits and by the collective ticking of America's biological clock, set ever later for having children. In 1970 Pergonal was still under study. That was the year that one volunteer, Margaret Kienast of New Jersey, gave birth to quintuplets. The publicity made infertile women frantic with hope. In Los Angeles Edward Tyler, MD (who happened to write for Groucho Marx on the side), had tried it on 300 patients but was still reluctant to recommend it for general use. The manufacturer, Cutter Laboratories, also believed the publicity was premature. One month after the Kienast births, the clinics testing Pergonal were booked solid and Tyler announced, "We don't have a vial in the house." Despite the hesitation of both the researchers and Cutter, the drug was approved that same year.

Today Pergonal has spawned a number of offshoots, including Humegon, Fertinex, Repronex, Gonal-F, and Follistim. In a recent interview, New Jersey fertility specialist Satty Gill Keswani, MD, (also a United Nations NGO delegate studying the environment's impact on fertility) described a close relative's near brush with death from a reaction to one of these ovulation drugs.

After trying to get pregnant for two years, Keswani's thirty-four-year-old relative, "Danielle," was diagnosed with endometriosis. "Everything was okay except that one of her fallopian tubes was problematic," Keswani told me. She did not want Danielle to go ahead with IVF. "With one healthy tube, and being under thirty-five, she still had a good chance without it," she said. "But many doctors press younger women to do IVF to increase their success numbers." Keswani does refer some of her own patients for IVF but notes that for those who fail after several tries, "it takes months to get the drugs out of their bodies." Keswani was attending a medical meeting in San Diego when Danielle, who had been on the ovulation drug for ten days, telephoned in tears. She had a pseudotumor in her brain. "This is a swelling that appears to be a tumor," Keswani says. "I ran for a plane and got home at 3:00 AM. We did an MRI of her brain. The accumulated fluid of the pseudotumor had to be removed by spinal tap. I asked Danielle's doctors to stop the drug and showed them studies that it can cause blindness. The spinal fluid pressure was 480, when normally it would be 250. Her doctors, all men, wouldn't listen to me. They didn't want to 'interrupt the cycle' and let their treatment go to waste."

About 5 percent of patients taking this family of drugs develop hyperstimulation syndrome, which often involves the rapid enlargement of the ovaries and can be fatal. Fluid typically accumulates in the abdomen and sometimes the lungs, cutting off the breath; if the ovary ruptures, blood also pools and clots can occur. With Danielle, who fortunately survived, the excess fluid collected in the optic nerves. Two days after her spinal tap, doctors removed nine eggs, and when they had two or three embryos, they implanted them into her womb. It didn't work. "She was so down," Keswani tells me, "and it took three months for her eyes to clear up from the swelling of the nerves." But the story had a happy ending. Danielle and her husband went on vacation to Italy, says Keswani, "and they came back pregnant the good, old-fashioned way."

If the risks of fertility drugs and treatments aren't clear, neither are the benefits. Add desperation for a child to the mix, and infertile women are in a difficult spot when it comes to making an informed choice about going high-tech.

Medical sociologist Joan Liebman-Smith, PhD, a former board member of the patient advocacy group Resolve, calls the examining table where IVF is done "the gaming table" because when you go for treatment, you are literally taking a gamble. The real odds of taking a baby home, however, remain elusive. Even when clinics don't blatantly inflate their success rates, the industry is rife with a more subtle kind of manipulation that skews the final numbers. Ninety-three-year-old Howard Jones, MD, who cofounded the Jones Institute for Reproductive Medicine of Eastern Virginia Medical School, points out that busy clinics bent on posting stellar rates are apt to turn away the harder cases. Jane Miller, MD, a fertility doctor in New Jersey, agrees that smaller facilities and solo practitioners have a difficult time cracking the high numbers if they welcome the big-clinic rejects. The Society for Assisted Reproductive Technology tracks success rates of clinics for the Centers for Disease Control and Prevention (results can be seen at cdc.gov). But these figures, by and large, depend on the accuracy and honesty of the self-reporting clinics, most of which are the society's members.

Whether a woman needs help conceiving in the first place isn't always obvious. When she goes in for a workup, the specialist may have little incentive to send her back to the drawing board, or bed, as the case may be. "Bear in mind that if you wish to develop a reputation as a fertility doctor, you don't want patients getting pregnant on their own," as one insider puts it. Last May the Medical College of Georgia's distinguished authority Paul McDonough, MD, speaking to a group of New York and New Jersey fertility specialists, urged his colleagues to "go after the low-hanging fruit," meaning the obvious causes of infertility—sperm problems, fallopian tube injuries (from STDs and abortions), and genetic or prenatal conditions—before they pull out their prescription pads. Prospective patients might also consider patience. Some research shows that couples up to their mid-thirties with no evident infertility factors have a better chance of success if they simply continue on their own.

The answers to all these questions will come one day. But for now, one can only proceed with extreme caution. For all the promise that reproductive medicine offers to those who dare to cross its threshold, with all the great joy it brings to a relatively small number of lucky seekers, it also breaks many hearts and bears risks that are yet unknown. In *The Empty Cradle: Infertility in America from Colonial Times to the Present*, two sisters, historian Margaret Marsh, PhD, and gynecologist Wanda Ronner, MD, wisely write, "Infertile women have served as both patients and experimental subjects." And for every one of us who follows in the footsteps of Liz Tilberis, that is still very much the case.

CHAPTER 6

Motherhood

IN THE 1970S, I WROTE A PROPOSAL for a book I never ended up writing. It would have been called *The American Mother: Whatever You Do, It's Wrong*. At the time, the women's movement—and the larger culture—was engaged in a fevered conversation about what it meant to be a good mother and a successful woman. Was it better to cultivate a career, putting aside the assumed 1950s role of housewife and mother? Or were you putting your children at a disadvantage in life if you weren't home raising them? Or could you do both? Of course in many ways we are still having the same conversations now, and I think it is more true than ever that as a mother in America you face amazing expectations, pressures, and criticisms. It can easily feel that whatever you do, it's wrong.

It is a little-mentioned fact that many (if not most) of the prominent second-wave feminists were mothers, and those who weren't often fought hard for the rights of those who were. The cultural stereotype of second-wave feminists was, quite inaccurately and unfairly, one that was antifamily and antichild. I was raising three children during the years when I wrote my first three books. I worked from home, trying to balance the needs of my small kids against the demands of my work. Sometimes when I think back, I'm not sure how it all got done.

The women's movement worked tirelessly—and continues to fight—for a world where women who have children also have choices. We fought for better access to day care, maternity leave, and other things that would make childrearing and maintaining a career possible. These conversations are more important than ever in a culture where the very people who claim to politically represent "family values" are often actively opposing things that would make raising families easier to do.

A certain strain of reactionary thinking has been gaining steam in the past few years. In September 2005, the *New York Times* published an article declaring "Many Women at Elite

Colleges Set Career Path to Motherhood." Author Louise Story explained that many high-achieving young women weren't aiming to be successful lawyers or doctors or CEOs—instead, they were hoping to stay home and raise children. In the controversy that followed the article, many young women came forward asserting it was their feminist right to stay home. I wouldn't disagree with them— I would say that no one has ever told a woman who has the means and wants to make motherhood her full-time commitment that she can't. However, women have been told consistently over the years— both in overt ways and through more subtle pressures—that they shouldn't be in the workplace if they are going to have kids. When people suggest, as one of the mothers in Story's article did, that women who work are being selfish and putting their children at a disadvantage, they are just re-cycling the old sexist (and ill-supported) theories. They are suggesting that there is only one way of parenting that works. They are also ignoring the fact that most women couldn't afford to stay home even if they wanted to—it's just not an option economically for most families. It also seems worth noting that this conversation rarely invokes the increasing numbers of young men interested in staying home and raising children.

My hope is that we will continue to create a world in which women (and men) can envision parenthood differently and that diversity is re-spected. Beyond cultural acceptance, I would dream of a world where social and political struc-tures support the many different types of families we have and choices we make.

Yes, We Have No Bambinos

MOLLY HASKELL

Molly Haskell, "Yes, We Have No Bambinos," *Viva*, March 1975. Reprinted by permission.

I recently moved with my husband from a small apartment in midtown Manhattan to a larger apartment on the Upper East Side, in what is fondly referred to by everyone except me as a "family neighborhood." Eleven floors below, back to back with our building, is a boys' school called St. David's which seems to have staggered recess periods. There is at least one class of little boys shrieking and yelling in the courtyard at all times. I never would have thought prepubescent voices could be so loud or carry so far. When I tell my friends about it, or they hear it for themselves, they smile benignly and say that these are "life sounds," or "the music of human voices." The best I'm able to say, I'm afraid, is that I've grown accustomed to the voices (they often make the day begin, all too literally, well before the alarm clock rings). The very constancy of the noise turns it from an off-and-on intrusion into a background din, but I don't suppose I'll ever exactly relish it, or think affectionately of the little dears as they release their youthful high spirits.

What's wrong with me? Am I a female W. C. Fields? An infantophobe? A Lady Macbeth? No, I'm just a nonmother with what I like to think is a healthy balance of hormones and perhaps an above-normal quotient of husband-love and pro-fessional drive. I write, of course, and my powers of concentration, as you may have guessed, are not those of Jane Austen, who wrote at her little desk in the middle of the living room, surrounded by a huge family (and even she didn't have a child to contend with). But aside from the demands of a career, there are other features of my life that I would have to surrender were I to become a mother. I like to stay up and watch the late show or go with my husband to the movies or to a restaurant on the spur of the moment. I like to read the paper through in the morning and eat the kind of food children would gag at and take walks and choose my friends because of a natural affinity rather than because they have kids the same age as mine. I like to spend money—not extravagantly, but without having to think about each penny. I like not having money arguments with my husband, and I like not being forced into a conservative philosophy because of concern for the "future well-being" of my children. I like the idea that if my husband and I ever did divorce, the height of acrimony would be over the division of books rather than human beings.

Of all the rumblings and murmurings, tremors and upheavals that have taken place in the last few years, both within the wake of the women's movement and as a distant echo, the most radical is that women, in something that could be described as *numbers,* are deciding not to have children. Not to have children! This, more than any technological breakthrough or political movement, is a revolutionary idea. It reverses, or at least questions, the whole process, thought to be both instinctual and immutable, by which the human race reproduces and multiplies and woman fulfills her destiny as a woman. It goes against the supposedly automatic, heaven-decreed assignment of woman to marry and give birth and consign herself to twenty years of being more or less at the disposal of her offspring. And yet this radical option is being discussed and adopted by women who are not freaks or witches or "selfish bitches" or even necessarily obsessive careerists, but who are well-adjusted, sane, happily married women, some of whom do and some of whom do not have professions. The reasons, as I discovered from talking to women around the country, range from genetic weaknesses inherent in one member of the couple to concern with overpopulation to lifestyle choices. And it has happened—that is, the idea has become socially acceptable if not widely applauded—within an amazingly short time.

In January 1963, Gael Green wrote an article in the *Saturday Evening Post* entitled "A Vote Against Motherhood," describing in quite reasonable terms the ways in which children had frustrated or crippled the lives of some of her friends and the reasons she and her husband had decided not to have any of their own. The resistance, the censure, and the horror that those around her felt at her decision was confirmed by the 3,000 pieces of hate mail provoked by the article.

Just four and a half years ago Betty Rollin wrote a piece entitled "Motherhood—Who Needs It?" that ran in *Look* magazine and drew a scandalized response. It was a lively, dispassionate, well-researched examination of all the myths surrounding and pushing women into motherhood. *Look* was inundated with what Betty says was one of the greatest floods of mail ever received, "most of which was hate mail."

Reaching the point where not having children has become an acceptable cultural choice couldn't have happened without the pressure of important social forces like inflation and overpopulation creating an atmosphere in which large families are discouraged. Sterilization has had an astonishing success with both younger and older couples as a way of limiting a family or preventing children altogether.

There is even a new organization dedicated to furthering nonparenthood. NON, the National Organization for Nonparents, brings together people who share an interest in curbing population either on a world scale or in their own homes, and in simply making the notion of nonparenthood acceptable.

But it is on married women in their early thirties that the burden of decision falls most heavily, for they (and we who have made the choice) must live with its consequences. There are feminists who feel, with some justice, that women shouldn't have to make such a choice. The *Ms.* ideal woman, for example, as analyzed by Hunter professor of communications Dr. Helen Franzwa, is a working mother *with* children. There is even a semantical feud with NON over whether women without children should be characterized as "childless (considered too negative by NON) or "childfree" (considered arrogant by *Ms.*)—hence my own positive-negative title for this article.

In a recent *Ms.* article, Ellen Willis expresses the opinion of certain feminists that an expansion of day care programs and an increased delegation of responsibility to the fathers would and should permit women to combine work and children. Nonmothers are characterized as "militant," elitist snobs (little difference here from the white-collar view of them as "selfish bitches"), or dupes of a sexist society, which forces a choice upon women that no man ever incurs. It is this last charge that rings true and is almost unanswerable unless we shift our thinking entirely towards a more communal, socially shared form of child-rearing. When you suggest, as Willis does, that many of the drawbacks of motherhood are the result of a patriarchal, capitalist society, then you must pursue the political corollary: that motherhood itself, as practiced in our society, a proprietary, bourgeois-individualist institution. The dream of giving birth—of having *one's own* child, of nurturing him/her with "every advantage," of hoping he/she will surpass his peers—all of this not only sits quite well with the patriarchal capitalist system but is its very foundation, its means of perpetuating itself.

Couldn't Ms. Willis and others like her participate in the rearing of others' children? Why must she, particularly in a world endangered by overpopulation, have her *own* child? This would take a certain reordering of habits and institutions. But even without any kind of socialized child care many of the women I talked to are finding ways to involve themselves in caring for other women's children, becoming, in effect, unofficial godparents. The point is, it's a very complex issue, and no one can prescribe for anyone else.

As Betty Rollin says, "Not to have children doesn't mean a life without children. I have a part-time child [her husband's by a former marriage]. Often the people who contribute the most to children have none of their own, and they can do this because they are free. Just think—if Anna Freud had had her own family, she might never have done her remarkable work in child psychology!"

The popularity of sterilization (both laparoscopy and vasectomy), enabling women to enjoy sex without fear of pregnancy, is an acknowledgment of something that ten years ago was inadmissible— that adult women, whether mothers or nonmothers,

continue to enjoy sex. One of the most crippling aspects of Momism (the cult of motherhood as it was defined in the fifties) was that the mother figure was purged of the "taint" of sexuality at precisely the time in her life when she might be expected to enjoy it most. In a culture obsessed with youth, a lusty, sexy woman in her thirties was an embarrassment, a figure of ridicule, and a woman's only claim to status was through her children. But women are fighting back, refusing to be prematurely put out to pasture by the next generation.

It is, perhaps, the image of motherhood as it has evolved in our society and been purveyed, rather unappealingly, in Hollywood films, that we are reacting against. We who identified with James Dean in *Rebel without a Cause* must suddenly cast ourselves in the roles of the villains—parents—or reject the part.

Several years ago, when there still seemed some hope that I might have children, my mother was trying to persuade me with the solace-for-your-old-age argument, emphasizing how much I'd meant to her.

"But, Mother," I protested, "how could I? We live 300 miles apart."

"It's just your being there, and my being interested in what happens to you," she said. But I kept thinking about her loneliness, made greater by the infrequency of our visits together. I happen to think I have one of the world's greatest mothers—so there's no reacting against a bad childhood on my part—and yet I have no desire to follow in her footsteps and bring up a selfish brat like me, who'll want to sprout wings and fly away at the first opportunity. If anything, it's not the model of motherhood that discouraged me from having children—it's the model of childhood . . . my own! And I think I'm not unlike many women in feeling, somewhere below the surface, this loss of connection between parent and child, a lack of concern for one's "elders," that might, one day, be turned against us as parents.

At this moment in history, both young and middle-aged middle-class couples seem to live in the worst of all possible worlds: close enough to parents to still feel the pressure of obligation and guilt, but not close enough to benefit from a sense of warmth and protection, or even the services they might offer.

We feel a pressure to "keep house" in the style of our parents, but without domestic assistance. And we feel social and psychological pressure to love and guide our children, to give them more attention than was given us, while we have less time to give. Our lives are completely different from our parents', but we continue to judge ourselves, or allow ourselves to be judged, by their standards and expectations.

In a scene from the Bergman film *Scenes from a Marriage* that burns a hole in the memory, Liv Ullmann, as a divorce lawyer, interviews an elderly woman who has made up her mind to divorce. Very slowly and methodically, the woman reveals that her relationship with her husband has been a sham for fifteen years, that she feels she is losing her ability to respond to life, and, finally, that she doesn't love her children.

"I have never loved my children," she says, "I know that for sure. But I've been a good mother all the same."

This woman has uttered the most shocking words a woman can say, the unsayable, the unthinkable. It is one thing for a child not to love his mother and father; it is even permissible for a father to acknowledge reservations about his children. But for a mother to make such an admission! Is mother love not an absolute? The answer, of course, is No, it is not. And the sooner we admit it the less hypocrisy there will be.

The beatific aura in which motherhood has been sold to us has intimidated women from expressing even minor reservations, for fear they will be thought monsters. Only once in a while will you find a woman who admits that life with children is a flawed affair, who even admits that if she had it to do over she might do without.

Yet even after all the rational arguments have been made, the name-calling level of debate re-mains. Part of the charge is the oft-touted "selfishness" of not having children—which seems to me a childish issue. A case could be made for family life as the most *self*-centered institution ever conceived. But it's like the religious debates my friends and I used to have in the sixth grade, when we argued that believing in God and doing nice things for other people were selfish because the only reason you did them was to make *you* feel good.

Well, I don't have children, and I feel good. Possibly, if I had them I would feel just as good, for different reasons. Still, I find that even the most emancipated woman is reluctant to say, definitively, that she is not going to have children. "Not for the moment," she will say, as I used to say, knowing in the back of my mind I probably wouldn't but wanting to keep an escape hatch open. At least that was the reason I gave to myself. Now I think it's because I was still afraid of What People Would Think. That I was a monster. And even perhaps, that what they were thinking about me, I was thinking about myself. Even now I haven't decided if I'm "right" or "wrong," "selfish" or "un-selfish"— only that whatever it is I can live with it.

And speaking of monsters, just listen to those voices—shouting, brimful of life, eleven floors below. I'm glad they're not in the next room.

Dr. Spock's Advice to New Mothers

ALIX KATES SHULMAN

Alix Kates Shulman, excerpt from *Memoirs of an Ex-Prom Queen*, New York: Knopf, 1972. Reprinted by permission.

We made Andrea in the new year and I bore her in the fall, entering the park world in the winter, bundled up. The books I had taken from the library in preparation proved to be mere parodies of life; but there was nothing else to go on. Child care was neither discussed in society nor taught in school. However contemptuous I'd been of the prospect of Spock, I was grateful for him now. He had the latest word and a good index.

It would be good news for every baby weighing 10 pounds or more to be outdoors, when it isn't raining, for 2 or 3 hours a day, as long as the temperature is above freezing and the wind isn't bitterly cold.[1]

The old lady who fed pigeons peered into the carriage, but otherwise I was alone on a deserted bench, paralyzed by the fragility of my overwhelming charge, afraid to move for fear of waking her, afraid to take my eyes off her lest she sleep and die. During her brief sleeps I studied her like a difficult text, trying to fathom each mysterious tremor and start, praying she would not wake too soon. When she did wake—always grievously ahead of schedule—I leaped to juggle the carriage as I had seen the neighbors do, trying to shake the sobs from her throat and the knots from my gut.

If you live in the city and have no yard to park the baby in, you can push him in a carriage. Long woolen underwear, slacks, woolen stockings, and galoshes make your life a lot more pleasant during this period.

In summer it would be different. She would be older then and I would not fear her death so much as her life. In my breast lay the power to soothe or torment her, but also dangers. If ten minutes of jiggling the carriage didn't get her back to sleep, that would be ten wasted minutes, six hundred useless sobs tearing at my raw conscience. It would take ten more minutes to get home from the park, and another ten to get the carriage up the stairs and our wraps and clothing off.

What do you do if he wakes as soon as you put him to bed or a little later? I think it's better to assume first that if he has nursed for 5 minutes he's had enough to keep him satisfied for a couple of hours, and try not to feed him again right away. Let him fuss for a while if you can stand it.[2]

The baby carriage turned out to be an unexpected aid in stopping traffic. But it was still a good half hour between whimper and feeding—a half hour that took months off my life and left yellow milkstains on my nursing bras.

It may start leaking from the breasts when you hear the baby beginning to cry in the next room. This shows how much feelings have to do with the formation and release of the milk.[3]

If I had stayed home with her instead of going to the park I could have put her to suck the instant she woke, forgot the clock and the dangers.

The treatment of fretfulness seems clear to me. . . . The baby should be allowed to nurse as often as every 2 hours, for 20 to 40 minutes.[4]

But I so wanted everything to be right for her, and the park was the preferred milieu. Constant feeding was contraindicated. If my breasts were never more than partially emptied, which could result from putting her to suck too often, then they would not be properly stimulated to fill up again and I would dry up with no comfort for my helpless daughter.

If the breast-milk supply is insufficient at all feedings, you will need a bottle at all feedings, whether you give the breast first or not.[5]

I knew I shouldn't be offering her bottles yet, but how could I risk starving her? Her life was in my hands. I nursed her around the clock every two hours for half an hour at least, watching her tiny fists clutch spasmodically at my long hair and her toes curl in the joy of sucking, until she fell asleep at my breast; then gingerly I tried to roll her onto her stomach without waking her.

There are two disadvantages to a baby's sleeping on his back. If he vomits, he's more likely to choke on the vomitus. Also, he tends to keep his head turned toward the same side. . . . This may flatten that side of his head. It won't hurt his brain, and the head will gradually straighten out, but it may take a couple of years.[6]

During the mornings and late afternoons, when I had the diapers and laundry, the bottles and bedding to do, I let her sleep on our bed between feedings. I carefully slipped rubber padding between her diaper and our sheet, sometimes leaving her bottom bare to help her diaper rash. ("Jesus, Sasha, isn't there anything else you can use on her diaper rash besides Destin® ointment? It smells worse than shit; our bed stinks of it," said Willy.) But at night, when I longed to share with her my brief interludes of sleep, I couldn't risk keeping her in bed with me. Even if Willy hadn't protested her little body coming between ours, it was a dangerous place for her. A carelessly flung arm could snuff out her fire like a breath on a birthday candle; not to mention the

> chance that he may become dependent on this arrangement and be afraid and unwilling to sleep anywhere else.[7]

No; better to follow the doctor's better sensible rule not to take a child into the parent's bed for any reason[8] (even as a treat when the father is away on a business trip); better to suffer now than later.

The conspiracy of silence about motherhood was even wider than the one about sex. Philosophers ignored it and poets revered it, but no one dared describe it. The experts who wrote articles for magazines ("Ten Steps to Restore Muscle Tone"; "Before You Call Your Pediatrician"; "Take the Time to Stay Interesting: Six Shortcuts to Keeping Informed") spoke in euphemisms; as to the real dangers, their best advice was to consult still other doctors. Why didn't the women speak? Evidently they were too busy. . . .

She purred and giggled as I suckled her. She had her preferences, did my daughter, and when something made her cry she broke my heart with her great stores of tears that flooded her enormous green eyes and overflowed their thick banks of black lash like swollen rivers. How, I wondered, could Willy bear to be away from us? Why did he leave us promptly every morning and return late every night?

"Sasha," called Willy, "she's started crying again. I was just sitting here with her and she started screaming for no reason."

I dropped the spatula and ran to the living room, oblivious of Spock's warning to parents who

> always anxiously pick him up when he fusses: . . . the more they submit to his orders the more demanding he becomes.[9]

"Give her to me, Willy, for God's sake, don't let her cry like that!"

> If your baby is sensitive about new people, new places, in the middle of his first year, I'd protect him from too much fright by making strangers keep at a little distance until he gets used to them, especially in new places. He'll remember his father in a while.[10]

I took my baby in my arms and walked her, patting her perfect back the way I had when she was a newborn. The sound of her crying was always absolutely unbearable to me.

> Many mothers get worn out and frantic listening to a baby cry, especially when it's the first. You should make a great effort to get away from home and baby for a few hours at least twice a week—oftener if you can arrange it. . . . If you can't get anyone to come in, let your husband stay home one or two evenings a week while you go out to visit or see a movie.[11]

The trouble was, Willy didn't get home most evenings till eight or so and couldn't have helped me then if he'd wanted to.

How could he relieve me if he left us in the morning and returned late at night, or if he were away, as the omniscient Spock had divined, on a business trip? . . .

Once every two weeks I hired a daytime sitter and tore myself from Andy as Spock advised. I planned to slip off to the library and read a book or arrange to meet a friend at the Museum of Modern Art. But somehow the hours were too precious to use up on personal frivolities, and instead I took to dropping in on Will for lunch (as in the old days), doing everything I could to live up to my photographs. Flat-stomached supermother uptown between feedings.

I took more care dressing for those office calls than when Will wrenched me away from Andy at bedtime to accompany him to the movies or a party at Hector's, where I watched the world go spinning on as though babies were a recent invention. Couples stood in line at movie theaters holding hands, oblivious of the consequences; old friends gathered at Hector's with new girlfriends to exchange news of charter flights and recent books, as though Dr. Spock's *Baby and Child Care* had not been written for them. . . .

That first summer I took Andy to the crowded playground every day, carrying her up the slide and sliding her down on my lap.

From a park bench I watcherd her at my feet intently tearing up a leaf, her mouth open and brows knit in concentration, her pudgy fingers moving with careful grace. Though I always took a book to the park I didn't dare read for the dangers; couldn't read for the distractions. Anyway, most books were now irrelevant. Instead, I searched around to see which of the other mothers, multiparous and knowing, could tell me things about my daughter I ought to know. Some of them were limber and accomplished, some foul-mouthed and acne-scarred, no doubt with mean lives and husbands to match. I hung on every casual comparison they made of Andy with their own like revelations. My daughter's life was in my hands. . . .

I began each day solemnly with resolutions:

Today I will make myself lunch; I'll brew myself a cup of tea between breakfast feeding and diaper delivery.

I will *not* pick her up whenever she cries today. I will be *calm* when she spits out her food.

The horror of my predicament was: everything counts. Each tiny mistake I made was destined to reverberate through all eternity.

The first time I yelled at Andy she looked at me unbelieving; betrayed. Her chin puckered, her lip trembled, then tears gushed from those green eyes all over her hands. I sank into a week-long depression.

> It's possible that you will find yourself feeling discouraged for a while when you first begin taking care of your baby. It's a fairly common feeling, especially with the first. You may not be able to put your fingers on anything that is definitely wrong. You just weep easily. Or you may feel very bad about certain things. One woman whose baby cries quite a bit feels sure that he has a real disease, another that her husband has become strange and distant, another that she has lost all her looks.[12]

Exactly as I had once imagined but forgotten, when my child was born my fate slipped through my fingers into the bay. I was hers now.

> If you begin to feel at all depressed, . . . go to a movie, or to the beauty parlor, or to get yourself a new hat or dress. . . .[13]

A new locale, a new hair style, could solve nothing any more. We swam around sifting plankton, hoping for some huge uplifting wave to come along and carry us high and wide; but there were only the usual ripples and currents and erratic seismographic disturbances to be recorded on the precision instruments of oceanographers. . . .

Thinking her still asleep in her crib at naptime I had gone next door to borrow some diapers from a neighbor. When I returned, I heard her screaming in her room. (Was it my fault? "Look, honey," Willy had warned, "this is the third time you've run out of diapers. What happened to the emergency supply I got you? You need better planning. If you won't increase the regular order, you'll just have to use the ones you have more sparingly.")

An accident? Had I forgotten to raise the side of the crib?

> A baby, by the age he first tries to roll over, shouldn't be left unguarded on a table for as long as it takes the mother to turn her back.[14]

I rushed to her room to find her standing in her crib clutching the bars terror-stricken, her fat knees buckling.

"Standing! Look at you!" I cried. She sobbed with exhaustion and victory. A star!

I unhooked her fingers one by one from the bars and scooped her up into my arms, my bumblebee, pressing kisses all over her shining face. "You can stand. You can do anything." I rejoiced. When she kicked to be put back again, I sat her down in the crib; then up she climbed on her little legs once more, crowing with pride.

She had learned to stand not for a moment or a day, but for all time. I knelt before her crib. She looked so much tinier upright than sprawled across her mattress. She was one of us now, though she didn't come up to my knees. As I knelt adoringly before her, trying to kiss her nose through the bars, she began to shake her little body furiously, rattling the bars, laughing until her chin puckered, her lower lip protruded toward me, and once again, the deluge.

Down again with my help to sitting, then up on her own. For an hour and more we did our joyful dance while the tide waited.

"William Burke, please."

"Just a minute, please." A new voice at the switchboard.

"Willy? She can stand up."

"Alone?"

"Yes. She holds on, of course, but she can get up by herself."

"Hey! That's great, Sash! Great! It's about time, isn't it?"

"No, Willy. She's only nine and a half months old. Spock says it happens any time in the last quarter of the first year. I thought you'd want to know about it."

"Sure do, honey. Thanks a lot for calling me."

When I hung up I chastised myself for having phoned him with the news. And when he finally did come home, I overdid it, searching his face for a joy that could not possibly appear. And filled up like a Hoover bag with resentments.

The experts would have agreed I expected too much of Will: infants' progress is news fit only for ladies' magazines. Andy's triumphs were everything to me—elating, exonerating—and only bonuses to him, which somehow diminished them. . . .

Willy tried. He brought home quince blossoms in the spring and roses often. But even with the living room a garden, he sat at the window and looked out. I could see he felt trapped inside with us, whereas I, trapped too, could barely be induced to leave.

On Sundays he was gallant, taking us to Central Park, first to the zoo cafeteria for pancakes, then to the carousel, where he waved to us from a bench each time Andy and I rode by. But in between, though I never actually caught him, I knew he looked at the carefree New York girls.

When I felt the flutter of life in me anew, I kept the thrill of it to myself. Something told me to be careful. I did my quota of nesting, washing Andy's outgrown layette and making extensive lists of details to attend to, but I was careful not to burden Will with them.

I did my best to avoid sensitive topics. I hid my child care pamphlets among my recipes as I had once hidden my beauty charts and *Seventeen*s. I knew they were considered vacuous, like the talk of formulas and play groups that blighted cocktail party repartee—unless it issued from some doctor. But they dealt with matters too important to leave to chance. I knew I risked the worst contempt for reading them, but I had more than my own ego to consider: there were the children's. How else was I to learn the pitfalls of sibling rivalry or the symptoms and cure of croup? I had no models, no advisers for child care. Like housework, it was something charming people didn't discuss and rich people didn't do.

Once I had tried to read Will an urgent paragraph from the "Parent and Child" feature in the Sunday *Times Magazine* supplement. Tearing it away from me he had cried, "Why do you read that trash and let it upset you? It's just bullshit!" as, during my earlier pregnancy, he'd forbidden me to read about the limbless thalidomide babies, saying, "You'd be a nervous wreck if you didn't have me to protect you."

I too was protective. But however carefully I spared him our disorder, he still used every excuse to come home late. No matter how endearingly Andy greeted him at the door, once home, it seemed, Will couldn't wait to get out of the house again.

> Men react to their wife's pregnancy with various feelings: protectiveness of the wife, increased pride in the marriage, pride about their virility. . . . But there can also be, way underneath, a feeling of being left out . . . which can be expressed as grumpiness toward his wife, wanting to spend more evenings with his men friends, or flirtatiousness with other women.[15]

Of all the experts I'd ever consulted, none—no Watson, Webber, or Spock—was unequivocally on my side. They made us do it, then blamed us for it, another case of damned if you do and damned if you don't. They found nothing more hateful than a clinging wife—except a dominating mom.

> Some fathers have been brought up to think that the care of babies and children is the mother's job entirely. But a man can be a warm father and a real man at the same time. . . . Of course, I don't mean that the father has to give just as many bottles or change just as many diapers as the mother. But it's fine for him to do these things occasionally. . . . Of course, there are some fathers who get goose flesh at the very idea of helping to take care of a baby, and there's no good to

be gained trying to force them. Most of them come around to enjoying their children later "when they're more like real people."[16]

From the confines of my cell I tried to thwart Willy's wanderings. It was my duty. And when I ran out of coffee or snapped at him in my regular early morning panic, I kicked myself for driving him off to Riker's Restaurant for breakfast, the *Times* tucked under his arm as he walked out the door. And when I finally went to the hospital to give birth to Jenny, I could no longer hide my obsessive conviction that once Will was free of us, with me away and Andy gone to stay with his mother and nothing in the world to keep him at home, he would simply pack up his things and leave.

NOTES

1. Benjamin Spock, *Baby and Child Care* (New York: Pocket Books, 1962), Section 244.
2. Ibid., Section 127.
3. Ibid., Section 102.
4. Ibid., Section 122.
5. Ibid., Section 126.
6. Ibid., Section 248.
7. Ibid., Section 250.
8. Ibid., Section 251.
9. Ibid., Section 282.
10. Ibid., Section 348.
11. Ibid., Section 278.
12. Ibid., Section 16.
13. Ibid.
14. Ibid., Section 349.
15. Ibid., Section 18.
16. Ibid., Section 20.

Lovely Me

BARBARA SEAMAN

Barbara Seaman, excerpt from *Lovely Me: The Life of Jacqueline Susann*, New York: Seven Stories Press, 1996. Originally published in 1987 by William Morrow. Reprinted by permission.

It was a strange, divided life Jackie led. They were spending around $2,000 a month on entertaining, making the rounds of Toots Shor's,

21, El Morocco, Sardi's, the Stork Club, the Little Club, Danny's Hideaway, and others. They were out so much at night that Irving figured it cost him close to $1,000 a year to check his hat, yet her days were spent worrying over Guy and dragging him to doctors. And mostly what she got was confusion, contradictions, implications that she had somehow caused his problems, or that she was failing to solve them. Irving's young assistant, a girl named Penny Morgan, recalls: "Guy was the most beautiful baby, and Irving just thought he was different. He had a face like sunshine. Jackie . . . focused all her energy on getting him well. She never stopped hoping that he would recover; she had constant anguish over it. Outwardly she coped with it well, but she would have traded anything she accomplished in life in return for Guy being normal."

In December of 1949 Guy turned three, and then his small vocabulary almost disappeared. Friends remember him screaming "Goddammit! Goddammit!" One afternoon the nurse brought him home from the park screaming, as had often happened before, but this time the blood-curdling screeches continued throughout the day and the following night, with breaks only when Guy gave in to exhaustion and slept fitfully. Irving questioned everyone in the park and even hired private detectives, but there was never a clue as to what had provoked the child. The screaming stopped in time, but Guy continued to withdraw. And now his condition was given a name: autism.

The word was used by Dr. Lauretta Bender, to whom Jackie's psychiatric journey had taken her. Dr. Bender was a petite and earthy woman who had originated the Bender Visual Motor Gestalt Test, a tool still in widespread use today as a means of evaluating "maturational levels of children, organic brain defects and deviations in function." She stood somewhat apart from her psychoanalytically oriented colleagues in that she was more inclined to look for physical, neurological bases for such disorders. She thoroughly disagreed with those colleagues who blamed the mother and "poor communication within the home" for autism. "I've had mothers come to me weeping and saying, 'I can't reach my child. I try every way I can but I can't reach my child.' Of course the mothers are very upset," she says, "*because* of the child's behavior. I have never seen one single instance in which I thought the mother's behavior produced autism in the child."

Dr. Bender was interested in Jackie's Uncle Pete, the *meshugge* dentist, and also in Irving's "peculiar" uncle, believing that there was often a pattern of schizophrenia in the family history of the autistic child.* She saw Guy's case as classic in many aspects, including his indifference to affection and his failure to communicate, his fascination with spinning objects, his rhythmic rocking and head banging, and his general withdrawal. She was not very encouraging, but she suggested a controversial approach—a series of shock treatments that might jar him out of his silent world enough so that he could benefit from therapy.

Shock treatments for a three-year-old? It seemed cruel, yet no one had offered anything hopeful as an alternative. Reluctantly, Jackie and Irving agreed to leave him in the Bellevue children's ward, in Dr. Bender's hands. They compared notes with other parents whose children were there, and were somewhat reassured to find them mostly upper-middle-class people who, like the Mansfields, sought only the best for their kids. One unhappy father, a physician, told her, "This is the last step before putting my little boy away for good."

Irving long regretted the shock treatments. "I think they destroyed him. He came home with no expression, almost lifeless." And now, the doctors advised that Guy be placed in an institution. Perhaps he might have a remission at puberty, Dr.

---

*Others, then and later, are less sure, and in fact so little is really known about autism that experts even now disagree about whether or not it is a form of childhood schizophrenia, from which it differs in several crucial ways.

Bender declared, but for now he needed the special care and supervision of an institution.*

They agreed, in the most heart-wrenching decision of their lives, and Guy was taken to his first of many institutions, a Rhode Island facility surrounded by rolling lawns. They left their son there, in one of the red-brick buildings of this strange place where he would be cared for but probably not loved. It was a decision they knew many among their relatives and friends could never understand or accept, so they agreed to keep it from all but a few of the people closest to them. To others, then and for the years that would follow, Guy was said to be attending a special school in Arizona because of a serious asthmatic condition. Jackie's explanation to those who knew the truth was that Guy might recover in his teens, and if so, she didn't want him "stigmatized."

The experience—not only the difficulties with Guy himself, but the grinder she'd been put through by the "experts"—took a harsh toll on Jackie. Autism, which afflicts about 350,000 people in the United States, most of them male, had first been described only a few years earlier, in 1943, by Dr. Leo Kanner of Harvard. At first he and most of his colleagues had blamed the condition on mothers: "refrigerator mothers," "schizophrenogenic mothers," or even—conversely—"smothering mothers." The influential Dr. Bruno Bettelheim had even gone so far as to advocate radical "parentectomy"—the complete and permanent separation of parents and child—as the autistic's only hope. In the intervening decades the tide has turned, and in 1975, a year after Jackie's death, Ruth Sullivan, director of information for the National Society for Autistic Children, would state: "There has probably been no group more crucified by the mental health profession than the mothers of autistic children. It is my own personal belief that it will rank high among the scandals of the twentieth century."

My Mother's Death: Thoughts on Being a Separate Person

JUDITH ROSSNER

Judith Rossner, "My Mother's Death: Thoughts on Being a Separate Person," *Ms.*, September 1974. Reprinted by permission.

I was born, I grew up. My mother died. She had no place in my everyday life, yet it is generally accepted as reasonable that my mourning should be deep and long. How long and how deep?

"I can't cry," she said in December.

Her face was soft and dry, and her voice was small and dry, and her hands were always cracked and dry—or at least she thought they were—even though she washed few dishes; I have used a huge jar of cream on my hands since January 9.

I cry often, but when I think of that most painful thing she said to me, that she couldn't cry, I cannot cry. Nor could she sleep. The first time that the last doctor gave her the last sleeping pills along with specific instructions for their use (two followed by cocoa, in bed, with a book—not television, which leads to catnaps—but a book), that night she slept for several hours but aside from that she didn't sleep for more than an hour or two each night, and for weeks at a time not even that, but only for a few minutes on the sofa or perhaps on the soft Moroccan rug in my house. My father slept for both of them. She lusted for sleep. She hoarded all the sleeping pills given her by all the doctors who need to get her pain out of their offices and only used them when she had enough to guarantee the kind of sleep she had wanted for so many years.

And the last doctor thought that he observed, when my father called him to the house, that she hadn't used the pills he'd given her, only the ones

---

*Even today, institutionalization is necessary for fully two-thirds of all autistic children, for whom no chemical or psychiatric therapies avail. Behavioral techniques have had limited effectiveness, particularly in cases where some language skills have been developed and retained, but the prognosis for the majority of autistic children is as bleak now as it was in Guy's infancy.

given her by the previous doctor; but he was wrong. And the previous doctor wanted to know if she'd been taking the antidepressants he'd prescribed during the time when she'd finally taken the others; he was fairly sure she'd stopped taking them or she wouldn't have done it, but he was wrong too. Both of them, finally relieved of her pain, did not want some new one of their own. All of which is irrelevant if I am a separate human being.

Item. I write a novel which I know isn't about me except in the inevitable sense. My mother reads it and says it is about her.

In December she asked me what reason she had to continue living. A literary slave of the truth, I told her that we were the reason. That while it was true it would be easier for her not to, it would be too painful for us to lose her. She watched my son loading cars onto his car carrier and told me she couldn't love him or any of her grandchildren. I said that I understood and didn't mind. I told her that her feelings would r eturn when this depression ended, and she said she was afraid this depression would never end. (I can't cry.) I put my arms around her.

"My God," she said. "Do you know how long it is since you've done that?"

But Mother, I thought, I'm not *supposed* to do it. There is a proper order of things. How could we all be so middle-class and yet never follow the proper order of things? On my wedding morning someone had to remind us that a bride was supposed to have a bouquet. There is a decorum that, when one is willing to subscribe to it, eliminates coarse possibilities like forgetting bridal bouquets and committing suicide.

What she wanted I couldn't give her. I could have tried harder, much harder than I did, and still not have given it to her. I began to withdraw.

Item. At quiet times my left breast hurts. Her left breast was cut off four years before she died.

Before we moved to this house we had a cat that had a litter of which we kept one kitten. When we moved two miles up the road to this house, mother cat and year-old kitten moved with us.

Mother cat and kitten were affectionate to each other, licked each other, nestled together, were abused by our children together. After a couple of months here, mother cat decided to return permanently to the other house. Kitten remained with us. If they were to meet now, they wouldn't even know each other.

Item. "I just put in a new bridge for her," said my mother's heartbroken dentist. "She was so pleased with the way she looked." Relevance. The way one looks is really important. You feel better when you feel as if you look good. "They were two beautiful girls," he said, remembering my mother and her sister at the City College fraternity party where he introduced my father to my mother. She was still pretty. Black hair her friends didn't believe she didn't dye until a pure white hair began to appear here and there against the others. Because I did not resemble my mother, I was thought not to take after her, but when closely examined, many of my faults and virtues turn out to be visible symptoms of her inner qualities or negative reflections of her outer ones.

Item. My mother took castor oil to induce my birth because she had struck a bargain with her best friend, who was due at the same time, that whoever gave birth first would have the services of a particularly fine maid who would be available. I took castor oil to induce my daughter's birth because an obstetrician who didn't want to risk being late for his vacation advised that the baby would be very difficult to deliver if it got much bigger. Same action, different reasons. A play instead of a novel. The actions show, the motives are hazy. Interpretations constantly change so that only the action remains.

She wouldn't have taken those pills if she believed in an afterlife. It wasn't life she was after. This is important. Aside from her one wildly symbolic gesture of accidentally sweeping the alarm clock off her night table that morning before my father left for his plant, a touch so obvious that it would be unusable in a work of fiction, there was no sign of disorder or regret in the room. Which I did not see until weeks later. She showered, and folded the towel afterward. She got into bed, the blankets were neat, the phone straight on the table and the receiver secure in its cradle.

Now my husband tells me, "The room was a mess when I first saw it that night. I straightened it up." And seeing my stricken face, adds, "Maybe the cops did it."

The cops don't mess up the bedroom of a middle-class white suicide. Maybe he means when they took her away. I don't ask. There is no way for me to face this new fact. I can only try to digest it by writing it down. My mother had the writer's consciousness without the writer's impulse. If she had been able to write, she might have digested the ironies of her life instead of letting herself be poisoned by them. Writing is my survival kit. My independence.

Item. A dream. I am looking at a hanging painting of a person sitting in a rocking chair. The painting is in a realistic manner but the person is hazy. "Who is that sitting in the rocker?" I ask a servant of the house. "There's no one sitting in the rocker," the servant says. "The rocker is empty." End of dream.

My two-and-a-half-year-old son brings me the bright-green ski sweater my mother knitted for him.

"Who brought this?" he asks.

I say, "Grandma made it for you, sweetheart." He says, "No. Grandpa bought it."

He was always closer to his grandfather, anyway. He is the first in our family to strongly resemble my father, with his blue eyes and fair hair, but there is more to it than that. My mother always seemed remote to him. Never hostile or domineering. Always gentle. But remote. She was a gentle person, but how much of her gentleness was violence rendered ineffectual?

"Grandma was never mean to me. She was *always* nice," says my daughter, who has to live with my temper but is certainly not aware that my mother entered a suicidal depression each time my sister or I became pregnant.

For my daughter, the loss is a serious one. For my daughter, who was born five years earlier in all of our lives than my son, my mother existed. For my son she always had the quality of those few dried-out autumn leaves that contrive to stay on the ground through spring.

"You'll write about me, won't you?" she said in December.

"Everything I write is about you," I said.

Take the Blame off Mother

PAULA J. CAPLAN

Paula J. Caplan, "Take the Blame Off Mother," *Psychology Today*, October 1986. Reprinted by permission.

Blaming mothers for their children's psychological problems has a long and, unfortunately, respected history, particularly among mental-health professionals. Sigmund Freud's work included some such trends, and the more recent coining of such key terms as "overprotective mother," "maternal deprivation," and "schizophrenogenic mother" swelled the mother-blaming tide. So, too, did theorists' obsessional overemphasis on the importance of mother-child "bonding" in the few days—even the first few minutes—after birth. With professionals leading the way, it's not surprising that mother blaming was legitimized in the layperson's mind as well.

Has the women's movement vindicated mothers and stemmed the tide of mother blaming? Critics of the movement say it has, hoping that feminists will pack up and go home, believing their work to be done. A few years ago, however, Ian Hall-McCorquodale, then a graduate student, and I decided not to take this assertion on faith. We studied a wide range of clinical mental-health journals published between 1970—soon after the feminist renaissance began—and 1982, when it was well into flower. During the twelve-year span, mother blaming did not abate; indeed, it continued in epidemic proportions.

Professionals have blamed mothers for a wide range of problems. In the 125 articles in our study, mothers were held responsible for seventy-two different kinds of psychological disorder in their children, ranging from agoraphobia to arson, hyperactivity to schizophrenia, premature mourning to homicidal transsexualism.

In the articles we reviewed, not a single mother was ever described as emotionally healthy, although some fathers were, and no mother-child relationship was said to be healthy, although some father-child ones were described as ideal. Far more space was used in writing about mothers than about fathers. Furthermore, fathers were often described mostly or only in terms of their age and occupation, whereas mothers' emotional functioning was usually analyzed (and nearly always deemed essentially "sick").

This collective portrait of pathogenic mothering, I believe, is not only scientifically implausible but also socially destructive. As long as mothering is assumed to be the only or primary cause of children's psychopathology, then all that remains to be done is to figure out which kind of bad mothering is to blame. This hurts not only mothers and children but also fathers, when we expect too little warmth, humanity, and involvement form them, assuming these to be somehow "unnatural" in men. Mother blaming also hurts psychology and society by preventing us from looking with fully open eyes at the total range of causes for children's unhappiness and psychological problems.

Why, then, does mother blaming by professionals thrive? One reason is that mothers are usually more visible to therapists than are fathers. Since fathers are frequently less involved than mothers in the family, when a child does have a problem, it is almost always the mother who takes the child to the therapist, making mothers—but not fathers—available for study and observation. It's easier to blame the person in the waiting room than to explore arduously what—and who—else might contribute to a child's problems.

Understanding the sources of psychopathology in children requires more than an intellectual knee jerk, because there are many possible causes, and their relative importance varies from case to case. For one child, the mother's behavior may indeed be the major source of trouble; for another, the father's behavior—or perhaps his absence—gives rise to problems. Yet another child may have had disturbing encounters with an adult relative, a caretaker, teacher, siblings, or other children or may be reflecting familial stresses and tensions stemming from difficult social or economic circumstances. Some children—such as those with a high activity level, autistic characteristics, or a genetic predisposition to mental illness—may be so innately vulnerable that they develop mental problems despite the best of parenting. In the studies we reviewed, such individual differences were rarely considered. To leap to the conclusion that flawed mothering made a child mentally ill is simplistic and unjustifiable; other explanations must be explored.

Mother blaming is also perpetuated by blind allegiance to past theories. In the articles we studied, attempts to question earlier mother-blaming theories or reports were distressingly absent. Instead, the authors we studied simply parroted them uncritically to their readers, ignoring the growing body of child-development research that challenges such simplistic interpretations.

Further fuel for mother blaming is the mistaken belief—held by professionals and laypeople alike—that because women give birth and lactate, they are better suited than men for child-rearing. This has had several repercussions. First, it has served to make women—not men—the main caretakers of children, despite the fact that all child care tasks but lactation can be done by people of either sex and a child can learn from either parent (or from other people, for that matter). Second, it has blinded us to the psychological importance of fathers in children's development and permitted or forced many fathers to be relatively uninvolved emotionally with their families. Third, it has created a vicious cycle of guilt and discomfort for women. Because mothers are made responsible for most child care, they become tense and worried about doing the best possible job and spending as much time as possible with their children. When a child has a problem and a mental-health worker blames the mother, she is likely to take her child's disturbed behavior as proof of her failure, thus reinforcing the professional who blamed her.

What can be done to stop the barrage of blame? First, both mental health professionals and mothers need to look before they leap to conclusions about why children develop problems. Mothers are unquestionably influential in children's lives, but so are fathers, other members of the child's world, and children themselves—a fact that often eludes both the blamers and the blamed. Mental health professionals need to face up to the complexity of child development, stop relying on old and often invalid parenting theories, and do the difficult but essential work of searching out and understanding the multiple influences on children's development.

Second, mothers would be less readily scapegoated and more often supported in standing up to professional "experts" who wrongfully berate them if their child-rearing successes were more frequently acknowledged. Our society usually fails to give mothers credit for the good they do, unless they are dead or described in the abstract, as in "apple pie and motherhood." Yet mothers, despite their anxiety and guilt, manage to raise millions of reasonably well-adjusted kids. They deserve far more credit for this than they get.

Third, we need to raise sons in ways that prepare them better emotionally for parenting, and we need to acknowledge the enormous personal and social importance and worth of parenting as a role for both women and men. When both sexes come to understand that there is no biological foundation for assigning child-rearing primarily to women and men are encouraged from childhood to develop and value their own nurturant abilities, we may set the stage for a more equal partnership in child care—and more equal responsibility for children's emotional well-being.

As one of novelist Robertson Davies's characters says: "I'm sick to death of people squealing about their mothers. . . . What's a perfect mother? We hear too much about loving mothers making homosexuals, and neglectful mothers making crooks, and commonplace mothers stifling intelligence. The whole mother business needs radical re-examination."

The Madonna's Tears for a Crack in My Heart

AUDREY FLACK

We're closing the house for the summer, leaving for New York. I am in the kitchen loading a huge straw basket, when my husband Bob holds up a picture in the *New York Times Magazine*, a full-page black-and-white photo of a young child.

"Do you think this could be Melissa?" he questions.

I lose my footing and stagger. It's a photograph of my daughter Melissa when she was five years old. The photo focuses on her beautiful eyes and nose, the rest of her face partially hidden by the back of a slatted chair, which she presses her lips against. She appears to be behind bars.

Oh, those eyes. Extraordinary, beyond belief . . . wide, green, and unbelievably huge, staring, looking blind yet seeing all, and seeing nothing. Her ethereal beauty was awesome, with delicately arched eyebrows, a finely chiseled nose, and a full mane of chestnut hair. Her eyes gathered the power of her muteness; she would eventually use them to speak for her. I was to find out, years later, that her strange stare was a classic symptom of autism.

The picture was taken at the height of Melissa's autism. Her anger, rage, frustration, and physical pain had run its course. It had ravaged her. She cried incessantly, mercilessly, uncontrollably, during her infancy. I brought her to pediatricians for help and was told I was nervous. After persisting in my cries for help, I was labeled neurotic. They could find nothing wrong—but there *was* something wrong and I knew it! She was in pain, maybe her limbs ached or her head throbbed, she screamed, and all I could do was hold her and watch, nothing alleviated her agony. I begged for help as I watched my beautiful child's body, soul, and mind devoured by a mysterious neurological demon. The next stage of devastation seemed to be a caving in, a giving way, a slide into a world of total bewilderment and confusion. She looked stunned, shocked, stupefied.

Whatever biochemical imbalance had taken place within her small, delicately boned body had affected her comprehension, hearing, depth perception, and motor coordination. She would freeze in panic in the middle of a stairway. Sounds of fear came from her throat, choking sounds, and then she'd collapse in a heap and shake, perched on a too-shallow step.

She would flinch and blink rapidly when my hand came close to her face, to feed her or comb her hair. To strangers it looked like she was an abused child. I learned to move slowly and never approach her peripherally. Her condition seemed much like Helen Keller's, only she was not blind and deaf, she only appeared to be. Just the opposite. Her peripheral vision is amazingly astute, almost like a bird with eyes on either side of its head. Melissa prefers to watch television from the side. Her hearing is uncanny, far exceeding the normal range.

If Melissa's hearing is truly as acute as I know it to be, and sounds, even minor ones, are amplified, it would follow that she had to find a way to turn them off, in order to survive. A bomb could explode in front of her, and she wouldn't blink. Doctors insisted she was deaf, I knew it was just the opposite.

I researched autism, searching out any program available, any information accessible, however pitiful, driving around and dragging Missy from doctor to doctor.

What incredible agony I felt when specialists told me their terrible stories. All were firmly committed to their contradictory diagnosis. She is absolutely deaf! Retarded! Brain damaged! She is incurable! Send her away! Forget her! She's not retarded . . . just wait until she's twelve years old, she'll straighten out. She's schizophrenic . . . deviant . . . mentally ill . . . hopeless!

Autism was an unknown entity until the late 1950s, when a Dr. Leo Kanner isolated a small group of children who could not be categorized. While their behavior lagged behind the norm, these beautiful and strange children did not appear to be retarded in the classic sense. While some spoke strangely, others stared off into space . . . even stared right through you. A great many, like my daughter, remained mute, unable to express themselves or make their wants known.

They seemed removed, wanting to be alone, they didn't play with other children and remained isolated, sitting in corners rocking, spinning tops, or mechanically stacking objects. Some stared at bare light bulbs, others covered their ears at the sound of certain noises as if in pain. Melissa did both. Many acted deaf. Some hit, scratched, and kicked. Some mutilated themselves, biting chunks out of their own arms, even gouging out their eyes.

A very few showed extraordinary skills, such as naming what day of the week a certain future date would fall on, photographically memorizing telephone books, and making extraordinarily detailed drawings after just one glance. The term "idiot savant" was changed to "autistic savant." The movie *Rain Man*, starring Dustin Hoffman, exposed the syndrome to the public. The main character was based on an autistic boy who attended Melissa's school. But only one in a million is a savant; the overwhelming majority are severely impaired and far from glamorous.

Most would walk in front of an oncoming car or out the window of a high-rise building. The medical establishment said these children wanted to commit suicide in order to get away from their intolerable cold, aloof, destructive mothers. All their abnormal behavior was unconditionally blamed on the mother.

Dr. Bruno Bettleheim, founder of the Orthogenic School associated with the University of Chicago, was the leader of the pack. He labeled us "refrigerator mothers" and unequivocally declared that because we were so cold, removed, and uncaring, our children developed the symptoms of autism.

I can think of no greater nightmare than to have a sick child, a child you have birthed, a child you love with all of your being, a child whom you would (and often did) sacrifice your life for, and be blamed for their condition.

In his book *The Empty Fortress*, Bettelheim compared the homes of autistic children to Nazi concentration camps and suggested that their condition stemmed from extreme frustration in the mother-infant relationship. He said we rarely cuddled or fondled our children, our behavior was mechanical and expressed no feelings of love or parental affection. A substantial body of the mental health profession accepted his position: mothers were a major "pathogenic" factor in contributing to the disorder.

In an odd way, I almost welcomed the blame. If I was the cause of Melissa's condition, then a change in my behavior could also cure her, and I wanted to cure her desperately. But none of this was true.

I was to find out that Melissa stiffened when being held because her skin was so sensitive. It hurt her to be touched. I had all this love, warmth, and affection for her, which she physically could not accept. She was not rejecting me psychologically, she was in *pain*. She bit and kicked me when I tried to dress her because clothing felt like sandpaper and razor blades scraping her skin. She could not say what she felt.

It is only within the past few years that a few older autistics have been able to describe their feelings. It never occurred to them to commit suicide by walking out a window or stepping in front of oncoming traffic. They tell us that a ten-story-high window can look as if it is on ground level, a car can appear to be miles away one minute or on top of them the next, or not there at all. Stairs can suddenly disappear or wave as they are walking down them. The pattern on an oriental rug can come alive, as if it's moving or jumping up at them. One mother whose child screamed and refused to walk on grass found out years later that he thought he would fall through the spaces between the blades of grass. It is clear that their spatial perceptions are distorted, they go on and off, working sometimes and blurring at other times.

Instead of the "refrigerator mother," the child herself may be doing the rejecting. She may not be able to recognize her own mother's face. How painful not to have your own child recognize you, love you, hug you, or speak to you, but imagine going for help and being systematically tortured and blamed. Most of us stoically took it. There was no other recourse. We learned to say what the doctors and social workers wanted to hear in order to get our children into the only programs available.

After numerous phone calls, researching, and networking, I found out that Lenox Hill Hospital had a special program for autistic children which met for one hour once a week. It was based on Bettelheim as well as Freudian psychogenic doctrine and promoted the theory of blame. The doctors and social workers were instructed not to talk to the mothers in front of our children because we were the cause of their problems and if they saw us talking, the children would not trust the doctors. Melissa was three years old and mute at the time.

Everyone (except the other mothers) blamed me. I was an outcast. I could not get help. I had no money. I went to a psychiatrist through a clinic. My behavior was analyzed. Why did I do it? Do what?

Melissa was uncontrollable; I was the only one who could handle her. She did not sleep for four years. She had to be watched every moment. She wandered around the house all night long, throwing everything down, turning on gas jets, taking knives, forks, and scissors out of drawers, putting them in her mouth and walking full speed ahead. I had to protect her from herself.

This meant that I did not sleep for four years . . . cat naps . . . one eye open, one eye closed, always in attendance. It got to the point where I didn't know whether I ate or drank. It was only if I felt faint that I realized I had not eaten for the entire day. I was consumed by Melissa. I couldn't bear to tie her to her bed, and there was no other way to keep her still. The fifty minutes I spent in the psychiatrist's office was the only peace I had all day and night. It didn't matter what was said, I could sit still for fifty minutes.

I always put on a smile as I pushed the stroller because Hannah, my younger daughter, needed friends, and if I showed my depression and desperation I was afraid no one would play with her. I kept up a front and maintained some degree of normalcy for Hannah's sake.

It was while waiting in the lobby of Lenox Hill Hospital that I got acquainted with and came to love the other mothers of these sick children. These loving, selfless women not only carried the burden of their sick children, but had to bear the guilt, blame, shame, and accusations heaped on them by the medical profession, including social workers and teachers, as well as an entire society that shows little empathy for those who don't fit in.

Families were destroyed. Husbands left and wives stayed behind, becoming alcoholic or dependent on pills given to them because they were "neurotic." Husbands who remained understandably escaped to their jobs, a relief for them, but not for the wives who were left to care for noncommunicative, mute, and uncontrollable children.

On the rare occasions when we were able to get together, we compared notes and found that we had all started talking to ourselves. Our looks faded, our hair went uncombed. Who had time for lipstick? Who had time for ironing? Food stained our clothing and stuck in our hair.

At least we had each other, as we sat holding or running after our children while waiting our turn,

on hard plastic chairs in the cold hospital lobby. We exchanged news about new developments in research, pharmaceutical medicines, and school programs. We understood each other's plight. In those few minutes we could comfort and support each other, offering hope, even if the doctors couldn't.

Our observations and opinions were dismissed as neurotic and therefore invalid, although we knew far more than any doctor about our children's condition, we learned to keep silent or say only what the authorities wanted to hear. We were alone, we didn't even have a group, just these happenstance meetings in the lobby, as we delivered our children and watched them come out of some test or special class, which we were kept unaware of.

Once a child was accepted, the program offered only a small playgroup, which was really for the benefit of the hospital's psychiatric department to conduct psychological studies using our children as specimens. Melissa was accepted and I was instructed to bring her to a private street-level entrance on Lexington Avenue, ring the bell, and wait. I followed the instructions, a door opened, a teacher took Melissa's little hand, and without a glance or nod of recognition, proceeded to close the door in my face.

The process of getting Melissa to the hospital was formidable. First there was the ordeal of getting her dressed. She fought, kicked, screamed, and bit. We hear now that the clothing may have hurt her exquisitely sensitive skin. My arms were scarred with bite marks from her desperate attempts to protect her skin, yet I couldn't let her go naked. No one knew the reason or understood the behavior until years later when older verbal autistic adults found ways to express their feelings. We have learned a great deal from people like Temple Grandin, who has written several books about what it's like to be autistic.

Getting Melissa to the program, a simple trip, presented problems of almost insurmountable proportions. I couldn't afford a baby-sitter and had to drag Hannah along with us. I carried one child and held the other. I had to drag Melissa by the hand. Sometimes I tugged so hard, I was afraid I might pull her arm out of its socket. Everyone looked, heads turned. The light turned green, but Melissa refused to walk. Suddenly, in the middle of oncoming Broadway traffic, she would drop, collapse in a heap, and stretch out flat on her back. Panic and terror seized me.

Finally I'd get Melissa up and into my other arm, and we'd get across the street. I now think that Missy must have been disoriented by the moving vehicles and dropped to the ground for safety, but we still don't know, she can't tell us.

The feat of getting Missy dressed and across town was nothing compared to the stockpile of other problems I had to deal with. Windows had to be locked to prevent her from walking out of them. I had to keep them closed even in the summertime when we had no air-conditioning. I had to keep a constant eye on her. Melissa destroyed the house every day. She turned chairs upside down, pulled cloths off tables, smashed dishes and glassware, unmade beds as fast as they were made. Everything had to be upside down. I now wonder if her retina couldn't reverse vision as normal eyes do, and in her own way she was trying to right things by turning them upside down.

Poor motor coordination made it impossible for her to take food or drink from the refrigerator without disaster. Pouring a glass of milk was traumatic. Sour cream, plop, ketchup, she managed to get the top off, then bang, splatter over the floor and the refrigerator door. She would bite into the cheese with the plastic wrap still on. I'd fight to pry her mouth open to prevent her from swallowing it. I tied a rope around the refrigerator door for sanity, protection, and survival.

One of the few things that kept her attention, and that she enjoyed, was looking down at the cars and passersby on Broadway. We lived on the second floor, and I would hold her for hours while she peered out the window.

I could never leave her alone. She needed to be protected from herself. I even took her into the bathroom with me. I was the basic vehicle for her simple survival. Missy was blessed with good health, but on the few occasions that she did get sick, her temperature shot up from normal to 105–106 degrees in an instant, with no other symptoms. I shook with fear.

Life was unbearable. I could no longer continue. I was forced to make a devastating decision. I sent my child away. I knew she needed help and I had to save the family, which was collapsing under the strain. The Rudolph Steiner School had a residence in Pennsylvania focusing on children with special needs. They followed Steiner's theosophical philosophy and were kind to the children. It was the best option I could find. I couldn't continue alone any longer, and I was very worried about Hannah, who had developed severe asthma. I wasn't about to kill the healthy chicken to make chicken soup for the sick one, and that was the choice.

I mourned for a solid year after Missy went away. What must that have been like for young Hannah? This was the first time my three-year-old had her mother all to herself . . . a mother in mourning.

We were not allowed to visit Missy for three months. The theory was that she needed time to adjust to her new surroundings and was not to be reminded of her family.

Can you imagine being five years old, in physical distress and mental confusion, unable to communicate, totally dependent on your mother, and having that connection wrenched away? It would have been difficult enough for a normal child, but for an autistic, who also needs to keep the same patterns in order to make sense of life, it must have been devastating. This information was not known at the time; research on the neurological aspects of autism was in its infancy. Melissa became seriously ill, would not eat, would not sleep. I was not told until months later, after she had recovered.

The anguish I felt was unbearable, a large crack had formed in my heart. . . .

I brought Melissa home after a year at the school to institute a program called "patterning" developed by a group that called itself the Institute for Human Potential. The theory was based on improper, missing, or defective brain development. The program involved retracing and reenacting the physical activities of infancy and childhood, such as creeping and crawling. The child was placed face down on a table. It required three people. One moved the child's head, the other two stood on either side moving both an arm and a leg, reproducing the act of crawling.

The procedure itself was simple, but the rules were rigorous. Patterning had to be done for twenty minutes every two hours. This meant finding people who could come to the house, stay for half an hour, and leave. I needed an army, and in fact I found many friends and neighbors who were willing to help. When someone canceled, Hannah handled Missy's head, when she was home from school. But it was a terrible strain to be always searching and always in need. I patterned for a year, maybe two. It dominated our lives.

My second husband, Frank, played the cello in pickup orchestras, and I sold a painting here and there. We desperately needed money. When Sid Tillim asked me to take over his drawing class at the Pratt Institute, I grabbed the opportunity. I rearranged my life in order to teach the very next day. It was the start of my teaching career.

It took an hour and fifteen minutes on the subway to get to an early-morning class at Pratt in Brooklyn, and another hour to get back and teach anatomy at New York University in Washington Square. I'd gulp down a cup of coffee and a jelly donut before making a wild dash back to Pratt to teach in the late afternoon. Teaching jobs were hard to come by, particularly for women. Even though I was an excellent teacher and my classes were filled to capacity, I was given the worst time slots and paid the lowest salary. A request for a raise was met with, "You're married, you don't need the job. Be glad for what you've got."

When I finished teaching I returned home to relieve the baby-sitter, clean up Melissa's mess (which was a hundred times worse than a normal child's), calm Hannah, cook supper, and feed the family. Frank would arrive in time to consume a brief dinner, between performances at Radio City Music Hall, where he worked as a cellist. Since there were four to five shows daily, he was rarely home. I washed the dishes, bathed the children, read to Hannah, and prayed that Melissa would fall asleep.

Eventually there came a better time, when Bruno Bettelheim's doctrines were disproven and invalidated, and autism was recognized as a neurobiological disorder that interferes with the functioning of the brain.

How shocked and disgusted I felt when I read *The Creation of Dr. Bettelheim*, a biography by Richard Pollack, whose brother had attended the Orthogenic School. It exposed Bettelheim as a fraud. Bettelheim had invented degrees he never earned. He told of being trained as a psychoanalyst, which he never was, and bragged about his relationship to Freud, whom he never met. He was bordering on psychotic.

The medical establishment backed off, and doctors who had previously blamed the mothers apologized publicly. A feeling of relief and satisfaction came over me when I heard that Bruno Bettelheim had committed suicide. Justice had prevailed, the evil man was dead, and I was, after forty years of torment, redeemed. Mountains of guilt collapsed like compacted garbage heaps but the emotional trauma remained.

Today I persevere, searching for an answer, but I am no longer alone. A strong body of passionately committed parents, many of them doctors and scientists, is united in their efforts to find the cause and a cure.

Back in the summer house, I look up and see Bob still standing there. He knows that I have been far away and has been waiting for me to return to the present, East Hampton, 1986. I must know for sure if it's Melissa's picture in the *Times*.

The next day I call the school where Missy lived twenty-two years ago, and through them I track down the photographer.

"Are you the person who took the picture of the little girl with the big eyes that was in the *New York Times* this Sunday?"

"Yes, I am."

"Could you tell me the name of the girl?"

"Melissa," he says slowly, "her name was Melissa."

With a heavy sigh of relief, and a flush of excitement, I tell him, proudly yet timidly, that I am her mother. Then, I flood him with questions.

He says he visited the school twenty-two years ago and noticed this incredibly beautiful child with huge, soulful eyes.

"I shall never forget her," he says. "You are her mother? Tell me, are her eyes the same? How is she doing?"

"Ironically, she is still in Pennsylvania," I reply, "near Paoli. She is doing well. She still cannot speak, but she has found other ways to communicate. And yes, her eyes are still as big. Would you like a picture of her?"

"Yes," he says, "and I will try to find a print for you. I am touched by your call. Several people have called me about that photograph today!"

Is this why I painted Dolores of Cordoba with a torrent of tears pouring down her cheeks, gritting her teeth in a grimace? The statue in Cordoba has an oversized, thick gold heart placed in the dead center of her chest. Twenty-five daggers pierce her heart, and blood gushes, drips, and spurts from the stab wounds. Some find Spanish Baroque passion sculpture extreme. I find it realistic.

Breastfeeding Revisited

MARGOT SLADE

Margot Slade, "Breastfeeding Revisited," *Child*, September 1998. Reprinted by permission.

When the American Academy of Pediatrics gave its definitive word [in 1997] on how long women should breast-feed, the message was hardly aimed at undermining American mothers.

But that's precisely the way many people interpreted the statement, which recommended that women nurse their children for a minimum of one year, preferably well into the second year of life.

"That sounds like a long time to me!" says Julie O'Shea, a mother of two and an attorney in New York City. O'Shea took pride in the fact that she had surpassed the AAP's earlier recommendation that mothers breast-feed for at least six months and ideally for a year after a child's birth.

Heather King, a regional trainer for Home Box Office in Amesbury, Massachusetts, considers herself a breast-feeding devotee, but she didn't reach the one-year mark with any of her three children. "I could see how some women could freak. A new mom might say, 'I can't make it through a full year, so why do it at all?'"

Interestingly, the AAP statement that shook up so many women was directed at a different audience. It was part of a larger paper, printed in a pediatric medical journal, that documented newfound benefits of breast-feeding and outlined the vital supporting role pediatricians can play in the lives of nursing women.

"Rather than put pressure on women, we hoped our recommendation would give them a mandate to breast-feed by showing there are reasons to do it for a few days, a few weeks, and even beyond a year," says Ruth Lawrence, MD, a professor of pediatrics and obstetrics and gynecology at the University of Rochester School of Medicine in Rochester, New York, who worked on the AAP policy statement.

The AAP revised its recommendation in response to growing proof that the benefits of nursing are cumulative. That is, the incidence of disease decreases among women the longer they breast-feed and among children the longer they are breast-fed. The more time a woman devotes to breast-feeding over her life, the less her risk of breast cancer, osteoporosis, hip fractures, and ovarian cancer, according to Lawrence M. Gartner, MD, a professor of pediatrics and obstetrics/gynecology at the University of Chicago and head of the AAP's breast-feeding policy committee.

Benefits for kids include lower risk of ear infections, digestive problems, some cancers, and chronic illnesses like asthma and juvenile diabetes, and possibly better intellectual performance.

An equally important part of the AAP recommendation—one that many overlooked—is the qualification that nursing should continue *as long as the mother and infant desire*. And part of the problem with breast-feeding in this country is that what mother and child want has long been beside the point.

On one side of the issue have been breast-feeding proponents so ardent that, mothers complain, they care only that women nurse, regardless of overriding health concerns or personal issues. "Women call me in tears and in pain, asking for permission to stop," says Fern Drillings, a lactation consultant in New York City. "They're having a bad time, but to quit would seem like they failed."

On the other side, women say, are individuals and institutions who don't necessarily oppose breast-feeding but don't support it either. Among them are mothers and in-laws who harp on the fact that "we bottle-fed our children and they turned out just fine" and employers who make provisions for smoking and coffee breaks but not for pumping milk.

AMERICANS LAG IN BREAST-FEEDING

This combination of pressure on mothers has left the United States lagging behind when it comes to breast-feeding. In 1997, studies found that America had one of the lowest breast-feeding rates and one of the highest infant mortality rates in the developed world.

In 1995, the AAP reported that 59 percent of women in the United States were breast-feeding

exclusively or in combination with formula at the time of hospital discharge. At six months postpartum, only 22 percent of mothers were still nursing.

Though breast-feeding rates in the United States are up (only 23 percent of new moms nursed in 1970), experts attribute the comparatively low rate to the following factors: the continued increase in the number of women in the workforce, the lack of support for the practice from employers, physician apathy, lack of prenatal education, and the aggressive promotion of infant formula through hospitals and advertising.

It hasn't helped breast-feeding's cause that many people still consider the practice to be vulgar, even obscene. In 1996, Dina Tantimonaco was nursing her infant daughter in her car in the rear parking lot of a Connecticut restaurant when a policeman said he'd charge her with breach of peace if anyone complained. But it was Tantimonaco who did the complaining, eventually leading state legislators to pass a law that "no person may restrict or limit the right of a mother to breast-feed her child."

Similar laws have been enacted in sixteen states, and more have bills pending, according to Elizabeth N. Baldwin, a legal adviser to La Leche League International, based in Schaumburg, Illinois. "These laws clarify that breast-feeding is not criminal and that women have the right to nurse anyplace they have the right to be with their baby," she says.

BIGGER ROLE FOR PEDIATRICIANS

If more women are going to meet the AAP's minimum one-year recommendation, it will take more than laws that, in effect, decriminalize breast-feeding. It will take proactive support, starting with the medical community.

"Our new recommendations state that a woman's ability to breastfeed is intimately linked to a child's health, and that it is therefore up to pediatricians to learn about breastfeeding so we can encourage mothers to nurse their children and to do so longer," says Dr. Gartner.

This doesn't mean pediatricians will become lactation experts. "I'd rather have a pediatrician who can deal expertly with my kids' asthma," says Ellen Kadden, an international board-certified lactation consultant in Fairfield, Connecticut. "But the pediatrician should be able to tell me where to go for lactation expertise or provide such expertise through his or her office," she adds.

Kadden advises women to beware of pediatricians who seem uncomfortable watching women breast-feed or who recommend formula as a supplement too soon when a breast-feeding problem arises.

WHAT NURSING LONGER MEANS FOR MOMS

Certainly, the AAP's intention is not to make mothers nurse out of guilt. But the academy's statement regarding the benefits of breast milk makes the argument in favor of nursing more compelling than before, Drillings says.

Nursing women tend to agree. Kathy Hayden, mother of an eighteen-month-old in Detroit, says nursing through a child's second year is probably impractical for a lot of women, "but the AAP information makes a strong statement about nursing as long as you can."

What would help ease the way for women who want to nurse is realistic information about what breast-feeding will entail, say lactation consultants, especially when a mother also wants to resume some of her prebaby activities.

Drillings, who breast-fed her son for fourteen months, explains that how much a nursing mother needs to adjust her behavior depends on what her lifestyle was like before she became pregnant.

"For example, I always ate healthfully, so that wasn't a concern," Drillings says. Nor was she chronically ill or on medication—factors that can affect how long, if at all, a mother can nurse. And when she went to a wedding and drank a lot of wine? "I pumped when I got home and tossed out the milk," she says.

Women should also keep in mind that nursing isn't an all-or-nothing proposition. A mother can breast-feed in the morning and evening and pump during the day so that her child is bottle-fed breast milk in her absence. Heather King altered her routine from full-time nursing during her twelve-week maternity leave, to part-time nursing and pumping at work, to eventually nursing only at night and supplementing with formula during the day.

Susan Danaher, a senior vice president at MTV Networks in Los Angeles, breast-fed each of her two children for eight weeks. "I couldn't see continuing in the context of my schedule," she says. Rather than offer apologies, Danaher focuses on the benefits her kids reaped from when they were breast-fed.

MORE SUPPORT FOR NURSING ON THE JOB

The new recommendations on breast-feeding have particular significance when it comes to the workplace, where obstacles and negative attitudes toward the practice are legion.

"But demographics are destiny," says Ellen Galinsky, president of the Families and Work Institute in New York City, noting that the American workforce is now 48 percent female. "So-called female issues like breast-feeding are becoming work issues that employers dare not ignore," she states.

Supporting mothers who breast-feed isn't just socially responsible, it's smart business. Data show that because breast-fed babies are less likely to get sick, absenteeism among mothers and general health care costs can decline. Companies that offer lactation support—and this can be simply a quiet, comfortable space in which women can privately express milk—have reported reductions in turnover and in the loss of workers who decide not to return from maternity leave.

Congresswoman Carolyn Maloney, Democrat of New York, is trying to foster more corporate support through legislation making clear that the Pregnancy Discrimination Act of 1978 covers breast-feeding and related activities on the job. Among other provisions, the law would give tax credits to companies that set up lactation facilities and would ensure that nursing mothers be given a year's worth of "milk breaks"—up to an hour a day to nurse or pump.

The message that must be spread is that "breast-feeding is the right thing to do and makes sense from a societal perspective," says Rona Cohen, MN, head of the Los Angeles Department of Water and Power's lactation program, perhaps the oldest and most comprehensive of its kind in the country.

"How parents feed their babies should be their choice," Cohen says. "It is up to corporations, doctors, health professionals, family, and friends to offer mothers accurate information and options so they can make informed decisions about what is right for them."

Moms in Dark about OTC Drugs, Survey Shows

FRANCES CERRA WHITTELSEY

Frances Cerra Whittelsey, "Moms in Dark about OTC Drugs, Survey Shows." © 1999. Original for this publication.

A survey by the Women's Consumer Foundation shows that many inner-city mothers are in the dark about basic aspects of choosing and using nonprescription drugs, exposing them and their children to the possibility of serious illness or death.

The survey showed, in fact, that taking more than the recommended doses of these medicines is far more common than drug manufacturers acknowledge. Further, it showed that many of the women take medicines without knowing what is in them. Specifically, the survey found that less than half of the mothers could identify the active ingredient in the most widely advertised nonprescription drug, Tylenol®, or even define the term "active ingredient" itself. (The active ingredient in Tylenol® is acetaminophen.)

"We have issues of human life at stake here," commented Dr. John Renner, founder of the Consumer Health Information and Research Institute. "Not knowing the ingredients in common pain killers, with as much publicity as some of these products get, is remarkable. And with the overdosing that was found, can lead to real trouble."

The survey found that one out of eleven of the women knew of an adverse reaction to an over-the-counter (OTC) medicine that had resulted in a trip to an emergency room or doctor. Forty-four percent of the women said they knew people who very often, or somewhat often, take more than the recommended dosages. Twenty-five percent admitted to doing so themselves.

The survey results have been collected into a report called "Brand Loyal But in the Dark about Over-the-Counter Medicines," which includes an analysis and recommendations for action. It has been forwarded to the US Food and Drug Administration, which is finalizing new regulations that will standardize the formats and improve the readability of over-the-counter drug labels.

Asked to comment on the survey findings, the Nonprescription Drug Manufacturers Association said that serious illnesses or deaths due to adverse reactions from OTC medicines are "extremely rare."

In a written statement, the Association said "No drug is without potential toxicity, but OTC's have a very wide margin of safety."

Further, the Association maintained that "dozens of nationally representative independent surveys have found that consumers are responsible in their use of OTC medicines; they do read and understand labels; and do not take more than the recommended daily dosage." The Association noted that the surveys focused on mothers living in New York City.

While deaths and hospitalizations due to mistakes or reactions to prescription drugs have been widely reported, there is evidence that nonprescription drugs can also be dangerous: Gastrointestinal complications caused by aspirin, ibuprofen, naproxin, and other nonsteroidal anti-inflammatory drugs (some of them available only by prescription) result in approximately 76,000 hospitalizations and 7,600 deaths annually, according to the American Gastroenterological Association. This death rate is comparable to that for asthma, cervical cancer, and melanoma. People who consume three or more alcohol-containing drinks a day can suffer liver failure even when taking only the recommended dosage of acetaminophen (two 500 mg tablets four times a day), according to Mike Cohen, president of the Institute for Safe Medication Practices. People with allergies to aspirin may unwittingly take popular pain relievers or sleep aids that contain aspirin, and suffer life-threatening reactions. The institute reported that an eighteen-year-old woman, for example, had to be resuscitated and admitted to the intensive care unit after taking Excedrin® Extra Strength tablets. She knew she was allergic to aspirin, but did not realize that Excedrin contains aspirin.

"It is not being alarmist at all," commented Cohen, to suggest that ignorance about OTC medicines can result in serious injury or death. Cohen's Institute monitors adverse reactions reported to the US Pharmacopoeia and to the FDA's Med Watch program, and issues advisories about them that are published in medical, nursing, and pharmaceutical journals.

Fred Mayer, whose 1990 petition to the FDA began the process that will soon lead to new regulations for OTC labels, said in an interview that a 1989 federal report on adverse reactions to both prescription and OTC drugs suffered by the elderly put the price tag at $10 billion annually.

"A lot of [the problem] is mixing prescription and OTC medicines," said Mayer, president of Pharmacists Planing Service, Inc. "It's an epidemic and no one's in control."

Barbara Seaman, founder of the National Women's Health Network, also noted that more and more people with chronic diseases like depression, high blood pressure, and high cholesterol are on maintenance regimens of prescription drugs. "They need to be more conscious of possible interactions of prescription drugs with nonprescription drugs," she said.

According to a report prepared for the Nonprescription Drug Manufacturers Association by the research firm Kline Company, Inc., American consumers spent $14 billion a year on OTC medicines in 1997.

By purchasing generic brands and single-ingredient, rather than heavily advertised or combination medicines, consumers could save 50 percent or more on OTC purchases, according to price checks conducted by the Women's Consumer Foundation.

But the survey showed that many of the women questioned are unable to follow thrift advice because they do not understand the meaning of "generic," and the concept of active ingredients. As a result, they unnecessarily spend their limited resources on higher-priced, widely advertised name brands and combination medicines.

Three-quarters of the women surveyed were raising their families in New York City on $35,000 a year or less in total family income.

The survey was a project of the Women's Consumer Foundation, a nonprofit, New York–based organization that also publishes the SIS Web site. It was conducted during the second half of 1997 at a Harlem health center and at a Brooklyn shopping mall. A total of 181 women, who identified themselves as mothers and the primary buyers of over-the-counter medicines for their families, answered thirty-five questions read to them face-to-face by a surveyor. The study was financed with a grant from the Shelley Donald Rubin Foundation of New York City.

Less than half of the women surveyed—only 43 percent—could correctly define the term "active ingredient." An overwhelming 77 percent did not understand the word *antihistamine*. Nearly half—

48 percent—did not know that acetaminophen is the ingredient in Tylenol® (they were given four possible answers from which to choose), despite the fact that Tylenol® was the drug that the women said they bought most often.

These findings become alarming when viewed in conjunction with the results showing widespread disregard for dosage limits, and that many mothers do not or cannot adequately read and understand OTC drug labels.

What were the consequences of this overdosing and difficulty reading and understanding labels? The survey did not establish cause and effect, but thirty of the women, or nearly 17 percent, said that they or a family member had suffered an adverse reaction from an OTC drug. Fifteen of the women, or 8 percent, said the reaction was severe enough to require medical attention.

The pharmaceutical industry spent $2.03 billion on all forms of OTC drug advertising in 1997, according to Nielsen Media Research. In a pivotal decision in 1983, the Federal Trade Commission chose not to follow the recommendation of an administrative court judge that ads for OTC drugs always disclose the generic names of their active ingredients. Instead, the Commission said such disclosure would be required only under certain limited circumstances.

The response of the pharmaceutical industry ever since has been to avoid those circumstances. Ads promise symptom relief without usually identifying the agents of that relief. This confuses consumers into believing that brand-name products are unique formulations worth their high prices, instead of heavily advertised versions of common, inexpensive drugs.

If consumers understood OTC drugs better, their savings could be significant. For example, store-brand pseudoephedrine HCL can frequently be found for one-half to one-third the price of the name-brand decongestant, Sudafed; generic versions of Nyquil cost 50 percent less. A single dose of TheraFlu, a combination product, costs eighty-three cents. If the three active ingredients in Ther-aFlu were, instead, bought separately, a single dose would cost twenty-eight cents.

Among the benefits of smarter self-medication, said the Foundation, are healthier children and adults; fewer absences from school and work; fewer adverse drug reactions; fewer trips to doctors and emergency rooms; more competition among drug manufacturers, and, consequently, lower prices for OTC drugs.

The Baby Contract

SUSAN JORDAN

Susan Jordan, "The Baby Contract and the Value of Motherhood," in *The Baby Contract*, forthcoming. Reprinted by permission.

> *Susan J. and I, Jesse L., as marital partners agree on this 3rd day of June, 1996, to hereby contract to raise our son in a manner that we have determined will be most beneficial for the child and all members of the family and that will not penalize the parent who forgoes working outside the home. Upon mutual agreement. . . .*

Mother. Spoken in the 1950s, that word evoked warm and fuzzy images of a smiling woman, holding a pie, surrounded by children. Spoken in the 1990s, the image is vastly different. The once cohesive concept of The Mother has splintered. In her place, we have the working mother, the stay-at-home mother, the divorced mother, the welfare mother, the single mother, the step-mother, the teenage mother, the unwed mother, the soccer mother; each subject to some degree of criticism and scorn. This fractured perception of motherhood is but one small measure of the staggering decline in status and legal rights of all mothers, regardless of their category.

Similarly, our definition of what it means to "mother" children has grown increasingly abstract. Now, mothers who stay at home are more likely to be seen as liabilities for their children—a view that is encouraged by questionable research that claims to show that children of working mothers fare better than those whose mothers don't work outside the home. If you factor in the rapid advances being made in reproductive technology and the spawning of unique surrogacy arrangements, you find not only are mothers poorly regarded and perceived as increasingly unnecessary but, in some cases, it is disturbingly unclear, even to the courts, "who" the mother is.

With gathering momentum, the devaluation and, perhaps, termination of the active role of the mother has begun. It's looking more and more like Aldous Huxley's *Brave New World*. Ironically, while many readers associate that novel with the description of test tube babies, few recall that the most degraded, despised, and superfluous role in the "new world" was the role of the mother.

There are many reasons for the rapid devaluation of the role of the mother. Anyone who tunes in to the greatest social dilemma of our time—balancing work and family—is familiar with the two most commonly cited co-conspirators: the globalization of the economy forcing real wages into decline, thereby increasing the need for two paychecks, and an American feminist movement that seeks equality through parity in the workplace and reproductive control (primarily access to abortion).

If the yardstick of progress is workforce participation then there can be no question that women have made tremendous advances and feminism deserves much of the credit. But at what price? Workforce participation for women is at an all-time high. By 1990, 75 percent of all women aged twenty-five to forty-four years old were in the paid labor force. But the majority of working women are not in fast-track, high-paying careers; they are in low-paying service sector jobs that lack adequate health benefits, paid leave, or retirement pensions. And, while it is a generally accepted fact that women have narrowed the wage gap from fifty-nine cents to seventy-three cents for every dollar men make, it is not so much because women's

wages have increased but because men's wages have been on a serious decline; from 1979 to 1991 the average woman earning median income saw her hourly wages increase only 1.3 percent while the equivalent man endured a 14.3 percent plunge.

But it is women with children who pay the worst long-term penalties, particularly if they take time away from their careers to mother their children; estimates are that a woman's earning potential drops by 19 percent with the birth of her first child. And the myth that women can move in and out of the mommy track without consequences is contradicted by a recent study by Professor Schneer of Rider University that suggests that women executives who take time off and then return to work permanently sacrifice career advancement and earning potential. This penalty is echoed in the findings reported by June O'Neill, Director of the Congressional Budget Office, who reported that "among women and men, aged twenty-seven to thirty-three, who have never had a child, the earnings of women in the National Longitudinal Survey of Youth are close to 98 percent of men's." It is the women who have children who drag the average down to the seventieth percentile.

The modern feminist movement, born in the 1960s, has been remarkably effective in getting society to address the gross inequities to which all women have been subjected. But as Barbara Katz Rothman put it, "Giving women all the rights of men will not accomplish a whole lot for women facing the demands of pregnancy, birth, and lactation." Thus, despite the fact that mothers are one of the most vulnerable segments in today's society, the feminist movement has been disturbingly silent when it comes to defending mother's rights. Feminism's ambivalence has prevented it from, as Christina Looper Baker so eloquently put it, "reinventing motherhood so that it does not eclipse feminism and redefining feminism so that it does not exclude motherhood."

Hamstrung by defining liberation and equality as "sameness" with men and focusing on equality in the workplace and the right not to have children (i.e., abortion and contraception), feminists have been reluctant to fight for the protection of women's differences. By lobbying primarily for remedies that facilitate women's quick return to the workplace (i.e., brief maternity leaves, government and industry-sponsored day care, etc.), feminists have failed to adequately question the viability and impact of programs and policies that separate women from their infants and small children, sometimes arguing to the extreme that day care is actually better for children. By insisting that being able to raise children at home is just a white, middle-to-upper class problem, feminists have missed the precise point that women in lower socioeconomic classes have already unequivocally lost the right to mother their own children. It's gotten to the point where the poorest mothers—those on welfare—can be threatened with a loss of benefits based on the number of children they have and no one raises an eyebrow.

However, the increasing separation of women from their children is not a signpost of liberation and equality but one of the most subtle and far-reaching forms of discrimination and repression affecting women today. In her book, *The Illusion of Equality*, Martha Albertson Fineman, a feminist scholar, painfully details the impact that this gender-blind stance has had on family law and credits feminism with facilitating the removal of gender-specific rules that protected mother's rights, including the "tender years" doctrine. In the early nineteenth century, mothers had essentially no rights when it came to their children; fathers retained an absolute right of ownership and control over their children and had the corresponding duty of supporting them. Court documents routinely depicted women as the "inferior parent." It wasn't until the late nineteenth century when early feminists fought for the rights of mothers and children that family law shifted its emphasis to the "best interests of the child." Though far from perfect, under this construct, women's special skills as nurturers were recognized and the presumption of maternal custody during a child's "tender years" became the norm.

The acceptance of a mother's essential bond to her child was a powerful and radical notion that has been slowly chipped away by reforms in family and divorce law that increasingly emphasize "equality" between the sexes and the rights of fathers and noncustodial parents. So much so that when there is a divorce (a more than 50 percent chance), the law which varies from state to state makes little or no economic allowance for the sacrifices and contributions that women have made for their families.

Most women remain unaware of the economic penalties and risks they face when they become mothers or the extent to which their legal rights have been eroded until their marriage or relationship dissolves and they find themselves in divorce court. By then, it is too late.

For example, if a woman has the misfortune to reside in a separate property state (forty-one states out of fifty), she is entitled only to a minimal child support award and if she is deemed capable of self-support by the court, she may receive no alimony or maintenance support whatsoever. Distribution of marital property is at the discretion of the judge and generally mirrors the degree of financial contribution each of the parties has made.

That's not the worst of it. Few women know that if they support their spouse through professional or graduate school they are less likely to receive alimony and, contrary to common lore, may not receive any reimbursement for their spouse's professional advancement or future earnings. And many are shocked to realize that in some states their spouse can petition to reduce maintenance support and child support payments in order to support a new or "second" family.

And despite all this talk about deadbeat dads, if a spouse fails to pay his support obligations consistently over time, he is often in a better position to have his "arrearages" forgiven; the court's logic being that if his family has managed to survive the months or years without it then they must not have needed it after all.

Most working mothers, in particular, think that they will be protected under "equitable distribution." But what the court defines as equitable is usually two-thirds to the higher wage earner and one third to the lower wage earner. If a woman's earned income is substantially less than her husband's, then she will receive substantially less of the assets that they have accumulated together as "partners" during the marriage.

Custody of the children, which most women assume will be granted to them, particularly if they have been the primary caretakers, is now up for grabs. True, women are still more likely to get custody. But when a father wants it, he wins 70 percent of the time. And because the law no longer presumes that mothers should be the legal custodians of children during their "tender years," men have become adept at manipulating pleas for physical custody in return for further reduced financial arrangements. Remember that child support ends at eighteen and that, in most states, noncustodial parents do not have to contribute to college education for their children, and it is apparent why so many women trade away their rights to future retirement income for upfront money to pay college tuition.

Why does this inequity prevail? It prevails because the legal system has, as Fineman points out, adopted a gender-blind stance toward women and their children. And while it may sound nondiscriminatory on the surface, it is often disastrous in application. Mirroring society, family law now requires that women and men be viewed as "situationally the same" regardless of the degree to which women have assumed the role of mother/caretaker. In the shuttered eyes of the law, "men and women are equal" and they deserve no more or no less regardless of the way they have functioned in the family over the years. But men and women are not the same. Women have babies and men don't. And while fathers are increasingly involved in their children's lives, it is most often the mother who makes the sacrifices in her career to mother their children.

In the face of a society that refuses to acknowledge the importance of the role of the mother, women must craft their own legal solution. Recognizing that every time a woman marries she signs a contract governed by the state, there is nothing to prevent her from negotiating the parameters of that contract with her partner. In fact, men and women do this all the time. Note the numerous pre-nuptials signed by the wealthy that are designed to shelter their assets and future income from a new and untested spouse.

But if one can shelter assets, one can legally affirm the intention to share them as well. A "baby contract," would offer women (and some men) the opportunity to modify the state-defined marital contract via a binding pre- or post-marital contract. Its purpose would be to explicitly recognize the implicit value of the role of the mother and ensure that individuals who actively mother their children are economically protected from the inequities of a system that penalizes them.

To accomplish this goal, the baby contract would redefine the family as one economic unit comprised of two partners who share equally in the ownership and access to all assets and earned income of the household while legally recognizing that the partner who assumes the role of mother is entitled to equivalent economic compensation in the future should the marriage dissolve. And while the baby contract would call for the valuation of the role of the mother, it need not and should not discriminate based on gender; men who choose to assume the role of the mother are subject to the same penalties and risks that women are and should be protected as well.

Working to correct the economic imbalance within the household while attempting to reform the inequities present in the current state-by-state patchwork of family law, the baby contract represents a major step forward in the continuing struggle for equality for all parents who want 'to mother' their children.

Monster Mommies

ERICA JONG

Erica Jong, "Monster Mommies," in Erica Jong, *What Do Women Want?* New York: HarperCollins Publishers, 1998. Copyright © 1998 by Erica Mann Jong. Reprinted by permission of HarperCollins Publishers, Inc.

> What is home without a mother?
> —Alice Hawthorne

Mommy Guiltiest? So reads the headline in the *New York Daily News*'s rehash of the "Nanny Case," which has riveted the media's public since everybody overdosed on treacly elegies to Diana, Princess of Wales. The *Daily News* has proved once again the old saying "Vox populi is, in the main, a grunt." The *News* is supposed to cater to the down-market crowd that doesn't read the *New York Times* or the *Wall Street Journal*, but in truth most people in the word biz read all three, as well as the *New York Post* and the *New York Observer*. But without the *News*, you can't possibly know all that's not fit to print. And, of course, that's what tells you about the vacillations of the zeitgeist. And the zeitgeist is currently into blaming mommies for the deaths of their kids.

For this is the lesson of the nanny trial; Louise Woodward may have been nineteen, inexperienced, drowsy in the mornings and moonfaced at night, but Dr. Deborah Eappen was really the one at fault, because she worked three days a week as an ophthalmologist rather than staying at home full-time with her baby. Never mind that she came home at lunch to breast-feed on the days she worked. Never mind that she pumped out breast milk on the other days. Never mind that she was an MD working a drastically reduced schedule—a schedule no intern or resident would be permitted to work. She is the one to blame for the heinous crime of baby murder.

In an age when most mothers work because they have to, it is nothing short of astounding that this case resulted in raving callers to talk shows who scream that Dr. Deborah Eappen deserved to have her baby die because she left him with a nineteen-year-old nanny.

So much for twenty-five years of feminism. So much for smug commentators who say we live in a "postfeminist age." The primitive cry is still "Kill the mommy!" She deserves to be stoned to death for hiring a nanny.

Of course, we Americans already knew that welfare mothers were monsters. Dear Bill Clinton, champion of women and children, signed the most disgusting welfare bill in American history—a bill more appropriate to Dickensian England, a bill basically reinstating the workhouse in millennial America. But, of course, we know the American poor deserve nothing. Poverty is, after all, un-American, America has abolished any definition of the worthy poor (children, mothers, the blind, the lame) and decided that they alone shall pay for the budget deficit run up by male politicians. After all, children have no votes—unlike savings and loan officers. Besides, the latter have lobbyists, and poor children naturally can't afford them. So we have no worthy poor in the country I so lavishly fund with my taxes, but neither have we any child care initiatives—let alone child care.

Even some reactionary countries—La Belle France, for example—have mother care, crèches, kindergartens, but in America we rely on nature red in tooth and claw, so crèches are seen as "creeping socialism," and nobody's allowed to have creeping socialism except the army and the non-tax-paying super-rich.

Okay—welfare mommies are monsters, but what about entrepreneurial MD mommies? What about women who delayed childbearing to finish school, had babies in their thirties and forties, and work part time? Well, now we learn that they, also, are monsters. Why? Because they don't stay home full time. Apparently all mommies are monsters—the indigent and the highly educated both deserve to watch their babies die.

Wait a minute. What happened here? Is this

1898 or 1998? It doesn't seem to matter. Where motherhood is concerned we might as well be in Dickens's England or Ibsen's Norway or Hammurabi's Persia. Mothers are, by definition, monsters. They're either monsters because they're poor or monsters because they're rich. Where mothers are concerned, everything is a no-win situation.

Poor Louise was nice but somewhat incompetent. Maybe she did shake poor little Matty—the medical evidence is inconclusive. After all, she was a Brit, and Brits love caning kids; shaking is nothing to them. But Deborah was even worse than Louise. She was a doctor's wife (and a doctor, but who cares?) who chose to work.

Both women have been thoroughly trashed. Nobody inveighs against the other Dr. Eappen—the one with a penis—and nobody screams that his baby deserves to die. Nobody talks about Matty either. He's just a dead baby. Dead babies have no votes and no lobbyists. No—what everyone carries on about is which woman is at fault.

The mommy or the nanny? The lady or the tiger? Women, by definition, are always guilty. Either they're guilty of neglect or they're guilty of abuse. Nobody asks about the father's role or the grandparents' role. If it takes a village to raise a child, as Hillary Clinton's bestseller alleges, then that village consists of only two people: monster mother and monster au pair. Everyone else is off the hook. (Including a government that penalizes working moms in its tax policies, its immigration policies, and its lack of day care.)

How must Dr. Deborah Eappen feel, first losing her son and then facing this chorus of harpies (for the women-haters are often women)? Imagine the trauma of losing your baby, the trauma of reliving the pain at the trial, only to face the further trauma of trial by tabloid. Dr. Deborah chose her job because it allowed flexible hours. So did her husband, Dr. Sunil Eappen, but nobody's blaming him. If we have come so far toward the ideal egalitarian marriage, then why does nobody discuss the couple? Only the women are implicated. Both nanny and mommy face death by tabloid firing squad.

If the nanny trial is used as a litmus test for social change, then we must conclude that very little change has occurred. No wonder generation Y is full of young women who want to stay home with their babies! They saw what happened to their weary boomer mothers, and they don't like what they saw. If all feminist progress is dependent on the mother-daughter dialectic (as I believe it is), then we are in for a new generation of stay-at-home moms, whose problems will be closer to our grandmothers' than our own. Betty Friedan's *Feminine Mystique* will be as relevant in 2013 as it was in 1963—and our granddaughters will have to regroup and start feminist reforms all over again.

No wonder feminism has been ebbing and flowing since Mary Wollstonecraft's day. We have never solved the basic problem that afflicts us all—who will help to raise the children?

They Came to Stay

MARJORIE MARGOLIES AND RUTH GRUBER

Marjorie Margolies and Ruth Gruber, excerpt from *They Came to Stay*, New York: Coward, McCann & Geoghan, 1976. Reprinted by permission.

In 1970, Marjorie Margolies decided at the age of twenty-five to adopt a Korean child. She encountered a variety of responses: her mother told her to get married and have her own kids, her boyfriend Seth threatened to end their relationship, and adoption agencies rejected her because she was single. They Came to Stay *recounts Margolies's experiences navigating the complicated world of adoption, the relationships she forged with what became two adoptive children—one from Korea and the other from Vietnam—and the difficult moral and identity issues she and her daughters were forced to confront. The power of this memoir is not only in Margolies's pioneering redefinition of the American family and defiance of sexist adoption policy, but in its honest, unglamorized window into American cultural arrogance, the paradox of assimilation, and the human need for reconciliation with the past.*

The idea exploded in my head.
I would adopt a child.

It was a hot July afternoon. A warm breeze blew the sheer curtains into my studio apartment.

But I felt chilled.

I would adopt a child no one else wanted. An abandoned child. Perhaps an orphan from Southeast Asia.

How would my mother and father react?

Like a sleepwalker, I found myself walking down the stairs of the old red brick house. Three blocks away, across Rittenhouse Square, my parents lived.

My mother looked through the peephole.

"Oh, it's you, Monkey. Come in."

I followed her through the foyer into the kitchen.

"Where's Daddy?" I asked.

"At a meeting in Camden."

It would be easier if he were here. I ought to wait.

"Mom"—I heard the words come out—"you remember the picnic I covered for the six o'clock news last week? The picnic of that Open Door Society—those families that adopt children and get together—"

"Mom," I blurted out, "I want to adopt a child."

"What?" She looked at me. "Repeat that. I don't think I heard right."

"I said I want to adopt a child—a child—like one of those hard-to-place children at the picnic."

She shook her head unbelievingly.

"You must be out of your mind. Look, Monkey. I'm like any other mother. I want to see you get married. Then you can have as many kids as you want."

"I may get married some day. But that's in the future. Right now I want to give a home to some child who's been abandoned or orphaned. When I think of the suffering some of these children have gone through—the tragedies they've known—I feel I want to help one of them. What's so wrong about that?"

"It's crazy, Margie. You've got an exciting television job. You're free to get up and go any time you want—anyplace in the world. Once you have a

child, that's all finished. You won't be free for the rest of your life."

I was unprepared for the intensity of my mother's reaction.

Her anger made me realize I must have touched a raw nerve, perhaps something out of her background, her own frustrations.

"Look, Mom," I said in a low voice. "I'm sure I can cope. You know how I love kids. Look at the kids I shepherded across the country on bicycle tours. The kids I took on summer trips—to Greece—to the kibbutz in Israel."

"Then have your own."

"I just have this feeling. If there's a child without a home, why wait?"

"You think you're some kind of superwoman—you can work and take care of a child at the same time?"

"Millions of women do. Why can't I?"

Her voice dropped. "I couldn't do both. I had to give up my work as soon as Phylis was born."

Was that the raw nerve I had touched? That she had been forced to stop her creative work as soon as my sister Phylis was born. Until then she had worked full-time as a commercial artist.

She paused. Her voice was softer, less strident. "I didn't resent having a baby. I didn't resent Phylis. I resented giving up my career. Maybe that's why this thing you've thrown at me—out of the blue—maybe that's why it bothers me so much. This isn't the way I see you fulfilling yourself. Just don't mess up your life."

There was a whole landscape of agencies for adopting children. One needed a kind of road map to find one's way. Even then one needed a set of law books to understand the codes.

Their questions on the phone were almost always the same.

"What kind of child do you want to adopt? Name? Husband's name?" No husband. I'm single.

"Sorry, we do not place children with single persons."

Some said it bluntly, some with hostility. One agency told me, "You must hate men. You're probably a women's libber. We don't give children to single people who might psychologically feed on children for fulfillment."

At work I rolled film in the darkroom. Pictures of children fleeing down burning streets in Vietnam. A little boy bending over a dead mother. Rows of children lying apathetically in orphanages in Korea. A frightened Korean woman abandoning a baby on the street in Seoul, looking around surreptitiously, then running away. A stranger handing the baby to a policeman.

The commentator was talking:

"Hundreds of thousands of abandoned children in Vietnam and Korea. What becomes of an abandoned girl? If she is mixed race, if her father was an American or a European, she is the object of ridicule. If she is lucky and can go to school, she will be ridiculed by all the children. If her mother associated with foreigners or was a prostitute, she will probably never go to school. Perhaps by nine or ten she may be on the streets as a prostitute herself."

I was more than ever convinced. There were special agencies that brought in children from Korea—the International Social Services, known as ISS; Welcome House, the agency Pearl Buck started in Bucks County, Pennsylvania; the Holt Children's Services in Oregon. I telephoned all of them. I wrote letters. I went to interviews. Always the same answer. The same stone wall.

The single parent syndrome.

I kept hearing the words in my dreams: No single parent wanted.

The obsession never left me.

Then, one day, visiting my mother, she said, "Daddy and I are planning to visit Japan at the end of May. How about joining us?"

Japan! Japan was a short flight from Korea.

Korea was where the Holt agency had its orphanage.

I called Roberta Andrews [an associate director of the Children's Aid], to tell her I might be going to Korea. Was there a possibility I might find a child and bring her back?

"Who knows?" she said, "We'll try."

Three days later, Holt answered. "You are welcome to look up Jack Theis, our director in Seoul, Korea."

I went back to New York, mulling over the letter from Holt. I telephoned Seth.

"If you really take off and go to Korea," he said angrily, "and if you actually come back with a child, I'll know you've made your decision about us."

My sense of inner direction was spinning like a compass in a magnetic minefield. Was I running away from Seth? Was I incapable of a real commitment? Did the trip to Korea mean I was preparing myself for a new kind of commitment? Should I go? Was I setting myself up for more roadblocks, more heartaches?

The next morning I telephoned Roberta.

"Go," she said. "You know how to get to people. Put yourself across."

How would I feel if I really got a child? Would I go instantaneously from being the child of my parents to the mother of my child?

"On February 25, 1970, a child was found by the Buk-ae-dong police box and had been protected for one month until her placement."

"What's a police box?" I asked.

"It's a small police station," [replied Jack Theis]. "Many Korean children are abandoned that way— left in front of a police station. Each year five to six thousand children are abandoned in South Korea. Some are left on the street or in front of a hotel or railway station. Whoever finds them brings them to the local police box. The police keep them in a reception center for a month in case the mother changes her mind or perhaps the child is lost and some relative may come looking for it."

He continued reading:

"Physical history: Fair-complexioned child, with slender build. Walking and running well, she seems to enjoy a normal progress. Social history: Responsive to questions. Gets along nicely with friends and is more of a leader. Tries to excel in everything, keeping her personal effects in good order."

"Bright and quick," I whispered.

He nodded.

I felt my hands begin to tremble. "Nothing negative?" I asked. I had waited so long.

He thumbed the file. "The next report was written a month later. It reinforces the first one. It just adds, 'She loves apples for snacks.'"

I laughed. "Apples. That'll be easy to supply."

His assistant knocked at the door. "Mr. Theis. She has not been assigned. She is available for adoption."

"You're in luck." He handed me a tiny snapshot of a little girl with a round face, pretty bow lips, and almond eyes that looked sad. It seemed to me the face of a child who had known much suffering and learned to contain it. It was a head-and-shoulder shot, like a hospital picture, with a white sign beneath her collar: Lee Heh Kyung, 3-15-63.

This was the little girl—if things worked out—the little girl I would know for the rest of my life.

I was still studying the snapshot when the door opened again. A tiny girl who scarcely reached my hip and who looked about four years old entered. She walked straight toward me, put out her hand, and said, "Haw doo yoo doo?"

My first impulse was to pick her up and hug her. Instead I held her hand. Even her hand felt fragile, vulnerable.

She looked at me quizzically and repeated, "Haw doo yoo doo?"

She was graceful as a dancer, amber-skinned, with penetrating eyes. She wore a short white dress with little red flowers and multicolored Korean rubber slippers. Her black hair was cut short with a kind of ponytail standing straight up on the top of her head.

"I'm fine, thank you," I said. "How are you?"

FOUR YEARS LATER, JUNE 1974

My doorbell rang. It was Ruth Gruber, my collaborator on this book.

It was scarcely an hour since Ruth had dropped her bags in her own apartment. She and her daughter had just returned from Korea and Vietnam where they had gone to research the past lives of Lee Heh and Holly [my second adopted daughter from Vietnam].

"Let's start with Lee Heh," Ruth said. "I met her brothers in an orphanage in Inchon—the town where General MacArthur landed during the Korean War."

Ruth handed me the photos of the two boys.

"Margie," Ruth said. "I think I solved the puzzle. The reason Lee Heh blocked out her past so completely, language and all, Lee Heh was warned [that] she must admit to nobody that she had a family. Brainwashed."

"Who brainwashed her?"

"Let me read you my notes. Kyoo Bok, Lee Heh's older brother is speaking."

"'Our little sister was born in Kwangju—it's about 300 miles south of Seoul. Our father was a sergeant in the army. Our sister was eight months old when he died. We were poor, poor. When our sister was a little over a year, our mother took us to live in Inchon. She worked very hard to feed us. She earned a little money, sewing Korean native dresses and cleaning people's houses. We three children went with her and helped her clean floors.

"'We moved every two or three months because we had no money for rent. Still, we were happy. We played with our little sister. Our mother loved us very much.

"'At last our mother found a job that paid well. Working as a cook in the Sung Rin Orphanage in Inchon. The director let her keep us with her in the orphanage. But one day the director found out that our mother had tuberculosis. He told her she must leave right away. He put her into the Inchon Provincial Tuberculosis Hospital, and she didn't have to pay.'"

I remembered how Lee Heh had described her

mother lying on the floor sick. Not permitted to kiss her, she told me, because her mother always had a cold.

So it was TB. The disease of poverty.

"Kyoo Bok told me they had an aunt—their mother's sister. She and their mother talked things over and decided to leave the two boys in the Sung Rin Orphanage and put Lee Heh up for adoption.

"Why would she put only Lee Heh up for adoption?" I asked. "Why would she want to get rid of her one little girl?"

Ruth put her book down. "I asked myself the same question. Korea is a Confucian male-oriented culture. Boys are much more important than girls. Their mother may have thought that her little daughter, with neither father nor mother, might be doomed to living on the street—maybe have to become a prostitute."

She paused. "A girl without a family in Korea is a nonperson."

"Kyoo Bok heard his aunt warn her [little sister], 'You must never tell anybody you have a mother who's living. Or that you have two brothers. You must tell everyone that you are an orphan.'"

I felt my voice constrict.

Ruth went on. "'Our mother cried and we cried. But our little sister was very obedient.'"

"By now their mother was very ill. The aunt took Lee Heh to the police box. The police kept her for a month and when nobody came, they put her in the Star of the Sea Orphanage in Inchon. That was March 20, 1970. The nun in charge decided Lee Heh was bright and pretty, and could be adopted, so after three days they sent her to Il San—the Holt Children's Center where you found her. Her mother died a year after she came to America."

Suddenly her behavior those first months became clear to me. Her refusal to speak any Korean. Her panic when she met my father's Korean friends. Her fear that if she did anything bad I would abandon her, send her back.

"She had to bury these memories. She had to wipe them out of her consciousness in order to survive."

I had scarcely said the words when we heard, "Hi, everybody." Lee Heh rushed into the living room, hugged me, and flung her arms around Ruth. "Welcome home."

"Ruth brought you pictures of your brothers." I handed her the photos.

She shouted, "That's my brother, Kyoo Bok. And my little brother, Kyoo Sik."

She placed the photos on the glass coffee table, knelt beside them, and stared at the faces as though she wanted to imprint them on her brain.

We watched her in silence.

Then Ruth asked, "Would you like to see yourself as a little girl with your mother and father?"

Lee Heh lowered her face to the photo on the table. She looked solemn. "This must be my father because he's wearing a soldier's cap and uniform." She stared at the father whose face she had surely long forgotten.

She drew her index finger gently around her mother's fine, sensitive face, frail and thin, as if TB had begun consuming her lungs.

She took the picture and taped [it] on our living room wall. She seemed to be drawing her mother and father into our home. We were one family.

[After Lee Heh had left, Ruth continued,] "Some of the things I found out about Holly are so painful, it's going to be hard for her to relive some of this."

I was apprehensive. "I know she's been traumatized."

"Our quest began the second we landed in Vietnam. [We went] immediately to the Holt Center. There we met a key person in our search, Loan."

She pronounced it Low-Ann. "Why do I know that name?"

"She signed some of the reports that were sent to you on Holly."

"Loan gave us our first real insights on Holly's life," Ruth said. She knew Holly and . . . a lot about children with American fathers. She first met Holly in August, 1973."

August. . . . Eight months before Holly came to me.

I could almost hear Loan speaking as Ruth read

her words, "'I was looking for a child to send to my good friend—American colonel in Utah. He want to adopt Vietnamese orphan girl. I hear about a lady who keep children of bar girls. Mrs. Thu. She like a baby-sitter; keep ten mixed-race children in her house. I saw this child. She was cute. Thu Nga. You call her Thu Nga also? Or she have American name?'

"'We call her Holly,' I told her. She liked that name.

"'Pretty name. From now on, she be Holly to me, too. This lady, Mrs. Thu, say I can take Holly for my friend in America to adopt. Her foster mother very poor; she want to give her away. I take her home. I think I will keep her about 10 days, and get all her papers right, and send her to Utah.'"

Ruth's voice grew muted. "The day she brought her home, Loan noticed deep red scars around her wrists. 'I ask her what are these scars. She says her mother get electricity with sharp ends. She wind the wire around Holly's hands. Tie them together. And shock her.

"'Holly tell me sometimes her mother hung her up by the hands from the ceiling, because Holly did something wrong. She hung Holly over [a] table five or ten minutes until Holly say, "Sorry for that." Sometimes she spanked Holly with a leather belt with a heavy buckle—like a man's belt. Holly show me her back. Big, big bruises.'"

Ruth's voice choked. She stopped talking.

I couldn't sit still. I went into the kitchen where I had prepared iced tea and brought the glasses to the coffee table. Ruth sipped slowly.

"Loan really wanted to help Holly go to America, get away from all the brutality. But there were problems with her own family: 'sorry.'

"'I take her back to baby-sitter, Mrs. Thu. I tell her I can't keep her. She don't want Holly back. Foster mother don't want her back. But I don't know anyplace else.'

"In October, 1973, she went to work for Holt. A month later Holly was brought to the Holt Center by the baby-sitter, Mrs. Thu, and Holly's foster mother, Mrs. Hieu.

"This is the story Mrs. Hieu told:

"'I worked in a bar in Nha Trang. One night my friend came over to me in bar and told me she pregnant. I told her I want the baby. She say okay. But then the baby was born, she said no, she wants to keep baby. Real pretty. Then after ten days, she come to me and says lots of people want to buy her. Some even pay $200. But I will give her to you because I know you take good care of her.'

"I questioned Mrs. Hieu closely. 'When you brought Holly to Holt you told Loan you found her in a garbage can. Which story is true?'"

"'The true one is what I tell you now.'

"'Why did you make the other one up?'

"'Because I don't want Holly to know her real mother is alive.'

"I was stunned," Ruth said. "'So her real mother is alive! Where is she? What's her name?'

"'I don't know her name. I don't know where she live. Maybe far away—in Qui Nhon.'

"'Did you know Holly's father?' I asked her.

"She allowed herself a rare smile. 'I know him very well. He was a contractor.'

"Mrs. Hieu said he was about forty," Ruth explained. "'He very rich but he drink a lot. He like Holly but he didn't pay much attention. I don't know his name,' she said very quickly, lest I ask her.

"I called Loan aside and said, 'I'm beginning to think Mrs. Hieu is Holly's real mother. First she made up the garbage can story; maybe she also made up this story of her friend the bar girl.'"

"Is she really Holly's mother?" I blurted.

Ruth shrugged her shoulders. "Loan insisted she wasn't. She said, 'When Mrs. Hieu bring Holly to Holt, she never once come back to see her. A real mother always come back.'

"I asked Mrs. Hieu if she would allow us to visit her.

"She agreed. 'When you come to my house,' she said, 'I give you a present for Holly.'"

Ruth took out of her tote a brown leather zippered pouch [a picture album].

I unzipped the pouch. There was Holly as a cuddly toddler in a bathing suit with a beautiful seductive woman also in a bathing suit and carrying a parasol.

"That's Mrs. Hieu," Ruth said, "in Nha Trang—before she lost her money and her job."

I heard the key in the door. I slipped [the album] under a pillow.

Holly rushed into the living room, kissed me, and then flung her arms around Ruth.

"I so glad you home again, Ruth."

Her English was improving with astonishing speed. "I miss you. You have a good time Vie'nam? You like Vie'nam?"

"I love Vietnam, Holly," Ruth said.

[Holly asked for permission to watch TV in the bedroom and left the room.]

Ruth lowered her voice. "Two days after we saw Mrs. Hieu I decided to fly to Nha Trang where she said she had lived with Holly.

"Nguyen Minh Chieu Street was a labyrinth of alleys winding into alleys alive with bars and brothels and—in the orphanages—mixed-race children born of the bars and brothels.

"We came finally to a two-story wooden house with an outdoor flight of broken stairs and found ourselves in the very room where Holly had lived. Mrs. Thu, the baby-sitter, greeted us. She was one of the smart bar girls. She had saved her money and put it into real estate. Now she lived in one room and rented out the others."

"We had tracked down the very house Holly had lived in. But where was Mrs. Hieu?

"'She leave you present,' Mrs. Thu said. 'She not pay rent many many months. I tell her she not able to lived here if she not pay. She go away just now. She sleep on floor someplace. I don't know where she go. She very very poor.'

"Honestly, Ruth, what do you think," I whispered. "Do you think Mrs. Hieu was her mother?"

"Let's suspend judgment until we see Holly's face when she looks at the pictures of Mrs. Hieu."

I sighed. "I'm not sure we should show her the pictures right now. She's beginning to make progress now. I'm so afraid these pictures could stir everything up again."

Ruth put her hand on my arm. "I think we ought to show them to her."

I hesitated.

Holly ran into the room. "TV finished."

"Holly, honey." I made up my mind. "Come look at these pictures Ruth brought you."

I held my breath as Ruth handed her the brown leather album.

"That's my ma-ma's picture book," she shouted with amazement. She unzipped it. "Look, Mommy. My ma-ma."

It was Mrs. Hieu.

She began to squeal and coo with pleasure. "Look, Mommy, me and my ma-ma in Nha Trang. On beach. Holly little baby. So cute."

She leafed through the other pictures and then cried out, "My sister Hong. I love her. My brother Phuc. Look, he big soldier. He love me very much."

Holly put the pictures into the album and hugged it to her as if she was embracing a child. Embracing the child she had been in Nha Trang.

There was no hysteria. She nestled in Ruth's arms. "You bring me real good present from Vie'-nam, Ruth."

"It was a present from your mother, Holly. She wanted you to have these pictures so you will never forget."

In the end I realized both [Lee Heh's and Holly's] mothers had behaved the way most mothers would behave when faced by death or starvation. Lee Heh's mother gave her up only when she knew she was dying of tuberculosis. Holly's mother gave her up when she could no longer cope with hunger and hopelessness.

Both mothers gave their daughters up, to be adopted in America, in the hope they could live with decency and dignity, without hunger and without fear.

For each of their mothers it was not only an act of desperation, it was an act of love.

An Adopted Daughter Meets Her Natural Mother

BETTY JEAN LIFTON

Betty Jean Lifton, excerpt from *Twice Born: Memoirs of an Adopted Daughter*, New York: McGraw-Hill, 1975. Reprinted by permission.

> I said, "Who am I?"
> Looking into the mirror my eyes
> searched for clues.
> There were none.
> Nor were there likely to be.
> For I am adopted.

You wouldn't know it to meet me. To all outward appearances I am a writer, a married woman, a mother, a theater buff, an animal fanatic—yes, I can pass. But locked within me there is an adopted child who stirs guilty and ambivalent even as I write these words. The adopted child can never grow up. Who has ever heard of an *adopted adult*?

For most of my life my adopted state was a secret I kept from everyone, a game I played. But now I'm ready to break the rules.

Just think, I was thirty when I made the unexpected discovery that the parents I had been told were deceased at the time of my adoption had been very much alive—indeed, still might be. I was seized with a longing to know who they were—who, as the Bible puts it, begat me.

And so I started out on that perilous journey that Oedipus took so long ago. I did not expect to be the king's daughter, but I knew I could not refuse that call to adventure, which is the call to self.

I went into the labyrinth and emerged with what I sought—my story.

It took a year to find my natural mother—a year in which I contacted the adoption agency and then, armed only with her maiden name, searched tediously through musty record offices in three cities for birth, marriage, and death certificates, consulted old phone books for previous addresses, and then, in desperation, put a lawyer friend in the role of sleuth.

We finally managed to locate my mother's brother, Oran, who became the go-between. But she was recovering slowly from a glaucoma operation and was startled to hear of my reappearance. I was a painful secret in her past. After a few months of tortured indecision, she agreed to talk with me at her brother's home.

The day I went to meet my mother I dressed all in black. I often wore black, but this darkness was unrelieved by color: a black suit, black hat, black hose, black shoes, black purse. Not even a bright scarf. Although I felt joyous inside, this was not a celebration. This was something dark and secretive to be acted out in shadows. My guilt toward my adoptive parents covered me, making me invisible as I moved toward the execution of this nefarious deed.

My uncle's house in Queens reflected the simplicity of his life as an accountant. It was an unpretentious ranch house, the kind one sees sprawling over all the suburbs of this land. When he had called, he said "weather permitting" he and his wife would not be home. But it was pouring rain, and they were at the door waiting for us. "We've pulled the shades in the living room to protect her eyes," they said. She too needed that darkness.

She was sitting in a chair on the far side of the room with large sunglasses covering her eyes. I could not look into them. She rose as my husband Bob and I entered.

She was much shorter than I had imagined she would be, large hipped and bosomed. We approached each other tentatively. I'm sure the possibility of our rushing into each other's arms must have crossed her mind earlier too, but now the impossibility of it seemed to reach us both at the same time. I put out my arm, and we shook hands indecisively. Her fingers lay cold, limp in mine. Then she returned to her chair, and I perched tensely on the edge of the sofa at the opposite end of the room. Bob sat near me.

My aunt and uncle paced in the doorway like heraldic lions guarding the entrance.

According to Jung, the desire to be reunited with the mother is the desire to be reborn through her. I sat and looked at the woman across from me and knew I would not have recognized her as my mother had we passed each other on the street. Jung says the mother is a symbol of the unconscious to which an individual wishes to return in order to seek a solution for his psychic conflicts. Now here she sat in the flesh, nervously twisting a handkerchief in her lap, as ill at ease as I was. Yet everything in my life seemed to have led irrevocably to this moment. Her voice was gentle and caring as she spoke the first words.

"Betty, I want you to know you are from a good family." She used my adopted name, not Blanche—as she had named me. Then she reeled off some of the prominent New York relatives and their various professions, placing herself and me socially so that I need not look down on her, or myself.

"I expected you to look me up some day," she added to fill the silence which followed. "But I did not think it would take this long."

She began to weep at this. It was only later, much later, that I understood the true meaning of her words. She had lived with the hope that she would one day hear her daughter had fared well and was successful—perhaps that would redeem her sin. But she had also been living in fear with this secret—fear that the phone would ring one day, or a knock would come at the door that would expose her to the world.

The phone had rung, and here I was.

She was not the big, strong, all-powerful mother ready to take the frightened child in her arms and dispel the demons. She too was riddled with demons. She too was afraid: afraid of her secret, afraid of that cold, domineering, loveless mother of her own. Afraid of me. She was a disconcerting combination of self-awareness and denial, but she told me the story I had come to hear as best she could. She was brave about that.

My mother was not married to my father. She had had only a few dates with him in Freeport, Rhode Island, when her family moved, according to prior plans, to Brooklyn to be near her rabbi grandfather. When she realized she was pregnant, her wealthy aunt in Freeport tried to persuade my father to marry her. She promised an immediate annulment: all that was wanted was his signature on a piece of paper. He was a few years older, already a man about town. He refused.

A few months before I was born, my mother was shipped off by her family to a shelter for unmarried girls in Staten Island. She went there alone, unaccompanied by a relative or friend. She went in exile to that island, the waters of whose narrow channel would seem to her as wide as the oceans that separated exiled emperors and generals from the shores of their homeland. Her grief and loneliness would be as great as theirs. And she was only seventeen years old.

When her time came, my mother went alone in a taxi from the shelter to the hospital. She does not remember the hour I was born. She stayed alone in the hospital with me and then returned to the shelter for five months to nurse me. She had no visitors.

My mother said she was determined not to give me up. She must have been a strong-willed person—then. She hoped to persuade her mother to see me eventually and to allow me into the home. But my grandmother refused to recognize my existence.

My mother admitted there was talk of sitting *shiva* for her, that ceremony of mourning that Orthodox Jews hold for those prodigal children who marry out of the religion or transgress in other equally unforgivable ways and who must forever after be considered dead.

However, there was no *shiva* ceremony necessary for her since everyone soon began acting as if I had never been born. She was finally allowed back into the house, alone. Still she must have gathered strength in her exile, for in spite of the advice of social workers and other family members, she refused to part with her baby. Rather than place me for adoption, she put me in an infants' home in the Bronx and visited me there on weekends for the next year and a half.

Once her father (also afraid of her mother) dared to sneak out secretly to visit me with her. But no one else ever saw me.

"I took a job in a dress firm to support you," my mother said. "And every Sunday during visiting hours I came with a little toy. I called you 'Bubeleh,' and you held out your arms to me. You had such a lovely smile."

Here she began to weep again, and my aunt cautioned her from the doorway that she would hurt her eyes.

"But when you were older and standing up in your crib, I would look at you surrounded by all those other homeless children, and cry. 'My child should have something better than this,' I told myself."

During this period my mother kept hoping my father would call. Once she actually visited Freeport and phoned his house. He was not there. She left her office number in New York, but she did not hear from him.

"I suppose I was hoping he would change his mind and marry me when he saw you," she explained. "Then I would have had a home to take you to.

"When you were two, you had to have a mastoid operation. They told me you would die if you did not get a family of your own. They encouraged me to let you go for adoption if I really loved you. I was afraid you would die or I would never have done it."

Again she wept, and again my aunt poked her head in to caution her.

Another aunt, the wife of one of my mother's successful uncles, knew about the adoption agency run by the Reform rabbi, Stephen Wise.

"She told me you would go to a wealthy family," my mother said. "That the agency knew just the right people for you."

And so my mother, at the age of nineteen, signed the papers that released her child from her care forever. She was never told where I went or to whom. And in keeping with adoption agency practice, she was never given a report as to my progress. So does society unconsciously punish women who produce offspring out of wedlock.

Or is it conscious?

Never in this life are they allowed to see or hear of their children again. The agencies say they are protecting the "privacy" of these mothers.

In losing the battle to keep her child, my mother was like the luna moth who lays her eggs and dies. One part of her died, the part that was spirited and had dreams. From that moment she must have begun to change into the conventional, frightened, submissive woman I saw before me now. The only thing she kept of me was her secret: and this secret was to grow in her until it became one of her vital organs.

My mother became docile, even dutiful toward her own mother, who continued to put her down. Two young doctors—not one, but two—wanted to marry her, she said. But she was afraid they would find out her secret. Doctors notice things like that. When she met her first husband, a year after my adoption, she married him because he "pressured" her with kindness.

A businessman wouldn't notice.

During those years of her first marriage, my mother continued currying her mother's favor, as if only this woman could give her absolution for her crime. Then her son was born.

Her husband thought it was her first child.

When my half brother was still in my mother's womb, my father called her at her office.

"When I heard his voice, I began crying hysterically," she said. "I told him it was too late and to leave me alone. To never call me again."

He never did. We'll never know what he wanted.

After her son was born, my mother lived like a well-to-do Jewish matron. She even had a special nurse for her baby. She worked actively in philanthropy.

"One night a whole congregation at the temple stood up to honor my work. But I thought: I am not worthy of this. If they only knew what I have done. Yet I had another thought: If this could happen, couldn't something nice happen too? If only my daughter could know about this honor I am receiving tonight."

Now she knew.

When my half brother was thirteen, my mother divorced his father and moved in with her mother. She worked in a dress shop on Madison Avenue for a while. Then she married a second time.

"He was a sport like your father," she admitted with a shy smile. He followed the races—but she married him in spite of her mother's strong disapproval. "He had a daughter in her twenties, just the age you would have been. I always felt distant from her. I could never forget that she might have been you, and that *you* might have been living with us instead of her."

Again she daubed her eyes.

"You asked Oran if I was happy," she went on. "I asked him if you had asked that. I knew you would. But I want you to know that I felt I could never be happy after giving you up. There was always something unsatisfied in me that nothing could feed. I would look at other women with their daughters on the street and wonder if any of them could be you."

She didn't see the contradiction as she added: "No one knows you called except Oran and his wife. And they will keep my secret. I must not let my husband know. Or my son until he's graduated."

There was a silence as the room was washed by the waves of that secret.

Now I asked about my father. He was like a presence holding us together and yet standing between us. Who was he? What was he like?

I was unprepared for her response.

She stiffened in her chair, and her voice became tense. "I have spoken to you honestly today," she said, "and told you everything I know. But you must *never* ask your father's name."

Bob interrupted here to help me out. "His name is not important," he said softly. "But maybe you could tell Betty something about him."

I added quickly that now that I had heard her story, I certainly did not feel any kindness toward my father; my sympathy was entirely with her who had been through so much those first years.

She seemed relieved to hear this, and now her nemesis having been brought down to size, she volunteered the information that had been haunting her along with the secret.

"No one must know this," she warned. "He was a . . . a bootlegger."

"A what?" I asked. I couldn't quite understand the word she muffled in her embarrassment.

"You know . . . a rumrunner . . . a *bootlegger,*" she repeated nervously, as if federal agents might appear at the door even as she said the word.

I wanted to laugh. A bootlegger! Just like Gatsby. How romantic. How incredible.

"I'm sorry to have to tell you this," she said mournfully.

I tried to explain to her that I did not care what my father was. I had not come to judge either of them, just to learn the truth.

I asked her nothing further about my father, who being the source of me, was the source of her pain. Out of loyalty to this woman who was my mother and had tried to keep me, I closed my heart to that nameless man. It would be many years before I could bring myself to search for this part of my story.

The table in the dining room had been laid with cold cuts and open-faced sandwiches, enough to satisfy all the grown babies in that infants' home had they arrived with me. During our talk my mother would occasionally interrupt to urge Bob and me to eat something. I could not think of food, and even though Bob can always think of it, he was circumspect enough to leave the table untouched.

Now, it being almost evening, it was time to talk of food again—in earnest. Although I was a secret from the past, she insisted on taking us to a restaurant near Oran's house. She wasn't afraid of being seen with me: but then this wasn't *her* neighborhood.

She was flushed and excited, and a bit unrealistic. She spoke of having me meet a favorite aunt of hers, one of those millionaires who seemed abundant in another branch of the family but whose abundance did not spill over into her modest circumstances.

"But how would you introduce me?"

"I could say you were a niece of my husband's."

She spoke of telling my half brother about me—as soon as he graduated. She began listing some other prominent aunts, uncles, cousins.

I said as delicately as I could that I did not want to meet relatives, not now, not disguised as someone else. (I wasn't sure I wanted to meet them at all—perhaps it would make my disloyalty to my adopted family even more official.) We parted promising to see each other again before Bob and I left for Japan.

This time we embraced warmly.

But we were still strangers.

This woman had given birth to me and so she was my mother, but she had separated from me, and so she was a stranger.

Yet her whole life had been retribution for having borne me. I had influenced this stranger's life just as she had influenced mine. She had carried her loss within her longer than she had carried me.

It was all very confusing, but I did not feel disturbed by it—yet.

I was coming to grips with some of the complexities of the human condition. My mother was locked as I was in the intricate tangle of the past: I was the darling baby, the lost child, the ache in her heart; but I was also the dark secret, the one who had almost ruined her life and threatened to again.

And for me this woman was the beautiful lost mother, but she was also the one who had abandoned me.

I kissed her on the cheek as we parted. I promised to write while we were in Japan but to address my letters to her brother, Oran, who would relay them to her, thus preventing her husband and son from ever seeing them.

I promised to help her keep her secret.

It was a light casual kiss I gave her, like the brush of a butterfly's wing.

What Do You Love about Being a Lesbian Mom?

CATHERINE GUND

Catherine Gund, excerpt from *Letters of Intent*, New York: Free Press, 1999. Reprinted by permission.

Today, many of my lesbian friends have kids ranging from newborn to ten years old. When I came out I didn't assume being a lesbian and being a mother were mutually exclusive. I never thought I couldn't or wouldn't have children. And so my lover, Melanie, and I have. Our baby girl Sadie Rain will turn three years old on November 1, 1999.

A few years ago, with four other couples, we had some informal dinners and ongoing conversations about choosing to have children. We talked about adoption, foster care, and pregnancy. Also about how to get pregnant, anonymous or known donors, known donors as daddies or uncles. We discussed using midwives or doctors, our parents' presumed reactions, which one of each couple would carry, how many kids we wanted, whose biological clock was ticking the loudest, whose relationships were solid enough for this calling, and so on. From that group, we now have two girls and at least five more babies twinkling in their mothers' eyes. In our little circle, as in the wider United States society, there is a veritable lesbian baby boom under way.

It's a cliché to say that many aspects of parenting are the same for everyone; we all change diapers, have nursing and feeding routines, bathe the little ones, create spaces and time for them to sleep and play, and consider their health, safety, intelligence, looks, and well-being. A cliché maybe, but all that is true. However, as lesbian moms, we have a good share of unique issues to deal with.

In our case, we have a known donor who lives nearby and will know our daughter and be part of her life. Since most of our friends have used anonymous donors, we didn't have a lot of known-donor role models (maybe the next generation will have that in us!).

On Becoming a Grandmother

FRANCINE KLAGSBRUN

Francine Klagsbrun, "On Becoming a Grandmother," *The Jewish Week*, February 19, 1999. Reprinted by permission.

As of this writing, my first grandchild, a girl, has turned a week and a half old. Even as I type that sentence, every part of it fills me with amazement: That I have actually become a grandmother, a status I have longed for but cannot yet fathom; that this tiny being has already passed the milestone of a week and a half of life; that I am able to use my fingers for typing when, to paraphrase the psalmist, all my bones cry out in joy, "God, who is like You?"

She was born on a Friday evening, not long after sundown. "Friday's child is loving and giving," the old nursery rhyme says. But a Shabbat eve child is something more, a gift delivered to this world by the Sabbath Queen. I wonder if her parents will remember to tell her that some day.

Right now they cannot stop marveling at the miracle of this person in miniature—the little hands with their surprisingly long fingers, the perfect head with its downy coat of hair, the feet that curl to the touch. "Can you imagine," my son-in-law says in awe, "that just a short time ago, this complete human being was inside her mother?"

I cannot imagine it. In spite of the billions of babies born on this earth, I still cannot imagine how from a microscopic speck of sperm and egg a human being develops. In spite of photographs and sonograms, I cannot picture how that being lives and thrives within its mother's womb. Like my daughter and son-in-law, I can only gaze in astonishment at our newest family member. To look at her is to see God's handiwork. To look at her is to witness Creation.

For me there is also another miracle, one the couple cannot recognize. It is the miracle of their immediate transformation from children to parents themselves. My daughter feeds her baby day and night tenderly, without a moment's impatience, although she's fatigued from childbirth and lack of sleep. My son-in-law reads and talks to the infant, knowing full well that she doesn't understand a word he is saying, yet reveling in every changed expression. In some ways they're like kids playing house.

But in more ways they see themselves fully as parents now.

And as parents have always done, they're ready to place their child's well-being above their own. That is surely the essence and miracle of human parenthood.

I'm not certain what the essence of grandparenthood is. Part of it, I know, is letting go of your grown children so they can exercise their own parental roles without interference.

After my daughter told me she was expecting a child, she went impulsively to her closet and pulled out an album of her baby photos. We looked through the pictures together for more than an hour, holding on tightly to the past before allowing ourselves to venture into the future.

But another part of grandparenthood is being available to help our children in rearing their children. In today's high-pressured world, where mothers and fathers juggle a million obligations, they need all the help and support we can give.

The trick, of course, is to balance being available with letting go, giving with nonmeddling. To a great extent that has always been the hardest challenge of parenthood. The balancing act just becomes more delicate now, when we must be parents to grown children who are parents themselves.

I've said little so far about the grandparent-grandchild relationship itself. That's because it is still a mystery to me.

My granddaughter will grow up in a world I cannot begin to foresee. She will never know a home or classroom devoid of computers. She may have friends who are clones of their relatives and eat genetically powered foods as yet uninvented. Bill Clinton and Monica Lewinsky will be ancient history to her, and my parents and in-laws only distant names on a family tree.

How will I relate to this unknown being? After my daughter was born, my father-in-law, who spoke Yiddish-accented English, took speech lessons because he wanted to communicate clearly with his granddaughter. I, too, will do my best to keep up with the trends and patterns of her world.

But like grandparents throughout time, I will also try to ground her in my world, in the art that I love and the Jewish texts that have been a passion of my existence. People say that grandchildren represent our immortality, our compensation for having given up the tree of life for the tree of knowledge. Our best assurance of that immortality as Jews is passing on our teachings to each new generation. That I hope to do.

Meanwhile, I will love and cuddle the beautiful being who has joined our family. The Midrash says that the soul of every newborn dwells in the Garden of Eden until the moment of conception.

This soul, released into our lives, has touched us with paradise.

CHAPTER 7

Menopause and Aging

IF THERE IS AN AREA OF WOMEN'S HEALTH that has epitomized several mechanisms through which sexism works in medicine, it is menopausal health. From the age-old desire to equate women's gynecological transitions with mental instability and disease to broadly prescribing under-tested drugs and preying on fears about aging and sexuality: You name it, and menopausal women have been subjected to it.

By the 1990s, Premarin, the most popular type of hormone treatment (HT), had become the best-selling drug in America. Doctors and journalists alike dealt with hormone treatment as if it were as natural a part of menopause as unpredictable periods or hot flashes. Large observational trials and small clinical studies touted unproven health benefits from fewer wrinkles to a healthier heart. And yet, despite the fact that Premarin had been on the market for nearly fifty years, there were still no randomized, double-blind long-term clinical trials of any decent size. This changed when Wyeth Ayerst—the maker of Premarin—sought to get the drug approved by FDA for preventing heart disease. Although it had been prescribed "off label" (without an official "OK" from FDA) for years for that purpose, Wyeth Ayerst had never "made it legal." The only official uses of the drug remained the curbing of hot flashes and vaginal dryness and the building of bone.

During approval hearings, it seemed all but certain that Wyeth would emerge victorious. Until Cindy Pearson stepped in. A lifelong women's health activist and the director of the National Women's Health Network, Pearson pointed out that no drug had been prescribed for heart protection in men—not even aspirin—that had not had to undergo serious clinical trials. Pearson's point highlighted the sexism inherent in many drugs prescribed primarily for women—that doctors and FDA were taking a "shoot first and apologize later" approach. Pearson's testimony and the guerrilla activism of Philip Corfman, a long-time FDA employee and friend of the women's health movement, led to the establishment of the Women's Health Initiative (WHI).

The results of the WHI shocked the world and overturned long-held menopause paradigms. It turned out that estrogen *hurt* the heart, as well as causing a host of other problems including cancer, strokes, blood clots, gall bladder disease, increased rates of Alzheimer's disease, and urinary incontinence. While interpreting the WHI results is still a matter of furious debate, one thing that is not is that long-term hormone supplementation in most older women is a bad idea. (Those who have undergone hyster- and oophorectomy are a notable exception and benefit from some hormone treatment.)

The shock that most women—and their doctors—greeted the WHI results with surprised me. In 1977, I wrote a best-selling book called *Women and the Crisis in Sex Hormones* in which I outlined a subject that was becoming familiar territory to me: the dangers of estrogen drugs including birth control pills, DES, and hormone and estrogen therapy (ET) for menopause. It was a different moment: The women's movement generally and the women's health movement specifically had raised women's awareness about serious health abuses they were being subjected to. Problems with birth control pills, DES, and other drugs had been recently revealed and women were ready to be skeptical about any drug that put forth claims that far outstretched its proven benefits. In 1975 the *New England Journal of Medicine* reported in a series of articles that the risk of endometrial cancer in estrogen users was five to fourteen times higher than nonusers, and the FDA responded by ordering label changes which warned of the potentially lethal effects of the drugs. In one of *Women and the Crisis in Sex Hormone's* final chapters, I wrote hopefully, "Nineteen Seventy-Five was a year of reckoning for the American Doctor . . . Nineteen Seventy-Five was also a year when the ERT patient, most particularly, discovered she was getting less that she thought, and more than she bargained for."

I hoped that women were finally wising up about hormones. I had good reason to believe that things had changed, that the tide had turned. And for a while I was right. The fact that HT and ET were able to mount such a successful comeback leads me to believe that activism on menopause will always be necessary to prevent us from reliving the mistakes of the past.

That said, menopausal women have come a long way from the days when doctors prescribed them opium for their symptoms and nice women didn't speak about such experiences even with friends. Today there is a menopause industry, with books, products, and even a musical. Talk shows like *Oprah* and major magazines like *Time* have made menopause their top subject. With such visibility comes new dangers—many of the over-the-counter products touted for menopause are little better than snake oil, and many of the sources of health information ersatz or worse—pharma-funded.

My hope is that we will learn from the WHI and move toward a more natural understanding of menopause that allows women to get through the transition with the greatest possible ease and enjoy what anthropologist Margaret Mead called "postmenopausal zest."

For years the physical process of menopause has been conflated with the larger process of aging. While the two are discrete, menopause is often the first time when women in our ageist society are given the opportunity to think long and hard about their health as they get older. As the baby boomers begin to navigate the passage between middle and older age, generations of women used to fighting for their rights are confronting and challenging new forms of discrimination.

The Veteran Feminists of America are not a group of women accustomed to remaining silent on any issue. When they gathered in the fall of 2006 to celebrate a new book—*Women Who Changed America, 1963–1975*—they came to share memories of years of activism, the successes and the failures. They also wanted to have a conversation about what battles they were still passionate about, what issues they still wanted to organize around. Some were familiar—continuing activism around abortion rights, the wage gap, even the ERA. The most popular new issue, by far, was the issue of ageism and cultural attitudes toward older women.

Former Boston Women's Health Book Collective member and one of the original authors of *Our Bodies, Ourselves*, Joan Ditzion, writes with passion about ageism, and about the experiences that led her to fight it. This is, unfortunately, an issue that needs much activism. Even as the Baby Boomer generation moves toward old age in the next couple decades and an unprecedented number of people approach seniority, we are increasingly a culture obsessed with youth, confronted with a host of pharmaceuticals as well as beauty and lifestyle products aimed at keeping our bodies young, many of which carry serious and ill-understood risks.

Flashback: A History of Menopause

LAURA ELDRIDGE AND BARBARA SEAMAN

© 2003 by Laura Eldridge and Barbara Seaman. A version of this article appeared in *The No-Nonsense Guide to Menopause*, New York: Simon and Schuster, 2008.

We probably don't need to tell you that human beings are special and different from other animals. But what feature distinguishes us the most? Our large brains? Our opposable thumbs? For women, there is another aspect of our biology that sets us apart from even some of our closest relatives in the animal kingdom. Although there is some debate in the scientific community, it is generally agreed that humans are among a *very* small set of creatures that live long after our sexual reproductive capabilities end.

Although some apes—chimpanzees and other close human relatives—have a maximum reproductive capacity of around twenty-five years, it is rare for those species to live more than a couple years beyond losing the ability to have babies. Lest you think that is simply a product of their harsh lives in nature, scientists have found that these animals' other organs, upon death, are worn by age in a way that human organs wouldn't be

until extreme old age. These primates aren't meant to outlive childbearing. Human females are.

There are a handful of other animals that may share this strange trait with us—among them certain whales and African elephants.[1]

So when did we become different from the other apes? When did menopause really *begin*? It is possible that when humans first evolved, women were able to keep having babies until they died. At some point this changed. It's hard to say exactly when, but fossils suggest it was a long time ago,[2] perhaps 1.6 million years,[3] before homo sapiens replaced their prehuman ancestors.

Perhaps it was because of environmental changes that required homo erectus (a prehuman animal that was different from both apes and modern humans) to seek out harder-to-get foods,[4] or maybe because infant brains had begun to grow and offspring required more and longer care. Regardless of the reason, women began to live for much longer periods of time than they could have babies for.

One popular idea about why this happened is called the "Grandmother Hypothesis," and it holds that women enjoy long postreproductive lives to give their offspring an advantage by providing additional caretaking for grandchildren. This allows a woman's daughter to reproduce at a younger age and to have more children with the confidence that they will receive proper care. Also in a time before books and written records, grandparents became repositories for carrying on important knowledge,[5] human libraries handing out survival tips long before the advent of recorded wisdom.

This idea has had its critics. Anthropologist Jocelyn Scott Peccei is prominent among them. She argues that the "Grandmother Hypothesis" has some pretty serious holes in it. First and foremost, Peccei points out, it ignores the role of men in both helping get food and aiding in childcare. She cautions that "one cannot overlook male investment in an explanation of menopause," and adds that older men, who remain fertile to varying degrees until extreme old age or death, would have been just as capable as their aging female counterparts of providing extra family support.

Instead, Peccei advocates a competing idea called the "Mother Hypothesis." In this version of the story, as humans evolved it took more and more energy to raise babies and keep them healthy and safe. Women who stopped reproducing at a young age were at an evolutionary advantage because they would have more energy to put in to their existing children.[6] It also increased the likelihood that they would live long enough to provide proper support to their young.

Regardless of which of these ideas is true (we will never know, alas) it seems that middle-aged women had a great value in their families and societies. Menopause in ancient times, as today, became a vehicle through which women could transform themselves and do important work to improve both their own lives and those around them.

Although historical evidence about menopause is scarce before the fifteenth or sixteenth century, references can be found. They don't tell us much about the experience of earlier women, but they do tell us some very important things. An ancient Egyptian medical papyrus tells of a woman who hasn't menstruated in many years and is suffering from a battery of physical problems including nausea, vomiting, and burning in the stomach. Deborah Sweeny writes, "the diagnosis is not that the woman is growing older but that she has been bewitched."[7] In 1250 BCE, a Hittite king named Hattusilis wrote to Ramses II for help with his aging sister. Didn't the Egyptian ruler have some sort of medicine that could help his sixty-year-old sibling bear children? Ramses replied matter-of-factly that at that age, there was probably nothing even his best doctors could do to help.[8] These examples reveal two equally important details: In the second story, it is clear from Ramses's response that it is common knowledge that aging women become infertile. The first story reveals that even millennia before the common era, menopause was already in the process of being medicalized and explained with ill-supported rationales. Witchcraft and hormone

deficiency disease are the answers of two very different moments to menopause, but they still represent attempts to pathologize this natural process.

By the late middle ages, it was commonly believed that menstruation was necessary for cleaning out the body. In twelfth-century Italy, a female doctor named Trotula of Salerno wrote about menopause, menstruation, and the differences between male and female health. Trotula believed that men and women were composed of converse but complementary biologies, with men bearing too much heat and women too much moisture. Her view—and it was the popular one for centuries to come—was that this excess moisture (later specifically blood) collected in the body at unhealthy levels when not alleviated through monthly bleeds. She notes that menstruation lasts "up to about the fiftieth year if (the patient) is lean; sometimes up to the sixtieth or sixty-fifth if she is moist; in the moderately fat up to about forty-five."[9] Even in the midst of a lot of incorrect ideas about menopause, the good doctor is observing something crucial: Lifestyle factors play a role in when and how periods stop.

Another Italian—the sixteenth-century doctor Giovanni Arinello—gives a laundry list of the potential problems awaiting a woman, including "pains . . . apostemata, eye disorders, weak sight, vomiting, fever."[10] Perhaps most shockingly, he adds, women desired sex more than ever. By this point, doctors believed that menstrual blood served an essential purgative function, cleaning the body of toxins and bad chemicals. Or perhaps simply getting rid of excess blood. Either way, when a woman failed to menstruate, these bad substances built up in the body and at best would make a woman sick. One theory held that the blood converted to fat, and that was why menopausal women gained weight. At worst, experts feared, the extra blood might actually kill the female patient. There were dissenters to this alarmist view: in 1582, a Frenchman named Jean Liebault observed that the change "does no harm to the woman's body."[11] Liebault writes of more benign symptoms including what he calls "petites rougeurs"—"little reds"—most certainly hot flashes.

By the eighteenth century, with the boom of print culture, the first menopause manuals were printed. They were exceedingly popular—it has always been very clear that when information is made available, women are hungry to receive it. This century also saw a boom in potentially dangerous pharmaceuticals: These preparations, including "Pills of Rufus," "Pills of Frank," "The Sacred Tincture," and "Elixier de Propriete" were wildly popular, despite the fact that doctors scorned them as the province of female health experts who were, in the opinion of most male physicians, little better than witches. The doctor's solution, it should be mentioned, was far worse than the mostly herbal and narcotic ingredients in early pills: bleeding was recommended in the hope that letting blood from other parts of the body would relieve pressure on the reproductive organs.

The word "menopause" is a relatively recent one. It was in the second half of the ninetieth century that the word became common parlance. It was originally coined by a French doctor named Gardanne in his book treatise *On the Menopause: or The Critical Time for Women*. At the time, menopause was known in English as "the dodging time."[12]

The concept of "climacteric," popular in the nineteenth century, was an idea applied equally to men and women. This notion more closely resembled our "midlife crisis," and had been in circulation in "educated circles"[13] since the middle ages. Some nineteenth-century doctors observed that while women experienced climacteric, it was much worse and much more pronounced in male patients.

After centuries of purgation and bleeding serving as the main treatments for a bad menopause, late nineteenth-century doctors, full of their own growing power and new knowledge, came up with what they thought represented a true advance in medicine for midlife women: the prophylactic hysterectomy. For a doctor like the American gynecologist Edward Curry, the growing popularity of "female castration" represented a leap into modernity, the opening of centuries of shuttered dustiness in women's medicine.[14] Curry became a great advocate for the procedure, explaining that if you were going to remove the uterus and fallopian tubes, you might as well take the ovaries too. This idea has had a particularly persistent popularity with modern doctors, who have often taken the attitude that "while you're in there" you should make sure you finish the job. Around the same time Curry was taking out his patients' organs, other doctors were jumping on the "pill" bandwagon, employing more traditional herbs and opiates as well as newer drugs based on animal reproductive organs.

In the early twentieth century, drug companies would take on this effort to find new and better ways to medicate menopause. We will learn more about this later in this chapter when we talk about hormone therapy.

Also in the twentieth century, the growing field of psychoanalysis offered its own answers about midlife women. Janice Delaney, Mary Jane Lupton, and Emily Toth explain, "Victorian medicine men knew in their hearts that during the menopause, a woman could expect to have mental problems."[15] No less an authority than Sigmund Freud wrote that women "become quarrelsome and obstinate, petty and stingy, show typical sadistic . . . features which they did not show before."

NOTES

1. Lynette Leidy Sievert, *Menopause: A Biocultural Perspective* (New Brunswick and London: Rutgers University Press, 2006), 47.
2. Ibid., 48.
3. Jocelyn Scott Peccei, "A Critique of the Grandmother Hypothesis," *American Journal of Human Biology*, 2001, 13, 434–452.
4. Mirkka Lahdenpera, Virpi Lummaa, Samuli Helle, Marc Tremblay, Andrew F. Russell, "Fitness benefits of prolonged post-reproductive lifespan in women," *Nature*, Vol 428, March 11, 2004,178–181.
5. Barry Bogin and B. Holly Smith, "Evolution of the Human Life Cycle," *American Journal of Human Biology*, 1996 (8): 703–716.
6. Jocelyn Scott Peccei, "A hypothesis for the origin and evolution of menopause," *Maturitas*, 1995 (1): 83–89.

7. Deborah Sweeney, "Elder Women in Ancient Egypt," Tel Aviv University, www.tau.ac.il/humanities/archae-ology/projects/sweeneyproj.htm.

8. Ibid.

9. *Women's Lives in Medieval Europe: A Sourcebook*, Emilie Amt, Ed., London: Routledge, 1993.

10. Michael Stolberg, "A Woman's Hell?: Medical Perceptions of Menopause in Preindustrial Europe," *Bulletin of the History of Medicine*, Vol. 73, no. 3: 404–428.

11. Ibid.

12. Margaret Lock and Patricia Kaufert, "Menopause Local Biologies and Cultures of Aging," *American Journal of Human Biology*, 2001, 13, 494–504.

13. Ibid.

14. Janice Delaney, Mary Jane Lupton, and Emily Toth, *The Curse* (New York: E.P. Dutton and Co., Inc., 1976),182.

15. Ibid.

16. Ibid.

The Changing Years

MADELINE GRAY

Madeline Gray, excerpt from *The Changing Years: What to Do about the Menopause*, New York: Doubleday & Company, Inc., 1953. Reprinted by permission.

You're in your fifties, your forties, or even your thirties, and you're worried. Lately, strange things have begun to happen to you.

You woke up with a start the other night, perhaps out of a deep, sound sleep. A great wave of heat was spreading clear up over your body to the top of your head, drenching your nightdress and making you run to open the windows wide.

Or you have been having a series of whole-day blinding headaches. Not the old kind of headaches a couple of aspirins used to chase, but nauseating "sick" headaches with pain so intense your footsteps seem to echo like thunder as you walk from the bedroom to the bathroom door.

Or there have been days where your heart beat so loudly it seemed the whole world could hear it. Or other days when you were so inexplicably tired you could hardly drag yourself to the grocery store four blocks away.

While that old business of menstruation has been acting up also—either skipping a month or arriving like a flood.

Then what has been happening to your private world where everything had been so comparatively serene? The other day, for instance, you actually cuffed your daughter hard in a crazy outburst of temper when she did something you'd been amused at the day before. Then the same evening at dinner you got furious at your husband for smacking his lips over his pork chops when for years you rather laughed at the habit, saying it proved he enjoyed your cooking if nothing else. And to top it all you'd bawled like a baby when Junior, to whom you'd said for months, "Isn't it about time you settled down and got married?" came home and announced he'd gotten the girl of his choice to say yes.

Why the strange physical upsets? Why the even stranger mental instability? Gradually it dawns on you: This is it! The menopause—the dreaded "change of life." It is happening to you at last.

And you may be quite worried by the situation—not so much by one thing as by the whole picture. A few passing aches and pains you can take in your stride. But suppose it adds up to permanent trouble? Loss of energy forever? Headaches and temper outbursts indefinitely? Maybe even loss of figure, loss of your sex life, loss of your husband's love, loss of your mind? All the old fears drawn from centuries of gossip and ignorance crowd in upon you. The picture looks dark indeed.

Well, you're not the only one to feel this way.

Every year in the United States alone about 18 million women are in the same predicament as you are—faced with what you are facing, asking the same questions that are tormenting you.

I asked them myself until recently. In fact, that's how I happened to write this book.

A few years ago I had what is known as a surgical menopause—a change brought on by an operation. That means I was thrown into the midst of this thing headlong. I had no time even to get mentally "set."

And as I lay on my hospital bed, hardly out of

the anesthetic, all the old fears crowded in on me a hundredfold. What was I actually in for? What would happen to me? I was afraid I'd grow a mustache and gain forty pounds at the very least. But really I hadn't the faintest idea.

The first chance I got I cornered the surgeon who had operated on me and plied him with questions. But while he was a distinguished man and had done an excellent job, he was both far too busy and too abrupt to bother with me. He answered that he'd done what he had to do, and that was that. As to my future worries, he curtly dismissed them by telling me to go home and forget about the whole thing. Besides, the worries were all imaginary anyway.

This answer got me twice as worried as before. As if one could forget what one didn't understand! As if there is such a thing as an "imaginary" pain! A pain is a pain. It may have a mental rather [than] a physical origin—that is, be caused by fear or misunderstanding, and so originate mainly in the mind. But that doesn't make it "imaginary" in the sense that you think you have a pain when you haven't. When you have a pain, you *have* one. And I had several at the moment, believe me.

So with my surgeon ruled out as a source of information I next tried questioning some friends of my own age. But they knew less than I did. Worse, they knew all the horror stories. "You know Sarah Y. down the block?" they declared to me in hushed whispers. "*She* went out of her mind during the menopause. Yes, positively out!" Or: "I hear Mary G. lost her husband Tom to another woman. And you could hardly blame Tom. After all, poor Mary had become quite useless in the realm of sex." Or: "Remember old lady Brown? She got both high blood pressure and arthritis during her change, and never was the same again."

My friends evidently enjoyed telling me these juicy stories. But they hardly improved my peace of mind.

So then I tried speaking to some older women who had gone through the menopause, figuring they might tell me something nearer to the truth. Alas!

The results were no better than before. Some older women harped also on the theme "all the troubles are imaginary." This seemed to be because they themselves had had no trouble, which is of course often the case. And some went to the other extreme and boasted how, instead of the troubles being imaginary, they had been tortured for years. While still others actually told me to *expect* suffering, "because suffering is the badge of all women." Didn't the Bible say, "In sorrow thou shalt bring forth children?" And didn't that apply to the menopause as well?

Next I looked for books that might help me. But there were none at the time that seemed to answer all my questions satisfactorily. None at all.

Finally, in desperation, I decided there was no other solution: I was a writer and a former teacher; I would have to tackle it from scratch and do a book myself. Moreover, I was right in the midst of the experience. If I could learn the truth about the matter it would solve my own problems and maybe help others as well.

Yet the job wasn't going to be easy. It would mean talking to dozens and dozens of doctors—not only surgeons, but general practitioners, gland specialists, psychiatrists; and not only in the United States, but also in England, Canada, wherever knowledge was to be found. Tracking down the whole elusive subject like a detective tracks down clues. Especially it would mean tracking down the answer to the most haunting question of all: Why does a woman get *over* her menopausal troubles if she has any? She surely does get over them—practically all older women are living examples of that. But why? What happens inside of her to make the adjustment? Why does she come out at the other end of the experience practically as good as she went in?

So I started to work tackling this and every other question that puzzled me. I worked at the Academy of Medicine in New York, I traveled around the country, spending long hours in clinics, talking to both women and doctors. And I wrote letters, letters, and letters. Hardly a morning went by without my hopping out of bed eagerly to see what the mail had brought.

At last, after four years, I was through. Through with my search and through with my menopause. And during that four years I found out the great principle at work within us—"the wisdom of the body"—which brings us back to ourselves. I also found out that we do not lose our sex lives, do not lose our figures, do not lose our husbands, and certainly do not lose our minds.

And as I found out these things I had this remarkable experience: knowledge completely cast out my fears. Even on my darkest menopausal days (and having had a surgical menopause some of those days were quite dark indeed, since surgical changes are much more drastic than normal ones)— even on my dark days I was optimistic. Not with the silly optimism of a Pollyanna or a Coué who blindly repeats "day by day in every way I am getting better and better," but an optimism based on fact.

I learned, for example, that prolonged menopausal suffering is almost unnecessary, since there is now, for the first time in history, blessed menopausal medicine to help. Our mothers may have had to suffer; not us. We are the first generation lucky enough to have this help.

I learned how to answer the people who argue that the Bible says we *must* suffer and not use menopausal medicine. For the same people used the Bible against the introduction of anesthesia in childbirth—used it until a witty Scotch doctor answered them with an equally good quotation: "And the Lord caused a deep sleep to fall upon Adam, and in that sleep brought forth Eve." Deep sleep is the best anesthetic in the world, the learned doctor pointed out. Surely the Lord intended people to have help from pain. So the skeptics should have been silenced once and for all. Though it still took Queen Victoria using anesthesia for the birth of her seventh child to make it fashionable, so fashionable that it was known for a long time as "the anesthesia of the Queen."

But, most important, I learned why the blessed menopausal medicine is often not even needed, for the simple reason that no menopausal trouble occurs.

For the menopause is merely another forward-moving step—like a step in a dance. It is not a disease, and brings with it no disease. As a result, many of us take this step so easily, so comfortably, we need no help from first to last. Our own "wisdom of the body" sees us through.

Promise Her Anything, but Give Her . . . Cancer: The Selling of ERT

BARBARA SEAMAN

Barbara Seaman and Gideon Seaman, excerpt from *Women and the Crisis in Sex Hormones,* New York: Bantam Books, 1978. Originally published in 1977 by Rawson. Reprinted by permission.

By 1947, a dazzling array of estrogen products, some combined with thyroid, were competing for a place on the American doctor's prescription pad. DES and other female sex hormones were available, from dozens of companies, by mouth, by vagina, and by long-acting and short-acting injection.

In ads in the medical journals, the early Premarin woman was shown waltzing with Arthur Murray's double, while the patient who liked her nightly "nip" could have Lynoral Elixir, "The Most Potent Oral Estrogen in a Pleasant-tasting Cordial" (and in a 14 percent alcohol base).

GUSBERG'S WARNING

In the midst of all these cheery advertisements— six full pages of the December 1947 issue of the *American Journal of Obstetrics and Gynecology* — an alarm was sounded by S. B. (Saul) Gusberg, who was then a young gynecologist and cancer researcher at the Sloane Hospital and Columbia University in New York.

"Another human experiment has been set up in recent years by the widespread administration of estrogens to postmenopausal women," Gusberg said. He went on to point out that the relatively low cost of oral estrogen and the ease of administration had made its general use "promiscuous." Uterine bleeding provoked in patients by this medication had become so commonplace that at Gusberg's hospital the expression "stilbestrol bleeding" was employed to describe those cases admitted for diagnostic curettage.

What did all these curettages (uterine scrapings) in Estrogen Replacement Therapy (ERT) patients reveal? The pathology reports showed that ERT overstimulates the endometrium, or lining of the uterus, producing among other effects, "crowding of the glands into a lawless pattern."

Gusberg speculated that it was not the dosage of ERT, not the specific product, but *long-term exposure* that causes harm. (Research completed in 1975 showed Gusberg to be correct on two points out of three: Duration of use and high-dose levels are both significant in producing cancer, while product differences appear to be inconsequential.) Early as it was in the ERT game, by 1947 Gusberg had collected twenty-nine cases of women whose endometria were profoundly disturbed by estrogen therapy—twenty with a possibly premalignant condition called hyperplasia, which often necessitates hysterectomy, and nine with cancer itself.

The scholarly gynecologists, those who had read the articles as well as the ads in their monthly journals, responded swiftly to Gusberg's work. They also collected cancer cases, and the promiscuous use of ERT slowed or at least stabilized . . . that is, until January 1966, when the M. Evans Co. published a book called *Feminine Forever*, by a handsome, avuncular Brooklyn physician named Robert Wilson.

WILSON VERSUS LIVING DECAY

Feminine Forever, which was excerpted in *Look* and *Vogue* and sold 100,000 copies in the first several months, promised that menopause could be averted and aging allayed with ERT.

Wilson was wholly dismissed as a quack by his more sober colleagues, but rarely in public and always off the record. Even good friends of estrogen, or at least the pill, were growling among themselves.

Sherwood Kaufman of Planned Parenthood fumed at a medical meeting: "The situation has gotten ridiculous. Women come in asking for the 'Youth Pill,' and they say 'Check my estrogen levels.' From what they've read, they think it's as simple as driving into a gasoline station and having their oil checked."

Wilson, in the short space of an article in *Look* magazine, listed twenty-six symptoms that the Youth Pill would avert. These included nervousness, irritability, anxiety, apprehension, hot flashes, night sweats, joint pains, melancholia, palpitations, crying spells, weakness, dizziness, severe headache, poor concentration, loss of memory, chronic indigestion, insomnia, frequent urination, itching of the skin, dryness of the eye, nose and mouth, backache, neuroses, a tendency to take alcohol and sleeping pills, or even to contemplate suicide.

"While not all women are affected by menopause to this extreme degree," Wilson conceded, "no woman can be sure of escaping the horror of this *living decay.*"

Reporters at the *New Republic* and the *Washington Post* called attention to the money Wilson received from drug companies. In a 1969 book, *The Pill, An Alarming Report*, Morton Mintz of the *Post* summarized:

"The Wilson Research Foundation, headed by Dr. Wilson . . . received, in 1964, $17,000 from the Searle Foundation . . . $8,700 from Ayerst Laboratories and $5,900 from the Upjohn Company."

By November 1966, the FDA was on to Wilson. They formally notified the Searle Company that he was unacceptable as an investigator for Enovid in menopause because he was disseminating promotional material claiming that the drug had been shown to be effective for conditions for which it had never been approved. *And to this day, neither the FDA nor any other scientific body has ever approved Premarin or other hormone products as a preventive to aging.*

When we interviewed Robert Wilson in 1976, he commented truthfully enough: "There are some people who don't like me. They say I shouldn't do what I'm doing. They say that menopause is a natural process. We should grow old gracefully and enjoy it."

Then he warmed to his topic: "They say we should do nothing to retard menopause. Just think of that. Isn't that dreadful? The estrogen regimen should start at age nine—*nine to ninety*. It's necessary to begin then, and to check your estrogen level all through life, so that it never leaves you. Don't allow it to."

We asked Wilson to comment on endometrial cancer. "That's the worst lie in the world," he said, "the worst fallacy. I have over forty doctors working all over the world, Switzerland, Czechoslovakia, all over the world, and we haven't seen one case of cancer."

THE SERVICE FOR MEDIA

Other pro-ERT books followed Wilson's, including *After Forty* by Sondra Gorney and Claire Cox, published in 1973.

On the jacket of *After Forty*, Sondra Gorney is identified as "Executive Director of the Information Center on the Mature Woman." What the cover fails to mention is that the Information Center, formerly located in New York City, and finally closed in 1976, was a "service for media" thoughtfully provided by Wyeth-Ayerst, manufacturer of Premarin.

The Pharmaceutical Manufacturers Association, to which Wyeth-Ayerst belongs, has a code of ethics which maintains that prescription drugs will not be directly promoted to the public. Wyeth-Ayerst, in violation of the code, hired the talented and energetic Ms. Gorney to provide free filler items, lauding ERT, to magazines, newspapers, and other mass media—rarely, if ever, with any indication that the source was a drug company.

A typical "background paper" from Wyeth-Ayerst states: "It was once believed that the change of life meant every woman had to resign herself to years of anguish and suffering. . . . When ovarian production stops, a woman's endocrine system is thrown into disarrangement. . . . Emotional problems can affect entire families. If not overcome, they can cause lasting harm to a woman's personality."

CLOUDS ON THE HORIZON

Wyeth-Ayerst's slogan "Keep Her on Premarin" succeeded.

Millions of normal woman were staying on Premarin for an average of a decade or longer. Most stopped only when they had to stop, because of side effects, such as the uterine bleeding noted so long ago by Gusberg.

Others, many others, were taken off Premarin because of changes in the breast tissue, or allergic reactions, or edema, or metabolic disturbances, or gallbladder disease. A standoff developed between the physicians who prescribed long-term ERT, most often gynecologists, and those who mopped up after it.

Even so, in all the years since Gusberg's brilliant early report, no well-controlled studies comparing cancer frequency in human ERT users and refusers has been completed. Thus, defenders of ERT argued that a cause-and-effect association had not been proven, and that the extent of risk, if any, remained unquantified. Cancer specialists knew it was just a matter of time.

THE BUBBLE BURSTS

The time came. In the fall of 1975 rumors were flying in the drug industry and among knowledgeable physicians and science reporters. The *New England Journal of Medicine*, it was whispered, was to publish a series of articles comparing ERT users and nonusers, and showing that the risks of endometrial cancer in the former increased five- to fourteen-fold!

However it came to them, Wyeth-Ayerst knew the specific content of the *New England Journal* articles before publication.

This gave Wyeth-Ayerst time to tool up its propaganda machine. Wyeth-Ayerst sent a "Dear Doctor" letter concerning Premarin to physicians across the United States.

The letter was reassuring, making it appear that the *New England Journal* articles were "weak studies," and that the link between ERT and cancer was not really established. Meantime the physicians who advocated the Youth Pill found it hard to retreat:

"I think of the menopause as a deficiency disease, like diabetes," a San Francisco gynecologist told the *New York Times*. "Most women develop some symptoms whether they are aware of them or not, so I prescribe estrogens for virtually all menopausal women for an indefinite period."

"Everything in life is a trade-off—there are risks and benefits, and you must weigh one against the other," said another gynecologist.

However, these male physicians, unlike their patients, were not personally at risk. We wonder: Would they take a drug—and for symptoms they were "not aware of"—that greatly increased their chances of cancer of the penis?

ERT AND CANCER

The 1971 findings concerning cancer and DES came from Arthur Herbst and his colleagues at Massachusetts General Hospital. By contrast, the 1975 ERT studies were the work of *many* investigators, which all coalesced, or came together, in December. So many scientists dot the cast of characters that a summary of the contributions of each seems the clearest way to tell the story.

1. PENTTI SIITERI, UNIVERSITY OF CALIFORNIA MEDICAL SCHOOL IN SAN FRANCISCO, AND PAUL MACDONALD, UNIVERSITY OF TEXAS SOUTHWESTERN MEDICAL SCHOOL: Since cancer is more prevalent in older than in younger women, it was formerly argued that high levels of natural estrogen might *protect* against it. Siiteri and MacDonald, with various associates, were first to demonstrate that postmenopausal women continue to manifest high levels of estrone (a type of estrogen), which is synthesized in body fats from precursors formed in the ovaries and adrenal glands. They later demonstrated that women with cancer produce twice as much natural estrone as healthy women.

Premarin, which stands for PREgnant MAREs'

urINe, is composed principally of estrone, the very estrogen that postmenopausal women who get cancer have too much of naturally. The work of Siiteri and MacDonald, which dates back to 1966, gives the lie to comforting theories, espoused by ERT promoters, that high levels of estrogen protect against cancer in older women. Siiteri and MacDonald provided the framework that helped all the 1975 studies to fall into place.

2. HARRY ZIEL AND WILLIAM FINKLE OF KAISER PERMANENTE MEDICAL CENTER IN LOS ANGELES: In a study that cost only $1,900, Ziel and Finkle gathered the hospital records of ninety-four Kaiser Permanente patients who had endometrial cancer. These were matched with 188 carefully selected control women—two for each cancer patient—who were much like the cancer victims in age, area of residence, and general health.

The records were evaluated by "blind" analysts who did not know which patients had developed cancer. Women who had used conjugated estrogens for seven years or longer developed endometrial cancer at a rate *fourteen times as high* as comparable women who had never used it at all. Women who had used such products for one to five years developed this cancer at a rate that was about *five and one-half times as high as non-users.*

The overall risk, including longer and shorter term ERT patients, was computed to be almost eight times as great as normal.

ERT, according to Ziel and Finkle's research, may be more dangerous than heavy smoking. If you smoke for twenty years of longer, your risk of lung cancer increases seventeen- or eighteen-fold. Your risk of endometrial cancer increases fourteen-fold *after only seven years of ERT use.*

Other key researchers whose work helped clarify the estrogen/endometrial cancer risks included:

3. DONALD SMITH AND ASSOCIATES AT THE MASON CLINIC, UNIVERSITY OF WASHINGTON, SEATTLE: Smith and his associates compared 317 endometrial cancer patients with an equal number of women who had other female cancers, concluding that ERT increases the odds of endometrial cancer most in healthy women who lack other risk factors. Thus it may be more dangerous to a slim woman than a heavier one, who has a greater risk to start with.

4. THOMAS MACK AND ASSOCIATES AT THE UNIVERSITY OF SOUTHERN CALIFORNIA: Thomas Mack and his colleagues studied the residents of a Southern California retirement community. Here again the odds of developing endometrial cancer increased eightfold among ERT users, the same average figure arrived at by Ziel and Finkle. And, like the Smith group in Seattle, the Mack group also noted that the dangers of estrogen therapy appear most striking in healthy women with no other risk factors.

While Ziel and Finkle brought in evidence concerning *length* of ERT use, the Mack group was interested in *dosage*. They report that higher doses of estrogen also enhance the risk. Thus, dose and duration of ERT are implicated in different studies.

We know now that the length of ERT use increases the risk of cancer, and that size of dosage adds to this effect.

5. DONALD AUSTIN, CHIEF OF THE CALIFORNIA TUMOR REGISTRY: Austin informed the FDA on December 16, 1975, that among white women fifty and over living in California, there was an 80 percent increase in uterine cancer during the years 1969–74. The increase was noted in seventy-five hospitals, and was most pronounced in areas of greatest affluence where ERT use is high. In Alameda County, Austin reported, the annual incidence of endometrial cancer has *tripled.*

This unfortunate trend is now confirmed in other states that keep good registries, including Washington and Connecticut. Since 1969, endometrial cancer has steadily and rapidly increased.

FDA spokesman Crout has commented: "The chronic users tend to be middle- and upper-income women, the kind of people who go to doctors and the kind of people who would most value the longed-for youthful appearance. It's an interesting example of the poor being spared, if you will, some of the adverse effects of estrogens that are now coming to the fore."

6. BRUCE STADEL OF THE NATIONAL INSTITUTES OF HEALTH, BETHESDA, AND NOEL WEISS OF THE SCHOOL OF PUBLIC HEALTH AND COMMUNITY MEDICINE, UNIVERSITY OF WASHINGTON, SEATTLE: In an elaborate study of Seattle area residents, Bruce Stadel and Noel Weiss estimated that 51 percent of all women over fifty had, by 1973 to 1974, used ERT for over three months' duration. Most amazingly, of those who first responded that they had *not* used it, more than a quarter were found to be ERT patients after all. This was established during personal interviews at which estrogens were identified by a pill display, and by further discussion with the women's doctors.

The women on ERT were more apt to have suffered troublesome hot flashes before taking it—about two out of five reported this complaint—while the frequency in nonusers was less than one in seven. Clearly then, the flashes drove some women to ERT, but not the majority who took it. Weiss and Stadel conclude that "the frequency of menopausal estrogen use . . . is much higher than the estimated frequency of severe menopausal symptoms. . . . It appears that physicians in King and Pierce counties do not follow a conservative approach to hormonal treatment of menopausal problems."

THE STORY OF E

The earliest report on vitamin E therapy for menopause symptoms, authored by Dr. Evan Shute, appeared in the *Journal of the Canadian Medical Association* in 1937. Shute and his brother Wilfred continued their studies and published their work in many influential journals, including *Lancet* and the *American Journal of Obstetrics and Gynecology.* Their research was confirmed by other less controversial investigators.

But in the 1940s vitamin E was far more costly than most estrogen products. And estrogens do curb flashes in women who fail to respond to vitamin E, or even to the more potent vitamin E, B-complex, bioflavonoids, evening primrose oil, and herbs.

We fear that another reason vitamin E was ignored by most doctors may lie partially in the way prescription and nonprescription remedies are regarded. Many women probably thought estrogen "better" than vitamin E because the hormone was available by prescription only. They may have been disappointed in doctors who told them to go out and buy a vitamin or eat wheat germ. In the wake of the Youth Pill craze, physicians forgot the research on vitamin E. Younger doctors may never have been introduced to it.

On the doctor's side, prescription drugs are sometimes more appealing because they give him or her *control*. Furthermore, vitamins, and especially vitamin E, fall under the same mantle of suspicion as some herbal remedies because they are claimed to have such a wide range of benefits. In his book, *The Heart and Vitamin E,* Evan Shute remarks: "No substance known to medicine has such a variety of healing properties." This, he concedes, is a major drawback to acceptance.

Finally, we must again refer to the second- or third-class citizenship status of the older woman. Her complaints do not attract the attention of many qualified researchers or the interest of many journalists. Thus, vitamin E's proven effectiveness in curbing hot flashes had been obscured by other dramatic claims for the vitamin, such as its possible benefits to the heart.

Vitamin E as a relief for menopause symptoms resurfaced almost by accident. In August 1974, *Prevention* magazine included a questionnaire on this controversial vitamin. Later, reporting the results, biochemist Richard Passwater, author of *Super-Nutrition*, explained:

"Actually, there was no mention of menopause on the questionnaire. *Yet 2,000 women volunteered that they found vitamin E to largely or totally relieve the problems of menopause.* The most frequent comments written in were (1) more energy and a better sense of well-being, (2) relief of leg cramps, and (3) relief of hot flashes and other problems of menopause."

Passwater searched the medical literature and found a number of studies that confirmed what *Prevention* readers said. One, written in 1945 in the *American Journal of Obstetrics and Gynecology,* reported that twenty-five women, all with severe menopause symptoms, responded to the vitamin E treatment and showed either complete relief or very marked improvement. No untoward after-effects were noted.

In 1949 another investigator, Dr. Rita Finkler, described vitamin E treatment of sixty-six menopausal patients in the *Journal of Clinical Endocrinology.* Good-to-excellent relief was obtained in thirty-one cases, fair in sixteen, and the remaining nineteen women evidenced no improvement. The dosages used by Dr. Finkler were relatively low—about twenty to one hundred units daily, the average being thirty. In seventeen cases, when the real vitamin E was replaced with dummy pills, symptoms soon recurred.

Exploding the Estrogen Myth

BARBARA SEAMAN

Barbara Seaman, excerpt from *The Greatest Experiment Ever Performed on Women*, New York: Hyperion, 2003. Reprinted by permission.

In 1993, in response to pressure by breast cancer activists from Nassau and Suffolk counties on Long Island, New York, Congress passed a law mandating the National Cancer Institute to undertake a massive study to identify "environmental and other potential risk factors contributing to the incidence of breast cancer," and to look specifically at water and air pollution, pesticides and toxic waste dumps, and other environmental agents as possible causes of the high rates of breast cancer among Long Island women.[1] Many of those who pressed for the Long Island Breast Cancer Study Project hoped the study would pinpoint controllable causes of the alarming rise in breast cancer rates. Nine years and $30 million later, the project published results assessing a handful of mostly banned toxic chemicals, none of which was tied to increased breast cancer on Long Island.

In 1996, Congress adopted legislation that called for the screening and testing of possible endocrine disruptors, chemicals that can interfere with the glands that regulate human fetal development, sexual maturation, reproductive function, and energy metabolism. The Environmental Protection Agency and the National Institutes of Health spent several years and a few million dollars investigating natural and synthetic chemicals that mimic hormones.

Shockingly, both these massive multimillion-dollar studies ignored the proverbial elephant in the room: the pharmaceutical and veterinary estrogens and other hormones that humans and animals have been eating and depositing into the environment for years—hormones that have been proven to be linked to hormone-dependent breast, uterine, ovarian, and testicular cancers. A decade earlier in 1993, Richard Sharpe of Edinburgh and Niels Skakkebaek of Copenhagen reported in *Lancet* that "humans now live in an environment that can be viewed as a virtual sea of estrogens."[2] In view of what was already known about the health risks of pharmaceutical hormones, the exclusion of such hormones from two supposedly scientific studies raises disturbing questions as to what the real point of the studies was.

The dangers of synthetic estrogens are not limited to the women who have taken them, nor to their male or female children. Perhaps even more disconcerting is the growing evidence that such hormones pollute our soil and water and have a cascade of effects on wildlife. The hormone analogues used commercially are specifically designed to resist stomach acid "degradation" in order to remain effective. It was this very technology, the gastric durability developed in 1938 by Sir Charles Dodds, that ushered in the hormone age. Unfortunately, this same gastric durability allows chemicals to pass out of the body in our wastes, into our water and soil. Some 3 million women who live near the Thames River in London currently take birth control pills. Residues from 900 million contraceptive pills a year now pass into sewage systems and are released into surface or ground water nearby. Scientists believe this may explain the increasing evidence of hermaphroditic fish being caught in the Thames (at rates of up to 40 percent where urban sewage flows into the river).

Of even greater public health concern are the vast amounts of hormones fed to and excreted by livestock in this country. As I reported in my book *Women and the Crisis in Sex Hormones*, diethylstilbestrol (DES) and other gastric-resistant hormones have been widely used in the livestock industry for more than half a century, from the 1940s through today. In sheer tonnage, the amounts of estrogen excreted by livestock and presumably seeping into our soil and water vastly exceed the amounts excreted by women taking physician-ordered contraceptives, fertility hormones, and menopause treatments.

Since the end of World War II, farmers have doled out massive amounts of DES and other synthetic estrogen to poultry, pigs, sheep, and cattle. Feed stores sold it by the truckload, scrambling to meet a veterinary demand that was far greater than the human one. At the time my book was published in 1977, up to 85 percent of American livestock was being raised on DES. Though DES supporters claimed the hormone was administered to animals at "safe levels," a number of health experts insisted otherwise. They pointed out that DES was an established carcinogen. They noted that the 1958 Delaney Amendment to the Food, Drug, and Cosmetic law stipulated that "no [food] additive shall be deemed safe if it is found to induce cancer when ingested by man or animal." While the law was later changed, if it had been enforced at the time it should have prevented DES from being so widely used.

Experts also noted that DES did little to improve the quality of meat. Some compared the fattening of animals with DES to certain practices that were a hanging offense in years gone by: the old-time farmers knew not to slaughter a female animal "in heat" because of the excess salt and water in tissues at that time. But some unscrupulous farmers gave their cows salt, followed by water, just before taking them to market. The stockyard operators soon learned to wait a couple of days until the cattle had excreted the salt and water before weighing the animals and paying for them. This process of salting and watering the stock, if discovered, was a crime, punishable by hanging in some areas of the country.

In the 1970s, DES was far from the only additive used to fatten up livestock. Nine other hormones were also in the mix. Many, like DES, had been banned from agriculture in other nations. These culprits included: chlormadinone acetate, permitted in feed for beef heifers and beef cows for synchronization of estrus (heat); progesterone, permitted for subcutaneous implantation in lambs and steers for growth promotion and feed efficiency; dienestrol diacetate, permitted in feed for broilers, fryers, and roasting chickens for the promotion of fat distribution and for tenderness and bloom; estradiol benzoate, used in combination with progesterone and testosterone; estradiol monopalmitate, permitted for injection under skin at the base of the skull of roasting chickens to produce more uniform fat distribution and improve finish; testosterone, permitted for subcutaneous ear injection in beef cattle to stimulate growth; testosterone proprionate, permitted for subcutaneous ear implantation in heifers to promote growth and increase feed efficiency; medroxyprogesterone acetate, permitted in feed for breeding cattle and ewes for the synchronization of estrus and ovulation; and melengestrol acetate, permitted in feed for heifers for growth stimulation, improved feed utilization, and suppression of estrus. However, since DES was the additive known to have the most harmful effects, it was the one on which health advocates focused their ire. At my urging, the National Task Force on DES rec-

ommended that the use of DES in animal feed be banned. With a nod from Dr. Lester Crawford of the Veterinary Bureau, the FDA withdrew its prior approval of the use of DES in animal feed, to become effective in the 1980s.

The victory proved to be a Pyrrhic one. The ban was a farce for two reasons: because some ranchers and poultry farms continued to use DES illegally, and because many started using other, less well-known estrogens or other growth stimulants in its place. Through the rest of the seventies—and through the eighties, nineties, and the dawn of the new millennium—I watched in horror as the use of estrogen and other hormones in livestock feed continued unabated. Today, many of the nine substances listed above are not only still in use but are being administered in major quantities. Today, farmers still commit the hanging offense of using hormones to pack livestock full of salt and water. In the year 2003, our meat may be steeped in even more hormones than it was when DES was banned in 1979. This reality greeted reporter Michael Pollan when he investigated the American cattle industry for a lengthy article that ran in the *New York Times Magazine* in March 2002. Pollan stared in awe as bleating calves were "funneled into a chute, herded along by a ranch hand yielding an electric prod, then clutched in a restrainer just long enough for another hand to inject a slow-release pellet of Reviar, a synthetic estrogen, in the back of the ear." Pollan learned that US farmers raise an estimated 36 million beef cattle—and give hormones to roughly two-thirds of these animals. Estrogen advocates told Pollan that hormones "get a beef calf from 80 to 1,200 pounds in the span of just fourteen months" and can boost an animal's growth by 20 percent. They justified using estrogen because it seemed cost-effective. A hormone implant costing $1.50, they said, could add fifty pounds to the weight of a steer and yield a return of at least $25.

However, on the downside, Pollan noted that hormone-laced feed can change the pH level of a steer's digestive tract from basic to acidic—one reason 13 percent of feedlot cattle have abscessed livers by the time they are slaughtered. And, he reported measurable amounts of agricultural hormones can now be found in our meat, and that these hormones "contribute to the build-up of estrogenic compounds in our environment, which some scientists believe may explain falling sperm counts and premature maturation in girls."

Pollan noted that "recent studies have found elevated levels of synthetic hormones in feedlot waters; these persistent chemicals eventually wind up in the waterways downstream of feedlots, where scientists have found fish exhibiting abnormal sex characteristics."[3] Indeed, reports of gender-bending aquatic animals are multiplying like minnows. When scientists from Britain's Environmental Agency examined fish in ten major rivers they found intersex males in every single one. Just under 50 percent of males had developed either eggs in their testes or female reproductive tracts. Researchers believed the main culprit was ethinyl estradiol, a synthetic estrogen used in the contraceptive pill. Dr. Charles Tyler of Exeter University, the lead researcher, said the hormone is "so exquisitely potent that some of the very concentrations where we are seeing effects on fish are below the detection limit that is presently in place for testing our drinking water."

Evidence of estrogenic effects also continues to surface in American waterways. For example, researchers from South Carolina's Clemson University discovered ponds affected by runoff from cattle farms contained male juvenile sunfish that were making the egg yolk protein normally produced by adult females, while scientists in New Hampshire found frogs with elevated levels of estrogen—and deformed reproductive organs. In 2001, other researchers caught "female" fish in the Columbia River in Washington state. When they analyzed the genes of these fish, they discovered the "females" were actually males.

The most damning proof of estrogen pollution came in the summer of 2002, when the US Geological Survey completed the first comprehensive study of chemical contaminants in our water. Researchers examined 139 streams and rivers in thirty states and found that 40 percent of waterways showed traces of estrogen or other reproductive hormones. When the results of the two-year survey were published, USGS scientist Herbert Burton noted that compounds with hormone-like properties "can affect the growth and development of aquatic life." Much of this pollution can be traced straight back to animal and human waste. When Andreas Daxenburger of the Technical University of Munich studied US feedlots he discovered that animals shed about 10 percent of their progestin feed additive in their feces alone.

At the University of Florida researcher Louis J. Guillete Jr. (who spent years studying undersized penises and other sexual abnormalities in Florida alligators linked to hormone exposure) tried to compare the runoff from feedlots that use hormones to the runoff from those that did not. The experiment failed because Guillete couldn't find a single cattle farm that didn't give growth-stimulating hormones to its livestock.

While not a single country has dealt with the issue of pharmaceutical or agricultural hormone contamination of water and soil, at least some of the world has paid attention to the problem of hormones found in livestock. The European Union, for instance, has banned the importation of hormone-treated meat since 1988. When synthetic hormones do surface, authorities act to put safety measures in place. In July 2002, Provera (medroxyprogesterone acetate, a synthetic estrogen used in Prempro) was discovered in pig feed sent to farms in fifteen European countries. The culprit was water waste from an Irish processing plant owned by US drugmaker Wyeth-Ayerst. When authorities learned that the grain was tainted, they forced thousands of farmers to halt production and carefully weeded out the contaminated feed. Health advocates made certain that meat consumers were not exposed to hormones—a precaution that is foreign to the United States.

While the Long Island and NIH studies were

profoundly disappointing in their failure to ask about environmental and pharmaceutical hormones, there are some signs that US authorities may be grudgingly waking up to the dangers of such contaminants. In May 2002, Representative Louise Slaughter (D-NY) introduced legislation that would boost federal research on hormone disruptors by $500 million. The NIEHS's National Toxicology Program published its tenth report on carcinogens, including *all* steroidal estrogen products as confirmed causes of human cancer. Davis told me recently, "We know enough now to restrict our exposures to synthetic hormones. Of course, we need more research. We always need more research. But we also know that we should reduce our uses of many growth-stimulating compounds throughout the environment today."

While we wait, evidence keeps mounting that confirms the worries of scientists from past decades. In her book, Davis painstakingly documents troubling patterns of hormonally related cancer and other diseases. Why are more baby boys being born with smaller penises and undescended testes? Why are more young men developing testicular cancer throughout the industrial world? Why are deer and bear and whales and other wildlife showing up with deformities of their reproductive systems? Could this be related to the combined effects of hormones in the environment, whether from agricultural or pharmaceutical uses, to those agents found in toxic chemicals that can act like hormones when ingested, to undetected exposures to radiation, or to some combination of all of these?

Science remains incomplete on these matters, in part because the science is difficult. But, it is also true, as Davis and others make clear, that sometimes we know less than we should, because powerful forces have worked to make sure we remain uncertain. Nobody can be sure whether environmental estrogens lie behind the quadrupling of infertility rates since 1965; if the sea of estrogens in which we live explains the fact that sperm counts are half of what they were in 1940; and if, like intersex fish and mutant frogs, male humans might begin to shed their broad shoulders and slowly morph into women. Faced with the possibility of an all-female planet, authorities might finally have to sidestep the pharmaceutical companies and take decisive action.

The Bitter Pill

LEORA TANENBAUM

Leora Tanenbaum, "The Bitter Pill," *On The Issues Magazine*, Winter 1998. Reprinted by permission.

Barbara Dworkin, sixty-one, is one of 8 million American women taking Premarin, an estrogen replacement that eases menopausal symptoms such as hot flashes and dry skin. Dworkin started on Premarin fifteen years ago and plans to take the drug for the rest of her life. Although studies have shown that Premarin may increase the risk of breast cancer by 30 percent, as well as cause fatal blood clots, the drug also offers protection against osteoporosis and decreases the risk of fatal heart disease by 53 percent. Besides, as a 911 operator living on Long Island, New York, she leads stressful days fielding emergency calls and feels thankful for Premarin because it "makes my life much more pleasant and secure."

But Premarin costs between $15 and $25 a month. If there were a generic version, Suffolk County, New York (which covers Dworkin's drug plan) could cut its costs by 30 percent, more than $3,000 for her lifetime. If you consider that millions of other women lack health insurance or prescription drug coverage, a generic could save them more than $300 million a year.

But economizing isn't the only reason to push for a generic. Premarin is derived from the urine of pregnant horses, a fact that concerns animal rights supporters and repulses many users. People for the Ethical Treatment of Animals (PETA) claims that the collection methods on "urine farms" are barbaric: some 80,000 pregnant mares are confined to stalls for six months out of the year so that their urine can be collected; the 65,000 foals born to them are slaughtered as unusable byproducts of these pregnancies. PETA advises women to switch to an alternative hormone treatment that doesn't harm animals.

An alternative, however, will not be forthcoming. The FDA announced in May 1997 that it will not approve a recently manufactured, affordable, plant-based generic form of Premarin, even though FDA research has shown the generic to be just as effective as the brand-name drug. Rather than heed the recommendation of its own Office of Pharmaceutical Science, the FDA appears to have bowed to political pressure at the expense of women. While there are several plant-derived, FDA-approved estrogen regimens such as Estrace and Estraderm, they have not been proven to offer long-term health benefits. Only those who can afford Premarin or whose insurance will pay will be able to relieve their menopausal symptoms, ward off heart attacks, and avoid bone fractures.

It's no surprise that the commercial interests of Premarin's manufacturer, Wyeth-Ayerst, have superseded health considerations, but the tactics involved are particularly outrageous. Wyeth-Ayerst cultivated influential supporters through financial contributions. Then, when the company needed them, it prodded its beneficiaries to take a stand against their competition. The result? Several highly visible politicians and advocacy groups who knew nothing about the issues involved testified before the FDA against the generic form of Premarin. In the end, the consumer's ability to get the best drugs for the lowest price was sacrificed. The saddest part of this whole incident? Feminist politicians and women's groups were key players.

DOCTOR, I WANT MY PREMARIN

You don't have to be menopausal to recognize the brand-name Premarin. No doubt you've seen the drug's fear-inducing magazine ads, which suggest that midlife women who don't take estrogen will be crippled by osteoporosis if they don't die from a heart attack first. The ads also intimate that midlife women who don't take estrogen can never hope to achieve the carefree, wrinkle-free look of the models depicted.

Premarin, of course, is merely one of dozens of prescription drugs aggressively advertised in magazines such as *Newsweek, Redbook, Mirabella,* and the *New Yorker.* In recent years, drug companies have bypassed physicians and marketed their products directly to consumers. Eli Lilly's multi-million dollar campaign for Prozac, for instance, includes ads in more than twenty magazines. Some magazines, like *Good Housekeeping* and *Ladies' Home Journal,* contain so many drug ads you might be tempted to double-check the cover to make sure you're not reading a professional medical journal. Which is precisely the point: Drug manufacturers want consumers to play doctor by asking their physicians to prescribe particular drugs. And 99 percent of physicians do comply with patients' requests, market research confirms. In this era of "managed care," when physicians are pressed to see as many patients as possible in the shortest amount of time, educated patients who know how they want to be treated are a dream come true.

A dream come true, that is, for physicians and drug companies—but not necessarily for the patients. We may believe that by asking our physicians for Premarin or Prozac we are empowering ourselves by becoming more assertive in our relationships with our physicians, because only we really know our bodies and what's best for our health. But in reality, the drug companies are taking advantage of our adherence to this *Our Bodies, Ourselves* credo. We are intermediaries in a loop of influence that originates in magazine ads and culminates in a prescription.

Last year alone, pharmaceutical companies spent nearly $600 million advertising prescription drugs directly to consumers—twice as much as they spent in 1995 and almost ten times more than they spent in 1991, according to Competitive Media Reporting, a company that tracks ad spending. None of that money, however, seems to be spent on factual research: more than half of the drug ads scrutinized last year by the Consumers' Union advocacy group contained misleading information on risks and benefits, and false claims about efficacy. In the end, the consumer's ability to get the best drugs for the lowest price was sacrificed. Feminist politicians and women's groups were key players.

POLITICS VS. SCIENCE

But as the case of the massively popular Premarin shows, the influence of drug companies goes far beyond false advertising. Wyeth-Ayerst Laboratories is a pharmaceutical Goliath that garners $1 billion a year in revenue from Premarin, the most commonly prescribed drug in America. Owned by American Home Products, Wyeth-Ayerst has maintained a monopoly on Premarin ever since it began manufacturing the estrogen replacement in 1942. Even though the patent expired more than twenty-five years ago, Wyeth has gotten the FDA to change its guidelines in determining bioequivalence in generics, making it difficult for competitors to match Premarin. A lot is at stake: sales could reach $3 billion within five years, with more than one-third of all women in the United States currently over the age of fifty, and another 20 million entering the menopausal years within the next decade.

Because of the size of that market, two small generic drug companies have decided to compete with Wyeth. After the FDA concluded in 1991 that an effective generic requires only two active ingredients (estrone and equilin), Duramed Pharmaceuticals Corp. and Barr Laboratories Inc. teamed up to develop a urine-free generic according to FDA guidelines. In response, Wyeth filed a citizens petition requesting that one of Premarin's ingredients (an obscure estrogen called delta 8,9 dehydroestrone sulfate or DHES) be reclassified as a necessary component. Duramed has not been able to replicate an equivalent of DHES and Wyeth holds the patent on the estrogen. Furthermore, in 1995 the FDA found

that based on clinical trials, there was no evidence that DHES was anything other than an impurity.

And so Wyeth shrewdly lined up the support of several influential women's and health groups by making donations to Business and Professional Women/USA, the American Medical Women's Association, the National Consumers League, and the National Osteoporosis Foundation, among others. Representatives of these groups testified before the FDA on the drug company's behalf, saying that they opposed the approval of a generic that lacks DHES, despite the FDA's own contention that the estrogen wasn't essential. The president of the Women's Legal Defense Fund also testified, although this group did not accept money from Wyeth. None of these groups had taken a position on DHES prior to being contacted by Wyeth.

The company also developed close ties to the White House and the Senate. John Stafford, chairman and CEO of Wyeth-Ayerst's parent company, American Home Products, attended an intimate seventeen-person White House "coffee klatsch" with President Clinton in November 1995. And in June 1996, according to the Federal Elections Commission, American Home Products made a $50,000 contribution to the Democratic National Committee. Several months later, Democratic senators Barbara Mikulski (MD) and Patty Murray (WA) wrote the FDA for assurance that "it has no intention of approving a generic version of Premarin that lacks the 'same' active ingredient as the innovator." According to her press secretary, Murray became involved in this issue after she "was contacted by women's groups. As a result, our office spoke with the manufacturer, who was in contact with the same women's groups."

Lo and behold, the FDA reversed its stance. Janet Woodcock, MD, director of the FDA's Center for Drug Evaluation and Research, announced on May 5 that "based on currently available data, there is at this time no way to assure that synthetic generic forms of Premarin have the same active ingredients as the [urine-based] drug."

No matter how you look at it, the FDA flip-flop

appears to be the result of Wyeth-Ayerst's considerable lobbying muscle. Of course, just because a decision is politically influenced doesn't mean it's wrong. But an internal FDA memo dated May 3 (two days before the decision was announced) supports the generic, saying that DHES is not a necessary component. Even the vice president of Wyeth-Ayerst's regulatory affairs department admitted to the *Wall Street Journal* that there's "probably nothing" special about DHES, and that "it's but one of many components in Premarin."

Consumer health is clearly the last thing on the minds of everyone involved in the Premarin debacle. "This decision is pure politics," fumes Cynthia Pearson, executive director of the National Women's Health Network, the only women's organization that publicly supports the generic. Coincidentally, the network does not accept donations from drug companies. The decision "was not backed up by science," says Pearson. "This never would have happened without political pressure orchestrated by Wyeth-Ayerst."

Duramed has challenged the FDA decision in an administrative appeal; the company intends to file a court appeal if it is turned down. But Wyeth is already a step ahead: it is busily working to ensure that no matter what happens, it will continue to dominate the estrogen replacement market. After all, Wyeth is the sole sponsor of an important "memory study" on Premarin's effectiveness in warding off Alzheimer's disease, a study conducted under the aegis of the government-sponsored Women's Health Initiative. If a correlation is found, physicians and consumers alike will naturally turn to Premarin as a preventative for Alzheimer's.

COMMERCIALLY SPONSORED MEDICINE

Wyeth is hardly the only drug company to use political leverage to protect its turf. In 1997, the *Journal of the American Medical Association* (*JAMA*) published results of a 1990 study on thyroid medications and reported that the maker of Synthroid, one of the drugs under study, had suppressed for years the fact that three other medications were equally effective. Like Premarin, Synthroid has long enjoyed domination in a lucrative market because its manufacturer falsely claims that its product is superior to the competition.

Ten years ago, in order to establish Synthroid as the most effective drug in its class, Flint Laboratories (then the drug's manufacturer) approached researcher Betty Dong of the University of California, San Francisco. Dong signed a contract with Flint to conduct comparative studies of the bioequivalence of Synthroid and three other preparations. When her research was completed in 1990, Dong submitted the results to Boots Pharmaceuticals (which had since taken over Flint). It turned out that all four drugs were bioequivalent, and that consumers who chose the other drugs over Synthroid could save $356 million annually. Boots became alarmed: After all, it is the leader in a $600 million-a-year market.

With so much revenue at stake, Boots did everything it could to publicly discredit Dong's research. It dishonestly claimed that the research was flawed in design and execution, and that Dong had breached research ethics. It then published Dong's results in a "reanalysis" that reached the opposite conclusion. Conveniently, Boots was able to prevent publication of Dong's own account of her research, since the contract she originally signed stipulated that nothing could be published without written consent from the drug company.

Finally, under pressure from the FDA, Boots (now part of Knoll Pharmaceutical) agreed to allow Dong's results to be published—seven years after the study was completed. Later, Boots/Knoll agreed to pay $98 million in a settlement to consumers who purchased Synthroid between 1990 and 1997.

A MATTER OF TRUST

The growing power of pharmaceutical companies is troubling on a number of levels. It is frightening how poorly we are informed about the appalling treatment of animals in drug manufacturing. It is wasteful to pay for needlessly expensive medications. Forget about President Clinton's 1992 plea to the drug companies to control their prices. In the last few years, big-name drug companies such as Merck and Hoechst have withdrawn from the generics field because they realized they could make far more money selling brand-name drugs. But the real bottom line is that the drug companies have robbed consumers of the ability to trust anyone in the area of drug research: commercialism has infected everyone involved. We can't trust those companies to which we entrust our health to accurately represent their products. We can't assume that the FDA has weighed all of the scientific research fairly. We can't even take for granted that the scientists who perform drug research are working independently.

Savvy consumers, of course, realize that drug companies are motivated by profit. But what about advocacy groups, including women's and health organizations? Aren't they supposed to be looking out for the public good?

"All medical organizations receive money from the pharmaceutical companies," rationalizes Debra R. Judelson, MD, president of the American Medical Women's Association, one of the organizations that accepted money from Wyeth and testified before the FDA on the same issue. "There are no virgins. We've all been lobbied by the pharmaceuticals on all the issues." The National Women's Health Network, the lone women's advocacy group to support the Premarin generic, must be the only virgin at the orgy.

But perhaps the ever-increasing power and determination of certain drug companies to quash their competition isn't so terrible. Look, if we all just took Prozac, it wouldn't seem so bad.

In 1999, Wyeth Ayerst finally lost its monopoly of the US market in conjugated estrogrens. Duramed got its product, called Cenestin, approved, though not as generic. As a result, the product is not likely to be as inexpensive as it could have been.

A Friend Indeed: The Grandmother of Menopause Newsletters

SARI TUDIVER

IN THE BEGINNING . . .

A Friend Indeed was first conceived in 1983 by Janine O'Leary Cobb, a Canadian mother of five who taught sociology and humanities in Montreal. Approaching fifty, Janine felt uncharacteristically tired, burned out, and increasingly unable to cope—symptoms that she finally realized were the effects of menopause. Her local medical library provided almost no helpful information. Janine vividly remembers coming across the printed lecture notes about menopause distributed to third-year medical students: "Well-adjusted women have no problem with menopause," it said. Just by asking a doctor about menopause, women would label themselves as maladjusted. Janine was outraged and decided to do something about it.

"I got the idea for a newsletter for menopausal women that could be both a source of information and a support group through the mail," Janine says. "Because menopause is a time when a woman often is in need, I called it *A Friend Indeed*. In April 1984, the first commercial issue of *AFI* was mailed to forty women. A year later, word had spread and the newsletter had become a full-time occupation.

Demand grew and subscriptions have increased to thousands across North America and other parts of the world. While menopause has now become a popular topic in research and the press, *AFI* is recognized as "the grandmother of menopause newsletters." Offering helpful, well-researched, and balanced information about the litany of subjects that matter to women in midlife— night sweats, gas and bloating, vaginal dryness, heart disease, menopausal migraine, hormone therapy, stress, and anger, among many others—

AFI continues to flourish because it has a unique approach.

THE EXCHANGE

A key to the newsletter's success is its commitment that the voices of menopausal women be heard and taken seriously. "The Exchange" is a popular forum where women ask questions, receive responses from the editor or other readers, share concerns and personal experiences. Over the past fifteen years, thousands of women have written to document their symptoms and feelings related to menopause and have described a variety of encounters with the health care system. The women's stories reveal frustrations, sometimes despair, along with creative approaches to solving problems. There is also a delightful and, at times, unexpected sense of humor.

The themes of the letters and inquiries have not changed dramatically over the years. For many women, there is relief at knowing others have felt the same way and that one's strange sensations . . . are not so strange after all:

> . . . With your help I feel that I have successfully navigated this particular "sea of troubles." I was fortunate that I was able to do so without additional help from the pharmaceutical companies, probably because I was aware that most of the strange things that were occurring were not unique to me. Others had gone through them and were still around to write about it. I now feel like a graduate with all the positive aspects of that term, and would like to thank you for your tutelage.

The women reveal a strong sense of respect for the normal, natural processes involved with the end of menstruation . . . a respect that is often lacking in the medical and research communities which commonly consider menopause a condition of hormone deficiency requiring treatment and manipulation. Women gain the courage to deal with care providers, to press for more details about a proposed test, hysterectomy, or a prescription, or to seek a second opinion.

> Several months have passed since I received your answer to my letter concerning my problem diagnosed as strophic vaginitis. I took your advice and made an appointment with a dermatologist. He advised me to stop using the cortisone and steroid creams. In his opinion the skin had become sensitive from prolonged use of the medications. He prescribed an anesthetic ointment. I followed those instructions and have had gradual but steady improvement . . . I very much appreciate your advice and especially for taking the time to write to me personally. I read every issue of *AFI* from cover to cover.

Over the years, women have posed many important questions that cannot be answered readily, given the limited state of research. These include queries on whether menopause might have unique effects on women with . . . chronic illnesses, cerebral palsy, or other disabilities. There are many questions from women who have experienced premature menopause (before the age of forty) and from women who have had severe menopausal symptoms induced by surgery, chemotherapy, or other treatments. These questions, grounded in women's complex medical and life histories, offer key insights into areas for future research. *AFI* offers a forum for women to share anecdotal insights and details about what therapies or approaches to self-care might have worked for them. As well, researchers and practitioners often write in with comments and suggestions.

Through "The Exchange" women are referred to other resources or are offered suggestions that they can explore on their own or with a care provider. While all letters are confidential, some women ask to be put in touch with others. If both agree, they correspond directly, and lasting friendships have emerged through *A Friend Indeed.* Each woman is seen as an individual who experiences menopause in her own unique way. This is in contrast to the blanket approach espoused by the pharmaceutical industry and many health providers who promote the latest pills for all, often unattuned to a woman's deeper concerns and needs.

Many women are able to solve some of their problems through research and reading. One woman described what she learned:

> I have found this publication to be extremely helpful and I have kept every issue so that I can share the information with my friends and doctors. While reading about other women and their problems, I began to realize that although we may all share some of the problems, every case is unique.

> I started feeling different when I was fifty-two. My periods were regular, but I was very tired all the time and would get anxiety attacks while working at my job. I started hormone replacement therapy at that time and continued for six years. Although I tried various brands of estrogen, each and every one caused the same side effect—nausea. I can only describe it as having morning sickness every day of my life. About eighteen months ago, I read your book *Understanding Menopause,* and there, on page 95, I discovered that every estrogen pill contains lactose. I am lactose intolerant. My doctors were totally unaware that lactose was used as a filler in these medications.

TRACKING THE RESEARCH

In addition to "The Exchange," there are lead articles and "Hot Flashes" (research updates) in each issue of *AFI.* These provide a more in-depth, documented look at a particular topic. Some of the most popular back issues focus on alternative,

nonhormonal approaches to menopause and aging, as well as the pros and cons of hormone therapy.

A Friend Indeed also helps track and explain the many unresolved controversies surrounding the research into and treatment of menopause. It offers women critical tools to better understand the "hard" science of clinical trials and research about hormones, breast cancer, heart disease, and osteoporosis; to separate sound science from promotional hype; and to sift through what is currently known with some confidence from claims where evidence may be weak. *AFI* urges women to be informed, careful consumers whether considering more mainstream or alternative, complementary approaches and to read media and promotional information with great care.

AFI has often been on the "cutting edge" in identifying important research. As one reader recently noted, *AFI* "scooped the mainstream *New England Journal of Medicine*" by publishing an article almost a year earlier about alternative approaches to treatment of thyroid conditions for people not responding well to standard treatments. The newsletter also takes a critical "watchdog" approach to the pharmaceutical industry and its marketing practices. *AFI* takes no money from the pharmaceutical industry.

LOOKING AHEAD

Menopause can be an interval,
a closure, a threshold, a gateway . . .
all of these things and more.
—Janine O'Leary Cobb

Menopausal women have a tremendous capacity to widen their horizons and understandings. The menopausal years can be a time to reassess one's life, lay aside unresolved issues, and look forward to what the future may hold. Ideally it should be a time to share pleasures with those we care about and to find humor in the challenges of daily life.

Women are faced with pressures from many sources urging them "to make decisions about hormones" and a wide variety of other therapies. There is a vast amount of information to evaluate and absorb. The challenge is to remain afloat in the sea of information and heavily promoted products: to carefully evaluate the claims to what is known in order to develop strategies for good health and well being. There are many things we already know that are good for us all: nutritious food, pleasurable activity and exercise, a safe environment free from violence and poverty and satisfaction in our personal relationships. *A Friend Indeed* is a resource supporting women along this path to a deeper understanding of ourselves as we age.

To find out more about *A Friend Indeed: The Newsletter for Women in the Prime of Life*, write to PO Box 260, Pembina, ND 58271-0260; www.afriendindeed.ca.

The Truth about Hormone Replacement Therapy: How to Break Free from the Medical Myths of Menopause

THE NATIONAL WOMEN'S HEALTH NETWORK

National Women's Health Network, excerpt from *The Truth About Hormone Replacement Therapy*, New York: Prima Publishing, 2002. Reprinted by permission.

EACH WOMAN EXPERIENCES MENOPAUSE DIFFERENTLY.

When Martha Correll hit age forty-two, her life got complicated. "Let's just say I had PMS, cramps, periods, hot flashes, insomnia, and a toddler," she says now. "It was a really hot summer, and at first I thought it was just the weather that was bothering me. I'd hang out with other moms at our kids' playgroup, and the heat just drove us crazy."

After talking with her older sister who's a nurse, Martha realized that her hot flashes and resulting insomnia meant that her body was getting ready for menopause, a natural process that every one of us will experience if we live long enough with

our ovaries intact. By contrast, Rosalyn Reich breezed through her menopause. "I think I had a hot flash once," she says. "It happened when I thought I had lost a chapter of my dissertation."

During the reproductive years, our ovaries are the main producers of estrogen and progesterone, and at relatively high levels. During the years leading up to menopause (the "perimenopause"), ovarian production of estrogen and progesterone begins to fluctuate, and ovulation and bleeding patterns change and become irregular.

Eventually, the ovaries almost stop producing estrogen altogether. Estrogen and progesterone levels drop below the minimum needed to continue menstrual cycles, and menopause—literally defined as the cessation of menstruation—occurs. Different women have different rates and patterns, which may explain the variations in how they experience menopause. With Martha, for example, it began at age forty-two—the same age as her mother and sister before her. Among Martha's friends, changes began anywhere from age thirty-eight to fifty-one.

THE UPS AND DOWNS OF MENOPAUSE

Although we often hear that ovarian estrogen production declines in a straight line, hormone levels actually fluctuate quite a bit. Some of the changes associated with perimenopause are the result of high, rather than low, levels of hormones as well as rapidly changing levels. An abrupt drop in estrogen levels is almost certainly associated with a more sudden onset of menopausal "symptoms," while a gradual drop usually accompanies a gradual appearance of symptoms.

After menopause, the ovaries continue to produce low levels of estrogen and androgens. The adrenal glands—small glands located above the kidneys—also produce both hormones. Androgens are also converted to estrogen by fat tissue.

Contrary to the popular description of ovaries dying and postmenopausal women having no estrogen, women continue to produce roughly 10 percent of their former estrogen after menopause and throughout the rest of their lives.

WHERE YOU LIVE MAKES A DIFFERENCE

The hormonal changes that accompany menopause vary among individual women and among cultures. Some women breeze through menopause, while others experience heavy and unpredictable bleeding, painful intercourse, and hot flashes that disrupt sleep.

Women whose menopause is induced by surgery, chemotherapy, or other medical treatment in which ovarian hormone synthesis stops suddenly often have more severe symptoms. Cultural conditions also play a role, with the incidence and type of symptoms varying widely in different parts of the world.

Research done on Japanese women, for instance, reveals a low rate of hot flashes and few menopausal complaints. In contrast, Greek women are more likely to experience hot flashes, although they don't seek medical care for them. Mayan women, whose diet and lifestyle are very different from women in industrialized countries, look forward to menopause and do not report any hot flashes or other bothersome changes.

While women in Europe and North America associate menopause with hot flashes, night sweats, irritability, and depression, women in northern Thailand associate menopause with headaches, and Japanese women associate it with shoulder stiffness and headaches, but not hot flashes or depression. About half of all US women experiencing natural menopause complain of hot flashes. In Japan, approximately 15 percent of women report hot flashes and 3 percent report night sweats.

A Scottish survey of eight thousand women aged forty-five to fifty-four found that 57 percent experienced one or more of fifteen symptoms commonly associated with menopause, but only 22 percent of these found such symptoms a problem. The women reported suffering hot flashes, night sweats, sleep problems, dry/sore vagina, painful joints, headaches, sore breasts, nighttime urination, palpitations, dizziness, irritability, memory problems, anxiety, depression, and feeling unable to cope. Hot flashes and vaginal dryness or soreness were the only symptoms the women associated with menopausal status. Women with surgically or medically induced menopause and HRT users were more apt to report problem symptoms.

SOCIAL AND MEDICAL FADS HAVE AN EFFECT ON MENOPAUSE

It's difficult to determine the importance of cultural factors. Variations in symptoms in different countries could be a result of diet, lifestyle, genetics, or many other factors. However, the fact that Asians respect age while Westerners worship youth makes it hard to escape the notion that menopause in the West might be very different if older women looked forward to an honored place in society rather than discrimination and, in many cases, poverty.

In fact, women's experience of menopause depends in part on the way a society views menopause and aging women. During the era in this country when women were thought to be ruled by their hormones and thus were inferior to men, menopause was a shameful secret. Many women were embarrassed to admit they were undergoing menopause or to seek advice for menopausal discomforts. As late as the 1960s, male physicians described menopause as the end of a woman's active life. Symptoms of aging such as wrinkled skin and memory loss are still falsely believed to be the side effects of menopause.

The modern woman's movement has changed these old perceptions. Today, much more information about menopause is available, and women now feel comfortable openly discussing the experience. Although some clinicians mistakenly dismiss all physical problems experienced by midlife women as "just" menopause, many are beginning to take women's reports of uncomfortable menopausal changes seriously enough to offer remedies.

The current fashion is for clinicians to treat menopause as a risk factor for long-term diseases, particularly osteoporosis and heart disease. Clinicians also see menopause as a cause of mood changes and mental problems. Ignoring the fact that post-menopausal women continue to make estrogen, doctors inaccurately describe them as estrogen deficient and tell them that, since estrogen is essential for bodily function, it needs to be replaced.

Particularly misleading is the fact that some physicians take blood samples and then diagnose "low" hormone levels in women whose hormone levels would be low for a twenty-year-old but are perfectly normal for their age. The results are then used to justify treatment that isn't really needed.

Some experts from the old school claim that nature never intended women to live past menopause. They point to the fifty-year life expectancy common at the early part of the twentieth century and allege that modern medicine has kept women alive past their natural lifespans and that a "natural" approach to menopause will not succeed in keeping post-menopausal women healthy. These experts are trying to justify treating menopause as a disease. They have taken menopause, a perfectly normal phase of a woman's life, and "medicalized" it.

Medicalized menopause is not useful to women. Postmenopausal women who have their ovaries are no more estrogen deficient than prepubertal girls. Even in the past, many women lived to a ripe old age. Just look at how our great grand-mothers survived childhood diseases and dangerous childbirth practices and lived well into their eighties. Natural menopause does not "cause" osteoporosis or heart disease, conditions that don't usually affect women until twenty or thirty years after menopause.

On Aging

JOAN DITZION

Joan Ditzion, "On Aging," 2008. Original for this publication.

As a founder of the Boston Women's Health Book Collective (BWHBC) I am forever grateful that I came of age in the second wave of the women's movement. A whole generation of women, of which I am a member, embraced our identities as women and a women-centered view of the world. Our bodies, as we move through our life journeys, are ourselves and the place from which we view the world.

Had anyone said to me more than thirty-five years ago, "Joan, you will be engaged and concerned with women's aging issues," I would have said "nonsense!" Then, I was in my twenties and, like many in my cohort, I was caught up with the second wave of feminism and issues of pregnancy, childbirth, sexuality, and reproductive rights. In fact I have grown up with *Our Bodies, Ourselves* and now, as a sixty-three-year-old menopausal woman, I am very much embracing, validating, and affirming issues of midlife and older women.

One of the things that truly shape my vision and sense of self as I age is my feminist value system. I embraced my identity as a woman in the women's movement when I realized that sexism was a social construction, based on a patriarchal view of the world, and was not biologically predetermined. Now, thirty-five years later, I embrace my identity as an aging woman in a multigenerational world. As I age and deal with changes in my body, my place in the generational hierarchy, and social responses to my age, bump into ageism. I keep repeating the mantra, "ageism is a social construction."

AGEISM

Ageism is a pervasive cultural attitude which idealizes the young and has a negatively discriminating attitude towards people over fifty, which commercial interests (pharmaceutical, cosmetic, and fashion industries) exploit and profit from. The discriminatory attitude towards us as we age, which eventually affects everyone who is lucky enough to grow old, is a social construction, reflecting the values of our culture, and is not intrinsic to the human condition. There are societies that value and honor people as they age, but we are not one of them. Our culture turns on us as we age. As a society we need to heighten our consciousness, because the bottom line is that aging touches everyone's life; at some point everyone will be demeaned and discriminated by ageism.

I think we are living through a potentially transformative time right now that may see a shift in women's and the public's attitude towards menopause, midlife, and the aging process. I personally feel very hopeful about this. Following the historic moments of the hormone debacle of 2002 and its aftermath, notions that we need a pharmacological fix to deal with menopause and aging are being dispelled in the context of tremendous demographic change. The current largest generation of baby boomers (now forty-two to sixty) has the potential to live more fully and healthfully than generations before it, and will change demographics so that by 2030 one-fifth of the population will be sixty-five or older. And so the current cohort of midlife women who have been through, are going through, or will be going through menopause, numbering at least 33 million, has the opportunity to reframe the issues, deconstruct ageist attitudes, reconstruct notions of a holistic view of aging, and advocate for a vision that will empower and improve the health, well-being, and status of midlife and older women and men.

The real problems we face as we age are the cultural, social, economic, and political forces which undermine our confidence, health, and well-being. We need to be alert as we go through our aging journey. There are four important issues that influence women growing older in the second half of life: ageism, medicalization, sexism, and the feminization of aging.

MEDICALIZATION

Medicalization is the view that aging is a disease and a medicalized event. As more of us live longer we change the content and definition of these years and gain a new sense of the range of normal aging. Our older years can be a good phase of life and many distinctions are made now among young old (sixty-five to seventy-four), older old (seventy-five to eighty-five) and oldest old (over eighty-five). There is much we can do to take care of ourselves. Some changes can be prevented, reversed, slowed, treated, or managed, but even if we take care of ourselves and are socially engaged, aging brings loss, decline, and illness, and we have to cope with new circumstances. Our challenge is to get beyond the medical model and pathologizing of the aging process and continue to grow and develop with as much a sense of self-esteem and personhood as possible, whatever the limits our bodies face. We should seek to live in environments that affirm our uniqueness and individuality and meet our long-term care needs.

SEXISM

Our society still values women for our youth, reproductive and sexual capacity, and our beauty, and desexualizes and devalues aging women more than men. Although society has changed a lot of its sexist attitudes, they linger and especially affect us as we transition into midlife years. Women are still valued largely for their reproductivity, and are vulnerable to age discrimination at a much earlier age than men, while anti-aging marketing pressure and cosmetic surgery plays on and exaggerates our fears and anxieties about our bodies as we age. Why do we live in a society that clings to the ideal of remaining forever young rather than aging well with courage, passion, and power?

FEMINIZATION OF AGING

Demographics show us that women outlive men.

The older cohort in our society has and will have more women than men. There are certainly benefits of longevity but more challenges as we face chronic illness, increased dependency needs, and long-term care financial constraints, loss of spouse, partner, friends, and relatives, and end-of-life issues. More women face these issues than men at a time when we are not able to advocate for ourselves. It's important for each of us to plan for our aging in midlife and before, and be proactive about it, as well as to advocate for systems to support women and men growing older.

In addition to these attitudes, our outlook, health, and well-being as we age is profoundly shaped by the social, economic, and political contexts that shape our lives. Our society has a long way to go to support us in our aging process. This means health insurance, a comprehensive health care system that is sensitive to the needs of women in the second half of life, decent work/family policies, retirement, economic security, and long-term and end-of-life care.

We have to be working on many levels at the same time, reframing issues that affirm our value, personhood, and potential for growth and development in the second half of our lives and in coping eventually with increased dependency needs and end-of-life needs. We will need to work for policies and programs that support this process and at the same time protect the policies that are already in place.

This means:

➤ Combating ageism, internalized and institutional, and fostering dignity, personhood growth, and development in our midlife and older years.

➤ Questioning the medicalization of the aging process which defines events based on a medical model with pharmacological interventions and solutions.

➤ Questioning sexism and the implications of the feminization of aging.

➤ Taking care of ourselves and taking a preventative approach to our health, becoming informed consumers and developing a critical perspective on medical treatments made available to us.

➤ Advocating for a health care system that is sensitive to the continuum of the health care needs of older women.

➤ Recognizing that our aging process is shaped by the economic, social, and political content of our lives. As individuals we can do so much and we need to know that our society supports us in the aging process. This means: health insurance, decent work/family policies, economic security in retirement, and long-term care.

The personal is political, to carry forward a theme from the sixties. So here we are on the brink of demographic changes and together we have the opportunity and potential to "seize the decade," to reframe issues and to construct a vision that resists ageism and will empower the health, well-being, and social status of midlife and aging women and men. I feel personally compelled at my age to advocate for changes so things will be better when I can't advocate for myself. Young women have a lot at stake in what we do as women in our second half of life, and their turn is coming. In our age-segregated, youth-oriented society, women at each stage of life need to be talking with one another. We have demographics on our side and the more conversations we have, and the more we resist ageist attitudes and the medicalization of aging, and the more we give voice to nonageist experiences and attitudes and everyone's place in the aging continuum, the more of a force we are for social change. And I think women, with our relational sensitivity, our full awareness of the age continuum and of our dependent and interdependent needs throughout the life cycle, are in a good position to lead.

CHAPTER 8

Gynecological Surgery

MADELINE GRAY WAS NOT A WOMAN accustomed to helplessness. A journalist and author of several books, Gray was still in her early forties when she underwent a total hysterectomy. In 1951 she would describe her experiences in a landmark book about menopause, *The Changing Years*: "A few years ago I had what is known as a surgical menopause—a change brought on by an operation. That means I was thrown into the midst of this thing headlong. I had no time even to get mentally 'set.'"[1] Frightened and uninformed, Gray's fears ranged from the small—would she suddenly grow a mustache and get obese—to the large—what was she really in for?

Like most people in the 1940s and '50s, Gray turned with deeply ingrained trust to her doctor for information. She was disappointed when he responded with dismissal: "While he was a very distinguished man and had done an excellent job, he was both far too busy and too abrupt to bother with me . . . as to my future worries, he curtly dismissed them by telling me to go home and forget about the whole thing. Besides, the worries were all imaginary anyway."

Next Gray turned to her friends. This time she met no resistance, but rather profound ignorance on all sides. Gray's qualms were answered with urban myths, horror stories, and more questions; but Gray wasn't one to take this lack of information sitting down. Instead she wrote a book that was the first patient-to-patient guide to speak frankly about menopause—both from a surgical and a natural perspective.

If we asked you to guess what one in three American women have in common by the time they die, what would you say? Perhaps you would guess a cholesterol that exceeds a certain level, or bones that have thinned. Would you be surprised to find out the answer is that they don't have a uterus?

It is estimated that around one-third of American women will undergo surgical removal of their uteri, and often their ovaries as well. That adds up to around 600,000 procedures a year, and a five billion dollar industry.[2] Many of these procedures are performed on women who are still getting periods, plunging them instantaneously into the discomforts of menopause.

Even experts are often astounded to find out that hysterectomy rates in the United States are still so high, assuming the days of routine uterine removal to have passed along with girdles and petticoats. But how many of them are really necessary? If we know so much more about both women's bodies and surgical procedures, why has so little changed?

Long-held assumptions have slowly begun to shift. In 2005, a California doctor named William Parker and his colleagues published a meta-analysis (a large analysis of over 200 previous studies) looking for increased mortality in oophorectomized women (those whose ovaries had been removed). What Parker and his colleagues found was shocking: Based on their model, if ten thousand women between the ages of fifty and fifty-four undergo a hysterectomy with oophorectomy, they will have forty-seven fewer cases of ovarian cancer by the time they reach eighty than a similar group who keep their ovaries. The oophorectomy group, however, will suffer 838 additional deaths from coronary heart disease as well as 158 more deaths from hip fractures. In other words, while a few lives are saved by preventing ovarian cancer, substantially more are lost to other chronic illnesses exacerbated by pulling out ovaries.

As more research becomes available, and more women question the wisdom of gynecological surgery, it begins to change the face of menopause and aging. If a hysterectomy was routine for most women through much of the twentieth century and extremely common for the rest, a new generation of aging women with their reproductive organs intact are in uncharted territory.

NOTES

1. Madeline Gray, *The Changing Years*, Garden City, NY: Doubleday, 1951, 12.
2. William H. Parker, MD, with Rachel L. Parker, *A Gynecologist's Second Opinion*, New York: Plume, 2003.

Needless Hysterectomies

MARCIA COHEN

Marcia Cohen, excerpt from "Needless Hysterectomies," *Ladies' Home Journal*, March 1976. Reprinted by permission.

In the United States in 1973, the most recent year for which statistics are available, hysterectomies were performed on 716,000 women. Only one other major surgical procedure—tonsillectomy—was performed more often. The number of hysterectomies performed increased by 25 percent in only eight years, between 1965 and 1973.

As the number of hysterectomies performed escalates, so does the controversy surrounding them. Women's groups, consumerists, and even many physicians are asking: How much of this surgery is really necessary? Are hysterectomies performed when less radical procedures would suffice? Are women fully informed of what a hysterectomy involves, and what other choices they may have?

WOMEN UNDER FORTY-FIVE

Most of us think of cancer when we hear the word "hysterectomy." But in fact, only 20 percent of all hysterectomies are performed to eliminate malignancies involving the cervix, the body of the uterus, or adjacent organs.

But what about the other 80 percent of hysterectomies, those that don't involve cancer? Why are they performed? Some of the most common reasons are fibroid tumors, prolonged or irregular vaginal bleeding or discharge, precancerous lesions (cell changes which may signal impending malignancy), "excessive" menstrual bleeding, uterine polyps, and sterilization. It is in these cases that controversy develops; here is where doctors themselves may disagree about the need for a hysterectomy.

FIBROID TUMORS

In usual practice, most gynecologists recommend hysterectomy when fibroid tumors have expanded the uterus to the size of a ten- to twelve-week pregnancy. But many women do not realize that fibroids do not *always* grow to such size, and that they *almost always* shrink after menopause. Elmer Kramer, MD, professor of gynecology and obstetrics at Cornell University Medical College, is an outspoken critic of the frequent use of hysterectomy for women who have fibroid tumors.

"WORKING" A PATIENT

"A doctor can 'work' a patient," contends Dr. Kramer. "He knows she'll get suspicious if he mentions an operation on the first visit, so he just says she has fibroids and gains her confidence. Then, by the third visit, he says: 'Your fibroids are growing. They should come out.' By that time, she figures he's very conservative. Of course her fibroids are growing. But by how much? Two percent a year? The patient could be just about to enter menopause—when the fibroids will suddenly shrink by themselves—and the doctor could talk her into surgery she doesn't really need."

Dr. Kramer's suspicions were given some statistical credence in a study published recently by Dr. Eugene McCarthy, associate clinical professor of public health at Cornell Medical College. In this study, 32 percent of the hysterectomies recommended by the original physician were declared unnecessary by a second, consulting physician. (Dr. Kramer served as one of the "consulting physicians" on the study.) The results—which Dr. McCarthy admits are preliminary—agree almost exactly with the Trussell report, a study made thirteen years ago of 239 Teamsters Union members and their dependents. The Trussell report also disputed the need for hysterectomies in one-third of the sixty recommended cases and concluded that "the grave suspicion of patient exploitation could be raised."

Both the Cornell study and the Trussell report have been challenged. The Medical Society of the County of New York countered the Trussell report with a study of its own members' practices showing only 3.2 percent of recommended hysterectomies to be unnecessary and 7 percent questionable, out of a total sample of 504 women in the study.

But Dr. Kramer remains convinced that physicians recommend surgery too quickly, partly because of the relative safely of surgical procedures today and because "they have to make a living." According to him, virtually all the women in the Cornell group whose recommended hysterectomies were disputed by other doctors had fibroid tumors. According to the "second opinion" doctors, those tumors were not sufficiently symptom-producing to require surgery in those patients.

Hysterectomy is, of course, not only a therapeutic measure but a totally effective method of sterilization. The Health Research Group in Washington DC claims that some physicians are "selling" hysterectomies to patients (particularly minority groups) without informing them that the process is irreversible.

The group's report also documents pressure on hospital interns and residents to secure patients for "training" operations. "Let's face it," one physician admits, "we've all talked women into hysterectomies they didn't need while we were residents and needed to learn."

CAVALIER ATTITUDE

Such a cavalier attitude might seem to suggest that doctors consider the uterus as dispensable an organ as, say, an appendix—and some feminists have accused the medical profession of just such callousness toward female patients. But if needless hysterectomies are being performed, the blame must be shared by patient and doctor alike.

"It never ceases to amaze me," said a doctor on the CBS program *Magazine*, "when a patient comes in who has never seen me before—they've picked my name out of the phone book—and after I've examined them and concluded that they would benefit from a surgical operation, they say, 'Okay, when do we do it?'"

Patients—particularly women, according to some physicians—simply don't ask questions. Whether this throne room atmosphere is created by the sexist power delusions of gynecologists, as some feminists claim, or by the timid dependency and undue modesty of women, as some physicians insist, the fact remains that it's unhealthy. . . .

UNQUESTIONING WOMEN

Given the seriousness of this surgery, it is amazing that so many physicians report that many women do not question their doctors closely regarding either the severity of the operation or what other options may be available.

A woman's own informed choice is the best protection against an unnecessary hysterectomy. That means ask questions about your condition, about its severity, and about the consequences of a hysterectomy compared to other forms of treatment.

FIND ANOTHER DOCTOR

If the answers are withheld or given grudgingly, find another doctor. And, most important, every patient facing surgery has the right to a second consulting opinion. Honest disagreement can be just that—honest disagreement. If that happens, she may want a third opinion.

Every one of the gynecologists who were interviewed for this article agreed that a physician who bristles at the suggestion of a second opinion is "not worth his salt."

And finally, the checkups. Every woman should have a yearly pelvic examination and Pap smear. For there is no controversy about the lifesaving value of hysterectomies where malignancy is involved. Any woman who neglects her checkups is not worth *her* salt.

So You're Going to Have a New Body!

LYNNE SHARON SCHWARTZ

Lynne Sharon Schwartz, "So You're Going to Have a New Body!" in *The Melting Pot and Other Subversive Stories*, New York: Harper and Row, 1987. Reprinted by permission.

I

Take good care of yourself beforehand to be sure of a healthy, bouncing new body. Ask your doctor all about it. He can help.

Your doctor says: "Six weeks and you'll be feeling like a new person. No one will ever know."

Your doctor says: "Don't worry about the scar. We'll make it real low where no one can see. We call it a bikini cut."

He says: "Any symptoms you have afterward, we'll fix with hormones. We follow nature's way. There is some danger of these hormones causing cancer in the lining of the uterus. But since you won't have a uterus, you won't have anything to worry about."

He says: "There is this myth some women believe, connecting their reproductive organs with their femininity. But you're much too intelligent and sophisticated for that."

Intelligently, you regard a painting hanging on the wall above his diplomas; it is modern in aspect, showing an assortment of common tools—a hammer, screwdrivers, wrenches, and several others you cannot name, not being conversant with the mechanical arts. A sort of all-purpose handyman's kit. You think a sophisticated thought: *Chacun son goût.*

You are not even sure you need a new body, but your doctor says there is something inside your old one like a grapefruit, and though it is not really dangerous, it should go. It could block the view of the rest of you. You cannot see it or feel it. Trust your doctor. You have never been a runner, but six weeks before your surgery you start to run in the lonely park early each morning. Not quite awake, half dreaming, you imagine you are running from a mugger with a knife. Fast, fast. You are going to give them the healthiest body they have ever cut. You run a quarter of a mile the first day, half a mile the second. By the end of two weeks you are running a mile in nine minutes. From the neck down you are looking splendid. Perhaps when you present your body they will say, Oh no, this body is too splendid to cut.

II

You will have one very important decision to make before the big day. Be sure to consult with your doctor. He can help.

He says: "The decision is entirely up to you. However, I like to take the ovaries out whenever I can, as long as I'm in there. That way there is no danger of ovarian cancer, which strikes one in a hundred women in your age group. There is really nothing you need ovaries for. You have had three children and don't intend to have any more. Ovarian cancer is incurable and a terrible death. I've seen women your age. . . . However, the decision is entirely up to you."

You think: No, for with the same logic he could cut off my head to avert a brain tumor.

Just before he ushers you out of his office he shows you a color snapshot of some woman's benign fibroid tumors, larger than yours, he says, but otherwise comparable, lying in a big metal bowl wider than it is deep, the sort of bowl you often use to prepare chopped meat for meat loaf. You nod appreciatively and go into the bathroom to throw up.

III

Your hospital stay. One evening, in the company of your husband, you check in at the hospital and are shown to your room, which is not bad, only the walls are a bit bare and it is a bit expensive— several hundred dollars a night. Perhaps the service will be worth it. Its large window overlooks a high school, the very high school, coincidentally, that

your teenaged daughter attends. She has promised to visit often. Your husband stays until a staff member asks that he leave, and he leaves you with a copy of *People* magazine featuring an article called "Good Sex with Dr. Ruth." This is a joke and is meant well. Accept it in that spirit. He is trying to say what he would otherwise find difficult to express, that your new body will be lovable and capable of love.

Your reading of *People* magazine is interrupted by your doctor, who invites you for a chat in the visitors' lounge, empty now. He says: "You don't have to make your decision about the ovaries till the last minute. However, ovarian cancer strikes one in a hundred women in your age group." Hard to detect until too late, a terrible death, etc., etc.

As he goes on, a pregnant woman in a white hospital gown enters the visitors' lounge, shuffles to the window, and stares out at the night sky. She has a beautiful olive-skinned face with high cheekbones, green eyes, and full lips. Her hair is thick and dark. Her arms and legs are very bony; her feet, in paper slippers, are as bony and arched as a dancer's. Take another look at her face: the cheekbones seem abnormally prominent, the eyes abnormally prominent, the hollows beneath them abnormally deep. She seems somewhat old to be pregnant, around forty-five. When she leaves, shuffling on her beautiful dancer's feet, your doctor says: "That woman has ovarian cancer."

The next morning, lying flat on your back in a Demerol haze, when he says, "Well?" you say, "Take them, they're yours."

You have anticipated this moment of waking and have promised to let yourself scream if the pain is bad enough. Happily, you discover screaming will not be necessary; quiet moaning will do. If this is the worst, you think, I can take it. In a roomful of screamers and moaners like yourself, baritones and sopranos together, you feel pleased even though you have only a minor choral part. Relieved. The worst is this, probably, and it will be over soon.

A day or two and you will be simply amazed at

how much better you feel. Amazed, too, at how many strangers, men and women both, are curious to see your new bikini cut, so curious that you even feel some interest yourself. You peer down, then up into the face of the young man peering along with you, and say, "I know it sounds weird, but those actually look like staples in there."

"They are," he says.

You imagine a stapler of the kind you use at home for papers. Your doctor is holding it while you lie sleeping. Another man crimps the two layers of skin together, folds one over the other just above where your pubic hair used to be, and your doctor squeezes the stapler, moving along horizontally, again and again. Men and women are different in this, if you can generalize from personal experience: at home, you place the stapler flat on the desk, slide the papers between its jaws, and press down gently. Your husband holds the stapler in one hand, slides the corner of the papers in with the other, and squeezes the jaws of the stapler together. What strong hands they have! You think of throwing up, but this is more of an intellectual than a physical reaction since your entire upper abdomen is numb; moreover, you have had almost nothing to eat for three days. Your new body, when it returns to active life, will be quite thin.

No one can pretend that a postsurgical hospital stay is pleasant, but a cheerful outlook should take you far. The trouble is, you cry a good deal of the time. In one sense these tears seem uncontrollable, gushing at irregular intervals during the day and night. In another sense they are quite controllable: if your doctor or strange men on the staff drop in to look at your bikini cut or chat about your body functions, you are able to stop crying at will and act cheerful. But when women doctors or nurses drop in, you keep right on with your crying, even though this causes them to say, "What are you crying about?" You also do not cry in front of visitors, male or female, especially your teenaged daughter, since you noticed that when she visited you immediately after the surgery her face turned

white and she left the room quickly, walking backwards and staring. She has visited often, as she promised. She makes sure to let you know she has terrible menstrual cramps this week, in fact asks you to write a note so she can be excused from gym. Your sons do not visit—they are too young, twelve and nine—but you talk to them on the phone, cheerfully. They tell you about the junk food they have been eating in your absence and about sports events at school. They sound wistful and eager to have you returned to them.

IV

At last the day you've been waiting for arrives: taking your new body home! You may be surprised to learn this, but in many ways your new body is just like your old one. For instance, it walks. Slowly. And if you clasp your hands and support your stomach from below, you feel less as though it will rip away from the strain inside. At home, in the mirror, except for the bikini cut and the fact that your stomach is round and puffy, this body even looks remarkably like your old one, but thinner. Your ankles are thinner than you have ever seen them. That is because with your reproductive system gone, you no longer tend to retain fluids. An unexpected plus, slim ankles! How good to be home and climb into your own bed. How good to see your children and how good they are, scurrying around to bring you tea and chocolates and magazines. Why is it that the sight of the children, which should bring you pleasure, also brings you grief? It might be that their physical presence reminds you of the place they came from, which no longer exists, at least in you. This leads you to wonder idly what becomes of the many reproductive organs, both healthy and unhealthy, removed daily: buried, burned, or trashed? Do right-to-lifers mourn them?

You sleep in your own bed with your husband, who wants to hold you close, but this does not feel very comfortable. You move his arms and hands to permissible places, the way you did with boys as a teenager, except of course the places are different now. Breasts are permissible, thighs are permissible, but not the expanse between. A clever fellow, over the next few nights he learns, even in his sleep, what is permissible.

Although you are more tired than you ever thought possible, you force yourself to walk from room to room three times a day, perhaps to show this new body who is in control. During one such forced walk. . . . Don't laugh, now! A wave of heat swirls up and encircles you, making you sway dizzily, and the odd thing, no one has mentioned this—it pulsates. Pulses of heat. Once long ago and with great concentration, you counted the pulses of an orgasm, something you are not sure you will ever experience again, and now you count this. Thirty pulses. You cannot compare since you have forgotten the orgasm number; anyhow, the two events have nothing in common except that they pulse and that they are totally overpowering. But this can't be happening; you are far too young for this little joke. Over the next few days it is happening, though, and whenever it happens you feel foolish, you feel something very like shame. Call your doctor. He can help.

A woman's voice says he is extremely busy and could you call back later, honey. Or would you like an appointment, honey? Are you sure she can't help you, honey? You say yes, she can help enormously by not calling you honey. Don't give me any of your lip, you menopausal bitch, she mutters. No, no, she most certainly does not mutter that; it must have been the tone of her gasp. Very well, please hold on while she fetches your folder. While holding, you are treated to a little telephone concert: Frank Sinatra singing "My Way." Repeatedly, you hear Frank Sinatra explain that no matter what has happened or will happen, he is gratified to feel that he did it his way. Your doctor's voice is abrupt and booming in contrast. When you state your problem he replies, "Oh, sweats." You are not sure you have heard correctly. Could he have said, "Oh, sweets," as in affectionate commiseration? Hardly. Always strictly business. You were misled by remembering, subliminally,

"honey." "Sweats" it was and, in the plural, a very hideous word you do not wish to have associated with you or your new body. Sweat, a universal phenomenon, you have no quarrel with. Sweats, no.

Your doctor says he—or "they"—will take care of everything. For again he uses the plural, the royal "we." When you visit for a six-week checkup, "they" will give you the miraculous hormones, nature's way. In the meantime you begin to spend more time out of bed. You may find, during this convalescent period, that you enjoy reading, listening to music, even light activity such as jigsaw puzzles. Your twelve-year-old son brings you a jigsaw puzzle of a Mary Cassatt painting—a woman dressed in pale blue, holding a baby who is like a peach. It looks like a peach and would smell and taste like a peach too. At a glance you know you can never do this puzzle. It is not that you want another baby, for you do not, nor is it the knowledge that you could not have one even if you wanted it, since that is academic. Simply the whole cluster of associations—mothers and babies, conception, gestation, birth—is something you do not wish to be reminded of. The facts of life. You seem to be an artificial exception to the facts of life, a mutation existing outside the facts of life that apply to every other living creature. However, you can't reject the gift your son chose so carefully, obviously proud that he has intuited your tastes—Impressionist paintings, the work of women artists, peachy colors. You thank him warmly and undo the cellophane wrapping on the box as if you intended to work on the puzzle soon. You ask your husband to bring you a puzzle of an abstract painting. He brings a Jackson Pollack puzzle which you set to work at, sitting on pillows on the living room floor. Your son comes home from school and lets his knapsack slide off his back. "Why aren't you doing my puzzle?" "Well, it looked a little hard. I thought I'd save it for later." He looks at the picture on the Jackson Pollack box. "Hard!" he exclaims.

V

Your first visit to the doctor. You get dressed in

real clothes and appraise yourself in the mirror—what admirable ankles. With a shudder you realize you are echoing a thought now terrible in its implications: No one would ever know.

Out on the city streets you hail a taxi, since you cannot risk your new body's being jostled or having to stand up all the way on a bus. The receptionist in your doctor's waiting room is noticeably cool—no honeying today—as she asks you to take a seat and wait. When your name is finally called, a woman in a white coat leads you into a cubicle just off the waiting room and loudly asks your symptoms. Quite often in the past you have, while waiting, overheard the symptoms of many women, and now no doubt many women hear yours. As usual, you are directed to an examining room and instructed to undress and don a white paper robe. On the way you count the examining rooms. Three. One woman—you—is preexamination, one no doubt midexamination, one is post.

When your doctor at last enters, he utters a cheery greeting and then the usual: "Slide your lower body to the edge of the table. Feet up in the stirrups, please." You close your eyes, practicing indifference. It cannot be worse than the worst you have already known. You study certain cracks in the ceiling that you know well and he does not even know exist. You continue to meditate on procedural matters, namely, that your doctor's initial impression in each of his three examining rooms is of a woman naked except for a white paper robe, sitting or leaning on an examining table in an attitude of waiting. He, needless to say, is fully dressed. You contemplate him going from one examining room to the next; the devil will not have to make work for his hands. After the examination you will be invited, clothed, to speak with him in his office, and while you dress for this encounter, he will visit another examining room. It strikes you that this maximum efficiency setup might serve equally well for a brothel and perhaps already does. This is a brothel realized.

Your doctor says you may resume most normal activities and even do some very mild exercise if you wish, but no baths and no "intercourse." "Intercourse," you are well aware, stands for sex, although if you stop to consider, sex is the more inclusive term. Does he say "intercourse" because he is unable to say "sex," or thinks the word "sex" would be too provocative in this antiseptic little room, unleashing torrents of libido, or is it an indirect way of saying that you can do sexual things as long as you don't fuck? This is not something you can ask your doctor.

The last item of business is the prescription for the hormones. He explains how to take them—three weeks on and one week off, in imitation of nature's way. He gives you several small sample packets for starters. At home, standing at the bathroom sink, you extricate a pill from its tight childproof cardboard-and-plastic niche, feverishly, like a junkie pouncing on her fix. Nature's way. Now no more "sweats," no more tears. Your new body is complete. What is this little piece of paper in the sample packet? Not so little when you open it up, just impeccably folded. In diabolically tiny print it explains the pills' side effects or "contraindications," a word reminiscent of "intercourse." Most of them you already know from reading books, but there is something new. The pills may have a damaging effect on your eyes. Fancy that. Nature's way? You settle down on the edge of the bathtub and go back to the beginning and read more attentively. First, a list of situations for which the pills are prescribed. Funny, you do not find "hysterectomy." Reading on, you do find "female castration." That must be it. Yes indeed, that's you. You try to read on, but the print is terribly small, perhaps the pills are affecting your eyes already, for there is a shimmering film over the fine letters. Rather than simply rolling over into the tub, you go back to bed, fully dressed, face in the pillows. No, first close the door in case the children come in. Many times over the past weeks you have lain awake pinched by questions, pulling and squeezing back as if the questions were clay, weighing the threat of the bony-footed woman pregnant with her own death—an actress summoned and stuffed for the occasion? Part of a terrorist scheme?—against your own undrugged sense of the fitness of things. Now you have grasped that the questions are moot. This is not like cutting your hair, and you have never even had a tooth pulled. The only other physically irreversible things you have done are lose your virginity and bear children. Yes, shut the door tight. It would not do to have them hear you, hysteric, *castrata*.

But of course the sun continues to rise, your center is hardly the center of the universe. Over the next few weeks you get acquainted with your new body. A peculiar thing—though it does not look very different, it does things differently. It responds to temperature differently and it sleeps differently, finding different positions comfortable and different hours propitious. It eats differently, shits differently and pisses differently. You suspect it will fuck differently but that you will not know for a while. Its pubic hair has not grown back in quite the same design or density, so that you look shorn or childlike or, feeling optimistic, like a chorus girl or a Renaissance painting. It doesn't menstruate, naturally. You can't truthfully say you miss menstruation, but how will you learn to keep track of time, the seasons of the month? A wall calendar? But how will you know inside? Can it be that time will feel all the same, no coming to fruition and dropping the fruit, no filling and subsiding, moist and dry, moving toward and moving away from?

VI

At nine weeks, although your new body can walk and move almost naturally, it persists in lying around the house whenever possible. And so you lie around the living room with your loved ones as your daughter, wearing an old sweater of yours, scans the local newspaper in search of part-time work. Music blares, Madonna singing "Like a Virgin," describing how she felt touched as though for the very first time. Were you not disconcerted by the whole cluster of associations,

you might tell your daughter that the premise of the song is mistaken: the very first time is usually not so terrific. Perhaps some other evening. Your daughter reads aloud amusing job opportunities. A dental school wants research subjects who have never had a cavity. Aerobics instructor at a reform school. "Hey, Mom, here's something you could do. A nutrition experiment, five dollars an hour. Women past childbearing age or surgically sterile."

A complex message, but no response is really required since her laughter fills the space. Your older son, bent over the Mary Cassatt puzzle, chuckles. Your husband smirks faintly over his newspaper. He means no harm, you suppose. (Then why the fuck is he smirking?) Maybe those to whom the facts of life still apply can't help it, just as children can't help smirking at the facts of life themselves. Only your younger son, building a space station out of Lego parts, is not amused. Unknowing, he senses some primitive vibration in the air and looks up at you apprehensively, then gives you a loving punch in the knee. You decide that he is your favorite, that one day you may run away with him, abandoning the others.

VII

The tenth week, and a most important day in the life of your new body. Your doctor says you are permitted to have "intercourse." If your husband is like most men, he can hardly wait. Proceed with caution, like walking on eggshells, except that you, eggless, are the eggshells on which he proceeds with caution. Touched for the very first time! Well, just do it and see if it works; passion will come later, replacing fear. That is the lesson of behavioral science as opposed to classical psychology. But what's this? Technical difficulties, like a virgin. This can't be happening, not to you with that hot little geyser, that little creamery you had up there. Come now, when there's a will.... Spit, not to mention a thousand drugstore remedies. Even tears will do. Before long things are wet enough, thank you very much. Remember for next time there's still that old spermicidal jelly, but you can throw away the diaphragm. That is not the sort of thing you can hand down to your daughter like a sweater.

VIII

Over the next month or two you may find your new body has strange responses to your husband's embraces. Don't be alarmed: it feels desire and it feels pleasure, only it feels them in a wholly unfamiliar way. In bed your new body is most different from your old, so different that you have the eerie sensation that another woman, a stranger, is making love to your husband while your mind, your same old mind, looks on in amazement. All your body's nerve endings have been replaced by this strange woman's; she moves and caresses the way you used to, and the sounds of pleasure she makes are the same, only her apparatus of sensation is altogether alien. There are some things you cannot discuss with your husband because you are too closely twined; just as if, kissing, your tongues in each other's mouths, you were to attempt to speak. But you cannot rest easy in this strangeness; it must be exposed, and so you shine a light on an experiment.

You call an old friend, someone you almost married, except that you managed in time to distinguish your feeling for each other from love. It was sex, one of those rare affinities that would not withstand daily life. Now and then, at long intervals, a year or more, you have met for several hours with surprisingly little guilt. This is no time for fine moral distinctions. He has often pledged that you may ask him for any kind of help, so you call him and explain the kind of help you need. He grins, you can see this over the telephone, and says he would be more than happy to help you overcome the mystery of the sexual stranger in your body. Like Nancy Drew's faithful Ned.

You have to acknowledge the man has a genuine gift, as regards women. From the gods? Or could it be because he is a doctor and knows his physiology? No, your knowledge of doctors would not bear out that correlation, and besides, this one is only an eye doctor. In any case, in his arms, in a motel room, you do rediscover yourself buried deep deep deep in the crevices of hidden tissues and disconnected circuits. It takes some time and coaxing to bring you forth, you have simply been so traumatized by the knife that you have been in hiding underground for months, paralyzed by any kind of penetration. But you are still there, in your new body, and gradually, you feel sure, you will emerge again and replace the impostors in the conjugal bed. You feel enormous gratitude and tell him so, and he says, grinning, "No trouble at all. My pleasure." Perhaps you will even ask him about the effects of the pills on your eyes, but not just now.

"Do I feel any different inside?" you ask. He says no, and describes in exquisite terms how you feel inside, which is very nice to listen to. This is not in your husband's line or perhaps any husband's—you wouldn't know. After the exquisite description, he says, "But it is different, you know." You don't know. How?

He explains that in the absence of the cervix, which is the opening of the uterus, the back wall of the vagina is sewn up so that in effect what you have there now is a dead end. As he explains, it seems obvious and inevitable, but strange to say, you have never figured this out before or even thought about it. (It is something your doctor neglected to mention.) Nor have you poked around on your own, having preferred to remain ignorant. So it is rather a shock, this realization that you have a dead end. You always imagined yourself, along with all women, as having an easy passage from inside to out, a constant trafficking between the heart of the world and the heart of yourself. This was what distinguished you from men. They were the walled ones, barricaded, the ones with such difficulty receiving and transmitting the current running between the heart of the world and the heart of themselves. It is so great a shock that you believe you cannot bear to live with it.

Watching you, he says, "It makes no difference. You feel wonderful, the same as always. You really do. Here, feel with your hand, so you'll know." With his help you feel around your new body. Different, not so different. Yet you know. Of course, with his help it became an amusing and piquant thing to be doing in a motel room, and then it becomes more love, wonderful love, but you cry all the way through it. A new sensation: like some *Kama sutra* position, you wouldn't have thought it possible.

"At least you don't have to worry about ovarian cancer," he says afterward. "It's very hard to detect in time and a terrible way—"

"Please," you say. "Please stop." You cannot bear hearing those words from this man.

"I'm sorry. I know it's hard. I can't imagine how I would feel if I had my balls cut off."

With a leap you are out of bed and into your clothes, while he looks on aghast. How fortunate that you did not marry him, for had you married him, after those words you would have had to leave him. As you leave him, naked and baffled, now, not bothering to inquire about the effects of the pills on your eyes yet thanking him because he has done precisely what you needed done. It will be a very long time before you see him again, though, before the blade of his words grows dull from repetition.

IX

Months pass and you accept that this new body, its torso ever so slightly different in shape from the old one, is yours to keep. Not all women, remember, love their new bodies instinctively; some have to learn to love them. Through the thousands of little acts of personal care, an intimacy develops. By the sixth month you will feel not quite as teary, not quite as tired—the anesthetic sloshing around in your cells must be evaporating. You resolve to ignore the minor nuisance symptoms—mild backaches, a recurrent vaginal infection, lowered resistance to colds and viruses. . . . Now that the sample packets of hormone pills are used up, you are spending about $15 a month at the drugstore, something your doctor neglected to mention in advance. Would he have told you this, you wonder, if you were a very poor woman? How does he know you are not a very poor woman? Foolish question. Because you have purchased his services. The pills cause you to gain weight, jeopardizing this thin new body and the ankles, so you run faster every morning (yes, it runs! it runs!), racing nature's way. One very positive improvement is that now you can sleep on your stomach. Your husband can touch you anywhere without pain. When he makes love to you, you feel the strange woman and her alien nervous system retreating and yourself emerging in her place. You will eventually overcome her.

And before you know it, it's time for your six-month checkup. You do not respond to your doctor's hearty greeting, but you comply when he says, "Slide your lower body to the edge of the table. Feet up in the stirrups, please." He does not know it, but this is the last time he will be seeing—no, seeing is wrong since he doesn't look, he looks at the wall behind your head—the last time he or any man will be examining your body. There is nothing he can tell you about how you feel, for the simple reason that he does not know. How can he? Suddenly this is utterly obvious, and as you glance again at the painting of assorted tools, the fact of his being in an advisory capacity on any matter concerning your body is both an atrocity, which you blame yourself for having permitted, and an absurdity, such an ancient social absurdity that you laugh aloud, a crude, assertive, resuscitated laugh, making him look warily from the wall to your face, which very possibly he has never looked at before. How can he know what you feel? He has never attempted to find out by the empirical method; his tone is not inquisitive but declarative. He knows only what men like himself have written in books, and just now he looks puzzled.

Why not tell your doctor? That might help. In

his office after the examination you tell him—quite mildly, compared to what you feel—that he might have informed you more realistically of what this operation would entail. Quite mild and limited, but even so it takes a great summoning of strength. He is the one with the social position, the money, and the knife. You, despite your laugh, are the *castrata*. Your heart goes pit-a-pat as you speak, and you have a lump in your throat. To your surprise, he looks directly at your face with interest.

He says: "Thank you for telling me that. But not everyone reacts the same way. We try to anticipate the bright side, but some people take it harder than others. Some people are special cases."

X

A few months later, you read a strange, small item in the newspaper: a lone marauder, on what is presented as a berserk midnight spree, has ransacked the office of a local gynecologist. She tore diplomas from the walls and broke equipment. She emptied sample packets of medication and packages of rubber fingers and gloves, which she strewed everywhere, creating a battlefield of massacred hands. She wrote abusive epithets on the walls; she dumped file folders on the floor and daubed them with menstrual blood. As you read these details you feel the uncanny sensation of déjà vu, and your heart beats with a bizarre fear. Calm down; you have an alibi, you were deep in your law-abiding sleep. Anyhow, you would have done quite differently—not under cover of darkness, first of all, but in broad daylight when the doctor was there. You would have forced him into a white paper robe and onto the examining table, saying, "Slide your lower body to the edge of the table. Feet up in the stirrups, please." Not being built for such a position, he would have found it extremely uncomfortable. While he lay terrorized, facing the painting of common tools, you would simply have looked. Armed only with force of will, you would have looked for what would seem to him an endless time at his genitals until he himself, mesmerized

by your gaze, began to look at them as some freakish growth, a barrier to himself, between the world and himself. After a while you would have let him climb down untouched, but he would never again have looked at or touched himself without remembering his terror and his inkling that his body was his cage and all his intercourse with the world was a wild and pitiable attempt to cut his way free.

XI

A year after your operation, you will be feeling much much better. You have your strength back, or about 80 percent of it anyway. You are hardly tired at all; the anesthetic must be nearly evaporated. You can walk erect without conscious effort, and you have grown genuinely fond of your new body, accepting its hollowness with, if not equanimity, at least tolerance. One or two symptoms, or rather habits, persist: for instance, when you get out of bed, you still hold your hands clasped around your lower abdomen for support, as if it might rip away from the strain inside, even though there is no longer any strain. At times you lie awake blaming yourself for participating in an ancient social absurdity, but eventually you will cease to blame as you have ceased to participate.

Most odd, and most obscure, you retain the tenuous sense of waiting. With effort you can localize it to a sense of waiting for something to end. A holdover, a vague habit of memory or memory of habit. Right after he cut, you waited for that worst pain to end. Then for the tears, the tiredness, and all the rest. Maybe it is a memory of habit or a habit of memory, or maybe the blade in the flesh brought you to one of life's many edges and now you are waiting, like a woman who after much travel has come to the edge of a cliff and, for no reason and under no compulsion, lingers there too long. You are waiting for something to end, you feel closer than ever before to the end, but of what, you do not push further to ask.

Keeping All Your Eggs in One Basket

BARBARA SEAMAN

Barbara Seaman, "Keeping All Your Eggs in One Basket," *O, The Oprah Magazine*, October, 2006. Reprinted by permission.

If you're a woman who stands up for your rights and doesn't believe that the doctor always knows best, I wish you could have met my friend Rose Kushner. Rose was a formidable breast cancer activist—one of the first, and one of the best. I watched in awe as she persuaded President Jimmy Carter and the National Institutes of Health through her writings and personal appearances to get behind massive clinical trials that could show us if radical mastectomy, the debilitating automatic treatment at the time, saved more lives than a less invasive option, lumpectomy. Rose won. Lumpectomy won. Even old-fashioned breast doctors took off their hats to Rose and agreed that the Halsted radical mastectomy was "the greatest standardized surgical error of the twentieth century."

We may have to amend that now. Yes, the Halsted was the greatest error above the waist, but what about below? What about our ovaries, if you please?

"Federal data from the late 1990s show that 78 percent of women between ages forty-five and sixty-four who underwent a hysterectomy also had their healthy ovaries taken out, even though most were not at a particular risk for ovarian cancer," says William Parker, MD, lead author of a study that roiled the gynecological community when it was published in the August 2005 issue of the journal *Obstetrics & Gynecology*. A clinical professor at the David Geffen School of Medicine at UCLA, Parker at one time believed it was "good prevention" for women forty-five and older to relinquish their ovaries when they went in for a hysterectomy. He has changed his mind. The results of his study show that for women who do not have a family history of ovarian cancer, keeping the ovaries until at least age sixty-five significantly saves lives by reducing the risk of dying from heart disease and complications of osteoporosis. In fact, at no age is there a clear benefit from taking them out.

OVARY POWER

It's no secret that, if you still menstruate, should you and your ovaries part ways, you might as well brace yourself for a wretched premature menopause and rapidly thinning bones. Less well understood is the fact that after menopause, your ovaries continue to make small amounts of estrogen for years, as well as testosterone and other androgens that help stimulate lust and desire—and that oophorectomy is another way of saying female castration.

The issue patients and doctors alike have been more concerned about is the specter of ovarian cancer, which is extremely difficult to detect, especially in its early stages, when five-year survival rate is a high 94 percent. The overall five-year survival rate—only 45 percent—is a testament to how rarely the disease is caught in time.

PARKER'S AHA!

What changed Parker's mind was a layperson who, much like Rose Kushner, had her own thoughts about women's health. In 1984 Janine O'Leary Cobb, a Canadian mother of five and professor of humanities and sociology at Vanier College in Montreal, started *A Friend Indeed*, which would become the grandmother of menopause newsletters. Parker says it was her review of his book, *A Gynecologist's Second Opinion*, originally published in 1996, that got him thinking. She'd liked it, except for his position on oophorectomy during hysterectomy (the old "take 'em out while you're in there" theory). She'd heard from too many newsletter readers who complained about loss of energy, concentration, interest in sex, and even interest in living after having their ovaries removed. "I never forgot your comments," he wrote her years later. "I want to thank you for putting some doubt in my mind that what I had been taught may not have been well thought out or true."

Parker got in touch with a former colleague, Michael Broder, MD, a gynecologist and expert on health outcomes research, who remembered from his medical school days "a youngish woman being wheeled into the operating room. She cried out to her surgeon, 'I don't want my ovaries out.' The doctor scolded her, 'What if you get ovarian cancer someday, and I would have been the one who left the ovaries in? That could be malpractice.'" As a student, Broder felt he couldn't say anything, "but I wanted to tell the woman to get off the operating table and run," he said.

Parker and Broder—working with Donna Shoupe, MD, Cindy Farquhar, MD, Zhimei Liu, PhD, and Jonathan Berek, MD—decided to take data from dozens of published studies and use a mathematical model to estimate the survival impact of leaving the ovaries in versus taking them out.

THE RESULTS

The findings were far more dramatic than any of the researchers had expected. Based on their model, if 10,000 women between the ages of fifty and fifty-four undergo a hysterectomy with oophorectomy, they will have forty-seven fewer cases of ovarian cancer by the time they reach eighty than a similar group who keep their ovaries. The oophorectomy group, however, will suffer 838 additional deaths from coronary heart disease as well as 158 more deaths from hip fractures. (These numbers reflect women who do not have estrogen therapy; with estrogen there's smaller survival benefit to keeping the ovaries, but that assumes staying on the drug forever.) "Forty-seven women are spared ovarian cancer but at a cost of more than 900 women's lives whose hearts and bones failed without the normal hormone support," says Parker. Unless a woman is at high risk of developing ovarian cancer based on genetic testing or family history, the study showed, there is no real advantage in removing the ovaries.

Berek is concerned that most patients do not know the symptoms of early ovarian cancer: unexplained change in bowel or bladder habits, including urinary urgency and incontinence; persistent indigestion or nausea; unexplained weight gain particularly in the abdominal area; constant pelvic and/or abdominal pain, discomfort, bloating, or feeling of fullness and fatigue. As terrible as ovarian cancer is, however, the lifetime risk is only one in sixty-nine—lower if you don't have a genetic pedigree. Compare that with heart disease and stroke, which kill nearly one out of two women.

Parker's research bears further study, but in the meantime, these numbers are important to keep in mind. And, as his story reflects once again, we should not be intimidated by a doctor headed for excavation. As the book *Women Talk About Gynecological Surgery* reminds us, you're "hiring a surgeon, not crawling to Lourdes."

CHAPTER 9

Abortion

"MOMMY, WHAT'S AN ABORTION?"

My youngest child, Shira, greeted me with the question as I walked in the door. I was weary after days of organizing and meeting. That night, I had been on television making public one of the most private decisions of my life—my choice to have an abortion when I was a teenager.

It was during the battle for legalizing abortion access in New York State that Betty Friedan came up with the idea: She overheard prominent black feminist Florence Rice and me discussing our illegal abortions. Mine had been relatively painless: A friend of mine had given me the name of a doctor who would do it for the then-princely sum of five hundred dollars. Luckily my boyfriend at the time came from a family that was well-off enough; he assembled the necessary cash, and it was done. Florence, on the other hand, found herself facing Harlem's back alleys and nearly died during a dirty procedure. What better way, Betty argued, to make the point that abortion would always be available to those who had the means. Keeping it illegal penalized poor women and subjected them to the very real possibility of injury, mutilation, and even death.

Together, Florence and I stood together on the steps of the Judson Memorial Church in Greenwich Village and shared our stories. Television crews were there to capture the moment. Opening up about something so personal wasn't easy—the questioning face of my little child brought home to me the broad implications of my decision. But I have no doubt in my mind that it was the right thing to do.

Flash forward thirty years and young feminist Jennifer Baumgardner was making the same point in an equally powerful way with her film, "I Had an Abortion." Until women talk openly about their experience, Baumgardner argued, we surrender our voice in the national conversation about choice to right-wing forces that would take away our rights. While we might wish for an abortion to be a profoundly private moment, as women, we cannot afford to "stay in the closet" on this subject.

Over the years, women have found different ways to tell their stories, be it in person, as I did and the young women in Baumgardner's film did, or in fiction, as Alix Kates Shulman did so movingly in *Memoirs of an Ex-Prom Queen*.

There is nothing simple about abortion rights. In 1994, Norma McCorvey (Jane Roe of *Roe v. Wade*) powerfully told her own story in collaboration with Andy Meisler. Later she reconsidered and changed her mind about choice, at least in part because of the generous emotional and financial support she received from anti-abortion women. The pro-choice movement has too many martyred heroes who never received the recognition they deserved. Another example is Lucinda Cisler: a key figure in New York activism, a full-time, brilliant volunteer for choice, an architect who gave up her practice in service of her cause, scraping to get by, and in the end having some of her best writing and other work appropriated by others without credit or compensation.

Abortion rights are under near-constant assault. As I write this, the increasingly conservative Supreme Court of Justice John Roberts has finished their first session. Among their key decisions: the upholding of a ban on so-called partial-birth abortion. In the lead opinion, Justice Anthony Kennedy argued that such a ban was necessary because women couldn't be expected to know how horrible the consequences of their actions in seeking such a procedure would be. In other words, the little ladies just don't know what's good for them and the big strong court will watch out for them and make the tough decisions. Old-fashioned patriarchal sexism re-packaged as judicial compassion. Most feminists despaired at the ruling, recognizing it for what it was: another chip in the already precarious cliff that the right to choose has become.

The good news is that young women have taken up the fight. New grassroots groups, funds, and organizations founded by shockingly young people have begun to crop up across the country providing money for poor women who can't afford proce-

dures, emotional support for those trying to make a decision about a pregnancy, and even housing for those who must travel out of state to receive second trimester procedures. In 2004, millions of women marched together in Washington to show their commitment to choice in an event reminiscent of 1970s activism. College women and those in their twenties came by the bus load and organized groups of friends to travel to the nation's capital and stand together.

There are, undoubtedly, dark days ahead for women on the issue of abortion access. We must learn from our past successes and keep fighting the good fight. And most of all we must keep raising our voices and telling our stories without shame.

I Am Roe

NORMA McCORVEY

Norma McCorvey with Andy Meisler, excerpt from *I Am Roe: My Life*, Roe v. Wade, *and Freedom of Choice*, New York: HarperCollins, 1994. Reprinted by permission.

In February 1970 I was Norma McCorvey, a pregnant street person. A 21-year-old woman in big trouble. I became Jane Roe at a corner table at Columbo's, an Italian restaurant at Mockingbird Lane and Greenville Avenue, in Dallas. I'd suggested to Linda Coffee that we meet there.

Columbo's is gone now, which is a shame. It was an inexpensive place, clean, and made very good pizza. The tables had red-and-white checked tablecloths—just like the one I'd bought for Woody back in California. Columbo's wasn't very big. When I walked into the place that evening, I didn't have any trouble figuring out who was waiting for me.

Linda Coffee and Sarah Weddington, sitting together, stood out in Columbo's. Both were older than me, and both were wearing two-piece business suits. Nice clothing, expensive looking. One of them was tall and dark and thin. Delicate. The other was short and blond and a little plump, her hair in a stiff-looking permanent. Her hairdo was old-fashioned, even for then.

I was wearing jeans, a button-down shirt tied at the waist, and sandals. I wore my bandanna tied around my left leg, above the knee. That meant I didn't have a girlfriend.

I walked over to their table. It was obvious to me even from across the room that these women hadn't talked to a person like me for a long time, if ever. For a second, I felt like turning around and running out the door, writing the whole meeting off, and starting over again. But I didn't. Instead, I thought, Norma, they're just as scared of you as you are of them. Looking at the nervousness and doubt in their eyes, I almost believed it.

"Hi. I'm Norma McCorvey," I said.

The shorter blond woman came to life.

"I'm Sarah Weddington," she said.

Sarah Weddington reached out and shook my hand. Linda introduced herself, too, but it was apparent right away that Sarah was the one who would speak for both of them. For most of that meeting—in fact, for most of all our meetings—it was Sarah who talked, and it was Sarah who listened to me with the most concentration.

"Thanks for showing up," I said.

I don't remember much else about the first few minutes. Small talk was awkward for us, considering how little we had in common. I talked about Henry and how much I liked him. Sarah agreed. She told me that she and Linda were lawyers, which I already knew. The conversation died down.

I went to order our pizza and beer at the counter. While I stood there, waiting, I worked up the courage to ask these women the only question I was interested in getting an answer to.

I brought the beer back to the table.

"Do you know where I can get an abortion?" I said.

"No," said Sarah, "I don't."

Son of a bitch! I thought. I sat up in my chair and got ready to leave. I didn't want to hear the adoption spiel again.

But surprisingly, Sarah didn't begin to give it to me. Instead—and this is what kept me from leaving—she went off in another direction entirely.

"Norma, do you really want an abortion?" she asked.

"Yes," I said.

"Why?"

"Because I don't want this baby. I don't even figure it's a baby. And I figure it's making my life pretty miserable right now."

"Yes," said Sarah. "Go on."

I looked closely at her to see if what I'd said disgusted her. Or made her dislike me. But no, all I could see was that she was interested in my story. And maybe, just maybe, interested in helping me somehow.

"See, Sarah," I said, "my being pregnant, I don't think I'll be able to find work. And if I can't get work, I can't take care of myself. I don't want to be pregnant. I don't want this thing growing inside my body!"

By the end of my answer I was almost shouting. But Sarah didn't seem to mind.

"Norma," she said, "do you know what the abortion process is? Do you know what women have to go through when they get one?"

"Not really," I admitted. "But I kind of have a general idea."

Sarah told me, roughly, what a doctor did during a regular abortion. It sounded awful. But the truth was, it wasn't much different from what I had imagined all along.

Sarah leaned forward. "Norma. Don't you think women should have access to abortions? Safe, legal abortions?"

For the first time I realized that Sarah and Linda weren't just ordinary lawyers. For the first time I realized how interested she was in what I was interested in. Abortions. And in my getting one, too? Despite everything, my hopes rose a little.

"Sure," I said, "of course they should. But there aren't any legal ones around. So I guess I've got to find an illegal one, don't I?"

"No!" said Sarah and Linda, together.

"Why the hell not?" I said.

I felt a little flare of anger. First they were for

abortions. Then they didn't want me to have one. What kind of mind games were these women playing with me?

"Because they're dangerous, Norma," said Sarah. "Illegal abortions are dangerous."

"Yeah, so?" I said.

Sarah shook her head. Then this woman in her nice suit, a woman I couldn't have imagined even going to a horror movie, began to tell me stories.

Terrible stories. Stories of women who'd had illegal abortions and lived to regret them. Or hadn't lived. Women who'd gone to gangsters, or shady doctors, and had their insides torn out. And who'd gone home and bled to death.

"These women were murdered," said Sarah. Then she told me about pregnant, unmarried women who had been so desperate to get rid of their babies that they'd tried to give themselves abortions with coat hangers. And killed themselves.

Then the worst story—one that made me shiver with fear. Sarah told me about a woman who didn't want anyone to know she had gotten the abortion—who was found, in a pool of blood, in a hotel room in New York City.

"They didn't find her for a couple of days," said Sarah. "And even when they did, she had no identification. So they didn't know who she was. They couldn't notify her family. All they could do was call her Jane Doe. And wait for someone to come forward and claim her body."

Jane Doe! That could be me.

An awful picture passed through my mind. Of me, alone—no friends, no lovers, not even a name—lying dead in that hotel room. Who would claim my body?

I began to cry, in front of strangers. Smart, rich strangers, who made me feel poor and ignorant. It was awful that they were seeing me cry. Embarrassing. Sarah handed me a Kleenex from her purse.

"Yes," she said, "it's really unfair and inhuman. And it shouldn't have to happen to any woman. Rich or poor. Anywhere." That's why, she said, she and Linda and some other people who thought just like them were working hard to overturn the Texas law against abortions. Their weapon was a legal project, a lawsuit, to challenge the law in the courts.

She wasn't sure if they would be successful, but if they could do it—and it would take a lot of hard work, plus a pregnant woman like me, who wanted but wasn't able to get an abortion, to put her name on their lawsuit—then abortions would be legal in the state of Texas.

"Would that mean that somebody like me would be able to get an abortion?" I said.

"Yes," said Sarah, "it would."

It would? New hope began to flood through me, even though I'd been crying my eyes out a few seconds ago.

"That would be great," I said, excited despite myself.

"Yes!" said Sarah, just as excitedly.

In her excitement, Sarah began describing the road the lawsuit would take—through district courts and appeals courts, state courts and federal courts. Early on, I lost the thread of what she was saying. But I kept nodding anyway. Sarah sounded so revved up, so intense, so passionate about her plans, that it was as if she were telling me her innermost personal secrets—instead of describing all sorts of complicated legal business, using words that I was certain only lawyers understood.

I thought, I don't really want to hear about courts. I've been in too many courts in my life. But I didn't want to interrupt her. This woman might be able to help me.

Finally, she stopped.

"That's great," I said, a little bit too late.

But I must not have fooled anybody, because there was an awkward silence. Then somebody, either Sarah or Linda, asked me to tell them all about myself.

Another silence. A longer one. All about myself? What would these women think about me if I told them all about myself? I didn't know much—anything at all, really—about their lives, but I was pretty sure they hadn't gone to reform school or dealt drugs or been beaten by their husbands or spent their days and nights in gay bars.

They might be shocked—or worse, maybe disgusted—by my story. On the other hand, they seemed to like me, wanted to connect with me, in their own way.

Would they still want to help me if I told them that my private life was none of their damn business? I took a deep breath and made my decision.

Over that red checkered tablecloth, I told them everything. Or almost everything. Louisiana and Dallas and Woody McCorvey. The whole miserable story. Over pizza and a pitcher of beer. While the people at the next table laughed and whooped it up.

Sarah and Linda hung in and listened sympathetically for a while. Then I got to the part of telling them I was a lesbian. That I liked girls. That I lived with women, get it?

Sarah and Linda looked at each other. They frowned. I felt the flashes of fear and doubt and confusion passing between them. I realized what they were thinking: how could this woman who says she's a lesbian have gotten herself pregnant all these times? It doesn't make sense. Maybe nothing she'd told us makes sense. But here's what does make sense: maybe she's lying to us. Or maybe there's something we don't understand about her. Something weird. Something dangerous. Something that will hurt our lawsuit. Hurt us.

No! Inside my head, I shouted back to them: You don't have to worry about my hurting you! I'm only dangerous to myself!

They didn't hear me. But how could I explain it all in words? I could sense them thinking about brushing me off and finding another pregnant woman. They were slipping away from me. And with them, my only chance for an abortion.

I panicked.

"You know," I said, "I was raped. That's how I became pregnant with this baby."

The horrible lie—this was the second time I'd used it—pulled at the insides of my stomach. But it got their attention. The two lawyers turned away

from each other and quickly said they were sorry to hear this. That rape is a terrible thing. A crime.

"Was the rapist arrested?" asked Sarah.

"No," I said.

"Did the police look very hard for him?"

"No," I said, sinking deeper and deeper.

"Did you report the rape to the police?"

"No," I said, burning inside with shame.

Sarah stopped quizzing me. I tried to figure out whether she thought I was lying. This time, I couldn't read her.

She looked at Linda again. They seemed to come to some sort of conclusion.

"Well, Norma," she said, "it's awful that you were raped. But actually, the Texas abortion law doesn't make any exception for rape. So it doesn't matter in terms of our lawsuit."

"Oh, that's too bad," I said.

"Yes, it is," said Sarah.

A long pause.

"Well, anyway, we would like to have you as a plaintiff in our lawsuit. Would you like to help us?"

"Sure," I said, trying to be as cool as I could. A plaintiff. What was that? Well, I'd look it up in the dictionary later. At least I hadn't lost this chance.

We drank a beer toast to our lawsuit. Before she left, Sarah explained to me that they'd need me to sign some legal papers. With my own name, if I wanted to, but under a false name if I wanted to stay anonymous.

"Great," I said.

Sarah asked me if I had any questions. I said yes, I did.

"How much will I have to pay you two for being my lawyers?" I said.

Sarah smiled. "Nothing, Norma. We're doing this case *pro bono*." That meant, she said, that they were doing it for free.

"Then when can I get my abortion?" I asked.

"When the case is over, if we've won," said Sarah.

I was two and a half months pregnant. I didn't know how late you could get an abortion, but I did know that it was better to do it as soon as possible. How long could a lawsuit take? I remembered some of the trials I'd seen on television. The times I'd been in court myself. None of those occasions seemed to have taken much time at all.

"When will that be?" I said.

Sarah looked at me closely. I can see her sitting across from me, right now.

"It's really impossible to tell you that, Norma," she said. "We'll just have to let due process take its course."

It was a couple of weeks until I heard from Sarah and Linda again. In the meantime, I stayed at my dad's. I didn't tell him, or anyone else, about what had happened at Columbo's. Why risk being held up to public ridicule if the whole thing failed and we lost, and I still had to have a baby? Or worse, what if it was all some kind of harebrained scheme—or even a scam?

That's what made me decide to stay anonymous. To not put my own name on the lawsuit.

By the time Linda called me to come down to her office I was cleaning my father's apartment immaculately, several times a day, as if I was possessed by cleaning demons. I went downtown, and in front of Sarah and Linda signed a piece of paper. Not as Jane Doe—that reminded me of the woman who had been killed giving herself an illegal abortion—but as Jane Roe. The whole thing took only a few minutes. Sarah and Linda seemed very excited about it all. And so was I, despite myself, despite the feeling that I shouldn't be getting my hopes up too high.

And that was the start of *Roe v. Wade*. The lawsuit that would allow me, and millions of other women, to be in control of our own destinies.

To me, it didn't feel historic. Just a little confusing . . . and intimidating.

I didn't even know who Wade—Henry Wade, the Dallas district attorney who would be fighting the lawsuit against us—was. But that was all right. Sarah and Linda looked as if they knew what they were doing.

They both thanked me and said I could go home and let them do the legal work.

And then I waited. . . .

It was a strange pregnancy. It was a strange time, watching and feeling this baby—no, this *thing* I didn't want happening to me—growing bigger and bigger inside me. Some days, I looked very pregnant. Others, for some reason, I didn't look pregnant at all. I was out of work. Alone most of the day in a little apartment. I had all the time in the world to think about things.

My moods swung up and down, usually by the day, sometimes by the hour. When I was up, I was way up—I was the smartest thing on two legs. I wasn't just sitting around feeling sorry for myself, after all—I had taken action. I'd gotten a pair of wonderful smart young lawyers, and I was going to win my case and be the first girl in Texas to get a legal abortion. . . .

I was six months pregnant by the time the trial was over. When I called in, Linda told me to come right over. She sounded excited. After I finally arrived, hot and tired, she said that she had both good news and bad news to tell me. The good news was that we had won the case.

"That's wonderful," I said, holding my breath for the second part.

The bad news was that I had lost.

Even though the judges had ruled that abortion was now legal in Texas, Henry Wade had announced he would appeal the case—and until that appeal was decided, he would prosecute any doctor who performed an abortion on a woman.

"Well, then, Linda, how long will the appeal take?" I asked.

"A while," she said. "But, Norma, what does it matter? An abortion has to be performed in the first twenty-four weeks of pregnancy, and it's clearly too late for you now."

The world stopped.

The Jane Collective

PAULINE BART

Pauline B. Bart, excerpt from "Seizing the Means of Reproduction: An Illegal Feminist Abortion Collective—How and Why It Worked," *Qualitative Sociology*, 10(4), 1987. Reprinted by permission.

The unique female capacity for reproduction has always been regulated. In no society and in no era have all women had control of their reproductive capacity. Yet, everywhere and in all times, women have attempted, with varying degrees of success, to obtain such control. Jane, or, the Service, began in 1969 as an abortion counseling and referral service, a work group of the Chicago Women's Liberation Union. Some of these women went on to do more than counsel and refer—they assisted the illegal abortionists. By the winter of 1971 they took over the entire process themselves. They decided to provide abortions for any woman, at any stage of her pregnancy, with or without funds.

Let us follow a woman through the steps she took to obtain an abortion from Jane.

1. A woman needing an abortion could get Jane's phone number from the Chicago Women's Liberation Union or personal networks or even Chicago police officers. She could call and leave her name and number on a message machine.

2. The messages would be collected every two hours and the call would be returned by a woman assigned to that task, called "Calling back Jane." She would take a medical history and advise the woman that a counselor would call her.

3. The woman would be assigned to a counselor by the administrator, "Big Jane." The counselor saw the woman either individually or in a group. The woman would then receive the appointment time, date, and address where she was to go.

4. The woman would go to an apartment called "the Front" with her significant other(s). The Front was set up so that nonmembers would not know where the procedures were taking place.

5. The women, but not those accompanying them, were taken by a Jane driver to an apartment where the procedure, including a pap smear, actually occurred.

6. They were returned by car to the Front.

In order to prevent complications and to treat any which occurred, the woman would phone her counselor during the following week. If she did not call, the counselor would call her, since it was important for an illegal organization like Jane to avert problems. Protection for "mistakes" available to physicians was not available to them.

The process for second trimester abortions varied. Leumbach Paste was inserted when available. Otherwise, the amniotic sac was ruptured or the umbilical cord was cut to induce labor. The woman was told to go to a hospital when labor started. She was given careful instructions on how to be admitted without the hospital calling the police. She was told her rights and what she did not have to reveal. Since women were "hassled" in spite of that information, a midwifery apartment was established with Jane women who specialized in delivering "long terms." The women aborted in that apartment.

A major logistic problem was disposal of the embryos and fetuses. At night "runs" were made to supermarket disposal bins. Sometimes this task was assumed by men who were friends, lovers, or husbands of the Jane women.

Women in the collective also served as assistants, giving shots, inserting speculums, and dilating cervixes. All these jobs, except abortionist, developed from the beginning of Jane's history.

WHY DID IT WORK?

The most important reason for Jane's effectiveness was the strong, radical, and feminist sentiment pervasive in 1969 when the Service was initiated. Police brutality vis-à-vis antiwar protesters at the Democratic Convention the year before had radicalized the liberal and radical communities, leaving them angry and disenchanted with exciting institutions. It was in this climate that the Women's Movement began to attain momentum in Chicago.

The first national Women's Liberation meeting was held in Chicago in November 1967. While many of the Jane women were not initially feminists and some were not "political," they wanted to do something for and with women. Since this was their first feminist activity, it was fueled by an enormous amount of energy, faith, and hope, as well as anger towards men and patriarchal institutions.

The original members were primarily housewives supported by their husbands and with enough free time to organize the Service before there was enough surplus money to pay them. Baby-sitting was performed by some childless members and also was shared. When Jane women took over the Service from the professional abortionists and created paying jobs, it allowed the participation of more women who were young, single, and radical, and who could devote time to the Service only if they were paid.

Engaging in illegal activities made the group cohesive in the face of a common enemy. More important, the illegality of voluntarily terminating a pregnancy convinced Jane members that it was absolutely necessary to perform abortions. Jane members followed the tradition of civil disobedience to unjust laws with they had learned through participation in the civil rights and peace movements.

Because the group was illegal, it was cohesive and efficient, according to the women. No time was spent in what they termed hassling with the licensing agencies or maintaining bureaucratic forms. When some of the women subsequently organized a legal women's health center, they found bureaucratic restrictions to be constraining.

In contrast to other groups of people with equal good will, members of this group could actually solve problems—the women would walk in pregnant and leave no longer pregnant. In contrast, a worker on a woman's hotline stated that there was little she could do for the battered women who called because at that time Chicago had no battered women's shelters.

The collective supported itself and could pay salaries. Although no one was turned away for lack of funds, the average fee received was fifty dollars. The fact that women could be paid enabled a group of women to put much time into the Service who otherwise would have had to work at what they termed "shit jobs." By earning money in productive feminist work they were able to lead totally radical feminist lives. Financial self-sufficiency also ended the contradictions some women felt when supported by their husbands. Moreover, no energy was required for fund-raising or for grant-writing.

ORGANIZATIONAL THEORY

1. *The Goal of Providing Safe, Humane Abortions on Every Woman who Needed One Was Not Diluted by a Concern for Organizational Survival.* Some organizations have a vested interest in the continued existence or even exacerbation of their "problem" in order to justify and expand their funding.

2. *Authority Resides in the Collectivity as a Whole.* Jane's commitment to consensus meant that although they sometimes had to spend more time than they would have liked hammering out lines of their agreement, their eventual agreement allowed them to work smoothly under pressure.

3. *Minimal Stipulated Rules.* Although Jane members followed strict rules of medical procedure—e.g., if a woman was feverish, she was given an antibiotic—they had few formal rules of collective behavior. Their openness to the ad hoc decision-making of each member allowed flexibility and a degree of autonomy for each member that helped them maintain their voluntary commitment of time and energy.

4. *Social Control through Homogeneity.* Jane's membership was homogeneous: over one-half of the women were between twenty and thirty years old, and all but two were white. Most were born and raised in urban areas, particularly Chicago. When the Service was operating, about one-half of its members were single and one-half married, with two divorced or separated. The ratio of Protestants to Jews was approximately one to two, and

four women were Catholic. The typical Jane worker had postgraduate education.

Distressed by their own homogeneity, Jane workers, with only slight success, tried to recruit black and latino workers, the ethnic and racial characteristics of large segments of their clients. Although the women claimed ideological diversity, the diversity was within feminist and leftist boundaries. Although they fought against it, the relative cultural homogeneity of the members of Jane was a blessing in disguise because it provided social cohesion.

5. The Ideal of Community. The search for community never replaced the goal of providing safe, humane abortions. Little time was spent "processing" relationships because of the urgency of the task of providing abortions.

6. Recruitment. The major pathway to Jane membership was through friendship networks. Some women became members after they or their friends had abortions with the Service. Recruitment procedures insured a relatively culturally and ideologically homogeneous group.

TRANSMITTING SKILLS

All skills were learned by observing other women and performing tasks under the supervision of women with greater skill. Skills necessary to perform abortions are not difficult to learn. One woman said:

> The thing itself [the curettage] was real easy. It's like making cantaloupe balls–the same motion with the curette. . . . The greater precision was in the handling of the dilator. You had to feel the woman's muscles through the instrument into your hand. So much of what you have to learn is sensitivity to the woman's body and that is what is unlearned in medical school.

Birth control information was offered and all the women received copies of *Our Bodies Our Selves, The Birth Control Handbook* and the *VD Handbook.* However, counseling was considered the heart of the procedure and everyone was supposed to counsel.

7. Solidarity and Personal Growth Incentives Primary; Material Incentives Secondary. Jane's appeal was in enacting symbolic values, such as a woman's right to control her own body. Moreover, all paying jobs paid the same, and many tasks, including counseling, were not remunerated at all. Because the Service was illegal, no one in Jane could use their experience in the organization to further their careers.

The individual autonomy and varied work that the organization provided had a major impact on the lives and self-images of the participants. In taking care of others, the Jane women fulfilled their own potential. Jane women also reported sharp increases in their feelings of identification with other women.

8. Social Stratification: Egalitarian. Jane had a strong commitment to equality. Consistent efforts were made to flatten the decision-making and status hierarchies, especially after the paid professional abortionists were no longer present.

9. Minimal Division of Labor. The goal was to have every member perform every task. The Service exemplifies Marx's belief that "Only in a community with others had each individual the means of cultivating his [sic] gifts in all directions; only in the community therefore, is personal freedom possible."

CONCLUSION

Jane illustrates both the characteristics of a successful movement organization and the possibility of making abortion a less alienating experience for the women having them and for the medical personnel involved. To use Ehrenreich and English's phrase (1973), these women seized the "technology without buying the ideology"; that is, they used antibiotics and medical equipment but did not adopt the hierarchical system or the sense of entitlement that characterizes physicians.

Since abortion has been legalized in this country, some physicians and nurses have expressed guilt over abortions they were performing. No women in Jane expressed such guilt, probably because they all had to counsel women who wanted the abortions and, therefore, knew the importance for the woman's life of not having a baby at that time.

When this research was begun, abortion was legal and poor women received third-party payments. Now, however, third-party payments for abortions are almost nonexistent and a strong lobby supporting a "human life" amendment is trying to make abortions illegal again. Perhaps knowledge of the success of Jane will do more than expand the sociology of medicine, the sociology of social movements, and organizational theory. Perhaps it will enable us to seize themes of reproduction.

The Abortion

ALIX KATES SHULMAN

Alix Kates Shulman, excerpt from *Memoirs of an Ex-Prom Queen*, New York: Knopf, 1972. Reprinted by permission.

Roxanne told me about a way to abort myself with a speculum, a catheter and syringe, sterile water, and a friend. (Not till months later did I learn it could be lethal.) "There's nothing to it. I've done it twice myself. You just have someone squirt a little sterile water into the uterus, you wait, and in a few days you abort."

"What if you don't?"

"Then you do it again."

When I told Willy, he hit the roof. "Are you kidding? That's insane! We'll find a proper doctor to do it, thank you."

"But Roxanne's done it three times," I said, exaggerating. "She says it's easy."

"Just thinking about it makes me sick."

"Come on, Willy. You'll help me, won't you?"

"Not that way. I'm going to find you a doctor."

Roxanne knew an intern whom she got to do it at his apartment in the Bronx. He pulled all the blinds and locked the doors while she boiled up the instruments.

"What a tight little twat you have," he said as Roxanne directed a flashlight between my legs. Each leg hung over a kitchen chair instead of being fitted into stirrups. I was ashamed. "It's a pleasure to work on you after the gaping smelly cunts that come into the hospital. If you could see them, you'd never want to have children."

"What do children have to do with it?"

"Believe me, having babies wrecks your plumbing. Now hold still a second. I don't want to hurt you if I can help it."

An instant of pain, and the catheter was in. "I wouldn't want to have children even if it was good for my plumbing," I said flatly.

"Don't you like kids?"

"I love kids. Other people's."

"Hey, will you relax? That's better. Don't you have any maternal instincts?'

"I have an instinct of self-preservation."

"You'll feel different when you fall in love. That's when they all want their babies. Now hold very still one more sec. Here comes the water."

"But I am in love."

"I doubt it," he said.

It was a familiar line, about love and babies. I'd been bucking it all my life. If it were true, as the scientists claimed, it would be smarter to live without love. The only power a woman had against a man was the possibility, never more than problematical, of leaving him; with babies even that defense vanished. No; plumbing aside, maternity was vulnerability itself, sentencing a woman at best to the plight of Mrs. Alport, and at worst to grubby isolation.

Sensation without pain, I felt the liquid enter me. "When I'm in love," I told him, "I rely on my convictions."

That very night, sometime after midnight, I awoke with unbearable cramps. I was exploding, coming apart at the seams. I rolled around and doubled up and moaned.

"What's the matter, Sash?" asked Willy in his sleep.

"Nothing. Go back to sleep."

I thought it was food poisoning or appendicitis. Then at last I felt I had to take an enormous crap.

"Where are you, Sash?" called Willy, feeling me absent from the bed.

I sat on the toilet and pushed and pushed. Then out it popped, my first baby.

I looked down. It was suspended over the water in the toilet bowl, swinging from my body, its head down.

"Oh my God! Oh my God! Oh Willy!" I cried. I covered my mouth and screamed.

A nightmare. I looked again. It hung there like a corpse.

"Willy, please! Come quickly! It's a baby!"

I couldn't understand what was happening. I had thought at two or three months it would be a fish with gills, or a tadpole. But it looked like a real baby, with a human head, only blue.

"Oh God! It's hanging here! Please help me."

"Now listen, Sasha," Willy was saying softly, "you've got to pull it out of you."

"Did you see it?"

"Yes."

"It's a baby, Willy!"

"I know honey, but you've still got to pull it out."

"Oh I can't." I was all atremble.

"You've got to."

"I can't."

It was too awful: the first baby I produced in this world I deposited like a piece of shit straight into the toilet.

"Try darling. Pull it out. Trust me."

At last, I pulled it out of me and dropped it into the water. It had always lived in a liquid medium. I couldn't look at it, my own child. I flushed the toilet. Then I dissolved on the bed in a shudder of tears and afterbirth.

"It was a baby. I can't believe it. It was a baby," I moaned. Will stroked my back as I wept and bled.

"Do you think you'll be all right for a few minutes while I get the car? I'm going to take you to a hospital."

"I'm all right," I sobbed. "I'll get blood all over the car."

"Fuck the car," said Willy.

"I'm all right," I repeated. "I don't need to go to a hospital."

"Do as I tell you!" he shouted.

When we got to the hospital, a doctor prescribed three kinds of pills and a bed in the maternity ward.

"Don't leave me here, Willy. I don't want to stay here."

"Don't worry, honey, I won't leave you."

"I'm sorry, sir, but you're not permitted on the ward," said the nurse. "You can visit her tomorrow."

"What are you going to do to her?" Will asked the doctor. "Can't you do something now so I can take her home?"

"Can't do anything till tomorrow," said the doctor.

"Why not?"

"I've ordered some pills to control the bleeding, and antibiotics and a tranquilizer. If she'll stop with the hysterics there may be a chance we can save your baby."

"But there is no baby, doctor," said Will. "She miscarried."

The doctor looked skeptical. "You sure?" he asked.

"Of course I'm sure. I saw the fetus myself."

"Did you bring it with you?"

"Bring it? No!"

The doctor shrugged and turned away.

"It's flushed down the toilet," said Willy frantically.

The doctor shook his head. "That's really too bad," he said, "If you'd brought it with you we might be able to clean her out tonight. But if she's not hemorrhaging and there's no fetus and I do a D-and-C at 3:00 AM with no one from the regular staff around, I could get into a lot of trouble. You understand. I wish I could help you out—"

"Take an X-ray," said Willy desperately. "You'll see there's no baby inside her."

"We can't take an X-ray."

"Why not?"

"An X-ray might damage the fetus."

Starting the New York Abortion Access Fund: Grassroots Activism on Abortion Rights, from Vision to Reality

IRENE XANTHOUDAKIS AND LAUREN PORSCH

Irene Xanthoudakis and Lauren Porsch, "Starting the New York Abortion Access Fund," 2008. Original for this publication.

Karen is a young woman from rural Pennsylvania living on a fixed income. When she found out she was pregnant and decided to terminate her pregnancy, the nearest clinic was four hours away and the procedure was $500. While Karen worked to put together $500, her pregnancy entered the latter portion of its second trimester—and the price of the procedure rose to $2000. In addition to learning that she needed an additional $1500, Karen found out that she could no longer get an abortion in Pennsylvania—she was now beyond the twenty-week point, after which abortions are not legal in her state. She decided to come to New York, where abortion is legal through the twenty-fourth week of pregnancy. After seven hours on a bus, Karen arrived at a clinic in New York City. After spending a day in the waiting room, she was sent back home—she hadn't put together the remaining $1500 and the clinic's social worker was not able to raise the full balance from abortion funds. She spent seven hours on the bus back home. A week later, she spent another seven hours to come back. This was Karen's last chance—she had reached twenty-four weeks and she would need to have the procedure in the next few days, or she would be past the legal gestational age limit in New York. The clinic social worker struggled to raise the money, and was finally able to put it all together after the New York Abortion Access Fund (NYAAF) received a $500 contribution towards Karen's procedure.

Although every woman's story is different, Karen's struggle to raise money to pay for her procedure is an experience shared by many low-income women who rely on Medicaid for their health care and live in one of the majority of states that prohibit Medicaid funding for abortion.

It was stories like this that inspired us, as young recent college graduates, to create and help sustain the NYAAF, a grassroots, non-profit organization that raises money to subsidize abortion procedures for low-income women and adolescent girls. Founded by coauthor Lauren Porsch in 2001, NYAAF is part of a larger network of abortion funds that respond to gaps in access to reproductive health care created by inadequate social policy.

So how can people who feel passionate about social justice issues identify a need and turn that insight into real activism for social change? What are some of the problems that are encountered on the long road between identifying a specific problem and beginning to provide an answer?

STEP 1: LOCATING A NEED

Passed by Congress in 1976, just three years after *Roe v. Wade*, the Hyde Amendment to the Labor/Health, Education, and Welfare Appropriations Bill effectively barred the use of federal Medicaid funds for abortion services. The impact of this piece of legislation was far-reaching, given that approximately 6 million women of reproductive age rely on the Medicaid system for their health care.[1] This meant that while the right to an abortion was now legally guaranteed, many women who required the procedure now had no way to pay for them.

Initial attempts by abortion rights activists to challenge the Hyde Amendment in federal courts were unsuccessful, culminating with the Supreme Court's 1980 decision in *Harris v. McRae.* The Court held that there was a difference between actively impeding the exercise of a constitutional right and passively refusing the resources needed to actualize this right. "Although the government may not place obstacles in the path of a woman's choice, it need not remove those not of its own creation," the Court stated. "It simply does not follow that a woman's freedom of choice carries with it a constitutional entitlement to the financial resources to avail herself of the full range of protected choices."[2]

After this decision closed the issue of Medicaid funding for abortion at the federal level, the decision to make abortion available to Medicaid recipients was now up to individual states, which had the option to pay for these services with their own funds.

By 1990, the number of states that denied Medicaid funding for termination of pregnancy had jumped to thirty-seven. Today in thirty-three states and the District of Columbia women cannot obtain Medicaid coverage for their abortions unless their pregnancy is the result of rape or incest or if a doctor argues that the pregnancy threatens a woman's life.[3] Of the remaining seventeen states, sixteen cover all medically necessary abortions. However, only four states—Hawaii, Maryland, New York, and Washington State—have chosen to do so voluntarily. The remaining thirteen provide the coverage as the result of litigation and one state, South Dakota, only provides coverage when the pregnancy threatens the woman's life, in clear violation of the already restrictive law.[4]

On a practical level, however, the administrative hurdles a woman must overcome to actually gain access to funding when she is eligible for it under these criteria are even more complicated and difficult than they seem. In Pennsylvania, for example, a woman must provide a police report verifying her claim of rape or incest in order to receive Medicaid payment for her procedure.

In New York City, one of the least expensive places in the country to get an abortion, the cost of the procedure ranges from $350 in the early first trimester to $2,000 at the end of the second trimester. Research indicates that Medicaid-eligible women living in states that do not provide Medicaid coverage for abortion are often forced to redirect money from basic living expenses in order to pay for their procedures. Women reported that they used money that would have gone to "rent, utility bills, food, and clothing for themselves and their children" to finance their procedures. In a survey published in 2000 by the Alan Guttmacher Institute (AGI), 60 percent of Medicaid-eligible respondents said that paying for their abortion "entailed a serious hardship," compared with only 26 percent of women not eligible for Medicaid.[5]

The irony behind restrictions on Medicaid funding for abortion, which are presumably intended to prevent abortion, is that they force women to have procedures later in their pregnancies. That the price of an abortion rises with increasing gestational age fuels a cycle in which women are, in effect, "chasing the fee." AGI research indicates that Medicaid-eligible women wait, on average, two to three weeks longer than other women to have an abortion because they have trouble raising the money to pay for it. Correspondingly, research looking at women's reasons for seeking abortion in the second trimester indicates that close to half of women who had abortions after sixteen weeks' gestation said they had "difficulty making arrangements" for the procedure, which included raising the money, finding a provider, and making the travel arrangements.[6] While approximately 88 percent of abortions in the US occur in the first twelve weeks of pregnancy,[7] low-income women make up a disproportionate number of those having abortions after twelve weeks. In its first two years of operation, 96 percent of NYAAF clients had an abortion past sixteen weeks' gestation.[8]

Ambiguity in Constitutional law compounds the problem by creating a situation wherein many women have to travel out of state to have their abortions performed, adding travel expenses and the cost of a hotel for at least one night to an already unaffordable bill.

Low-income women face two major hurdles in obtaining a timely procedure, the first of which creates the other and compounds itself: first, they are unable to raise the money, and then, because of the time taken to compile funds, they have the added difficulty of getting a procedure at a later state in the pregnancy, which is not only more expensive but something that is possible in fewer states. So in addition to financial burdens, women now have geographic and travel issues to contend with.

STEP 2: STARTING NYAAFF

The New York Abortion Access Fund is a grassroots, volunteer-run organization in New York City that raises money and provides financial assistance to women's health clinics on behalf of low-income women who cannot afford the cost of their abortion procedure. The organization has no staff or office, and functions with almost no overhead. The organization was founded in 2001 by coauthor Lauren Porsch. Coauthor Irene Xanthoudakis served on the board in different capacities for four years.

The inspiration for NYAAF came during the winter of 2000 when we were among a group of college students volunteering as escorts at a New York City abortion clinic. The group learned that a patient was unable to obtain an abortion because she could not pay for it—the woman did not have enough money to pay for the procedure herself, but she was not "poor enough" to qualify for Medicaid. The students, all members of the Barnard/Columbia Students for Choice (SFC) organization, transformed their frustration into action, deciding to make their next project a fundraiser.

The initial plan was to hold a fundraiser on campus and give the proceeds to a reputable clinic, asking that it be used as a subsidy for other women who needed the support. Several months later, however, SFC Co-President Lauren Porsch met a representative of the National Network of Abortion Funds (NNAF), a national coalition of organizations that did what SFC members aspired to do. Among other things, NNAF produced a manual with the information and guidelines necessary for establishing a non-profit abortion fund. Wanting to make a more sustainable impact than a single fundraiser, NYAAF was born.

That summer, Porsch began the process of incorporating as a 501(c)3 non-profit organization, recruited a board, and began actively raising funds. Involved in the original fundraising projects, Irene Xanthoudakis became a founding member of the board of directors. We (Porsch and Xanthoudakis) spent several years on the organization's board—two and four respectively—before moving on to complete graduate school. The work that we and other early board members did established an infrastructure that enabled operations to continue, well after the founding members had left.

One of the most interesting lessons we learned through our involvement with NYAAF was that the day-to-day work of social change is about as unglamorous as it can get. While there was a certain amount of cache that came with being involved in a start-up organization focusing on a controversial social issue, the work itself was rarely exciting and was often tedious in the way that administrative work often is: With the help of a pro bono attorney, Lauren spent hours filing incorporation papers and drafting bylaws, and board members designed operating procedures, opened bank accounts, and entered donor information into a database.

STEP 3: WHAT WE LEARNED

We often found that basic concepts that we had considered important for organizational success—leadership and diversity, for example—were as important as we had believed, but meant something different from what we expected.

NYAAF's continued success was rooted in our ability to maintain focus on a very narrow, single project: raising money to subsidize abortions for women who needed them. Although this seems straightforward, it was in fact one of our biggest challenges, and one of the biggest contributors to our successes. We were often faced with the opportunity to participate in projects that were vital to the women's health movement as a whole, and exciting—but that would have taken time, energy, and/or money from our primary purpose. Although we spent considerable meeting time debating the merits of joining coalitions advocating for increased access to emergency contraception and other similar projects, we pushed ourselves to remain focused. Constantly wary of "mission creep," we realized that what we did was unique. Other, larger organizations had the resources to effectively design and launch advocacy campaigns, but at the time, we were the only independent abortion fund in the state of New York. We repeatedly opted to focus on improving and expanding what we already did well, rather than drain limited resources by participating in a project we were not equipped to successfully complete.

While our primary goal as an organization was always to work to make abortion more accessible by financing individual women's procedures, we had a secondary commitment that was an equally important element of our organizational identity. Although we were conceived of as a response to a specific social problem, much of what motivated us to work for NYAAF's success was that we had created a space where young women's voices could be heard. Many of NYAAF's founders were recent college graduates or young professionals who were drawn to work where we were intimately involved in decision-making, an opportunity we lacked in the other portions of our professional life. We found that while the older leaders in the reproductive rights movement often lamented the supposed apathy of younger women towards abortion rights activism, many of these leaders did not allow younger women opportunities to help set the agenda within the movement.

NYAAF, not unlike many other grassroots feminist organizations, struggled to create an organization that was diverse in terms of race/ethnicity, class background, and life experience. With few exceptions, board members were white, college-educated young women working professional jobs (albeit in entry-level positions). The most glaring problem with this arrangement was that we were not representative of the women we served, many of whom were women of color, and who, as a whole, were poor and lacked meaningful educational and professional opportunities. We were conscious of the ways we differed from our clients and reached out to as many different sources as we had at our disposal. But the networks we reached out to were comprised of people similar to us, perpetuating the problem. Because clinics were the intermediary between our work and the clients who received our grants, we had almost no opportunities to engage them in our work. Ultimately, this is a challenge that we repeatedly faced and were not able to address as successfully as we had hoped.

Racial and economic diversity was not the only kind of diversity important in NYAAF's work. Much of our early success came from the Board's recognition that we needed a wide range of skill sets in order to run the organization and recruit as diverse a pool of donors as possible. Because we realized this, we were able to actively recruit people who had strong financial management skills, attorneys who could advise us as laws regulating abortion access changed, and people who had experience writing grants and planning events.

STEP 4: KNOWING WHEN TO SAY WHEN

We began this project believing that we were committed to its mission. Because we were committed, we reasoned, we would work hard and the organization would succeed. But as we each left NYAAF we came to realize that knowing when to step away from an organization is as important an indicator of commitment. Working hard, sometimes at the expense of our own personal needs, did not do a service to the organization (or to ourselves). We recognized in ourselves decisions that in the short-term allowed us to get more done but in the long-term compromised the strength of the organization. For example, rather than training other board members in basic administrative procedures we would push ourselves to do them knowing we could complete them more quickly. This left us exhausted and overburdened, and left NYAAF without anyone who had the experience necessary to push the operations forward on a day-to-day basis in our absence. In a bigger sense, deciding to leave the organization was a leadership challenge to both of us. When Lauren resigned as president, she had spent a year getting the organization off the ground and two years leading it. When Irene resigned, two years later, she had been on the Board for a total of four years, two as president. We had put considerable time and energy into the organization, and the choice to leave cut us off from work that had been a big part of our lives. Despite the conflicting feelings, leaving the organization created space for new leaders and the creativity, spirit, and energy they brought with them.

NOTES

1. H. Boonstra, "Rights Without Access: Revisiting Public Funding Of Abortion for Poor Women," *The Guttmacher Report on Public Policy*, April 2000.
2. D. Roberts, *Killing the Black Body*, New York: Vintage, 1997, 231.
3. P. Levine, A. Trainor, and D. Zimmerman, "The effect of Medicaid abortion funding restrictions on abortions, pregnancies, and births," *Journal of Health Economics* 15 (1996): 555–578.
4. See http://www.nnaf.org/NNAF_Policy_Report.pdf and http://www.reproductiverights.org/pub_fac_portrait.html.
5. Boonstra, *The Guttmacher Report*.
6. Ibid.
7. Ibid.
8. Ibid.
9. See http://www.reproductiverights.org/pub_fac_portrait.html.

Lesbian, Bisexual, and Transgender Health

THE RELATIONSHIP BETWEEN women's health activists and LGBTQ communities has never been simple. Despite the significant portions of the women's health movement who are lesbian, bisexual, and transgender, the needs of these communities have sometimes been ignored or at best misunderstood.

In the landmark book *Stone Butch Blues*, transgender activist Leslie Feinberg describes some of these contradictions. Feinberg writes a fictional account of a person named Jess who has lived as a butch lesbian and has taken steps toward transitioning. Exiled to New York City in the 1970s from Buffalo, Jess is barely getting by in the city. After taking antibiotics for a cough, Jess develops a yeast infection. Rather than seeking treatment, she secretly hopes that it will heal itself. When this doesn't happen, Jess seeks treatment at a local women's health clinic only to meet ignorance from the staff, who assume she is just a crazy man. An angry receptionist berates Jess, saying, "You may think you're a woman, but that doesn't mean you are one." At the moment that Jess is surrounded by hostility, a kind female doctor decides to write a prescription and offer reassuring words, encouraging her to return for a gynecological exam. In the early days of the women's movement, strict ideas of what it meant to be a "woman" and to come together based on that identity often led to the exclusion of people who didn't neatly fall under one sexual banner or another.

To the credit of the movement, it has responded to such criticisms and continues today to address the changing needs of various queer communities.

In their book, *Sappho Was a Right-On Woman*, authors Sidney Abbot and Barbara Love sought to describe the experience of being lesbian in America in the 1970s. The book that resulted became an early touchstone for women struggling with sexual identity. In 2007, Sidney Abbott reflected on the book, saying, "we weren't worried about health exactly. Well maybe mental health. We were trying to stay sane."

Today there are new debates and concerns. Jennifer Baumgardner takes up the issue of bisexuality, arguing that this substantial part of the queer community is often still invisible or even derided by the mainstream gay and lesbian (and straight) populations. Lauren Porsch writes about the urgent need to improve transgender health resources, still one of the most underserved parts of the population.

Sappho Was a Right-On Woman

SIDNEY ABBOTT AND BARBARA LOVE

Sidney Abbott and Barbara Love, excerpt from *Sappho was a Right-On Woman*, Stein and Day, 1972. Reprinted by permission.

SANCTUARY

Living in an environment that is hostile or indifferent, lesbians find themselves floundering for validation. They feel alien, uprooted—no longer able to count on acceptance from anyone or in any place. They feel that they don't count, don't exist, in a system whose social institutions and resources do not include them.

Not knowing what to do or where to go, not knowing even what it is that she wants, a lesbian may escape the tensions of feeling different by daydreaming, taking long walks, or seeing endless double features. In another mood she may seek release in driving fast or a reckless run down a ski slope.

But it is almost impossible for human beings to live without community, the sense of belonging to something. Sooner or later, the lesbian begins to see her carefully constructed and valued seclusion as forced upon her. Isolation drains her will, her conviction of the rightness of her love, even her passion and feeling. Her ingenuous feelings of love for another woman now present a new problematic face. For relief from the sustained concentration of exacting pretense, she seeks a sanctuary, a place where she will be protected enough to feel free.

Sanctuary has customarily been offered by the church, but for the lesbian sanctuary is often found in the anonymity of the urban night, the amorality of the mafia, which runs the bars for women, or the secretive sociability of the Daughters of Bilitis (DOB), the first national lesbian organization.

For heterosexuals, finding a partner has elements of a twenty-four-hour-a-day game of chance. A lover or a potential spouse can appear at work, at church, on the bus, or in a supermarket, or be a friend of your brother. But there is no everyday way to meet other lesbians.

One cannot—yet—look in the yellow pages for a gay computer dating service, or even buy a guide to gay bars, without first knowing where it is sold.

Night becomes a longed-for sanctuary. There is a sense of relief at the end of the day. With dusk, lines between conventional morality and immorality, rejection and acceptance, begin to blur, much as the hard edges of the buildings and streets lose their definition. Whatever destination she has in mind, the lesbian is able to disappear into the hiding place of the night.

Perhaps dressed in dark tones or in black, in the fashion of old gay custom, the Lesbian blends into the environment, camouflaged like other life forms that develop protective coloration in hostile environments. By day she must contain her feelings in a dark closet; but protected by the night she feels she can allow her lightest moods to emerge. Day and night reflect the split in her identity that divides who she pretends to be and who she is.

One woman said that she began her hunt for others like herself by following women who looked gay down the street. Another said it took all the courage she had to ask a cab driver; and even then she was not sure of the right words: "I want to go to a place where only women go." "What do you mean, lady . . . the YWCA?" Frantically, "No." Pause. "Oh."

In many American cities there is at least one such place—inevitably a bar—and the lesbian knows she must find it: this is where she belongs.

The bars are usually hidden away in warehouse districts, in lofts and cellars. Spooky at best, the deserted streets, with papers and bottles blowing in the dark, heighten the excitement of the forbidden. Often a bar is not marked; the entrance is unlighted, signless. Looking through the windows or through a peephole in the door, one can see very little. The door is frequently locked; if there is a bouncer at the door, he looks over each customer before admitting her. If the bar is called a private club, he asks for her card, which is usually signed with a pseudonym.

When the lesbian enters a bar, she feels as though she is being let in on a secret.

> *I felt when I entered that I should give a secret handshake or a special code word. I did not know these women, but they were my sisters. I felt something like I was visiting another chapter of my sorority.*

Inside the bar, the décor is often barren and seedy: red lights, wallpaper imitating brocade, a jukebox. The bartender on the scene, often a woman, has heard it all, seen it all, done it all. It seems a worn-out, grimy place.

Prices for watered-down drinks are high: You pay for protection. Order right away and pay before you're served. The need to keep drinking in order to be allowed to stay in the bar means that patrons drink slowly or hold a warm beer in their hands for hours.

Just how much security or protection does a bar offer?

In New York, bar after bar opens or reopens under a new name with the same management. Bars exist today, in 1972, but they still serve as reminders of an underground life.

A well-known lesbian bar that flourished in New York in the late 1960s featured a back room for dancing, open only to regular patrons. Although nothing went on there but dancing and talking at tables, this room was protected by a bodyguard, as was the street entrance. Police visits were signaled to back-room clients by sudden bright lights and the silencing of music. Women would stop dancing and return to their seats. The police would look around for the owner, presumably to collect a payoff. Payoffs seemed to be a part of bar life. When politicians are running for office and threaten to "clean up" the city, there are sometimes raids.

Fear of arrest keeps people away for a while, and then they come back or turn to another, safer bar, perhaps with still higher prices. The money from the patrons goes to the management and to the police, who function in the gay underground as oppressors and exploiters.

There is always the rumor, if not the probability, that in a raid the names of those arrested might be published in the newspaper. This is a threat that plagues the patrons who are always sensitive to police cars out front, or to the presence of policemen in the neighborhood. A kind of puritanical terror hangs over the clients of a gay bar, the clandestine, guarded nature of the bars heightens the fear of consequences. The feeling prevails that, should her excursion be known, a woman could be branded for life. The atmosphere of an illegal den of iniquity is promoted deliberately and with mastery by the management. It gives them power through fear, born of guilt and isolation.

The bar exaggerates the sense of the forbidden, and at the same time makes the protectiveness of the bar seem all the more necessary. The sanctuary is in many ways a trap.

Lesbians have strong reactions to their first visits. Many say they were "freaked out." Some found it "repulsive, but exciting." One woman said it seemed "sophisticated, hip, exotic." Another said, "It was revolting. I started to cry and ran out." But they soon learn that if you are a lesbian, this is the most you can hope for. And so they arrive from the suburbs, from other states, from miles away. The bars attract all ages, all socioeconomic groups, all races, colors, and creeds.

There is something in the bar in addition to the mystique of sexual vibrations. There is the need for identity; it is affirming, comforting, just to talk with others who feel the same way about their lives. There is a need to discuss, although the noise and the flirting leave little opportunity for discussion. There is a need to strengthen self-image, although the pressures of the atmosphere and the games of conquest often act to diminish one's dignity.

Sometimes a lesbian finds in the bar a solitary kind of renewal. She comes simply to be alone among other lesbians. She will sit by herself or stand leaning against a wall just watching. Or she may not even look around but stare at the jukebox or at her drink, with no intention of meeting anyone.

The bar is the only relief I have from pretending. I can dress the way I want and think the way I want. I can truly relax for a few hours. I need this to carry on during the day, which has become increasingly exhausting.

After a while she may have enough verification, or whatever tonic it was she needed. She is satisfied that it is still there, a hard-to-define part of her she sometimes hides so well she loses the sense of its reality. It is still there because they are still there—other lesbians. The minimal level of need has apparently been filled, and she leaves alone, perhaps without having spoken a word to anyone.

At first the bar, like a drug, can give a high: a moment of reassurance, a sense of security, a surge of confidence. But the security is false, the confidence dissipates, and the reassurance is groundless. The beneficial effects wear off quickly, leaving the hard facts of the lesbian's isolation unchanged.

After their initial experiences in the bars, few lesbians really expect to find anything positive there. Although they come for renewal, most of them learn to accept despair; at least it is a despair they do not suffer alone. They do not really escape society's hatred in the bars; they bring it in with them.

Because there are drinks and loud music, the bar is a way to reach a state of semi-consciousness. Here the lesbian can let herself slip down to the bottom, where she can rest or give up. Just let her mind drift with the music, watch the smoke patterns, the motions of bodies swaying, and listen to the music, the voices and the glasses clinking. Perhaps for a moment the scene may even appear exotic; the lonely women may seem energized and happy.

For many the bar is an attempt to find a community. There is a desire to feel a part of the "in" group, the bar clique. Some lesbians make a point of getting to know the bartenders, bouncers, and waitresses by first names, and talking to the bar elite.

The support in the bar is superficial and so are bar friendships. Both vanish as quickly as the mood of a movie when you're out on the street again.

Bar life is centered around cruising, or looking for a sex partner, as the neophyte soon discovers. Traditional values don't count: the bar has its own set of values. Because there has been no other place to meet lesbians, their homosexuality is the only common denominator.

The lesbian couple may be ensconced in homes in the suburbs, the country, and summer places in spots like the Hamptons on Long Island near New York City. There are vacation places where the emphasis is not so much on couples. One is Fire Island, now nearly a legend, where female couples may go together, but both have summer romances or weekend romances while there in the luxury of sunshine. Another is Provincetown, on Cape Cod. There are lesbian couples there of course, but there are masses of younger women who may not be in couples. They surge through the town, fewer in numbers than the gay men, but sufficient to open two or three new lesbian bars at the peak of the season. Dancing, picnicking, going to the beach, parties in houses, and sailing constitute the fun. The atmosphere is relaxed; there is excitement in meeting and talking to people you will never see again. Lovers can walk down the street holding hands, and openly acknowledge each other in many ways. Even though homosexual visitors are the largest source of income for the pretty town, they are still confined to a gay ghetto, separated from the townspeople. Being free to be gay stops at a certain block on Main Street.

Lesbians with adequate incomes find the country a fresh-air sanctuary where people—and therefore prejudices—can be escaped. In the city or suburbs, lesbians must always be conscious of what the neighbors will think—and do—but in the country, with the seclusion of a farm or a house off the road, a lesbian couple can be spontaneous. They can invite friends up from the city or entertain other gay women from the area. There is often enough distance from the public to entertain out of doors, with barbecues, or play volleyball, or swim, or just socialize in the sunshine. Warm sunshine and soft grass make lesbian life seem more positive, simply because the necessity of hiding is reduced.

Sanctuary is also a circle of friends who share the same standards of discretion. The lesbian subculture is fragmented into thousands of groups of friends. A careful lesbian with a stake in the system will choose her friends as much for their ability to pass for straight as for more positive qualities. The pickings are apt to be slim, for cultivating new friends means dropping your cover and exposing yourself and friends to danger. The hiding lesbian, though she may know some lesbians with masculine habits from the bars or the beaches, rarely encourages their friendship. She will usually shrink from any contact with them outside exclusively gay precincts. They represent a terrible threat to her, and the prospect of being publicly associated with a tough, unmistakable dyke is the stuff of nightmares. Even when she is quite obviously homosexual herself, she may think of her deception as more successful than it is and, ludicrously, avoid contact with lesbians who are scarcely more detectable than she.

The cell-like structure of lesbian society leaves intact the self-hatred that a woman usually brings with her into a gay subculture. As she has been contemptuous of the lesbian in herself, she learns from other lesbians to be contemptuous of the lesbian in others.

Lesbian society is notoriously inbred. The line between friends and lovers is a wavering one, so that lesbian friends may represent a real threat to an established relationship. This varies, to some extent, and, of course, with the individual and with the group. Some women are naturally more monogamous than others, and some groups have strong taboos on "home-breaking." It is not unusual, though, for a lesbian to have had love relationships with several members of her group. It is a characteristic of lesbians that their relationships with one another are not well diversified or delineated: Every friend tends to become a lover. With a small field of choice, and acting on society's vision of them as primarily sexual creatures, lesbians often go to bed together when they really want to be friends, come on sexually when they mean to be sympathetic, take on a sexual partnership when it is a working relationship that interests them most.

There are destructive forces always at work to drive lesbian lovers apart. There do exist in lesbian life those dark creatures of the stereotype who feast on intrigue and who seem interested only in women who are already involved in love relationships. And even the best-intentioned lesbian may find that without being aware of it, she has drifted too close to her best friend's lover.

In lesbian society, where there is no marriage, no social or legal sanctions to help sustain relationships beyond the initial period of romantic love, insecurity and jealousy have a field day. On the other hand, those relationships that do last are usually very strong and deep, and very loving in the fullest sense of the word.

Some lesbians find that the safest friends are former lovers. After the wounds of parting have healed, whatever originally drew the lovers together, and the good experiences they share, may survive, along with the tenderness that lingers after sexual intimacy, as a friendship of remarkable closeness and warmth for which there is scarcely any counterpart in the heterosexual world.

Even with gay women's bars and organizations growing in numbers, you could not count the lesbians by going to these places—you could only estimate their numbers. It may be that the majority never approach a gay meeting place.

Passive by education, the woman who is a lesbian is often too insecure to take her life into her own hands and experience even the periphery of the gay subculture. Some women say it took them ten years to get up the courage to walk through the door of DOB. The risk is too great. A lesbian might be seen there by a teacher or a student, a client or an employer, a friend or a colleague. And so the same is true of the bars, the beaches, the restaurants, the bookstores. "What if someone were to see me?"

Many lesbians frown on organized gay life and refuse to enter a community of gays. They live in isolation and somehow solve—or don't solve—their loneliness in the straight world. For example, suburban married women are finally forced to write notices in underground newspapers with box numbers and pseudonyms. Others take the risk of approaching a desired woman in the "straight" world. Entering the gay community with body, face, and name, seems to be too risky.

Neither sanctuary, nor straight culture, can give the lesbian all that she needs. She cannot live in a gay bar, on a gay beach, or even in the DOB center. Recreation spots do not make a life. For most of the lesbian's life, she has to walk the same streets, go to the same schools, work in the same companies, and shop in the same stores as heterosexuals. She is always in the midst of others who may hassle her if her lesbianism is not tucked in.

The conflict between society and sanctuary is agonizing when one needs both. For necessities and opportunities in *life*, the lesbian clearly needs to participate in the system; for nourishment in belonging and opportunities for *love*, she needs sanctuary. Often it seems decisions involve the difficult questions of integration or segregation, adaptation or individuality, compromise or integrity, hurting others or hurting oneself, social respect or self-respect, pretense or peace of mind.

Most lesbians are intensely aware of the limitations of their gay resources. Sanctuaries—inadequate, temporary, often sordid—act as reminders of their dilemma and dramatize the need to make it in the larger world, or to create a larger world.

Putting Lesbian Health in Focus

VIVIEN LABATON

Vivien Labaton, "Putting Lesbian Health in Focus," *Ms.*, September/October 1998. Reprinted by permission.

During the heady days of the gay liberation movement in the early 1970s, Joan Waitkevicz, MD, learned all too quickly that lesbians were not receiving adequate medical care despite gaining greater visibility: "Someone I knew of developed inoperable cancer of the cervix because she didn't feel she could go to a regular doctor for a Pap test."

Since 1974, when Waitkevicz and seven other lesbian health activists founded the St. Mark's Women's Health Collective in New York City—one of the first community-based clinics in the US to offer care by and for lesbians—she has made it her priority as a physician to provide gay women with safe and comfortable medical environments. Today, she is the director of a first-of-its-kind hospital-based health center, the Gay Women's Focus (GWF) at Beth Israel Medical Center in New York City.

"Despite advances made in the private sector in the last twenty-five years, important barriers to health care for lesbians in the US still persist," says Waitkevicz. Some include: homophobia and bias in doctors' offices and within institutions, fear and reluctance on the part of the patients to disclose their sexual orientation, and lack of training for health care providers on lesbians' particular health needs, such as donor insemination and treatment of sexually transmitted diseases. "For lesbians, the risk of sexually transmitted infections is different—not higher, but different," says Waitkevicz. "We have to ask a patient's sexual history in a nonjudgmental way, because ultimately, it's saving lesbian lives."

Run by three physicians and three staff members, GWF has seen approximately 2,000 patients since opening in 1997. On the future of GWF, Waitkevicz comments: "We're a little too new to start counting our successes, but I hope our work enables others to see its importance. I will be very happy when it's no longer needed, because that means we will have done our job educating our colleagues."

Lesbian Health Gains Long Due Attention from Institute of Medicine

AMY ALLINA

Amy Allina, "Lesbian Health Gains Long Due Attention from Institute of Medicine," *The Network News,* January/February 1999. Reprinted by permission.

In early January, the Institute of Medicine (IOM) released a study looking at the knowledge base and gaps in lesbian health research, *Lesbian Health: Current Assessment and Directions for the Future.* The IOM is a prestigious agency which carries great weight within the academic research community, and lesbian health advocates believe that the study will help establish the legitimacy of the field of lesbian health research. The fact that the IOM convened a committee to study lesbian health was in itself hailed as a breakthrough by lesbian health advocates. Though the committee's conclusion that more research into lesbian health is needed is not new to those who have followed the development of the lesbian health movement, it is ground-breaking for a mainstream institution to call for increased research attention to lesbian health.

HEIGHTENED RISK IS NOT ASSOCIATED WITH SEXUAL ORIENTATION ALONE

While noting that there is only limited research data available for a comparison of the health of lesbians with heterosexual women, based on the information that exists, "the committee did not find that lesbians are at higher risk for any particular health problem simply because they have a lesbian sexual orientation."[1] Though some health problems may, in fact, be more prevalent among lesbians than heterosexual women, the committee asserts that increased incidence, where it exists, may be explained by other risk factors. The report cites several examples of this:

➤ Breast cancer is more common in women who have not had children, and lesbians may be less likely than heterosexual women to bear children.

➤ Lesbians often avoid seeking regular health care due to the homophobia they encounter from health care providers, and this reduced access could lead to an increased risk for some health problems.

➤ As a result of their exposure to the stress effects of homophobia, lesbians may be more likely to experience stress-related health problems.

METHODOLOGICAL LIMITATIONS OF EXISTING LESBIAN HEALTH RESEARCH

The committee identified a number of methodological limitations with the research that has been done to date on lesbian health. First, and foremost, the lack of standard definition of what constitutes a lesbian limits the ability of researchers to compare findings from different studies. The IOM study notes that researchers working on lesbian health must consider the definition they will use in designing their studies and points out that "it should not be assumed that racial and ethnic minority cultures share views of lesbian sexual orientation identical with those of the dominant culture."[2]

Another limitation of existing research on lesbian health is that most studies have been conducted using small samples of people who researchers found at bars, festivals, or through organizations. Most people in the studies have been white, middle-class, well-educated, and between twenty-five and forty years old—not representative of the general lesbian population. Finally, very few studies have included control groups that would allow researchers to compare lesbian health to that of other subgroups of women, and there is almost no data tracking lesbian health over time.

HOMOPHOBIA CREATES ADDITIONAL CHALLENGES

In addition to the methodological challenges, the committee notes that homophobia creates another set of barriers to lesbian health research. Research institutions, research scientists, and research participants, all may fear being associated with a study that includes information about sexual orientation. Homophobia makes it difficult to find institutional support for lesbian health research, and there is very little money available for the work. There are few researchers working in the field, and those who are may have difficulty finding colleagues and mentors.

Researchers have reported political obstacles to conducting work on sexual behavior and have found it difficult to get their findings published. Homophobia also makes the confidentiality of research participants of critical importance, and lack of confidence in research confidentiality makes it harder to recruit people for studies.

PRIORITIES AND RECOMMENDATIONS FOR FUTURE RESEARCH

The committee established three priorities for future research on lesbian health. These are to gather more information about the physical and mental health status of lesbians, to determine how to define sexual orientation in general and lesbian

orientation in particular, and to identify possible barriers to access to health care services for lesbians as well as ways to increase their access to these services.

Specifically, the committee recommended:

➤ More public and private funding for lesbian health research, including a long-term federal commitment.

➤ Finding for methodological research to improve the definition of lesbian sexual orientation.

➤ The routine inclusion of questions about sexual orientations on data collection forms in relevant behavioral and biomedical studies, with pilot studies conducted first to assess the feasibility and impact of these types of questions.

➤ When designing lesbian health research studies, researchers should consider the full range of racial, ethnic, and socioeconomic diversity among lesbians, include members of the study population in the development of the research, and give special attention to protecting the confidentiality and privacy of study participants.

➤ Funding for a large-scale probability survey to determine the range of sexual orientation among all women and the prevalence of various risk and protective factors for health, by sexual orientation.

➤ Increased dissemination of information about the conduct and results of lesbian health research.

➤ The development and support by federal agencies, foundations, health professional associations, and academic institutions of mechanisms for information dissemination about lesbian health.

➤ The development of strategies to train researchers in conducting lesbian health research.

You can obtain a copy of the IOM report by contacting the National Academy Press at 800-624-6242. Their Web site is www.nap.edu.

NOTES
1. Andrea L. Solarz, ed., *Lesbian Health: Current Assessment*

and Directions for the Future, Institute of Medicine (Washington DC: National Academy Press, 1999), Executive Summary, 5.

2. Ibid., 3.

Look Both Ways

JENNIFER BAUMGARDNER

Jennifer Baumgardner, "Look Both Ways," 2008. Original for this publication.

The first time I kissed another girl, other than pre-junior high exploratory sessions, I was twenty-three. I had never thought I was gay, hadn't spent my teen years pining for my gym teacher or feeling like a deep secret was burning in my core. My affable, popular boyfriends in high school (John and Tim) dominated my thoughts and yet our conversations and laughter paled in comparison to my deep, caring, stay-up-all-night-talking friendships with Seana and Kerri. At my Wisconsin college, I became a sort of schizophrenic feminist (quoting bell hooks by day, partying at the frat house in a scant skirt by night). I slept with Brady, my rakish Sig Ep boyfriend with the washboard stomach and the tendency to go home with other girls, while cultivating intellectual affairs with women (Marianne, who was hilarious and addictive; Lucia, who was heartbreaking and vulnerable; Kate, who was beautiful and competitive). By the time I graduated and moved to New York City to take a low-level magazine job that I loved, the separation between people I related to (women) and people I had sex with (men) was sharp.

One night about a year into my tenure in the big city, my friend Anastasia (raven-haired and gorgeous) and I found ourselves in a straight bar called Tom and Jerry's on Houston and Elizabeth Street, drunk and with me practically sitting on her lap. It was 2:00 AM. "Me and Bobby McGee" was on the jukebox and I was beerily singing "freedom's just another word for nothing left to lose" a little too intensely in her ear, as if I were, in fact, Janis Joplin. I kissed her. Minutes into this session,

I felt a tap on my shoulder. A woman said, "I don't think this is the safest situation for you," and gestured at the arc of guys making no effort to conceal that this was also a show for them. We stumbled out of there and made our way to our separate homes, laughing really hard at the spectacle we had made.

I blush a little thinking about that escapade, from the absurd singing to the fact that performing for those guys (imagining that they found it sexy) was part of the fun to me. Despite that clichéd beginning, Anastasia and I went on to date off and on for nearly three years, providing me with my first orgasms. After her, I fell for a witty older writer named Steven, seemingly my perfect match—a straight man who shared my admiration for Burt Bacharach and Sandra Bernhard. Sublime in some ways, the relationship left me frustrated at his grumpy, withholding side—and having dated Anastasia (who literally baked bread and brushed my hair for me) put our disconnects into relief. I felt like a doormat, and I longed to pull the rug out from under him. The best time in my relationship with Steven was just after I met Amy. Amy was an activist and musician who, in her butch way, was twice the man Steven had been (great with cars, guitars, and sex), and also *primo* at the talking and connecting I had gotten with Anastasia. For four incredible weeks, I was with him yet I didn't respond to his moodiness; I had a sexual confidence with him that stemmed directly from how appreciated I felt with Amy. Fearful of going back to a problematic old relationship with him, I forged ahead with an exciting new one with her. Until I met Gordon. . . . When it comes to looking for love, I look both ways.

I'm not alone. Have you noticed that many women who, perhaps thirty years ago, would have "just been straight" are falling in love and having relationships with other women? I think this is due to two happy reforms—feminism, which raised our expectations of what a good relationship should be (caring, equal, orgasms for all) and the obvious successes of the gay rights movement (check your TV guide for reflection that same sex love is becoming, yes, normal in our culture). Common as women with women is, it is also rebelling against convention, against the idea that our worth is reflected glory derived from men, and against the trope that we need to be good girls. And within that rebelliousness, there are two types of women—"the ones that are doing it mainly because it is a straight man's fantasy," said my friend Marianne, "and ones who are doing it because it's *their* fantasy."

It's performing vs. exploring. I have been on both sides of the fence and while certain scenarios make me cringe, I don't judge, not even the women who drunkenly make out during spring break for *Girls Gone Wild* videos. "I think some of the attraction is exploring what it is like to kiss someone who is just like me, building a confidence in my sexual identity," says Constance, a twenty-three-year-old staffer at the ACLU, who estimates that 75 percent of her female friends have had relationships with women. "One of the reasons I'm fearful to make a commitment to my boyfriend is that I don't want to miss out on having a deeper relationship with women." I think that some women might just be kissing because they think it's what their boyfriends want to see—which isn't so deep, but has its own power. But other women, my fellow explorers, are getting a lot more from these relationships than our culture, saddled as it is with bi anxiety, might apprehend.

Bisexuality can reveal unasked questions about sex, for instance. Until Anastasia, my way of compensating for sexual insecurity—the openness that intimacy needs—was performing. Up until that point, I felt if I was a vixen, my partner's pleasure proved my allure, but I remained fuzzy and perplexed about my own pleasure. Of course, men don't necessarily think these performances are so great and an evolved guy would rather be connecting. Gordon once described an ex of his as having a very "practiced" blowjob, one with the hand and the mouth and the big hair all swinging around. It took me a moment to realize that he didn't think of it as a good thing.

Marianne recalls that she always felt like she was pretending around men: "To me 'sexy' was something that was so outside of me, if I could imitate Angelina Jolie or if it seemed like I was driving him wild, that was titillating to me." But being with Megan, her best friend in college, "removed the self-consciousness that I felt around sex," says Marianne, age thirty-six, "so that I could actually start enjoying the feelings." Letting go of the performance with Megan led to Marianne eventually finding a way to be in the moment with a man. Similarly, I managed to take what I learned with Amy to my next relationship with Gordon, a man who liked to begin and end each date with a romp. My first night in bed with Gordon, I couldn't remember what I was "supposed" to do. It had been five years since I had been around a penis in any appreciable way and it looked bizarrely large to me. I looked down and then said, "Um, your penis is really big." He glanced at me to see if it was a practiced remark and then he replied, "It's not, actually." "Oh," I paused and then smiled. "I don't really know what I'm doing." And it was one of the most genuine sexual moments I have ever had and led to some quantum leaps forward in my sexual awakening.

Gordon was the first time I allowed myself to be openly unsure sexually around a man. I fumbled for a while with Anastasia after that first incredible kiss, and I actually allowed myself to fumble, rather than retreat to some routine I thought was what sexpots did in bed. Sex with women taught me that the fumble is crucial to getting to the good stuff. Which brings me to what I have learned from men: the importance of having an inner Lothario. "For a lot of women only dating women, it takes longer to arrive at the decision that you really want sex to be aggressive," says Liza, a married writer. "I think you get there eventually but when I first started having sex with women, I remember thinking, 'I really like this but I kind of want to be a little more attacked and objectified.'"

"Objectified" is, of course, one of those words that a penetrating feminist movement in the seventies rendered entirely negative (along with the word "penetrating"). But that might not be totally true: as Helen Gurley Brown once said to me about being a sex object, "sometimes it's just wonderful!" Certainly there is a power and a pleasure to it—and it seems to me the dangerous thing is not being objectified occasionally, but being reduced so that you are *only* a sex object. Raised, as my generation was, with critiques of sexism and the advent of Brazilian bikini waxes—with the example of on-top Madonna rather than tragic Marilyn—I think we are well-positioned to manage sexual complexity.

I made peace with my desire to be desired a while ago, but honestly dealing with the female competition I often felt with friends was harder for me to square with my feminist values. One of my worst nights with Marianne was one in which a guy we'd both been flirting with asked me to dance—my choosing of him and patronizing sympathy for her made for bad feelings that rattled our friendship. "He didn't make me feel ugly," I remember her saying, "as much as you did." Of course, I have been on the side of not being the chosen one, too, and that feeling is, if anything, worse to me. An undercurrent of competition and distrust trembles below many wonderful friendships and when women date other women, that nasty sense of competition evaporates. Witness Anastasia, who in high school was curvy, wore high heels, had long hair and got tons of attention from men. "Because of the jealousy I felt from women sometimes, it was hard to have friendships," recalls Anastasia, "and I did find myself drawn to sexual relationships with women because it was a way to have the closeness with them and to eliminate the competition—you know, 'how about we don't compete with the men and just be together?'"

I know what I get from both women and men, but I still can't believe how hard it is for other people to hear that I look both ways. "Oh, yes, people say insulting things, even people who love you," Lana, a twenty-seven-year-old health writer told me, shaking her head. "Like 'hey, you're back on *our* team!' This sides mentality. . . . it's a problem, largely, because it's not true and forces the bisexual woman to claim that huge swaths of her life were 'just a phase' or otherwise not valid."

"I'm bisexual," the late poet June Jordan once said to me, just after she had removed herself from an anthology entitled *My Lover Is A Woman*. "I resent this resistance to complexity." Ain't it the truth? We women believe in the variety and endless interestingness of sex—that three-letter word merits a million cover lines. And yet when people say that part of their complexity includes attraction to both men and women, our sense of possibility stops—we have to *choose* and there are just two choices.

Looking back, if all I got from that first drunken night with Anastasia was an incredible kiss, I got a lot.

Women's Health/Transgender Health: Intersections

LAUREN PORSCH

Lauren Porsch, "Women's Health/ Transgender Health: Intersections," 2008. Original for this publication.

As a feminist and sexual and reproductive health activist, I have always felt that transgender rights, and transgender health activism in particular, were naturally aligned with my activist goals. The transgender fight for the right to express oneself outside of the restraints suggested by anatomical sex is but an extension of feminists' historical struggle for the right to occupy social roles traditionally reserved for men. The movement for women's reproductive rights, in particular, has long centered around a woman's right to bodily integrity and self-determination, an issue at the heart of the transgender experience. Further, some of the most pressing issues confronted by the larger women's health movement, such as educating and empowering individuals to take charge of their own health, creating a more compassionate health care experience, and working to break down the model of medical professionals as gatekeepers to care, are concerns that are currently being addressed by the nascent transgender health movement.

One of the most palpable points of historical common ground between the women's and transgender health agendas has been the overarching intention of each to increase women's and transgender individuals' participation in and satisfaction with their health care encounters. Spurred by the growing number of women speaking out about negative experiences they had had with their doctors, feminist health activists took on the hierarchical, paternalistic model of medical care that dismissed women's knowledge about their own bodies. With the goal of empowering women to become active participants in their health care, feminist health activists argued that women themselves, not physicians, were the experts on their own health care needs. They aimed to ensure that laywomen's voices were included in any discussion about women's health in the public or policy arenas.[1] Women's health activists also encouraged women to educate themselves about their bodies and to enter a health care encounter with their own expectations laid out, rather than defaulting to a provider-focused agenda that left them passive receivers of care that didn't meet their needs. When the mainstream medical establishment was not able to provide the type of care for which they were advocating, they organized among themselves, establishing gynecological self-help groups, feminist health centers, and in the pre-Roe days, networks of safe and ethical underground abortion providers.

In many respects, the newly emerging transgender health movement has followed a similar trajectory to that of the early women's health movement. Listening to transgender individual's powerful stories of negative health care encounters, which ran the gamut from provider ignorance and insensitivity, to purposeful humiliation, to the actual denial of care, community activists and allies have begun organizing to confront trans-

phobia in health care and to empower the transgender community to advocate for their own needs in the health care setting. Central to these goals is the belief that the voices of trans people must be at the forefront of efforts to formulate a specific trans health agenda. As transgender community activist Leslie Feinberg puts it, "we are experts on our own lives and what we need as patients."[2] Some of the early products of grassroots transgender health activism have included the delivery of training sessions for health care workers in basic transgender sensitivity protocols, the development of local referral lists of transgender-friendly health care providers, the distribution of educational materials for the trans community on topics such as safer sex and sexually transmitted infection screening and prevention, breast and chest health, and hormone therapy, to name a few.

Another area of common concern for women's and transgender health activists has been the issue of medical professionals as gatekeepers to care. This phenomenon transcends a single health issue and boils down to the right of an individual to retain ownership of his or her body. In the years prior to *Roe v. Wade*, desperate women seeking abortions in a hospital setting were forced to undergo humiliating evaluations by physicians and mental health professionals to determine whether they had a medical or psychiatric condition which would make an abortion permissible. Recommendations were then made to a hospital ethics committee, which would make the final decision about whether or not the woman could obtain an abortion in the medical setting. Many women were turned down, and no doubt some of those women were forced to seek abortions through unsafe means. Similarly, according to current widely used guidelines, transgender individuals who have chosen to begin a physical transition with hormones and/or surgeries are required to first be given a diagnosis of "Gender Identity Disorder" by a mental health professional, a designation which marks transgender identities as pathological, rather than normal expressions of human diversity. Aside from the requirement of a problematic diagnosis, these guidelines place mental health professionals in the position of being gatekeepers to transgender hormone therapy and surgeries, and there is no guarantee that a provider will decide that an individual qualifies for care.[3] This process presents such an obstacle to some transgender individuals that many decide to seek hormones through disreputable sources, placing themselves at risk of medical complications from exposure to contaminated preparations and improper dosing.

A current and pressing issue of concern to feminist groups and the transgender community alike is the issue of gender-based violence prevention. While the term "gender-based violence" is often used to mean violence against women, I would argue for an expansion of the definition to include violence perpetrated against individuals because of their gender identity or expression. Incidents of violence against transgender individuals are most often directed towards those who visibly transgress gender boundaries, such as trans people who do not "pass" as a man or a woman, or whose gender expression doesn't fit either side of the socially imposed gender binary. The phenomenon is troublingly reminiscent of violence used against women as a form of control, a means of keeping women physically and metaphorically in their place when they step outside of socially proscribed gender roles. In reality, both women and trans individuals find themselves on the front lines of a social struggle to enforce strict gender codes, falling victim to interpersonal violence at the hands of those who are disturbed by their transgression of "acceptable" boundaries. In 2004, the National Coalition for Lesbian, Gay, Bisexual, and Transgender Health released an updated report on transgender health priorities in the United States, naming violence and murder prevention as the number one priority towards improving the health of the transgender population.[4] This recommendation was supported by data, collected by both academic researchers and community advocacy groups, which illustrated an epidemic of violence against transgender people that shows no signs of abating. While there is still much long-term work to be done on a societal level to eradicate gender-based violence, in the short-term, the very tangible need of providing support and advocacy services to women and trans survivors of violence provides an excellent opportunity for cross-movement collaboration.

NOTES

1. J. Norsigian, et al., "The Boston Women's Health Book Collective and Our Bodies, Ourselves: A brief history and reflection," *JAMWA*, 1999: 54, 1.
2. L. Feinberg, "Trans health crisis: For us it's life or death," *AJPH*, 2001: 91, 6.
3. National Coalition for Lesbian, Gay, Bisexual, and Transgender Health, 2004.
4. Ibid.

Gender and Medicine

FOR MANY WOMEN'S HEALTH activists back in the 1970s who had been burned by male doctors who treated them like children, the prospect of women becoming doctors in larger numbers offered hope for creating a medical profession in which patients, particularly female patients, found themselves respected and treated as adults by their health care providers.

It has been a long and thorny road for women doctors. A year before the famous nineteenth-century Seneca Falls convention became the first modern statement of the American feminist movement, Elizabeth Blackwell became the first woman to enter an American medical school in Geneva, New York.

Women continued to enroll in medical school, but for over a hundred years, the numbers stayed very low. In 1969, less than 8 percent of medical students were female. By 1979, the figure tripled to over 25 percent. Why did this radical change happen? Well, it wasn't the sudden enlightenment of medical schools.

In 1972, Dr. Mary Howell, the first female dean at Harvard Medical School, set out to raise awareness about the sexism and discrimination against female medical students. Then serving as dean of student affairs, Howell distributed a questionnaire to students. The results, which contained stories of harassment and unequal treatment, enraged her and brought back memories of her experiences as a young medical student in the 1950s. Under the assumed name Margaret Campbell, Howell published *Why Would a Girl Go Into Medicine?* (1973).

Also in 1972, Congresspeople Edith Green and Patsy Mink (who had struggled unsuccessfully to become a doctor during her youth, applying and being rejected from twenty-five medical schools despite exceptional qualifications), spearheaded Title IX, the Women's Educational Equity Act, which stated, "No person in the United States shall, on the basis of gender, be excluded from participation in, be denied the benefits of, or be subjected to discrimination under any education program or activity receiving Federal financial assistance." Designed to ensure that federally funded institutions would be required to treat boys and girls equally, it is usually associated with girls' sports. However, the full implications of the act were far more drastic than equal funding for athletics. In fact, it required the dropping of quotas and the opening up of medical school admittance to women. The number of female doctors quadrupled in America between 1970 and 1990 from 25,400 to 104,200.[1]

In 1995, it was reported in the journal *American Demographics* that one out of five physicians was a woman. The American Medical Association noted around the same time that 40 percent of medical students were women.[2] Harvard Medical school reported that 50 percent of its 1999 class were women and that 52.8 percent of its 2000 class.[3] The number of female gynecologists has been following a similar trend: as of 2001, about one third of American gynecologists are women. The number of residents planning to enter the field was high enough at that point that Cornell University Medical Center predicted that by 2012, half of ob-gyns would be women.[4]

The report also noted that women tended to enter primary care in larger numbers and to devote more time to each patient, scheduling fewer patients to begin with. A study at Massachusetts General Hospital in Boston found that female doctors spent an average of seven and a half minutes longer in office visits with patients.

A 1993 University of Minnesota study found that of 25,000 women in a certain health plan, those who had women as primary care doctors were "twice as likely to have an annual Pap smear as those whose internists were men. They were also 41percent more likely to have a mammogram than those with male doctors."

All of this is despite the fact that the wage gap is larger between female doctors and their male colleagues than the national average. According to the American Medical Women's Association, the average female doctor makes only 63 percent of what her male counterpart makes, a gap that seems to be growing, not declining.[5]

It is also possible that patients, particularly female patients, are just more comfortable discussing personal health problems with other women. In one study, women were nearly one-third more likely to speak in visits with female doctors. As one expert at Harvard explains, "Most studies show that women are more successful than men at involving patients in decisions and explaining medical terminology."

Dr. Erica Frank, in her ambitious Women Physicians' Health Study published in the *Journal of the American Medical Association*, found that despite the importance of feminists in getting women into medical school and the continued gender disparities in central issues such as pay, most women doctors declined to call themselves feminists. This was despite the fact that Frank found nearly half of her respondents had experienced harassment based on their gender (including things like being called "honey" in front of patients or being lectured that medicine is "not a career for women.") These same women, made so uncomfortable by the "f" word, had no similar problem with questions about potentially more personal issues such as sexual orientation.

Frank also found that while women physicians were generally happy in their careers, 31 percent said that if they could do it all over again, they would have chosen another job. The *Journal of the American Medical Association* noted, "Those who reported the most dissatisfaction were likely to be younger and have the least work control, most work stress, or have experienced severe harassment."[6]

While female doctors seem to be making some positive changes in the doctor/patient dynamic—giving more time, doing a better job (on average) listening, and being more likely to advise against unhealthy behaviors—there are other, less positive changes. Drug companies have been incredibly successful at exploiting what is basically a great thing—that female patients feel more comfortable talking with and sharing with their female doctors. This "girl talk" dynamic between doctor and patient has become the subject of a series of drug campaigns for gender specific drugs. A recent example, a series of ads for the birth control patch (Ortho-Eura) feature a pretty young doctor who assures her patients, "I'm not just speaking as a doctor here—I'm also a birth control user." In another one, a female patient asks her questions in a nonoffice environment, sort of Sex in the City–style restaurant setting, and the young physician responds like a friend offering advice on love life problems. If the old paradigm of the male physician relied on the metaphor of the stern father offering dictums and prescriptions, this new one exploits the trust women have—rightly and wrongly—in each other.

For their part, female doctors are not always the best advocates for their patients in terms of standing up against dangerous drug company propaganda. During the heady days of hormone prescription in the 1990s, when many doctors worshiped at the altar of estrogen replacement, female doctors were among the most enthusiastic devotees. An *Annals of Internal Medicine* study, published in 1998, observed that "female doctors who have undergone menopause seem to believe in hormone replacement therapy more than their patients: They are twice as likely as other postmenopausal women to take hormones . . . overall, 47 percent of the doctors surveyed were on HRT versus a national average of 24 percent."[7] There are many incredible female doctors who we would wholeheartedly recommend, and we would also say that if seeing a woman is a more comfortable medical situation for you, than do it. But don't assume that because your doctor is female that she is more trustworthy or less likely to prescribe dangerous drugs.

NOTES

1. *University of California Berkeley Wellness Letter*, March 1995.
2. *Harvard Women's Health Watch*, vol. II, no. 9 (May 1995).
3. "Doctors from Venus and Mars: How they Differ," *Harvard Health Letter*, May 2001.
4. "Your next gynecologist could be a woman," *Cornell Women's Health Advisor*, July 2001, 2.
5. "Gender Discrepancy in Physician Salaries," *AMWA Connections*, vol. XXVI, no. 5, September 2004.

6. *The Archives of Internal Medicine*, 159 (1999): 1417-1426.
7. *The Johns Hopkins Medical Letter: Health After 50*, vol. 10, is. 2 (April 1998): 1.

Why Would a Girl Go into Medicine?

MARGARET A. CAMPBELL

Margaret A. Campbell (aka Mary Howell), excerpt from *Why Would a Girl Go into Medicine?* New York: Ann E. O'Shea, 1973; and Old Westbury, NY: Feminist Press, 1973. New introduction by Ann E. O'Shea, 1999. Reprinted by permission.

In 1973, ten years after the publication of Betty Friedan's *The Feminine Mystique*, nine years after passage of the 1964 Civil Rights Act, which prohibited discrimination in employment on the basis of sex, four years after Barbara Seaman's book, *The Doctors' Case Against the Pill*, rocked the medical-pharmacutical industries, and one year after Congress enacted Title IX of the Educational Amendments Act, which banned discrimination against women in all federally supported educational institutions, a typewritten, 113-page book entitled *Why Would a Girl Go into Medicine?* by Margaret A. Campbell mysteriously appeared. The book, which the author described as "a survey of discrimination against women in US medical schools, written to inform and encourage women medical students of the past, present, and future and to promote radical change in medical education and in the care of patients," began to circulate just as the women's movement and its outspoken feminist health advocates converged with the passage of dramatically far-reaching federal legislation making discrimination in employment and education against women and minorities illegal.

I was three years out of college and working with Barbara Seaman at *Family Circle* magazine. Barbara gave me a copy of the typewritten manuscript and asked if I would help her distribute it for the author, whose real name was Mary Howell, a dean at Harvard Medical School. This was an extraordinarily radical document, which detailed the insidious discrimination faced by women medical students at the most prestigious American schools, including Harvard. The need for a pseudonymous author was apparent, as was the need for an underground method of distribution. The feminist publications advertised the book and let readers know that copies could be obtained for $2 by writing to me at my New York City apartment. I remember making hundreds of photocopies of the book—many on *Family Circle*'s copying machines—and convincing Alan Handell (who would later become my husband) to run off hundreds more copies at his newly established printing company. I became the ersatz publisher of a radical underground book describing the discrimination suffered by women medical students and suggesting the larger issue of discrimination suffered by women consumers of health care. Mary Howell's book, together with Title IX, revolutionized medical education in the United States.

—ANN E. O'SHEA, 1999

Why "girl"? The title of this booklet requires a word of explanation. It is a direct quotation from a woman medical student: "I have often been asked, "Why would a girl go into medicine?" It was chosen to symbolize the themes of this report. The wonder expressed in the question—that anyone of the female sex would want to, or could, become a competent physician—is half of the problem. The other half of the problem is found in the word "girl." Of course, one does not expect of "girls," nor of "boys," the maturity one hopes for in a physician. The denigration of the term "girl" used to describe a woman, an adult, tells us how we have all been socialized with regard to stereotypes of gender-role. This report is an attempt to inform all who are concerned about health care about the relationships between the prejudice that describes women as "girls," the effects of the prejudice on women being trained to become physicians, and the inappropriate attitudes and

assumptions that color the behavior of many physicians toward their women patients.

We all know that discrimination against women exists, although we sometimes deny that knowledge because discrimination is painful to experience. Trying to change the sources of discrimination is a long, hard process, and in the meantime we must keep from being destroyed or poisoned as a consequence of what some people would have us think about ourselves. I believe the first three lines of defense are (1) information about the specific forms of discrimination in any situation, so we are never taken by surprise, (2) an understanding of ourselves and how we react to discriminatory attitudes and practices, and (3) strong support of each other, in formal or informal networks. That is what this document is about.

INTRODUCTION

This document has been assembled to assist women in selecting and surviving a medical school education.

Most of the information that students need to have before choosing a medical school is of course equally relevant and equally available to men and women. One set of questions has, however, been very difficult to answer: What is it like to be a woman student at X medical school? Are the various medical schools significantly different in their dealings with women? How do women who are now medical students feel about their experience?

The information collected for the report is "case study" data from women medical students. An exploratory questionnaire composed of open-ended questions was widely but nonsystematically sent to many (but probably not all) of the 107 degree-granting medical schools in the United States. Seventy-six questionnaires were returned from 146 women students at forty-one medical schools. All data were collected between February and September of 1973.

What follows is an unremitting recital of Bad

Things. Of course, there are also many positive aspects in the experience of being a woman medical student, as illustrated by the fact that 140 of the 146 student respondents urge other women to join them at their schools. This can in no way excuse the occurrence of the instances of discrimination cited here. These things should not happen.

INSTITUTIONAL DISCRIMINATION

The instances of discrimination described in this and following sections are only those that students are aware of and thought appropriate to describe. Evidence of institutional discrimination is difficult for students (or anyone else) to document, probably because it is blatantly illegal.

RECRUITING Because of the very large numbers of students now applying for a relatively few places in US medical schools, little recruiting is done. Many schools do recruit (and compete for) students representing racial and ethnic minorities, and often some informal recruiting is done by faculty and alumni to attract especially attractive white male applicants. There is little or no school-supported recruitment of women, although women students sometimes organize among themselves to encourage women applicants.

> Recruiting policies are not equal. Women are a minority in the school: twelve out of 125 in our class, equal or smaller percentages of previous classes. There is an active recruitment program for blacks and chicanos with the goal of equalizing population and enrollment percentages.*

ADMISSIONS Students have very little accurate information about admissions policies in action. In order to assess the possibility of discrimination in the admissions process we need to know, for each school, the qualifications of the applicant pools and of the accepted students, and the criteria used to judge students.

Until this information is made available, the

AAMC data on admissions is limited but suggestive: we know only the proportion of women in the entering class of each school, and the proportion of women in the combined entering class of all schools taken together (the national mean). Schools that admit women in proportions less than this national mean may be presumed to be discriminatory until they supply data to disprove this presumption.

The admissions formula (compiled from weighted averages of grade point average, points for type and place of degree, MCAT scores, extracurricular scientifically related activities) is equal on the surface. However, one's acceptance also depends on how the applicant impresses two interviewers, who are of course male faculty members; this is probably the place where the discrimination takes place.

"MOTHERSTUDENTS" Only sixteen schools—fifteen percent of the total number of schools offering MD programs—are known to have admitted nine or more women students who were mothers in the years between 1956 and 1972. A discriminatory policy cannot be ascertained unless we know about the applicant pool and the number of "fatherstudents" admitted, but we should inquire whether those schools at which few or no motherstudents have been admitted have not made discriminatory prejudgments about applicants' capabilities based on traditional and stereotypic views of women and family life (i.e., that mothers care for children but fathers do not, that children cannot thrive unless their mothers care for them full-time, and that mothers cannot also be competent students and workers).

FINANCIAL AID Information about financial aid is also closely guarded, and students generally do not know how aid is distributed with regard to need; they could begin to find out, of course, by asking each other.

> One of the women could not get aid that would include her husband as dependent, although men with wives in the same po-

sition have no problem. Getting financial aid for children was almost impossible. They seemed to think I was asking for maid service, and that I was lazy.

LODGING The most frequent instances of discrimination against women have to do with on-call rooms at school-affiliated hospitals. Often the women students, with admirable flexibility, offer to make do by using the men's facilities—but the usual result is that the men students become angry and upset at the women.

> We asked for a lounge for women doctors and students because we can't go in the surgeons' lounge (they dress there) and it is not always comfortable to spend on-call nights sleeping in a long row of beds fully dressed between several undressed males. We have no place to leave purses and coats and, unlike the men, no place to shower. We were stalled and stalled and we never got the lounge.

> Female restrooms for students and house staff are nonexistent in our hospital.

ATHLETIC FACILITIES The principal examples of discrimination fall in the general category of "forgetting" that there are women students, or of counting the women's needs as less important than the men's. Lack of equipment for women, inequitable access to facilities, and absence of showers and locker rooms are the problems most frequently described.

HEALTH SERVICES: GYNECOLOGICAL CARE The student health service provides more than health care: for medical students it is one of the few examples they see, during their years of medical education, of physicians in action, the "real world' of clinic practice as opposed to the theoretical or ideal taught about in school and in the hospitals. For this reason, the quality of health care provided by the health service is of special importance.

Our first question is whether the female sexual reproductive system is included within the range of general medical care. Alternatively, are women told by implication that this part of their bodies is exceptional and aberrant, and must receive medical care under unusual (often more inconvenient and expensive) circumstances?

Most departments of medicine argue and teach that examination of the female sexual reproductive system is part of a general physical examination, and that care of "routine, uncomplicated" health problems in this area falls within the province of the generalist physician. In the real world, internists, family physicians, and other generalist physicians often do not consider themselves to be responsible even for simple matters relating to the female sexual reproductive system. Although they will examine eyes and offer advice and treatment for simple ophthalmologic problems—sending a patient to a "specialist" only when the problem is complex or otherwise warrants additional expertise—they may refer all matters relating to the female sexual-reproductive tract to the gynecologist. (The reasons for this refusal to care for "female problems" as part of general medical care are complex and probably include such personal dynamics as disgust about female genitals, sexual anxiety, and denigration of the importance of the special health care needs of women.) The effect is to tell the women patient that her genital system is not part of her body in the ordinary sense, but a special, bothersome (offensive?) part of her that has to be shipped out for special care.

If complete general health care is offered to men, but women must go outside the health service (physically, financially, or by delayed appointment) for care for uncomplicated medical problems of the sexual-reproductive system, this is discriminatory.

HEALTH SERVICES: PSYCHOTHERAPY All women in our society live in "special circumstances," different from those of men. These special factors include (1) a socialization that rewards dependency and passivity and discourages autonomy, (2) a cyclic physiology and the ability to bear children, and (3) a social expectation that they will be subservient to men. Women training in a "man's" profession (by traditional definition) may well have many questions and some anxiety about the conflict between the professional role and the stereotypic female role. While many women find support from each other or from individual faculty members to be adequate in managing these questions and anxieties, some may wish to seek regular counseling or therapy. A health service that provides psychotherapy "appropriate to individual needs" will recognize these needs of women students.

DAY CARE Institutional "support" for day care means financial support, since no high-quality day care arrangements can be paid for by parents—except the wealthy—if caretakers are to be paid an adequate wage. While day care is a problem for parents (and not for women alone), some medical student parents are single-parent women, so the matter has been included here as an instance of discrimination against some women. I believe that the need for institutionally supported day care is great, and hope that men and women together will work for this cause as an acknowledgment of their responsibility as (current or potential) parents.

AFFIRMATIVE ACTION PLANS The executive orders of 1965 and 1967 and the 1972 law that bar federal contractors and educational institutions from discrimination on the basis of sex require all institutions that receive substantial federal funds (including all medical schools or the universities of which they are a part) to (1) describe the discrimination that presently exists and (2) outline the affirmative steps they will take to reduce discrimination.

That few medical student respondents know what an AAP [affirmative action plan] is reflects the institutional and governmental apathy surrounding this possible remedy to existing discrimination. While an AAP is no panacea, it does signify that the institution has responded formally to the executive orders rather than exhibiting open defiance or simply ignoring the presence of minorities and women.

Working to help one's school develop an AAP offers a focus for energies and an opportunity for a group of women from diverse backgrounds to share a common set of goals. In addition, the information collected to fulfill the first part of the requirement (the documentation of present discrimination) is enormously revealing, and the entire project has high publicity value. We must, however, be cautious in hoping that the existence of an AAP will bring significant and sweeping changes in the near future.

REPRESENTATION OF WOMEN ON FACULTY AND ADMINISTRATION The AAMC lists information about minority faculty and administrators by school but without denominators so that one could calculate proportions. No such listing is provided for women faculty and administrators.

Students generally remark that they see very few women faculty or administrators. Only statements that include some numerical information (or estimate) are included here—again, without denominators it is difficult to calculate the precise significance of these numbers.

The number of senior women at an institution is of course important information for the senior women themselves. For women medical students, these statistics have two kinds of significance: (1) senior women serve as "role models" and counselors for students, and (2) the proportions of women hired by the institution instruct students about the breadth of possibilities for their own future careers.

There are two women pediatricians who are

---

*These statements are taken directly from student questionnaires.

attending staff. We have no women who are full professors, administrators, or advisers. Our hospital has one female intern out of fifty spaces and somewhat more female residents.

The majority of the teaching staff is male (80 percent).

MISCELLANY There are other instances of institutional discrimination that do not fit neatly into categories.

Social activities are geared to the single men—like inviting nursing students to parties.

Surgeons' lounge—with a sign on the door saying "Surgeons and Medical Students Only"—is off-limits to female students, in spite of the fact that a certain amount of relaxed, informal teaching is done there.

All parties and social events require a woman student to sign up for refreshments—however, some of us refuse to volunteer before each of the other [male] classmates do KP (kitchen patrol) first. The number of class parties has declined.

OVERT DISCRIMINATION

The "culture" of the medical schools apparently promotes certain (traditionally) "male" attitudes and behaviors and often is supported by a men's club atmosphere. Open discrimination against women (serious and "in fun") is encouraged by this atmosphere and promoted in the process of professional enculturation. The varieties of overt discrimination against women can be described as baiting, belittling, hostility, and backlashing.

BAITING The occurrence of baiting conveys the men's sense of social support for and approval of discrimination against women: It may, of course, also signify a deep and uncomfortable personal insecurity that can be slightly assuaged by denigrating others.

"Because of you a man probably went into chiropractic school."

On one ward a resident called his male students "Dr." and his female students "Ms."

BELITTLING The largest number of overtly discriminatory comments cited by students seemed to fall in this category. The belittling comments noted here are only those with reference to professional women or women physicians; see the section on "Women as Patients" for comments demeaning of all women as patients.

Quote of our new dean: "I don't think women belong in medicine anyway." This sums it up.

"A woman doesn't belong in the OR [operating room] except as a nurse."—chief of ob-gyn.

A cardiologist said, "It will be interesting to go to your twenty-fifth reunion and see how many of the women have done a full day's work."

HOSTILITY While baiting remarks seem designed to evoke a reaction from the women to whom the remarks are directed, hostile comments appear to be undisguised and open expressions of free-floating anger against woman-as-colleagues. As is always true with discriminatory attitudes and behaviors against any group, a contagion develops that thrives on group support. The interaction between male students and faculty in this regard is apparent. Some women believe that discriminatory remarks are more often made in large lectures because of supports and approval from male students; others (perhaps in more "liberal" areas of the country) say that discriminatory remarks are more frequently made in small groups, especially by instructors who have the power to give grades and comments on the student's performance and personality.

In the first two years of medical school, when large lectures were the rule, it was very common for lecturers to begin sessions with little jokes, invariably with women as the butts, in an attempt to gain rapport. This, of course, encouraged the men in my class to adopt a similar attitude toward women, and whenever any attempt was made by women in the class to point out these humiliations, they were further belittled.

An example of the private remarks, from a student: "Well, if the women don't like it [the use of "nudie" slides in required lectures], they don't have to come to class."

The head of the ob-gyn department tells obscene degrading jokes while performing surgery and considers it his right to tease black nurses about bizarre sexual habits in front of ten other people during surgery.

BACKLASHING In medical schools, as in almost every other social environment, the recent surge of feminism has brought out a particularly nasty kind of male anger, apparently as a reaction to a sense of threat. To a degree this backlash may only offer men an excuse or justification for doing what they would have done anyway, but it is also possible that backlash may promote even more overt (and covert) discrimination than might otherwise have occurred. In medicine, of course, men are reacting to feminism in the general sense (which may, for instance, affect their marriages) but also to the specific changes that are bound to come to their profession as a direct result of the admission of more women students.

A dean advised several women in our class not to "band together," since there are now so many of us (twelve women out of 125) that we don't need each other for support

and protection. We were told that we must learn to work with our male colleagues.

SUBTLE DISCRIMINATION

OSTRACIZING Women physicians are often viewed as "fake men," and therefore as imposters. The message conveyed by ostracizing forms of subtle discrimination is that women really do not belong in the profession of medicine and that our very presence is jarring. Both ostracizing and forgetting (see below) must require a fair amount of energy in defense of the delusion that medicine is an all-male profession, since there have been successful and visible women in medicine (about 10 percent) for many decades. One of the ways women are ostracized from membership in a profession is by treating them—and expecting them to act—like dependent daughters, pampered sisters, nurturing mothers, help-meet wives or seductive playmates. It is apparently very difficult for many men to relate to a woman as a colleague; it may also be difficult for women to assume the relationship of colleague, because we have been trained to fill the familial roles.

When residents talk with male students they talk about diseases, patients, and other medical subjects, but when women students are around, conversation is always slanted toward "women in medicine" and "women's lib."

On several different occasions of small-group discussions led by several different obstetricians, I'm repeatedly excluded from the group—no one-to-one eye contact, referred to as "honey" (like a patient, all of whom are referred to as "gals" or "girls"), excluded from the camaraderie of the "fellows, who hang their stethoscopes around their necks to impress the chicks" with their prowess and status as docs.

One woman student was requested to wear a lab coat while making rounds with her tutor (three other male students were not) so that she would "look more like a doctor" to patients.

FORGETTING Even more frequently, the presence of women students in the medical school environment seems to be totally overlooked or forgotten. Even in classes in which the proportion of women is as high as 25 percent, instructors and administrators "forget" that there are any women present.

> Activities of the wives' club always exclude the women of the class, married or not, but special invitations are sent to the single men.

> Professors have refused to call on women students raising their hands for questions in class and have neglected answering women's questions after class.

SPOTLIGHTING It is nearly equally uncomfortable to be constantly spotlighted as it is to be forgotten. One way to deal with what is perceived as an aberration is to call attention to the phenomenon with a vigor that may reflect kindly interest, amusement or anger. Some men in the medical school atmosphere are apparently so puzzled, or discomfited, by the notion of a *woman* medical student that they always remark on the presence of a woman in this role.

STEREOTYPING I Attribution to women as a group of the traits of dependency, lack of intellectual interest, lack of competence and ambition, and all of the traditional stereotypic characteristics of femininity constitutes the first variant of stereotyping. This "social shorthand" disregards individual talents, interests, and traits by setting a mindlessly rigid standard for appropriately "womanly" behavior: if the object-person is of the female sex she must fit the appropriate mold, and if she does not fit the predictable mold she is not feminine.

This first form of stereotyping is exercised against women medical students either by the expectation that they are all alike (and like all other women) in their interests and capabilities, or by the implication that since they have chosen to come to medical school they cannot be like other women and must therefore be deviant and unfeminine. The alternative sex role options available to women medical students are a neutered role, denying femininity, or a pseudomasculinity ("being more like the men than the men themselves"). The sum and substance is a denial of the wonderful variations of humanity that occur in female form.

> In one class, all analogies were directed to the men, and if a woman asked a question he related it to baking bread or milk cartons.

> Female classmate being told by a male colleague after she gave a tutorial report, "You'd make a good fourth-grade teacher."

> The most common is a very confused male asking how I will ever be able to be a good mother and a good doctor.

> I have often been asked, "Why would a girl go into medicine?"

STEREOTYPING II The second form of stereotyping is based on assumptions about the "proper" roles of women in relationship to men. A woman is expected to be (in some combination) servile, seductive, grateful, admiring, tolerant and patient, respectful, a comfort for wounded pride, and an external superego and keeper of morality. If she does not "keep to her place" in her relationships with men but is independent, positive, even argumentative, and refuses to acknowledge and take part in seductive and flirtatious sexual games, she is looked upon as "inappropriate," "abrasive," or "bitchy"; by a process of escalation she may be described as "castrating." Admissions interview questions often reflect these attitudes.

> [In an admissions interview] I was asked repeatedly if I could perform in a class of

all boys [sic], if I was looking for a husband, and if I was "really" serious.

One administrative higher-up talked with a female prospective applicant for fifteen minutes and asked nothing about her interests and career plans, only whether her husband knew she was there and wasn't this just a passing fancy.

MALE SEXUAL PRURIENCE The "men's club" atmosphere of medical school is never so apparent as in the laugh-getting comments and pictures about female sexuality. Comments about female sexual practices, habits, and preferences are given as embroidery overlaid on factual material related to the clinical practice of medicine. It is assumed that any man has the right to regard any woman— colleague or patient—as an object of sexual interest.

> The slide of a nude female with arms outstretched was used to illustrate the shape of an IgG molecule.

> "The only significant difference between a woman and a cow is that a cow has more spigots."—lecturer.

> Every description of pathology [in ob-gyn lectures] is accompanied by graphic descriptions of the sex life of a woman with that particular pathology.

HOW DO WE COPE?

There are three broad patterns of response. One may deny the very evidence of discrimination; react with anger; or seek, and give, constructive support to and from other women. These three are not mutually exclusive, and probably all of us use all of these coping mechanisms from one time to another.

Thirty of the seventy-six questionnaires were completed by students who said that there was virtually no discrimination against women at their school. Nineteen of these then described three or more incidents (many of them quoted in the preceding sections) that have in this analysis been counted as discriminatory. Of the remaining eleven students who said there was little or no discrimination against women at their school, nine were countered by other respondents from the same schools who reported three or more discriminatory incidents and believed that discrimination against women was a general pattern; the remaining two were the only respondents from their schools.

Women medical students who utilized the energy-conserving adaptation of protective denial were most certainly in the majority in the recent past, and may still be the majority today. There may be a trend over time, however, for first-year student respondents were much less likely than students from upper classes to describe their experiences in this fashion.

Those who feel that there is essentially no discrimination against women in medical school, or who agree with the premises of the discrimination they perceive, often believe that women who react differently are "immature" or expect special favors. They often do not understand the questions in the questionnaire about "self-support," deny that they need support with respect to their status as women medical students, and may be angered by the implications of the questionnaire.

> It is usually the reverse: a department chairman will be carefully explaining the mechanism of X in the care of the patient, and I find myself thinking: I'm just a girl and he's taking all this time to explain it to me!

The first step in seeking support during the process of a medical school education is usually among status-peers—other women medical students and older woman physicians. The comments quoted here reflect some of the anger and frustration of these students, and some sense of loneliness. When status-peer groups work well, the sense of strength derived therefrom is also evident.

The women in the freshman and sophomore

classes got together on their own twice this year and invited women MDs from the [city] community. One was a pediatrician who is married and has three children. The other is a gynecologist who has not married (age about forty-two). We felt that we learned much from speaking to these women especially in the realm of what to expect and not expect from our colleagues in later years.

[We have] great support for women by other women of all classes—great ombudswomen. Several married women, some with children. Pretty good place for women, actually, though much improvement is needed.

Students who described a reaction of constructive support usually declared themselves as openly concerned with the matter of social equity for all women. They believed that they gained more strength by declaring their devotion to the cause of all women than from trying to please a group of men who seemed never to be pleased by their very presence as real persons. Concern for other women was often expressed by this group as concern for the medical care that women patients receive. Several students indicated that women—often, but not only, women who were declared feminists—were effective class leaders, especially in the role of organizers rather than as elected class officers. Some noted that consequent peer cohesiveness and support served to temper the process of "professionalization" by reducing students' dependence on teachers for support.

WORKING FOR CHANGE

We shall consider four ways to work for change: private negotiations, public "displays," organizing as an action group, and school-endorsed committees or task forces.

PRIVATE NEGOTIATIONS Most student respondents believe that judicious, politic, and carefully planned "confrontations" with persons who have acted in a discriminatory manner can be useful in bringing change. Some commented that one should never go alone—that the male-female, student-teacher dynamics were so well established that even polite protest was likely to backfire if one were alone. Students who felt confident that two women together more than doubled their strength were not disturbed by remarks about the "timidity" inferred by their support for each other.

Many noted that discriminators confronted in private were most likely to change if their discriminatory behavior had been unplanned, and if the discriminator had some reason to alter his/her behavior (incidents that we have categorized as subtle discrimination). In instances of overt discrimination, some students wonder if the slim chance of bringing change is worth the risk of being scolded, criticized, or formally reprimanded, as by a poor grade. Others feel that the registration of protest accomplishes some purpose in and of itself, and in some instances private negotiations with instructors and administrators have clearly brought changes in behavior, and perhaps even in attitudes.

We have just begun to speak to the doctor using [nudie slides] to explain that we think it is dehumanizing and that it makes us uncomfortable.

Sometimes we feel comfortable answering back, depending on how receptive we feel the lecturer is to criticism. Most of the time we feel that answering back will only reinforce their view of us as "women's libbers."

PUBLIC "DISPLAYS" Public "displays" are not "ladylike" and so have a kind of shock value that can be both very informative to witnesses and very gratifying to those who carry them out. While most women medical students are hesitant to use this method of urging change, it is apparent that it can have tremendous psychological impact. Those at whom a "display" is directed may be angry or hurt by the performance; others who observe are often surprised and in some way depressed; and those who perform (especially in a group) can be exhilarated by the sense of group solidarity, the audacity of their performance, and the strength of their statement for a cause.

Most "displays" described by students seem to result from careful political calculation, taking into account the instructor, the mood of the class, and concurrent events in the school.

> The women [students] also now have, of their own, a library of male nude slides [made up from a homosexual magazine]; although the idea is to have no confrontation, if need be, we will slip some of the slides into the lecturer's carousel of slides.

> We have in response to [discriminatory comments about women as medical students and as patients] (1) walked out of one class (2) confronted several teachers and presented our position (in one instance a professor harassed a woman in front of the class as a result of this).

ORGANIZING: GETTING OURSELVES TOGETHER A unified program to promote change comes most easily through an organized group. The energy derived from anger about discrimination (directed at one's self or at other women) provides a massive impetus for such an organized effort. Why is it so hard? So many of the women medical students tell of fledgling efforts to get together with each other, with older women physicians, and with other women, efforts that are not sustained. There are special skills of organizing that are often unfamiliar to women and to professionals. We are also terribly busy: Medical students and physicians have very heavy demands on their time, and employed or student wives have been shown to have little time for their own personal interests.

As women and as professionals we are brought up to mistrust other women; we learn in the pre-professional years to be individualistic and competitive with our peers; we are urged during professional training to act autonomously; and as women we are forced to compete with each other for "scarce-resource" jobs, research grants, and the favor or approval of our male colleagues. Thus it is difficult for all women professionals, students and graduates alike, to work in a sustained cooperative and sharing fashion toward a common set of goals.

It is typical of women in medicine that they are unwilling to stay long enough—much less give the kind of time and energy needed to make the group work. Perhaps if we as individuals understood what we hoped to get from belonging to a group, we could undertake group membership with a greater sense of its value.

SCHOOL-SPONSORED GROUPS Committees, task forces, and caucuses that have the official blessing of the institution usually have simultaneous positive and negative effects. Some changes are likely to come about through the actions or recommendations of an officially designated body mandated to study the status of women at the institution; it is not clear, however, that this is ever the best or only mechanism to bring such changes. School-sponsored groups often have a built-in conservative drag, either by virtue of membership—the inclusion of persons known to be conservative or not overly sympathetic to women, in order to give the group "credibility"—or by virtue of an agenda established by the institution. While small changes (on the order of increasing the number of ladies' restrooms) can be effected, it is less probable that major changes (such as objectifying and publishing admissions criteria or publishing salaries and salary criteria) will come through the efforts of such a group.

There is the further hazard that committee members will be co-opted by the philosophy of the institution. Appointment to the group is something of an honor as well as a chance to "do good" through established channels, and is difficult to refuse. One then becomes privy to the reasoning of the institutions about priorities, as expressed by masters (male or female) of persuasion. It is easy to forget our own goals and priorities. I believe that all institutions must develop such committees; unless they are totally co-opted they serve to raise the consciousness of the institutional community. The very existence of the group is an admission that some matters may need change. But one should be cautious in the belief that school-sponsored groups can be effective in bringing the kind of root-level changes that are necessary. And such groups are much more likely to function effectively both in their internal dynamics and in their communication with the community if they are made up of persons who begin by seeing the problems in a similar light.

WOMEN AS PATIENTS

It is widely believed that there is pervasive discrimination by professional health workers against women as patients. While some of this discrimination is expressed as inappropriate medical care (unnecessary hysterectomies, missed diagnoses because of assumed "psychogenic" or "hysterical" etiology, and so on), an equally serious and more widespread form of discrimination arises from assumptions about women that restrict them (more severely than male patients are restricted) to roles of dependency and uninformed reliance on the physician's authority. We are only beginning to document the extent and consequences of this discrimination against women patients.

It is clear that there is a direct interrelationship between discrimination against women as medical students and as patients: the one supports the other. We have seen that the medical school environment permits or encourages some kinds of blatantly discriminatory attitudes, behaviors, and policies to a degree that would not be considered permissible in other areas of life. Women medical students themselves are often aware of the relationship between their teachers' attitudes toward them, and attitudes toward women patients.

It seems likely that women physicians might be the best advocates for women patients; it seems unlikely, considering the prevailing views about women in medical schools, that very many men will be able to comprehend the force of those discriminatory attitudes and their damaging consequences. If women medical students learn to accept those attitudes (probably excluding themselves as "special" women) they will be less able to work for change in the care of patients, or even to conduct their own practices with women patients in a significantly different manner than that directed by their medical school teachers.

SELECTING A MEDICAL SCHOOL

It should be apparent that no clear differentiation can be made between the various medical schools with regard to discrimination against women medical students. The data collected here are neither sufficiently extensive nor complete (school-by-school) to rank schools as better or worse for women to attend.

One chooses a medical school for reasons of excellence of instruction, curricular emphasis on aspects of medical research or practice of particular interest to the individual student, and geographical considerations; one chooses to apply to schools at least partly because admission seems probable. Discriminatory attitudes and behaviors toward women must be at best a secondary criterion.

SURVIVING (AND THRIVING) AS A MEDICAL STUDENT

Only six of the 146 students completing questionnaires failed to encourage and invite other women to join them at their schools. The message, I believe, is that we feel a deep need for the support of other women, a strong hope that the presence of more women at medical schools will help bring change, and a belief that initiation into the profession of medicine is exciting, satisfying and worthwhile.

It's probably no worse than most med schools. Be prepared for a very ingrown atmosphere and some antiwoman feeling.

It's not as bad as I had expected (believe it or not). Come if you can find out how many women there are—and only come if there are ten or more because otherwise your chances for a good friend are slim. . . . If my experience is any guide, you will find good and true male friends.

Academically it is fine and the prevalent attitude toward women medical students is tolerable even though we are such a deplorable minority.

Please come. We need more women. The only way to change things is to have a larger number of women visible everywhere: in lecture halls, hospital corridors, labs, etc.

Be aware that discrimination exists and that you will run into it, both from your peers and faculty members. Don't let this discourage you. Also be aware that pronouncements or declarations from the administration aren't always the last word and can often be worked around.

A Woman in Residence

MICHELLE HARRISON

Michelle Harrison, excerpt from *A Woman in Residence*, New York: Ballantine, 1993. Originally published in 1982 by Random House. Reprinted by permission.

I am a thirty-nine-year-old physician. I graduated from medical school in 1967. As a feminist, family physician, and medical school faculty member, I was one of many people in the late seventies who were challenging the way in which women were being treated by the health care system. Attending home births, writing and lecturing, presenting testimony in Washington for HEW, the FDA, and consumer groups, I still felt limited by my lack of specific expertise and training in obstetrics and gynecology—even though I had my board certification in family practice.

At the age of thirty-five, when my daughter was five years old, I left teaching and practice to become a resident in obstetrics and gynecology at Doctor's Hospital, a prestigious teaching institution in Everytown, USA. I had sought and found a part-time position, which required my working up to seventy hours a week for half salary, or $8,000 a year. Part-time residencies had been developed to help physicians who were mothers obtain further training and still take care of their children.

Irv Warren likes to challenge me, I think. This morning scrubbing at the sinks before a delivery, he asked, "You don't approve of what I'm doing, do you?"

He's right. I don't. He had been screaming at the woman in the delivery room, yelling, "Push! Push!" then, "You lazy female, push!" When she whimpered, "I'm trying," he yelled, "You're not trying hard enough. Now push!" and his large round face became red and his belly puffed out, making him a fearsome figure.

At the sinks I responded to his question, "Well, that's not how I would do it," and shrugged, trying not to show how strongly I felt.

He stopped scrubbing for a moment and in a patronizing way said, "Michelle, when people are in a subservient position, sometimes you just have to tell them what to do."

"A twelve-week-sized uterus is about the size of a grapefruit," I was telling Caroline, the medical student also scrubbed in on the hysterectomy with Dr. MacDougal. He was teaching me as we did the hysterectomy, and I was passing on what I knew to the medical student. This woman had a fibroid tumor which had enlarged her uterus to the size of a twelve-week pregnancy. The three of us were busily working at tying off vessels, probing, chatting, when Dr. MacDougal, holding one ovary gently in his hand, showed us a small cyst on the surface and said, "I just might take it out. She doesn't need two."

Suddenly worried that this woman's ovary was

being so easily discarded, I tried an oblique way to argue for its being left in place. "Dr. MacDougal, I've heard of women's having hormonal problems after a hysterectomy even when both ovaries are left in. What causes that?"

"I don't really know, Michelle, but it happens. I personally think that even if we are careful there is still a cutting off of some of the blood supply to the ovaries when we take out the uterus. They just don't always work as well as before."

Glancing at Caroline, hoping she understood what I was trying to do, I said to MacDougal, "But if it's possible that this surgery will hurt her ovary, then if we take one out, she is more vulnerable to any damage done to the one left in."

Just then Johnson, the fertility expert, walked in and said, "Mac?"

"Yeah," Dr. MacDougal answered. "Hi there. What's up?"

"I was just wondering if you were planning to take out any ovaries this morning. I need some for culture."

"Well, I was thinking about it. Let me think about it some more," he said and turned to me. "You know they don't work as well after hysterectomy."

"Yes, but if you take the one out with the cyst, she might end up with none working."

"Maybe you're right."

"She's only thirty-two, and I think she still wants them," I added.

Johnson shrugged and said, "I don't want to push you. I was just asking," and left.

Later Caroline and I overheard Johnson taking with Enders out in the hall. "I see you have a hysterectomy later today. Are you taking out the ovaries on her?"

"Well, I hadn't made up my mind yet, John. Why?"

"I'm looking for ovaries. I need some."

"Well, I guess I could." Enders paused as though to say more.

"Don't do it for my sake," Johnson interjected, but he had his arm on Enders's shoulder, their closeness making evident the danger to Enders's patient's ovaries.

This last day on OB [obstetrics] was fourteen hours long, spent primarily with Jackie, my chief, and Hilda Cameron, the attending for the majority of women in labor throughout the day. Jackie, Hilda, and I spent much of this fourteen-hour day talking.

During the day Esther, a seventeen-year-old Puerto Rican, tall and massively obese, arrived on the floor. She said, "I'm here to have my baby today. My baby was due last week and I want it now."

She'd had no recent prenatal care, and didn't plan to return after today. She was adamant that she would have her baby today and that we were to make it happen. After asking her some questions, I tried to examine her, but she was terrified and would not let me touch her. I said I had to examine her, and the nurse backed me up. "When Esther let herself be uncovered, I could see huge warts covering her labia; it was difficult even to finger her vaginal opening. As I tried to insert the speculum she pulled her whole body away from me, up toward the head of the bed. When I tried to reach her, she pulled farther away, her eyes bulging. She looked like a cornered caged animal, and I stopped.

I called Jackie, who I knew would want to examine her anyway, so my exam would have been superfluous. I also expected Jackie to do better than I because people, like veins, sometimes know who has more authority and respond differently.

When Jackie tried to examine the girl, however, she had no more success. Esther, still terrified, pulled back, drew her legs together, and would not let herself be touched. Jackie was obviously getting angry, and after two tries, ripped off her gloves and left the room. Once outside, she turned to me and to the nurse and said, "Women like that prove that no woman can be raped unless she wants to."

Realizing how shocked the nurse and I were, she qualified that by saying, "Well, maybe with a gun or a knife. . . ." Jackie calls herself a feminist. She is known as a feminist physician. Women will come to her because they believe she is different from men.

I wanted especially to do well with Hilda today, since she was the attending with me on my first day on OB. Today I delivered a patient of hers with an episiotomy, then did the repair as Hilda wanted it. She complemented me on my skills and then went on to tease me about my trouble doing an episiotomy the first day.

I have finally mastered running the pH analyzer as well as calibrating it for accuracy, something I've been working on for a while in spite of Richard's insistence that I didn't need to know how, since he could run all the samples.

Hilda had a woman in labor today who had a questionable monitor tracing, so she tried to get a pH sample. The woman was in heavy labor and kept moving onto her side, trying to find a more comfortable position, but Hilda had to keep moving her onto her back. Using the disposable pH kit, Hilda took the long tube, shaped like a megaphone and about 8 inches long, and inserted the narrower end into the woman's vagina. She tried to get it through the slightly dilated cervix, which was especially difficult because the woman moved a lot whenever she had a contraction.

Hilda was unable twice to get the tube set right on the baby's head. After her second attempt she handed the tube to me while she got ready to do it for a third time. When Jackie happened to walk into the room, Hilda turned to her and asked if she would try. As Jackie opened a new kit, and got ready to try, she said to me, "Michelle, the reason you had so much trouble getting a sample, . . ." thinking because I was holding the tube I was the one that had failed. Hilda did not set her straight.

It wasn't until the day was over that I realized it had been a day spent mostly with women doctors, and yet it had been no different from other days at the hospital.

Last year, teaching at the medical school, I was on a panel about women's health. I was asked by an angry obstetrician, "Are you trying to say that OB-GYN should only be practiced by women?"

"No, I'm not saying that, " I responded, much to his surprise, "because the women in the field are not unlike the men. The problem is with some of the basic practices and basic assumptions about women that are an integral part of the profession. The same system, with women replacing the men, would not change it significantly."

Although I said those words, I had not been without some hope that it really would be different if the doctors were women.

Venus and the Doctor

BETTY ROTHBART

Betty Rothbart, "Venus and the Doctor," *Hadassah,* June/July 1999. Reprinted by permission.

> I attribute much of our modern tension
> To a misguided striving for intersexual
> comprehension.
> It's about time to realize, brethren,
> as best we can,
> That a woman is not just a female man.
> —Ogden Nash

At the dawn of the twenty-first century, medical researchers at last are realizing that woman is indeed not just a female man. The new discipline of gender-specific medicine is the most compelling trend in women's health, as researchers discover a startling array of sex-linked differences in how men and women respond to disease. As society moves steadily toward an ever more enlightened era of equal opportunity in jobs, paychecks and dishwashing duties, the medical community is reminding us that physiologically, equal doesn't mean "the same."

Recent research indicates that women's and men's brains function differently and their feet aren't the same, either; to help women avoid stress on their joints, shoemakers need to rethink women's footwear design. From saliva-flow rates (men's are twice as fast) to motility of food through the digestive tract (three times slower in women) to bone breakdown and buildup (different patterns in men and women) to the behavior of liver cells in tissue culture (different metabolism and responses to medications), the list goes on and on. But the bottom line is the same: "The hormonal influence is more profound than we'd ever thought," says Marianne J. Legato, MD, director of the Partnership for Women's Health at Columbia University and member of Hadassah's Health Advisory Council.

Why has it taken so long for researchers to address gender differences? Vivian W. Pinn, MD, director of the Office of Research on Women's Health, National Institutes of Health, cites several reasons:

➤ *A unisex mindset.* Researchers believed that any findings about men automatically applied to women, too. This approach has a certain efficient appeal, but it just doesn't work.

➤ *Women's distracting baggage.* Researchers regarded women's hormones as mischief-makers that interfered with the purity of data. Take the menstrual cycle, for example. Women's monthly fluctuations are a virtual symphony of rhythmic hormonal play. Instead of taking estrogen's peaks and valleys into account, researchers exasperatedly referred to women's cycles as confounders. Men, in other words, were easy; women were confusing.

➤ *Potential complications of pregnancy and childbearing.* Medical disasters such as thalidomide-linked birth defects and the increased incidence of clear-cell carcinomas in the uteri of daughters of women who had taken DES during pregnancy were among the events that led to the establishment in the 1970s of the National Institutes of Health Office of Protection from Research Risk.

WOMEN AS NO-SHOWS

Researchers complained that even when they wanted to include women, they were harder to recruit and retain. Men seemed to have fewer problems with transportation and scheduling; they were more likely to drive and less likely to have family obligations that interfered with their ability to keep appointments.

CHANGING COURSE

By the 1980s many grassroots views of women's health activists had moved into the mainstream. In mid-decade, an NIH task force urged a stronger government focus on women's health, and the NIH enacted a policy recommending inclusion of women in clinical studies it funded. However, a General Accounting Office study in 1990 revealed that researchers often ignored the policy and that compliance could not be ascertained since there was no system in place for documenting how many women participated in studies.

In 1993 Congress passed the NIH Revitalization Act, which mandated inclusion of women and minorities in National Institute of Health-funded studies of conditions that affect both women and men. Dr. Pinn points out that women often didn't participate because they didn't know about the studies and their doctors didn't refer them. The ever-growing popularity of the Internet has alerted more women to clinical trials and led to numerous self-referrals. Researchers also are incorporating more "women-sensitive factors," such as providing or supporting child care and transportation, and establishing support groups that keep women involved and interested. Epidemics of AIDS and breast cancer have given rise to a vigorous advocacy, which has made people more aware of the advantages of participating in clinical trials.

LOOKING AHEAD

Fine-tuning for females. It used to be thought that adapting a drug for women simply meant administering a smaller dose. It is more complicated than that. More research is needed in pharmacokinetics and pharmacodynamics: how the body handles drugs, how drugs affect the body, and how drugs interact with each other. Researchers are also studying the effects of estrogen and administration of a drug at different points in a woman's monthly cycle.

STREAMLINING WOMEN'S HEALTH CARE

For years women have been frustrated by a fragmented approach to health care, cluttering their calendars with appointments with different doctors for reproductive, general, and mental health.

"When a woman goes to a doctor she wants to be seen as a total person," says Dr. Pinn. "A postmenopausal woman may think she doesn't need a pelvic exam or a Pap smear. An internist may assume she gets a Pap smear from her gynecologist. Or she may not go to a doctor at all, although with women more in tune with screening exams and wellness care, that is not as much the case any more. It is important that doctors recognize how important it is to do comprehensive exams. Most women don't have the luxury of seeing a specialist for everything."

Women's health advocates have helped drive health care professionals toward a new awareness of women's needs as medical consumers. Primary care ob-gyn is a new specialty that acknowledges women's needs for one-stop shopping. The best doctors, says Dr. Pinn, "not only understand the importance of their practices to the lives and health of women, but the importance of women to their practices. Women play a major role in deciding on health care for their families."

FILLING IN THE GAPS

Of course, research must continue in heart disease, cancer, autoimmune disorders, and other areas that have gotten closer to their fair due in recent years. But many other areas remain woefully underexplored. Among those on Dr. Pinn's wish list are better understanding of endometriosis and fibroids, which contribute to the need for hysterectomies; exploration of sex-linked differences in

gastrointestinal disorders, e.g., how hormones affect irritable bowel syndrome; better ways to detect ovarian and other cancers early.

Dr. Pinn is especially excited about the testing of a vaccine to prevent transmission of human papilloma virus, a sexually transmitted disease that increases a woman's risk of cervical cancer. She urges support of urogynecological research into key areas such as pelvic floor disorders, including pelvic prolapse and its relationship to childbirth, exercise, obesity, and sexual dysfunction. Urinary and fecal incontinence also deserve more attention; for many women they make the difference between independent living or a nursing home.

TO A LONG LIFE

Now that the value, indeed the necessity, of including women in research is established, researchers are also reaffirming the importance of examining health issues within the context of the full life span, from the prenatal intrauterine environment, infancy, and childhood, through the teen years, the reproductive years, peri- and postmenopause, the elderly, and the frail elderly.

"With longer life expectancy," says Dr. Pinn, "we must pay attention to women's health beyond the reproductive system. As women speak up to ask for information on preventing disease and improving the quality of life, they spur the medical community to come up with the answers."

Woman Doctor

FLORENCE HASELTINE AND YVONNE YAW

Florence Haseltine and Yvonne Yaw, excerpt from *Woman Doctor*, New York: Houghton Mifflin, 1976. Reprinted by permission.

When I finally had a chance to get to bed, at about midnight, I didn't go home to my apartment, of course, but slept in the on-call room, where the interns who are on duty sleep between calls. There were two sets of metal bunk beds side by side in a small room, and hooks on the wall for clothes. I always slept with all my clothes on, however, except for my shoes. All the interns on duty on this part of the service had to sleep in this room, and it was assumed that they were all male.

My sleeping here bothered the men more than it bothered me. One guy glared at me every time I stumbled in for a nap when he was there. He looked like murder was in his heart. He mumbled about how his wife wouldn't like this. Once, as I fell onto the cot, I said, "Don't worry, I wouldn't rape you. I'm too tired."

I don't know whether he ever got any sleep. I was too exhausted to notice, and was always out like a light.

This time, though, I couldn't get to sleep. I had been on straight since Saturday morning; here it was Monday, with never more than two hours of sleep at a time in between; I had to be up bright and early for rounds that morning; all my duties on Medicine for the first three weeks had flooded me with fatigue—and I couldn't afford not to sleep. I turned from side to side, squeaking the cot springs, trying to find a comfortable position, hearing the heavy tired breathing of my friend Ted Gilman and then his beeper going off and him getting dressed in the dark. I couldn't sleep. When I finally gave up trying, I just lay there and thought in a confused reverie about everything that had happened to put me here on a sagging cot in my wrinkled whites in a small dark room that was filled with snoring men.

I decided to be a doctor when I was twelve. I was very clear about it. When I think of that twelve-year-old and her decision, I seem to look through her eyes again while she is sitting high in an apple tree in the spring. I see a whole orchard. In climbing up, I have shaken the limbs and bruised the blossoms. The pollen has brushed all over me and covers me with gold. The owners of the orchard don't want me to climb their apple trees, under-standably, so I've had to sneak. Now, when I get up here, I can see all the trees covering the hillsides like clouds, and they smell sweet while the limbs are dark and the blossoms are white and the petals are thinner than skin and curled at the edges and cool.

That orchard is all built over now, of course, even though it's been only twenty years since I climbed there. Things change fast, and I changed too. Nothing was ever that simple again, even my desire to be a doctor.

What happened in between then and now was just what happens to everybody. Many things you learn get layered over a promise like that, and you almost forget it. Finally, right after college, I married a man who was going to become a doctor. (What you want at twenty-one is more prudent than the crazy dream of a kid.) I had majored in zoology, so when I graduated and got married, I got a job as a lab technician to put my husband through medical school. I liked being married. For one thing, it relaxed me. As a teenager I'd been very tense. Now even my looks seemed to improve. I have slightly auburn hair and hazel eyes, and I wear glasses or contact lenses. I always used to wish my eyes were brown or blue, and not an in-between, all-mixed-up color, and I didn't like how thin my nose was. But being married helped me ignore what I thought of as imperfections. I enjoyed the challenge of turning out delicious food on our budget, and I became a gourmet cook. My husband began to have a good reputation for entertaining.

Of course, the students and the professors he brought home to dinner talked about medical cases. I was fascinated. I kept asking them a lot of questions until my husband told me that it made him tense when I did that. None of the other wives asked questions; they were all off having their own conversations, and I was the only female hanging around the men.

"But I'm interested!" I protested.

"Well, be interested in a more subtle way," he told me.

That was hard. With my background I under-stood most of what they were talking about, and I couldn't ask just those lay questions like, "How do you feel about socialized medicine?" The deeper he got into medicine, the deeper I fell, too. I began to read from his texts and to eavesdrop on those conversations as if I had a secret vice.

Then one evening, at the home of one of my husband's professors, after dinner his wife took me aside and said, sadly, "My dear, you want to be a doctor yourself, don't you?"

I gazed at her in astonishment. Suddenly I felt open, full of fresh air, like a child again, and humbly grateful to her for permitting me a revelation, as though she were the queen. But I didn't reply. I think she went on to talk about herself, but I don't remember anything she said.

Then I became very anxious, and for months denied the whole episode to myself, until the strain was obvious even to my husband and I had to have it out with him. We had intended our marriage to be a straightforward one in which each of us was free to do what he or she wanted and to be what he or she was. After a lot of discussion and argument it was decided that I could go to medical school, but that I would wait until he was finished and making money before I withdrew my financial support. I was pleased and thought we were being very logical and fair. Then he chose plastic surgery as his specialty, which meant an eight-year residency.

I could see that my desire might wear out before he was finished and I was terrified, both of his inexorability and of my own wild rebellion. I *had* to go ahead and apply.

With the help of recommendations from two of my college professors and my lab supervisor at the medical school, I got in. That was the end of our marriage. To become a doctor, I myself felt that I divorced myself from the human race, in a way. I was an outlaw, self-serving and aggressive. It never occurred to me then that I condemned myself unjustly for traits that were good in a man. When my husband and I broke up, I believed there were no hard feelings, and I shut out any pain. We both assumed I would go it alone.

Medical school was wonderful. Within the first two weeks I got my cadaver, and the minute I put my hands in that body, I knew this was where I should be. I felt like a kid again, with engrossing projects as exciting as building a complete village with blocks, or doing a chemistry experiment with beautiful, precise method. I went through medical school invigorated by what I was learning.

Because I was one of the few women in my class—thirteen out of 130—it was sometimes implied that I was there as a favor to my ex-husband, even though medical schools make sure no such influence is brought to bear on an application. It was uncomfortable that I was now divorced, for it suggested that I had gotten in under false pretenses, using my husband until he was no longer necessary. But I was so busy and happy that I ignored the few innuendos. I didn't want to believe anybody could be nasty, and I didn't want to be troubled by such fleeting misgivings.

It was when I went for my internship interviews that I began to notice how the male doctors reacted to my sex. Perhaps their attitude was stronger because the internship shows that you really mean business; until then, you can easily drop out at any time, and a few of the women who got into medical school did. For example, a friend of mine in college had gotten into the best medical school in the country. She had had all A's and was truly brilliant. But she got pregnant halfway through her first year and dropped out to get married, move away, and start a family. I know now that that kind of sabotage of herself must have come from what has been documented as the female "fear of success," but at the time it was taken as proof that women were not professionally serious or worth the investment. As a matter of fact, a larger percentage of men than women drop out of medical school.

I almost didn't get an internship at all. My applications were lost by the secretary of the medical school office. I found out about it only when one of my professors came up to me in the hall and said, "You know, it's after the deadline, and I thought you were going to apply for an internship at Grey's."

"I am. I sent it in."

"Well, we haven't gotten it. Better make out a new one. Send it return receipt requested this time, or take it over to Grey's in person. I'll try to reopen the admissions procedure for you."

In order to reapply, I had to get another copy of my grades, and when I went to the office for that, the secretary found my original applications, to three different hospitals, filed with my student chart. I was shaking so hard when she handed them over that all I could say was "Thanks." She apologized for accidentally filing them, but I was remembering how she'd sent all my material to my home address instead of my student address so I got my notices later than everyone else, and I couldn't trust myself to say anything. I wasn't paranoid; I found out later that she made such "mistakes" when dealing with any woman who came through the school.

When I came across town for my interviews, the sky was a blank, cold gray; an edgy wind was blowing, and dirty patches of icy snow remained in the corners of curbs and up against the buildings. I walked up the three broad front steps of Grey's and into the cavelike porch, chilled to the bone.

For a general, or rotating, internship, you have an interview with the head of each department you are going to work in. Although I was too old, I thought, to want a residency in Surgery—it would add another five years to my training—I knew I should have a Surgery rotation. I wanted a Medicine service, thinking I might go into private practice as an internist, and I would add Obstetrics, Gynecology, and Pediatrics as background for a general practice.

I was sitting out in the corridor, waiting for my interview with the head of Surgery, when it seemed to hit me all at once that I was doing something strange; I became very nervous. The head, Dr. Cohen, came to the door and invited me in. He was smiling.

"Come in, Mrs. Donnan!" That had not been my married name, and I was Dr. Donnan now, but he rushed on, almost boisterously. "Another woman to grace our halls, eh?" He laughed. "Well, whenever a woman comes along, I've always found her to be a conscientious student, very conscientious. Congratulations on getting this far!"

I smiled and nodded.

"You're a little late in applying, however . . ."

I had to say yes. I wasn't willing to offer the excuse.

"Well, well, well," he chuckled. "A little scatterbrained, eh?" He looked at a copy of my application. "A rotating internship is what you want? You're sure now?" He laughed again.

He laughed so often that I had a hysterical impulse to giggle whenever he chuckled, but fortunately, when he went on to talk about his surgical service, he became serious. "One of my surgical residents this year just happens to be a woman, you know. A very careful mind, very painstaking—which is all to the good in Surgery, of course. I often ask her to sew up my patients. It takes her only half as long as these men who've never held a needle in their lives, and her stitches are works of art. I'm transferring her to my lab, just where we need that kind of precision."

I was intimidated, for transfer to the lab was tantamount to being kicked out of the program.

He was still talking. "We need more women in Surgery, actually; I wish more would apply. I want you to know, however, that I've found it is most difficult for women to do the rotation. It requires immense physical strength, of course, not to mention stamina." He sighed. "My wife, as a matter of fact, began her career as a pediatrician—hard work, that, you'd never guess it. She's working in my lab now, too; the hours are regular."

I nodded and expressed the opinion that that was certainly a consideration. I was dazed. I had never withstood such an onslaught of condescension before.

My Obstetrics and Gynecology interview had a

different twist to it. The panel of three men seemed almost identical to me: they were all sandy-haired, rotund, and amiable-looking.

One said, "I remember that your husband interned at University several years ago, Mrs. Fairleigh."

"My name is Dr. Donnan now," I corrected him.

"Oh, ah. Yes. So, you changed your name. I remember your husband. Interesting record. What is he doing now?"

"He has finished up a residency in Plastic Surgery at Mencken," I said.

"Plastic Surgery!" one cried, and all three of them leaped upon the topic as if it were a godsend at a cocktail party. They spent fifteen minutes questioning me about my ex-husband's specialty and the techniques plastic surgeons were using nowadays and discussing the Elizabeth Taylor movie they'd seen.

These two interviews bewildered me with their shallowness. They weren't quizzing me on my abilities or my plans.

At the end of this one, one of the doctors said, "By the way, speaking of husbands, do you think we ought to pay women as much as men?"

I smiled broadly and said, "No. I think you ought to pay them much more!"

An intern's pay was eight hundred dollars a month. Only a few years before that, interns had earned one hundred dollars a month. I knew what they were asking, and at last I'd been able to speak up—on time.

Next I talked to a woman resident who was finishing up that year. She spent most of her time warning me about things, and she especially told me not to have a baby while I was working there, since that would put a burden on all the other interns and residents.

"I don't intend to," I said.

"That's what they all say," she retorted.

"But I'm not even married anymore!"

She went on to tell me about a woman several years earlier who, she said, had caused the hospital to be short one resident by leaving when her husband had to transfer.

She told me a long story, and as it unfolded I could see that what had happened was actually not the woman's fault. She had notified the hospital in December that she would be continuing elsewhere, and they had filled her place; then, in the middle of June, right before the medical year began, a man had decided that *he* wasn't coming after all. When people were moved about like dominoes to fill up that gap, the vacancy had ended up in what was originally the woman's specialty, so she was blamed for the shortage of one important staff member.

I was beginning to wonder whether this hospital in particular had been the right choice for me after all. By the time I got to my interview with my professor, Dr. Poirier, who was chief of Medicine, I felt knock-kneed and cross-eyed. However, he encouraged me.

"This is a wacky hospital, my dear," he said. "But then, all hospitals have a neurotic spirit; otherwise, they wouldn't have enough energy and stubbornness to do the job. We get the best interns and residents, and the best work out of them. You'll find yourself increasingly loyal to the place. After a while you won't even notice its quirks. It's like a beloved old autocrat, full of wisdom—and orneriness. You'll forgive him everything."

I got my internship, probably thanks to him.

Essays on Women

EDITH STEIN

Edith Stein, from *Essays On Woman*, 1996. Reprinted by permission.

Edith Stein is known as one of the most brilliant and controversial women of the twenty-first century. At the time of WWI, she was recognized in Germany as a very well-respected philosopher, and she is the author of several books, including Essays on Woman, *from which this excerpt is taken. Stein was a leading feminist in Germany fighting for women to have opportunities of every kind, especially as professors. She was born into an Orthodox Jewish family in 1891, but converted to Catholicism after reading the autobiography of St. Teresa of Avila in 1921. Upon her conversion she took on the name of Teresa Benedicta of the Cross. It was Edith Stein who wrote to Pope Pius XI urging him to take action against the Nazi Regime. In 1942, Stein and her sister were arrested and sent to Auschwitz where they were killed in gas chambers. She was canonized as a saint by Pope John Paul II in 1998. She is often referred to as "Saint Edith Stein." —The Editors*

If the care and development of human life and humanity are women's specific duty, so the specifically feminine vocations will be those in which such efforts are possible outside of marriage as well. I do not wish to enter here into the question of domestic service because here it is not a question of specifically feminine work, and in many respects it produces tasks other than those which the woman of the house must fulfill. It is more important to clarify the significance of occupations outside of the household, occupations which were denied women for some time and have only become available for women gradually through the struggles of the feminist movement.

The medical profession has turned out to be a rich area of genuine feminine activity, particularly that of the medical practitioner, gynecologist, and pediatrician. There have been severe objections to the admission of women into this profession: a young lady may encounter many things in her medical studies which would otherwise be kept away from her; a serious objection has been that the studies make extraordinary demands of bodily strength and nervous energy, and professional practice even more. Indeed, professional practice requires a particular zeal necessary for the assumption of the difficulties unique to that profession. Such misgivings are dispelled when these stipulations are respected. Of course, one will always be grateful to encounter the untroubled, innocent beauty which moves us, and which is completely unaware of the seamy side of human nature. Today it is hardly possible, but in former times how many women who were so protected in their innocence until marriage were suddenly robbed of all their ideals, in the cruelest manner, in marriage itself! In this respect, could one not say that the matter-of-fact and objective, scientific approach is still one of the most accepted methods, if not the absolutely best one, to become acquainted with natural data? Since most women are obliged to come to grips with these data, should not individual women who have the calling and opportunity make all sacrifices in order to fulfill this calling and stand by their sisters' side?

Experience indicates that this has happened in large degree. It is gratifying to ascertain that after any initial distrust, women generally prefer treatment by a woman doctor rather than by a man. I believe that this is conditioned not only by the patient's modesty but even more so by the specifically feminine manner of empathy which has beneficial effects. The human being, especially the invalid, needs sympathy in his total condition. The widespread method of modern specialization does not satisfy this need in treating a limb or organ while disregarding the rest of the person, even though the specific treatment is pertinent. (Also, in many cases, specialization is not the best method because most illnesses are illnesses of the total human being even if they are manifested in only one organ; the patient needs treatment in his individual peculiarity as a whole organism.) Counteracting this abstract procedure, the specifically feminine attitude is oriented towards the concrete and whole person. The woman doctor has only to exercise courage in following her natural inspiration and liberating herself whenever necessary from methods learned and practiced according to rule. (Of course, it must not be denied that it often happens as well with masculine specialists, although not generally—in earlier times the house doctor typified this total approach.) It is not only a question of summoning up the patience to listen to much which is absolutely irrelevant to the subject. The intent must be to understand correctly the whole human situation, the spiritual need which is often greater than the corporal one, and perhaps to intervene helpfully not only by medical means but also as a mother or a sister.

So conceived, the medical profession is a truly charitable one and belongs together with other social professions. These professions have been developed for the most part only in recent years, and they are specifically feminine vocations as rightfully as the housewife's. In all such vocations, it is a matter of actions which are truly maternal in the care of a large "family": parishioners, the poor or sick of a rural parish or of a municipal precinct, the inmates of a prison, endangered or neglected youth. There is always the potentiality, and basically the necessity, of understanding and helping the whole person whether one initially encounters these human beings to care for them in bodily sickness or to assist them financially, or to give them legal counsel. Demands here on the power of love are even greater than in one's own family: the natural bond is lacking, the number of people in need is greater, and preponderantly there are people who repel rather than attract by their disposition and frame of mind.

Susan Wood, October 2007

INTERVIEW BY MEGAN BUCKLEY

Megan Buckley, interview with Susan Wood, 2007. Original for this publication.

Dr. Susan F. Wood has been and continues to be a key advocate in the women's health movement. She began her education at Southwestern at Memphis University in Memphis, Tennessee, now known as Rhodes College, where she graduated with a BS in biology and psychology. She went on to get her PhD in biology at Boston University in 1989. Shortly after, Dr. Wood began Research Fellowship Training in neuroscience at Johns Hopkins University School

of Medicine. As a member of the Congressional Caucus for Women's Issues on Capitol Hill (1990–95), Dr. Wood changed direction from biology to dedicating her time to researching health and science policy. In more recent years (2000–05), she joined the Food and Drug Administration (FDA) Office of Women's Health (OWH) as Assistant Commissioner. In August 2005, Dr. Wood resigned from the FDA because of her opposition to the FDA's continuous delay in approving Plan B, an emergency birth control pill often referred to as the "morning-after pill," for over-the-counter distribution. Currently Dr. Wood is a Research Professor at George Washington University School of Public Health and Health Services.

MB: How did you come to be an advocate of women's health?

SW: It came about from a range of factors. One of course, was sort of personal, having to do with my family growing up and also experiences and learning about women's health in college. But professionally it started in the 1990s when I began work on women's health policy as a staff person and then as professional staff for the Women's Caucus on Capitol Hill and working directly on expanding research in women's health, including women in clinical trials, access to preventive screenings, and other sorts of legislative and policy work to advance women's health.

MB: Do you think that clinical and scientific evidence was ignored in the decision to delay over-the-counter access to Plan B?

SW: Yes. I think that unfortunately it is quite clear that the evidence was ignored and that the process that normally is used to assess any sort of decision made by the FDA—whether it is to bring a new drug onto the product or, in this case, to take an already approved product and bring it over the counter—was interfered with and distorted such that under normal circumstances it would have been a fairly routine approval. Because the evidence is strong, clear, and there are no safety concerns, it should have been a fairly straightforward action by the FDA but it wasn't—it was a process that took years of being denied a series of times and then ultimately now finally available to those eighteen or older which is still not an entirely correct decision but in the right direction.

MB: Right. Did Congress have any role in the FDA outcome?

SW: They did and they didn't. The role of Congress is important to recognize and the role of anyone outside the FDA is important to the extent that they, through law, set the priorities and the mission of the agency and this is administered through government agencies and the administration is to carry out those laws. So in this case, it's not Congress's role, nor is it, in my opinion—you know those people high up in the administration—it's not their role to tell the FDA to make a particular decision but rather to help ensure that it has the ability to carry out its job properly. Whether that's providing resources (which is a separate subject) or whether it's sort of a mandate to set certain scientific standards and then to abide by them.

Congress's role in this particular case was—and this was specifically Senator Hillary Clinton of New York and Senator Patty Murray of Washington State—was at different times to hold the FDA's feet to the fire and insist that the FDA essentially do their job properly. And I think the senators were very careful not to tell the FDA what decision to make, but rather to keep insisting that the FDA make a decision and make a decision in a proper fashion. And in this case, since the evidence was so clear I think I knew what the proper decision should be, but the senators were very careful not to be directive.

MB: The Office of Women's Health (OWH) was not directly part of the choice to delay the decision over Plan B, so how were you involved in the overall process?

SW: The OWH is part of the Office of Commissioners, not part of the review chain of any medical product. That's done within the Center for Devices and Radiological Health for medical devices or the Center for Drug Evaluation and Research for drugs. But I was watching it very carefully because the OWH was designed to help ensure that policies such as inclusion of women in clinical research studies were implemented and the data was evaluated. We were there to focus on the funding research in areas that were overlooked but were important for FDA regulatory decisions. We also carried out educational campaigns on things like hormone replacement therapy but also things like heart disease and diabetes and so forth. So, we were the face of women's health at the agency, the public face, as well as doing our work inside the agency. So, I was involved as someone who was trying to keep close tabs on what was happening best I could because I knew this was an important issue for women's health—it's just one piece—but it's an important piece. And I knew that it was somehow deemed a controversial decision.

MB: Were there other cases similar to this one while you were at the FDA or is this whole situation rather unusual, to ignore the advice of both the committee recommendations and professional staff recommendations?

SW: Well, I think this sort of stands out not necessarily as unique but as extremely unusual to have that kind of ruling and it's much more visible. I think there have been, over the last number of years, broad issues of morale at the FDA because of science, and public health doesn't seem to be the forefront of the priorities of the agency. And so there have been concerns raised in other aspects not necessarily of ideological intervention but perhaps industry having either too much of a role or being too much seen as the primary customer of the agency. There have been a host of issues like that where people feel, I think, that professional staff have suffered from sort of a loss of confidence and morale. The Union of Concerned Scientists did a survey about a year or so ago now asking these questions of FDA scientists and there were some fairly disturbing results about both the pressures and the interference that the scientific staff at the FDA feel. So, this is a very unique and visible case but at the same time it serves as a red flag for other problems within the agency.

MB: When was the moment, the final straw, when you said to yourself "enough" and made the decision to hand in your resignation?

SW: It was at the end of August 2005. I mean it really was right before I resigned and it was the decision announced by the Commissioner of the FDA that rather than approving Plan B for those seventeen and older—which was the recommendation by the Center of Drugs at that time—that instead the agency was going to open a process called "rule-making," to figure out how they were going to implement this two-tiered system of keeping it a prescription drug for one group and over-the-counter for the other group of folks. That to me, as someone who worked in government for a long time, I knew that going in to that kind of "rule-making" process traditionally takes many years to complete and so by putting this decision into that process and not allowing it to go over the counter for anyone it was essentially saying "no" without technically saying "no." No one was going to be allowed access to this over-the-counter, not even adult women, and it was being hidden under this veneer of "oh we're going into this process and we'll get back to you." And that was such a combination of ignoring the science and the medical evidence and ignoring the normal process by which the FDA makes decisions and ultimately disregarding women's health by not allowing anyone access to it over-the-counter in a timely fashion (which is important for this particular kind of product). And it was not something which was defensible. And if I combine that with my role as sort of the "face of women's health," it was clear that I wouldn't be able to explain this decision to the public. I wouldn't be able to work from the inside to make a difference because they were putting it into this process and I wouldn't be able to speak

with any kind of credibility in any area of women's health because this sort of very obvious decision had been made and I would have to defend it as an FDA staff members. So, I figured at that point, it was in the next couple of days from the announcement, that it was time for me to move on.

MB: Do you have any regrets about leaving?

SW: Not regrets about leaving. I still think it was the right thing for me to do. And if it was useful in helping to clarify the problem at the FDA, which I think it was, then that's a good thing. And then I think that other people picked up the issue and helped move it forward to where we are today and that's great. The only thing I feel badly about was having to leave the OWH itself and the FDA itself because there were and are a lot of really good people there who are really working to the best of their ability to accomplish the mission of the FDA, who really believe in what they are doing. And I felt that while I miss having them as colleagues I also felt that in the case of OWH I was sort of leaving them in the lurch and I had concerns about whether they would suffer the consequences of my departure.

MB: How do you feel that it (Plan B) should be advertised to the public? For example, do you think it should be compared to other birth control pills so as not to seem too "radical" like the abortion pill, making it more comfortable for general use?

SW: Well I think it is very important to say that this is just one more form of hormonal contraception and it works using the same mechanisms as regular birth control pills. And I think it is *very* important to distinguish it from RU-486, the abortion pill, because in fact, they are very different in terms of how they work and when they work—as terminating a pregnancy or preventing a pregnancy.

MB: On the Plan B website (www.go2planb.com), it suggests making sure to call your pharmacy if you live in Alaska, California, Hawaii, Maine, New Mexico, New Hampshire, Vermont, Massachusetts, and Washington to inquire whether or not the pharmacy carries the pill. Are these the only states that women can obtain Plan B directly from a pharmacy?

SW: No. Those are the states that, if you are under eighteen, are "pharmacy access" states, meaning that the pharmacist has the ability to essentially act as the prescriber for a woman under the age of eighteen if she needs it and if the pharmacist has gone under whatever the requirements are for that state. Many of the pharmacies in those states can provide emergency contraception to those under the age of eighteen without them going to a physician or a clinic to get a prescription.

It's over-the-counter for those eighteen and older in every single state because of the FDA's decision. In every state it should be available and I believe all of the major chains should be carrying it—pharmacists are getting training on dispensing it. There are problems: sometimes they don't stock it—that could be for business reasons that they haven't seen any apparent demand or it could be an individual pharmacist who objects to dispensing it and there are various issues around that as well.

MB: Are they allowed to refuse sale based on moral or ethical beliefs?

SW: It depends on the state and this is still in flux in a number of states. I think, for example, in the state of Florida, pharmacists can refuse to dispense contraception—they have sort of a right of refusal. In other states it's deemed unprofessional if you don't dispense a legally prescribed product or over-the-counter product. And I think what people want to make sure happens is that if a woman is seeking emergency contraception and if there is someone who has a personal objection at the counter, that that personal objection doesn't limit the access of the patient to the product that they need. So there needs to be a system in place so that a pharmacist may not have to engage in dispensing, but there is someone there that can assist in a professional manner so that it is sort of seamless to the patient even if there is an objection behind the counter. But it really depends state by

state in terms of what the rules are. States regulate pharmacy practice.

MB: Are there presently any efforts to change the law requiring women under the age of eighteen to get a prescription in order to access emergency contraception over-the-counter?

SW: This would not be a change in the law but rather a change in the FDA's decision and at this stage I don't know of any real efforts to do so. The company would have to come back in with a new request to the FDA, and the FDA would have to review that request either with new information provided by the company or based on existing information and then make a determination. I think it's an important question because everyone hopes that eventually prescription requirements for those under eighteen will be lifted and so one presumes the company is considering when is the best time to do that and whether they need to bring in more studies or not.

MB: In a Center for American Progress speech you gave back in 2005 you suggested there needed to be increased "independence in the scientific decision-making of the agency from some sort of outside pressure." Have you seen any changes in the agency's decision-making in the past two years that you know of?

SW: There's been some changes in the FDA law itself that just were signed into law a couple of weeks ago and which had to do primarily with providing continued user fees from industry to pay for review of medical products, but it also added on some provisions, which I think do try to address some of those issues. So, for example, there's a lot of drug safety provisions in there which I think are important; but also it makes sure, for example, that the packages containing all of the reviews and opinions of the scientific staff are promptly posted and made available to the public. There's a clinical trial results database which has to be implemented fairly quickly where results of all studies done by industry have to be posted publicly on the web and this is very new. There are provisions to ensure that the scientists at the FDA have the right to publish their scientific conclusions and opinions in the literature. There are new limitations on financial conflict of interest of FDA advisory committees. So there is a number of sometimes incremental, but nonetheless important changes that have been put into the law that direct how the FDA is to do business, which I think can help strengthen the science and the scientific independence of the agency.

MB: Can you speak as to how the OWH is now? Who is running it and do you have any lasting ties or connections with the department? Do you know anything about how it is being run?

SW: They've got a new director, Dr. Kathleen Uhl, who is doing an excellent job. And a number of the same people who have been at the FDA and been at the OWH for several years are still there and still doing fabulous work. Last winter (2007) the commissioner tried to essentially cut the budget of the Office of Women's Health, but Congress restored it. Hopefully they'll actually be getting an increase for this year's budget, and it will continue to produce and be important there.

MB: While your resignation from the FDA may be the action most associated with your career, what other issues were important to you while you worked at the Office of Women's Health? What did you work on that you are most proud of, other than resigning from the FDA?

SW: Well one of the things that stands out was the development of information in response to the Women's Health Initiative. When the Women's Health Initiative results came out on hormone therapy for menopause there was a lot of reaction, a lot of concern, and the FDA had a really important role to play. The agency had to work with the companies to change the labeling on hormone products to reflect the new data and put on warnings about heart disease risk and breast cancer risk. And the role that the OWH took on was to help pull together

information for women about what this all meant because the results were hotly debated but also caused massive changes in how women were using hormone therapy. What we tried to do at this time, with very little resources, was to pull together individuals and organizations with extra keys or with large grassroots constituencies to help develop an agreed-upon set of informational materials including questions for your doctor, a basic fact sheet—both English and Spanish—and try to get those distributed widely. We had differences of opinion but we could come together and put out information to help women talk about this and think about it for themselves, and have the tools to talk about it with their doctors from a trusted source, from the FDA, I think that was important work that we did and it helped clarify what we knew and what we still didn't know and what women had to decide for themselves about the risks and benefits that they wanted to take on.

MB: What do you think is the most important or most critical women's health issue today? What are you currently working on or concerned with?

SW: Obviously the broadest issue of getting women access to quality and affordable care whether through health insurance or through other means, I think, is critical. So health care reform is a big women's health issue and is at the forefront of everyone's mind at the moment. I think it's because there's hope we could have some movement on that in the next few years. In terms of other sort of non-active issues, you know, the fact that we have such an aging population and that women either as caregivers or in need of care make up the majority of both of those groups of people. Women are living longer; we want to make sure they are living healthier lives and that's going to take both more knowledge and more education and more prevention as well as the resources to take care of people as they age. So that's going to be—and continues to be a real issue for women.

MB: What are your hopes for the future of women's health care and also the future for Plan B?

SW: I'm always an optimist, truly, even on my most cynical days. I'm always an optimist so I'm hopeful that we can continue to move forward. I mean it's always a step-by-step process. I never expect a revolution but I hope that in this case, we still have to turn things around before we move forward. But, I think we are starting to turn, I think people are starting to understand that we have to focus on important health needs. We have to focus on prevention, we have to focus on getting people the care they need. It will take years—I don't expect a dramatic change overnight—but I do expect step-by-step we'll keep learning more and we'll keep improving things and we'll tackle the health care issues.

IN CONCLUSION, IN MEMORIAM, IN HOPE

IN FEBRUARY 2008, the women's health movement lost one of its mothers, and I lost one of mine. Barbara Seaman, the coauthor of this book and a tireless activist on behalf of women's rights, died of lung cancer at her home in Manhattan. After her diagnosis in April 2007, Barbara was determined to write her memoirs, to put to paper her various experiences working to reform women's health care, to offer advice and tales of victory and caution for young women who would fight the next generation of battles for better, safer lives. She never got the chance.

During the summer of 2007 I conducted a series of interviews with Barbara, asking her to talk about different points in her great career. She never could decide which moment or experience first put her on the path to a life of health advocacy. Was it the death of her Aunt Sally from hormone treatment (HT)–induced cancer, or the time a doctor ignored her stated intentions to breast feed and gave her postpartum drugs that leeched into her breast milk and poisoned her infant son? I like to think that, at least subconsciously, it was the moment when Barbara was seventeen and a doctor, in response to her queries on how to lose weight, put a free sample pack of cigarettes in her hand and told her to have one or two after dinner instead of dessert.

She was similarly undecided when asked about her greatest accomplishments. Some days she would say that her best contribution was her book *Women and the Crisis in Sex Hormones*, which predicted the HT debacle following the resolutions of the Women's Health Initiative in 2002. In other moments, the *Doctors' Case Against the Pill* and the resulting hearings, protests, and the world's first patient packet insert occupied her thoughts. In the end she decided it was a tie between her grandchildren (including two feminist granddaughters) and the creation of the National Women's Health Network.

On her greatest regret, she was decided. It was her inability to stop women from suffering the unnecessary side effects and even irreparable harm of bad drugs. She saw it as a recurring pattern: undertested drugs were pushed by irresponsible profit-hungry pharmaceutical companies on a population of women, and the damage was done before the truth could emerge. She saw it happen with the birth control pill, and again with DES, HT, Norplant, and fertility drugs. In recent years she worried about menstrual suppression drugs, bisphosphonates, statins, and the HPV vaccine Gardisil. Barbara saw the connections between these situations and was frustrated and discouraged that others couldn't. Each time we read or heard a story about a woman with a tragic outcome or an avoidable cancer or simply a serious life disruption, Barbara despaired that she had failed. She wondered how, after decades of activism and reporting, she was unable to prevent the same sorts of health tragedies that inspired her to begin her immense work. This was ironic to me, because Barbara was someone who refused to accept individual credit for her successes, preferring instead to spread the accomplishments around to other activists, writers, doctors, and feminists, yet she wanted to bear the responsibility for the movement's failures herself.

Barbara Seaman's greatest legacy, as dozens of people like myself rushed to eulogize, was her tireless work to mentor, educate, and encourage young women toward their own great works. I met her during my junior years of college when I was a directionless, restless young woman desperately searching for opportunities to work for positive change in the world. Barbara taught me to be passionate about health care and feminism. She gave me the skills and opportunity to write about these subjects, and introduced me to great thinkers and activists with whom I could work, organize, improvise, and theorize about how to continue the projects of the women's health movement. This book shows what Barbara always believed—that there is continuity between the generations, and that even as a young woman answers the questions of those who came before, she poses a new set that those who follow her will have to work to address.

Barbara originally imagined *Voices of the Women's Health Movement* as a comprehensive women's health manual organized around parts of the body. This sort of organizational scheme appealed to her. The book's unique structure is like the body—fluid, complicated, and gloriously disorganized. The process of grieving and letting go of Barbara is much the same. I think it is interesting that since she has died, I, and others who love her, have tried to reassemble a portrait of her, to recall each detail or preference, to try and build a more complete whole. We tell stories that capture her unique sense of humor, or recite poems she liked, or ruminate on new health problems that had started to occupy her thoughts. For all of these reasons, I am glad the book has taken the form it has. In a way, it is the memoir my dear friend never found the time to write.

Barbara's joy in her work was contextual—it always came from seeing her personal accomplishments alongside the work of others. Talk to her about her groundbreaking book on birth control, and she would start to describe Alice Wolfson's protests of the Senate pill hearings. Compliment her book *Women and the Crisis in Sex Hormones*, and she would detail the courageous scientists who helped underline the dangers of HT, or the work of a brave lawyer like Sybil Shainwald who helped get legal justice for DES victims. Barbara was never looking for individual attention, which is another reason I think this book constitutes a fitting biography of its author. Barbara's private stories appear alongside the great writings of her "heroic antecedents," peers, and intellectual and political daughters and granddaughters.

The heart of it all, while often personal and anecdotal, is fundamentally communal, instructional, and political.

There are so many health battles facing young women today. In the United States, our crumbling health system has created a world where very few, regardless of sex or gender, can receive adequate health care, and the drug companies have worked hard to see that those who do are full of dubious long-term drugs. Hysterectomies are still performed too frequently, despite strong evidence that un-necessary gynecological surgery shortens the lifespan. The right to a safe abortion, of course, continues to suffer constant assault. The rights of lesbian, gay, bisexual, and transgender people continue to be abused and curtailed. The political challenges of childbirth and motherhood continue unresolved, and even as younger women reap the expanded educational and career opportunities earned by second-wave feminism, they struggle to navigate a society that treats women and men, mothers and fathers differently, and always asks women to make fantastically difficult choices and suffer in a vocational world that is, sadly, still rife with sexism. Teenage and preteen women must contemplate a society where drug makers insist that periods are unnecessary and that the burden of STI prevention is still a predominantly female enterprise. More troubling still is the erosion of comprehensive sexual education programs and their replacement with "abstinence only" curricula that prevent young women from receiving basic information about their bodies and sexual health. In this world we must define and fight the new health care battles of the twenty-first century and carry forth the women's health movement. My hope and my belief is that the example, memory, and inspiration of women who have come before us, including Barbara, will help us to keep fighting.

—Laura Eldridge, November 2011

ABOUT THE CONTRIBUTORS

MARGOT ADLER is a correspondent for National Public Radio (NPR) and the author of *Drawing Down the Moon*, the classic study of contemporary paganism, *Goddess Spirituality*, and *Heretic's Heart*, a memoir of the 1960s. Since September 11, 2001, she has focused much of her work on stories exploring the human factors in New York City, from the loss of loved ones, homes, and jobs, to work in the relief effort. She is presently the host of *Justice Talking* and she is a regular voice on *Morning Edition* and *All Things Considered* on NPR.

AMY ALLINA is on the board of directors and the executive committee of the Guttmacher Institute, an organization that advances sexual and reproductive health through research, policy analysis, and public education. Prior to joining the National Women's Health Network (HNWHN) in 1999, Allina worked for the Reproductive Health Technologies Project and on other women's health policy issues at the consulting firm of Bass and Howes. She was also a political organizer for the Maryland affiliate of National Abortion and Reproductive Rights Action League (NARAL) and an associate editor at *Multinational Monitor*, a monthly magazine founded by Ralph Nader.

CHARON ASETOYER is currently the executive director and founder of the Native American Women's Health Education Resource Center and the Native American Community Board. Asetoyer has served on the board of directors for the Indigenous Women's Network, the Honor the Earth Campaign, and the National Women's Health Network.

BYLLYE AVERY co-founded the Gainsville Women's Health Center and co-founded Birthplace, an alternative birthing center in Gainsville, Florida. She moved to Atlanta in 1981 to begin the NBWHP, a nonprofit organization committed to defining, promoting, and maintaining the physical, mental, and emotional well-being of African-American women. Avery has received the MacArthur Foundation Fellowship for Social Contribution, the Essence Award for community service, and many other awards and honors. She was honored by *Women eNews* as one of "21 Leaders for the 21st Century."

LORI BARER, originally from New Jersey, is a graduate of the University of Michigan and a PhD candidate for public health at the University of Michigan.

PAULINE BART is professor emerita of sociology and women's studies in the department of psychiatry at the University of Illinois. Her most recent books are *Stopping Rape: Successful Survival Strategies,* coauthored with Patricia O'Brien, and *Violence Against Women: The Bloody Footprints,* coauthored with Eileen Moran. As an activist in issues of violence against women and women's health, fields which have recently substantially converged, she considers her task to demystify the world for women.

CYNTHIA BASEMAN, born and raised in Los Angeles, California, began her career as a motion picture and television development executive selling stories to studios and networks including TNT, ABC, and NBC. In 1995 she suffered the loss of her daughter, who was stillborn. Devastated, Baseman struggled to find meaning in life again. In *Love, Mom,* Baseman gives a first hand account of her experiences in order to help others find the tools to search for happiness in the wake of misfortune.

SHARON BATT is a breast cancer survivor and the founder of Breast Cancer Action Montreal. She has been a journalist, author, professor, advocate, and university chair. She lives and works in Canada.

JENNIFER BAUMGARDNER is a New York–based writer and activist. Once an editor at *Ms.,* she has written for *Bust,* the *Nation, Jane, Out, HUES, Glamour, Marie Claire, Z,* and *Ms.,* among other magazines. She is the coauthor of two books on the state of feminism and activism, *Manifesta: Young Women, Feminism, and the Future* and *Grassroots: A Field Guide for Feminist Activism* with Amy Richards. In 2007, Baumgardner published *Look Both Ways: Bisexual Politics.*

KAREN BEKKER studied Judaic studies and art at Oberlin College. She served on the board of New York National Organization for Women (NOW), and has been actively involved in the feminist movement for several years. Her writing includes several articles in *Lilith.* She received a JD degree, magna cum laude, from the Benjamin N. Cardozo School of Law, where she served as senior editor on the Law Review Editorial Board. Bekker is an associate at Satterlee Stephens Burke & Burke LLP, where her practice focuses on commercial and first amendment litigation.

SUSAN BROWNMILLER is the author of *Against Our Will, Femininity, Waverly Place,* and *Seeing Vietnam.* Her most recent book is *In Our Time: Memoir of a Revloution.* She is an adjunct professor of women's and gender studies at Pace University in New York City.

MEGAN BUCKLEY interned with Barbara Seaman in 2006. She graduated from Gettysburg College in May 2008, and is currently working at Special Ops Media, a full service interactive marketing agency.

CAEDMON MAGBOO CAHILL is a graduate of Barnard College and the University of Washington Law School. She currently works as a public defender in Seattle and has been active on the issue of military tour lengths.

PAULA J. CAPLAN was named an "eminent woman psychologist" by the American Psychiatric Association. She the author of several books including *Don't Blame Mother* and the best-selling *The Myth of Women's Masochism.* She is a clinical and research psychologist.

CARRIE CARMICHAEL is a writer and performer living in New York City. She is the author of the classic *Non-Sexist Childraising, How to Relieve Menstrual Cramps and Other Menstrual Problems* with Marcia L. Storch, MD, and three other books. Carmichael won broadcast awards for her work on the NBC Radio Network and has contributed to numerous magazines and broadcasts.

NELL CASEY is the author and editor of two anthologies, *An Uncertain Inheritance: Writers on Caring for Family* and *Unholy Ghost: Writers on Depression.* Her writing has appeared in the *New York Times, Slate, Salon,* the *Guardian, Self, Fitness, Cookie,* and *Elle.* She is a mental health journalism fellow at the Carter Center. She lives in Brooklyn with her husband and son.

MICHAEL CASTLEMAN is "one of the nation's top health writers" (*Library Journal*). He is the author of over fifteen books, most recently *Great Sex: A Man's Guide to the Secrets of Total-Body Sensuality, There's Still a Person in There,* and *Blended Medicine.* Castleman has also written for dozens of magazines. He has taught medical writing at the University of California, Berkeley, Graduate School of Journalism. He is the husband of a breast cancer survivor.

VERONICA CHAMBERS is the author of several books including *Having it All?, Mama's Girl, The Joy of Doing Things Badly,* and *Kickboxing Geishas.* She is a former culture writer for *Newsweek* and has written for *Premiere, Savoy, Glamour, O, The Oprah Magazine,* and the *New York Times.* She lives in Philadelphia.

DEBORAH CHASE is the author of seven books, including *Terms of Adornment* and *The Extend Your Life Diet.* She is an alumnus of Bronx High School of Science, a winner of the Westinghouse Science Talent Search, and graduated from New York University with a dual degree in science and journalism. She has done research at the National Cancer Institute and the New York University School of Medicine.

ARIEL CHESLER is a lawyer living in Manhattan.

PHYLLIS CHESLER, is an emerita professor of psychology and women's studies at City University of New York. She has lectured and organized political, legal, religious, and human rights campaigns in the United States and in Canada, Europe, the Middle East, and the Far East. Dr. Chesler is co-founder of the still-ongoing Association for Women in Psychology (1969) and the National Women's Health Network (1974), and is a charter member of the Women's Forum (1973–74). Dr. Chesler's thirteen books and thousands of articles and speeches have inspired people on many diverse issues.

SUZANNE CLORES is the author of a children's book, *Native American Women,* and the books *Memoirs of a Spiritual Outsider* and *The Wisdom of the Saints.* She is a professor of writing at DePaul University.

MARCIA COHEN is an editor and writer whose work has appeared in the *New York Times Magazine* as well as many other national newspapers and magazines. She is the author of *The Sisterhood,* a Book of the Month Club Featured Alternate. She is also coauthor, with Dr. Gilbert Simon, of *The Parents' Pediatric Companion* and the author of *Gender and Groupwork.*

VICTOR COHN was a former science editor of the *Washington Post* whose long-time coverage of science and medicine won him many of journalism's highest honors. His contribution here is drawn from his book *News & Numbers: A Guide to Reporting Statistical Claims and Controversies in Health and Other Fields,* now in an eighth printing and in use at many journalism schools. Cohn died in 2000.

GENA COREA is a writer, dancer, co-founder of the Feminist International Network of Resistance to Reproductive and Genetic Engineering (FINRRAGE), and a certified focusing trainer. She gives workshops on creating a first person science of reproduction and also on developing a relationship with body symptoms. Her books include *The Hidden Malpractice, The Mother Machine,* and *The Invisible Epidemic.*

PHILIP CORFMAN, a graduate of Oberlin College, Harvard Medical School, and obstetrics and gynecology residencies at Harvard Hospital, practiced his specialty at one of the first HMOs in the county, the Rip Van Winkle Clinic in upstate New York. In 1968 he became the first Director of the Center for Population Research. During this period, he was at the World Health Organization (WHO) and served on several of its advisory committees. In 1984, he was detailed full time by the National Institutes of Health (NIH) to the Human Reproduction Programme to reorganize and direct its research and development activities. In 1987, at the end of his WHO assignment, Dr. Corfman moved to the FDA to be in charge of the medical review of drugs for contraception, fertility, obstetrics, and gynecology. He retired from the FDA in late 1997 and is now doing consulting work.

BELITA COWAN is president of the Lymphoma Foundation of America, Inc. She is the author of *Health Care Shoppers Guide: 59 Ways to Save Money, Nursing Homes: What You Need to Know,* and *Women's Health Care: Resources, Writings, and Bibliographies.* She has testified before the US Senate, the US House of Representatives, the US Food and Drug Administration, and the District of Columbia City Council.

SUNNY DALY is a student with a committed interest in international women's movements, activism, and reproductive health. She has a bachelor's degree in history from Reed College, where she wrote her thesis, "Changing Images of the Birth Control Pill, 1960–1973." She is currently pursuing master's degrees in both political science and gender and women's studies at the American University in Cairo.

ANGELA Y. DAVIS is a radical black activist, feminist, organizer, and author. Her advocacy on behalf of political prisoners led to three capital charges, sixteen months in jail awaiting trial, and a highly publicized campaign, then acquittal, in 1972. During this period, an international Free Angela Davis movement grew, and Davis used the momentum to found the National Alliance Against Racist and Political Repression, an organization that remains active today. Davis has taught in all fifty states, as well as throughout Europe, Africa, the Caribbean, Russia, and the Pacific. Through her teaching and writing she remains a powerful role model and inspiration for social movements, as well as a prominent figure in the struggle against the death penalty in California.

ANSELMA DELL'OLIO is a writer, lecturer, founder and director of the New Feminist Theater, and associate producer of *Woman* on WCBS-TV in New York. She currently lives and works as a journalist in Italy.

JOAN DITZION is a founder of the Boston Women's Health Book Collective and a coauthor of all editions of *Our Bodies, Ourselves* and *Ourselves and Our Children.* She also contributed to *Ourselves, Growing Older.*

BETTY DODSON, artist, author, and sex educator, is an international authority on women's sexuality. In 1974, Betty Dodson wrote, illustrated, and self-published her first book, *Liberating Masturbation: a Meditation on Selflove,* which by the eighties had become a feminist classic. Her bold, innovative teaching methods have been documented in a series of videos. Her latest book, *Orgasms for Two,* was published in 2002. Dodson has a private practice in New York City.

CAROL DOWNER has become a legendary figure in the women's health movement. In the early seventies she pioneered the concept of vaginal and cervical self-examination as a key to self-empowerment. A lawyer, she is the founding executive director of the Federation of Feminist Women's Health Centers. She has served on the Board of Directors for the National Abortion Federation.

MARTA DRURY is a donor-activist with a focus on women and children of color. Her activism led her to a nomination for the Nobel Peace Prize as part of the project entitled, "1,000 Women," an effort to rec-ognize the efforts of 1,000 women all over the world working for peace and equality.

ANDREA EAGAN was the author of the first feminist advice book for girls, *Why Am I So Miserable If These Are The Best Years Of My Life?,* and the author of *The Newborn Mother: Stages of Her Growth.* She was the editor of the National Women's Health Network series for Pantheon Books and president of HealthRights, a nonprofit organization. She was the founding president of the National Writer Union and a founding board member of the Writers Room in New York City. She died in 1993.

BARBARA EHRENREICH is the author of fourteen books, including *Nickel and Dimed: On (Not) Getting By in America* and *Bait and Switch.* Most recently she published *Dancing in the Streets: A History of Collective Joy.* Ehrenreich has contributed to *Harper's* and the *Nation* and was a columnist for the *New York Times* and *Time Magazine.*

MARVIN S. EIGER is a nationally known pediatrician who practiced in New York City for thirty years. Educated at Harvard University, Dr. Eiger received medical training at New York University School of Medicine and served his residency in pediatrics at Bellevue Hospital. Dr. Eiger is the father of two children and lives in Manhattan with his wife, Carol.

ARLENE EISENBERG was the author of several best-selling books, including *What to Expect When You're Expecting, What to Eat When You're Expecting, What to Expect the First Year,* and *What to Expect the Toddler Years.* Updated every six weeks, the "expect" books are in their seventy-fifth printing. Together they have sold nearly 17 million copies and have been translated into twenty-one different languages. Arlene Eisenberg died in 2001.

VICTORIA ENG lives and works in New York City. She earned an MFA in creative nonfiction from Columbia University.

DEIRDRE ENGLISH is the coauthor (with Barbara Ehrenreich) of the classic feminist work *Witches, Midwives and Nurses: A History of Women Healers.* She is a former editor in chief of *Mother Jones* and has been a public affairs commentator for San Francisco Public Radio.

SAMUEL S. EPSTEIN, M.D. is professor emeritus of Environmental and Occupational Medicine at the University of Illinois School of Public Health, and Chairman of the Cancer Prevention Coalition. He has published some 260 peer reviewed articles, and authored or co-authored 11 books including: the prize-winning *The Politics of Cancer* (1978); *The Safe Shopper's Bible* (1995); and *GOT (Genetically Engineered) MILK! The Monsanto rBGH/BST Milk Wars Handbook* (2001).

BARBARA FINDLEN was an editor-at-large for *Ms.*, and is the editor of the anthology *Listen Up: Voices From the Next Feminist Generation*, and coauthor, with Kristen Golden, of *Remarkable Women of the Twentieth Century: 100 Portraits of Achievement*.

PHYLLIS L. FINE is a psychotherapist in private practice and the co-founder of Midwest Support, an organization formed specifically to work with victims of professional abuse. She is also a founder of Families Against Sexually Abusive Therapists and Other Professionals (FAST).

SHULAMITH FIRESTONE was a founder of the Women's Liberation Movement in the late sixties and author of the classic *The Dialectic of Sex: The Case for Feminist Revolution*. More recently she has been writing fiction, notably *Airless Spaces*.

AUDREY FLACK is one of the world's leading photorealist painters. Her work is in museums around the globe. In recent decades she has turned to sculpture, where, in particular, she has been "searching for the Goddess." Flack has been called the feminist conscience of the College Art Association.

ANNE ROCHON FORD has worked in Canada as a writer and activist on women's health issues for the past twenty-four years. She co-founded several national, provincial, and local women's health groups, including the Canadian Women's Health Network and DES Action Toronto. A particular focus of her work has remained the issue of women and pharmaceuticals.

JANE P. FOWLER was diagnosed with HIV at the age of fifty-five. Recognizing a need for awareness and support for older women affected by HIV, Jane formed HIV Wisdom for Older Women in 2002. She has spoken hundreds of times since 1995 and has been a guest on *Oprah* and a contributor to *Our Bodies, Ourselves: Menopause*.

ELLEN FRANKFORT was the health columnist for the *Village Voice* and the author of several books. She was one of the key journalists who popularized the women's health movement. In the early 1970s, she served as a trustee at the Women's Medical Center on Irving Place in New York City, the first freestanding legal abortion clinic in the Western world. She died in 1987.

LUCINDA FRANKS is a winner of the Pulitzer Prize for National Reporting (1972) and many other awards. She has written for the *New York Times*, the *New Yorker*, and *Talk* magazine. Franks is the author of *My Father's Secret War, Waiting Out a War*, and *Wild Apples*.

SARA GERMAIN has a Bachelor of Arts degree in English and women's studies from the State University of New York College at Geneseo. She is one of many young women who have been mentored and influenced by Barbara Seaman, and she looks forward to many more years of study in women's health. An avid reader and writer, Germain hopes to make an influence, as her mentor did, with her pen.

JENNIFER GONNERMAN has been a staff writer for the *Village Voice* since 1997. She covers the criminal justice beat and has reported on prisons, drugs, gangs, domestic violence, and the courts. Her stories have also appeared in *Vibe, Ms., Glamour, The Source*, the *New York Observer*, and the *Nation*. She earned a 2004 National Book Award nomination for *Life on the Outside*.

LOIS GOULD has written eight novels, two works of nonfiction, two satires posing as children's fables, and a collection of personal essays. A frequent contributor of articles and reviews to the *New York Times*, she created the personal column "HERS." Her memoir about her mother, the fashion designer Jo Copeland, titled *Mommy Dressing: A Love Story*, was published in 1998. Gould died in 2002.

MADELINE GRAY published one of the first patient-to-patient menopause manuals, *The Changing Years*, in 1951. Gray was a writer and editor who lived and worked in New York for decades.

TARA GREENWAY is a mind/body practitioner with a private practice in Brooklyn Heights, New York City. Tara was trained in Theta Healing by Eric Brumett and by Vianna Stibal, the founder of the Theta technique. She is a member of MBS Connect, an organization which brings wellness speakers and practitioners into Fortune 500 companies. With collaborator/director Ariane Brandt, Tara has written and performed *Missionary Position*, a play about one woman's fight for sexual and spiritual freedom, which premiered off-Broadway at the Grove Street Playhouse in New York City after its original workshop production at the HERE Arts Center.

GERMAINE GREER is a journalist and scholar of early modern English literature, widely regarded as one of the most significant feminist voices of the later twentieth century. Greer's ideas have created controversy ever since her groundbreaking book *The Female Eunuch* became an international best seller in 1970, turning her overnight into a household name and bringing her both adulation and criticism. She is also the author of *Sex and Destiny: The Politics of Human Fertility*, *The Change: Women, Ageing and the Menopause*, and most recently *Shakespeare's Wife*.

RUTH GRUBER is an American journalist, photographer, writer, humanitarian, and a former United States government official. At age twenty, she received a PhD in one year, becoming the youngest person in the world to receive a doctorate. In 1935, the *New York Herald Tribune* asked her to write a feature series about women under Fascism and Communism. In 1944, she was assigned a secret mission to Europe to bring one thousand Jewish refugees and wounded American soldiers from Italy to the US. Gruber has received many awards for her writing and humanitarian acts, and she has published two autobiographies, *Ahead of Time: My Early Years as a Foreign Correspondent* and *Inside of Time: My Journey From Alaska to Israel*.

CATHERINE GUND is a film/videomaker, writer, teacher, and activist. Her media work—which focuses on the radical right, art and culture, HIV/AIDS, and gay and lesbian issues—has screened around the world in festivals, on public and cable television, at community-based organizations, universities, and museums. She was the founding director of BENT TV, the video workshop at the Hetrick-Martin Institute for gay, lesbian, bisexual, and transgender youth.

DORIS HAIRE is best known for *The Cultural Warping of Childbirth*, a well-referenced analysis of worldwide obstetric practices published by the International Childbirth Education Association in 1972, while she was the president. Haire, a consumer activist and pioneer in the area of informed consent, has also authored *The Pregnant Patient's Bill of Rights*, *How the FDA Determined the "Safety" of Drugs: Just How Safe is Safe*, and *Drugs in Labor and Birth*. She has observed obstetric care in seventy-two countries and continues to lecture worldwide.

MICHELLE HARRISON, is a physician, writer, teacher, and leader in women's health. She consults and lectures internationally about women's health and other related health policy issues. Harrison is the author of *A Woman in Residence*, *The Pre-teen's First Book About Love, Sex, and AIDS*, *Self-Help for Premenstrual Syndrome*, and *A Safe Place to Live, A Story for Children Who Have Experienced Domestic Violence*.

FLORENCE HASELTINE is currently the director of the Center for Population Research. Dr. Haseltine has served as the director of the Center for Population Research since 1985. She is an obstetrician and gynecologist (OB-GYN) trained in reproductive endocrinology and genetics. Dr. Haseltine received a medical degree from the Albert Einstein College of Medicine. She did a residency at Boston Hospital for Women, and was on the faculty at the Yale University School of Medicine before assuming her current position.

MOLLY HASKELL is a film critic and has written for the *New York Times*, the *New York Times Book Review*, the *Nation*, and *Film Comment*, among other publications. She lectures on film at numerous universities and is a member of the New York Film Critics Circle and the National Society of Film Critics.

JUDITH HERMAN, is associate clinical professor of psychiatry at the Harvard Medical School and director of training at the Victims of Violence Program at Cambridge Hospital. She is the author of several books including *Trauma of Recovery* and *Father-Daughter Incest*.

SHERE HITE's groundbreaking Hite Reports have had a profound and lasting influence on generations of readers—countless millions all over the world. The four Hite Reports have been translated into fifteen langugages and published in thirty-five countries, receiving numerous academic and professional awards and honors. The initial Hite Report was named as one of the one hundred key books of the twentieth century by the *Times* in 1998. In 2006, Hite published *The Shere Hite Reader*, a collection of some of her most notable writings.

MARY HOWELL, also known as MARGARET CAMPBELL, was a co-founder of the National Women's Health Network and a contributor to the Boston Women's Health Book Collective. She had a law degree as well as a medical degree, and a PhD in child development, besides being the author of many books. In 1973 she was the first woman ever hired as a dean at Harvard Medical School.

RUTH HUBBARD is a professor of biology at Harvard University. Ruth Hubbard is best known for her challenges to colleagues who promote sociobiology and her criticisms of those who justify discrimination against women on the basis of genetics. She is the author of several books, including *Exploding the Gene Myth*.

JANE WEGSCHEIDER HYMAN is a researcher and writer on women's health and contributed to both *Ourselves, Growing Older* and *The New Our Bodies, Ourselves*. She is author of several books, including *I Am More Than One*. During her graduate studies in psychology, she specialized in mental health problems that primarily afflicted women.

ERICA JONG is the author of eight novels, including the international best seller *Fear of Flying*. In print in twenty-seven languages, this modern classic has sold eight million copies in the US alone. Jong's latest book is *Seducing the Demon: Writing for My Life*. Jong lives in New York City and Weston, Connecticut.

SUSAN JORDAN is a former partner of Dresner, Sykes, Jordan, and Townsend, a nationally known political and commercial research consulting firm. A lifelong feminist, she worked on a successful seven-year campaign to legalize the cervical cap in the US. She cur-

rently defends all types of criminal cases in State and Federal Court. Jordan was recently honored by being sworn in as the first tribal judge for the Hopland Band of Pomo Indians. She is listed in *The Best Lawyers in America*.

SUZANNE WHITE JUNOD is a medical historian with a PhD from Emory University, and she is employed by the US Food and Drug Administration. She has a special interest in women's health issues and is currently working on a published history in the field.

PAULA KAMEN is the author of what is widely noted as the first and still the only journalistic book on young women and feminism, *Feminist Fatale: Voices from the "Twentysomething" Generation Explore the Future of the "Women's Movement."* Her writing has appeared in about a dozen anthologies, the *New York Times, Washington Post, Chicago Tribune, Salon*, and many other publications. Her new book, *All in My Head*, addresses the idea of framing chronic pain as a "woman's issue."

STEPHEN R. KANDALL retired in 1998 as chief of neonatology at Beth Israel Medical Center in New York and professor of pediatrics at the Albert Einstein College of Medicine. During his professional career he lectured widely nationally and internationally and published more than ninety articles and book chapters. His book, *Substance and Shadow*, grew from his advocacy efforts on behalf of women prosecuted for drug use during pregnancy.

ANNE S. KASPER is a founding member of the US women's health movement, and has been an advocate, sociologist, researcher, and public policy expert on women's health for more than twenty years. Anne was health editor for *New Directions for Women* for five years and on the editorial board of *Women and Health* and the author of its health and public policy column for five years. She has also written for a number of other women's publications. Her new book, *Breast Cancer: Society Shapes an Epidemic*, examines the transition of breast cancer from a medical to a societal issue.

TANIA KETENJIAN is a journalist, documentarian, and sound artist. She has contributed nationally to PRI's *Studio 360*, APM's *Weekend America*, NPR's *Day to Day* and PRI's and BBC's *The World*. She has contributed internationally to the BBC and the BBC World Service in England, CBC in Canada, ABC in Australia, and RTE in Ireland. Tania hosts and produces a half-hour weekly program on the arts called *Sight Unseen* which airs in the San Francisco Bay Area and London. She has spoken with artists and thinkers as wide ranging as John Waters, Charlie Kaufman, and His Holiness the Dalai Lama. She has produced several long format audio documentaries including *The Pursuit of Happiness, Birth*, and *Born*. She has written for *Paper Magazine, Dazed and Confused, The Times* (UK) and *Icon Magazine*. Tania is a member of an artist's collective, Quorum, where she contributes sound pieces for exhibitions, and she shares a studio space with artists collectively called Compound 21. Tania lives in San Francisco with her husband, Philip Wood, with whom she co-founded *The [Un]Observed: A Radio Magazine*.

FRANCINE KLAGSBRUN is the author of more than a dozen books and often writes and lectures on feminist issues. Her most recent book, *The Fourth Commandment: Remember the Sabbath Day*, was a National Jewish Book Award Finalist. Her column, "Thinking Aloud," appears monthly in the *Jewish Week*.

ROSE KUSHNER was a pioneer in the field of breast cancer activism. She first gained national recognition in 1975, when she wrote about her battle with breast cancer in the book *Why Me? What Every Woman Should Know About Breast Cancer to Save Her Life*. She was the founder and director of the Breast Cancer Advisory Center in Kensington, a member of the National Breast Cancer Advisory Board from 1980 to 1986, and was appointed to the American Cancer Society's Breast Cancer Task Force. At the time of her death in 1990, Kushner was lobbying to encourage the Federal Government to require that health insurance companies cover mammograms.

VIVIEN LABATON was the founding director of the Third Wave Foundation. She is curently a fellow at Atlantic Philanthropies. A graduate of Barnard College, Labaton earned her JD at NYU Law School. She is the coeditor, with Dawn Lundy Martin (a Third Wave co-founder), of *The Fire This Time*, a collection of essays by young activists on the future of feminism.

SONIA LANDER is a midwife and nurse living in New York City. She graduated from Barnard College and earned an MS in nursing from Yale.

BERNARD LEFKOWITZ is the author of *Our Guys: The Glen Ridge Rape and the Secret Life of the Perfect Suburb*. He has written three previous books on social issues. He died in 2004.

BARRON H. LERNER is a medical historian and internist at the College of Physicians and Surgeons of Columbia University. Dr. Lerner, who is the Angelica Berrie Gold Foundation assistant professor of medicine and public health, is the author of *Contagion and Confinement: Controlling Tuberculosis Along the Skid Road* and *The Breast Cancer Wars: Hope, Fear, and the Pursuit of a Cure in Twentieth Century America*.

NICOLE LEVITZ is a recent graduate of Boston University, where she co-founded the Coalition for Consensual Sex, a student group which brought sexual assault survivor services to the Boston University campus. She is currently the program associate for the Lawyers Alliance for New York and has worked at the Center for Reproductive Rights and the Boston Area Rape Crisis Center.

CHARLOTTE LIBOV is an award-winning author and professional speaker specializing in women's health issues. She is the author of *Beat Your Risk Factors: A Woman's Guide to Reducing Her Risk for Cancer, Heart Disease, Stroke, Diabetes and Osteoporosis* and *The Woman's Heart Book*, and lives in Bethlehem, Connecticut.

BETTY JEAN LIFTON is an author and psychologist, and has an adoption counseling practice in New York City. Her adoption books include: *Twice Born: Memoirs of An Adopted Daughter; Lost and Found: The Adoption Experience; Journey of the Adopted Self: A Quest For Wholeness;* and the picture book *Tell Me A Real Adoption Story*.

MEIKA LOE is an assistant professor of sociology and anthropology and women's studies at Colgate University. She is the author of *The Rise of Viagra: How the Little Blue Pill Changed Sex in America*.

BARBARA LOVE is an editor, writer, and journalist. She is the author of *Foremost Women in Communications* and the co-author of *Sappho Was a Right-On*

Woman (with Sidney Abbott). She is on the board of the Veteran Feminists of America and co-authored the book *Feminists Who Changed America, 1963–1975* (with Nancy F. Cott).

DR. SUSAN LOVE is an author, teacher, surgeon, lecturer, researcher, and activist. *Dr. Susan Love's Breast Book* has been termed the bible for women with breast cancer; released in 1997, *Dr. Susan Love's Hormone Book* (updated and re-published in 2003 as *Dr. Susan Love's Menopause and Hormone Book)* provides an equally authoritative range of information about menopause.

MICHAEL LOWENTHAL is the author of the novels *Charity Girl, Avoidance* and *The Same Embrace*. His short stories have appeared in *Tin House*, the *Southern Review*, the *Kenyon Review*, and *Esquire.com*. He has also written nonfiction for the *New York Times Magazine, Boston Magazine*, the *Washington Post*, the *Boston Globe, Out*, and many other publications. Lowenthal teaches creative writing in the low-residency MFA program at Lesley University.

HELEN LOWERY attended the American University Washington College of Law in Washington, DC. She is interested in women's advocacy and has worked on issues of women's health, sexual assault, and reproductive justice. In her free time, Lowery is a baking enthusiast and likes to dance. She received her JD in May 2009.

KRISTEN LUKER is professor of sociology and a professor in the Jurisprudence and Social Policy Program (Boalt Hall School of Law) at the University of California, Berkeley. She is the author of many scholarly articles, as well as three books: *Taking Chances: Abortion and the Decision Not to Contracept, Abortion and the Politics of Motherhood*, and *Dubious Conceptions: The Politics of Teenage Pregnancy*. She is currently at work on her fourth book, tentatively entitled *Bodies and Politics*.

HARRIET LYONS was an original editor of *Ms.* She was a recipient of the Women in Communications' Clarion Award for "The Decade of Women: A *Ms.* History of the '70s in Words & Pictures." As a *McCall's* and *Redbook* senior editor from 1993 to 1997, she edited cover profiles, articles concerning social issues, and

human interest stories. She is currently Special Sections editor at the *Daily News*.

CAROLYN MACKLER is a young adult novelist living and working in New York City. Her books include: *The Earth, My Butt, and Other Big Round Things, Vegan Virgin Valentine, Love and Other Four Letter Words*, and *Guyaholic*. Mackler was a contributing editor at *Ms.*, and her articles and essays have also appeared in publications including the *Los Angeles Times, HUES*, and *New Moon*.

ARTEMIS MARCH has been evolving her own brand of narrative nonfiction for twenty years without realizing it was preparing her to write *Dying Into Grace*, a book about caregiving relationships and her mother's death. A sociologist by training, she first got into the storytelling business at the Harvard Business School where she designed dozens of teaching case studies, many of them bestsellers, for students and executives. Her consulting practice focuses on patient-centered care at every stage of life.

MARJORIE MARGOLIES served one term as a Democratic member of the US House of Representatives from Pennsylvania. She graduated from the University of Pennsylvania in 1963 and was in broadcast journalism for over twenty-four years, winning five Emmy Awards for her work. She currently serves as the founder and chair of Women's Campaign International (WCI), a group that provides advocacy training for women throughout the world. She is also a professor at the Fels Institute of Government at the University of Pennsylvania.

HELEN I. MARIESKIND has been active in women's health issues since the early 1970s. She is author of the landmark *Evaluation of Caesarean Section in the United States, Women in the Health System: Patients, Providers and Programs*, and the founder and editor for six years of *Women & Health*. She lives in Washington, DC and works as a writer and editor for the Office of Juvenile Justice and Delinquency Prevention, Office of Justice Programs, US Department of Justice.

NORMA FOX MAZER is the author of over thirty novels for children and young adults, plus two collections of short stories. She has edited an anthology of women's poetry and contributed articles, essays, and short stories to numerous journals and anthologies. Among her awards are a Newbery Honor, the California Young Readers Medal, a Christopher Medal, and an Edgar.

NORMA MCCORVEY has worked as a crisis counselor in a Dallas women's clinic. She is a frequent speaker on abortion rights and women's issues. She lives in Dallas, Texas.

JEAN BAKER MILLER is a clinical professor of psychiatry at Boston University School of Medicine and director of the Jean Baker Miller Training Institute at the Stone Center, Wellesley College. She has written *Toward a New Psychology of Women*; coauthored *The Healing Connection: How Women Form Relationships in Therapy and in Life; Women's Growth in Connection;* and edited *Psychoanalysis and Women.*

MARCIA MILLMAN is a professor of sociology at the University of California, Santa Cruz and a social psychologist. She is the author of several books including *Such a Pretty Face: On Being Fat in America, Kind Hearts and Cold Cash, The Unkindest Cut: Life in the Backrooms of Medicine,* and *The Perfect Sister: What Draws Us Together, What Drives Us Apart.* She lives in the San Francisco Bay area.

PATSY MINK was a third generation Japanese-American graduate of University of Chicago Law School (1951). Her lawsuit, *Mink vs. EPA et al.,* established the core principles of the Freedom of Information Act. An environmentalist, advocate of consumer rights, individual rights, and civil rights, Mink made her mark first as an opponent of the Vietnam War. She died in 2002.

THE NATIONAL WOMEN'S HEALTH NETWORK is an independent, member-supported organization dedicated to safeguarding women's health rights and interests by providing accurate, unbiased health information to women and advocating for national health policies that address women's health needs. The director of the Network is Cynthia Pearson, and the founders are Barbara Seaman, Belita Cowan, Phylis Chesler, Mary Howell, and Alice Wolfson.

MARYANN NAPOLI is a co-founder and the associate director of the Center for Medical Consumers in New York City. She writes *Health Facts,* the Center's monthly newsletter.

HEDDA NUSSBAUM was abruptly thrown into the public spotlight in November 1987 after her longtime partner, Joel Steinberg, assaulted and killed their daughter, Lisa. She went on to become an advocate for other battered women. A former senior editor at Random House and the author of children's books, Ms. Nussbaum has written a memoir about her experiences, *Surviving Intimate Terrorism,* which was published in the fall of 2005.

SALLY WENDKOS OLDS has written extensively about relationships, health, and personal growth, and has won national awards for both her book and magazine writing. Her college textbooks on child and adult development, *A Child's World* and *Human Development,* coauthored with psychologist Diane E. Papalia, PhD, have been read by more than two million students and are the leading texts in their fields.

SUSIE ORBACH has written extensively about women's psychology and the construction of femininity, gender, the making of the body, psychoanalysis and social policy, eating difficulties, obesity to anorexia, women and brands, globalism and body image, and emotional literacy in business, education, and government. She has been consultant to The World Bank and is currently consultant to the National Health Service (NHS) and to Dove®. She is the author of several books, including *Fat is a Feminist Issue.*

LESYLE E. ORLOFF founded Ayuda's unique domestic violence program, dedicated to serving the interrelated legal and social service needs of battered latina and immigrant women and children. Ms. Orloff was a co-founder of the National Network on Behalf of Battered Immigrant Women and is the Washington, DC spokesperson for that organization. In 1999, Ms. Orloff joined NOW Legal Defense and Education Fund's Washington, DC office as the director of the Immigrant Women Program and senior staff attorney.

AMY PAGNOZZI writes for *New York, Vanity Fair, Glamour,* and *Penthouse.*

CINDY PEARSON is executive director of the National Women's Health Network. She has worked at NWHN since 1987 and has coordinated the internship program, managed the information clearinghouse, and directed NWHN's program and policy work. Cindy became NWHN's executive director in May 1996.

She is currently the president of the board of directors of Women's Health Specialists in Northern California and is the treasurer of the National Breast Cancer Coalition.

JOANNA PERLMAN is a marketing and public relations specialist at the law firm Skadden, Arps, Slate, Meagher and Flom. She is a former press secretary for the New York City Department of Finance. She is a graduate of Barnard College and has also worked for NOW and the television station New York One.

REBECCA PLANTE is an assistant professor of sociology at Ithaca College. She is the author of *Sexualities, Identities, Behaviors and Societies* and *Sexualities in Context: A Social Perspective*. She has also worked as an evaluator of various state level HIV/AIDS education programs.

LETTY COTTIN POGREBIN is a writer and lecturer. Among her books are *Growing Up Free, Stories for Free Children*, and *Getting Over Getting Older: An Intimate Journey*. She was a founding editor of *Ms.*, and a former president of the Author's Guild. Most recently she has written her first novel, titled *Three Daughters*.

LAUREN PORSCH is the founder of the New York Abortion Access Fund, a nonprofit organization that provides financial assistance to low-income women who cannot afford the cost of an abortion, as well as being actively involved in health promotion and access to care campaigns for Lesbian, Gay, Bisexual, and Transgender communities.

AMY RICHARDS is a writer, researcher, organizer, and fundraising consultant. A co-founder and executive committee member of the Third Wave Foundation, Richards was profiled by *Ms.* in 1997 in "21 for the 21st: Leaders for the Next Century." She is the coauthor of *Manifesta: Young Women, Feminism and the Future* and *Grassroots: A Field Guide for Feminist Activism*. Richards's most recent book is *Opting In: Having a Child Without Losing Yourself*.

HELEN RODRIGUEZ-TRIAS was a founding member of both the Committee to End Sterilization Abuse and the Committee for Abortion Rights and Against Sterilization Abuse. In the 1980s she served as medical director of the New York State Department of Health AIDS Institute, where she worked on behalf of women with HIV. In the 1990s, she focused on reproductive health as co-director of the Pacific Institute for Women's Health, a nonprofit research and advocacy group dedicated to improving women's well being worldwide.

ESTHER R. ROME was a founding member of the Boston Women's Health Book Collective and coauthor of its best-selling book *Our Bodies, Ourselves*. For most of the 1980s she served as a consumer representative to a task force of the American Society for Testing Materials, which after many years of meetings, and due largely to Esther's persistence, finally enacted a uniform standard for tampon labeling. When confronted with breast cancer, Esther persistently and energetically researched treatment options and shared what she had learned with all who were interested.

JUDITH ROSSNER is the author of such best-selling novels as *Looking for Mr. Goodbar, August*, and *Emmeline*, on which the opera by Tobias Picker is based. She died in August 2005.

BETTY ROTHBART is a health columnist for *Hadassah* magazine and the author of a number of books on health and parenting. She is the author of four curricula on HIV/AIDS and abuse prevention for the New York City Board of Education, where she conducts teacher trainings on health and sexuality education. She coauthored her most recent book, *Healthy Teens, Body and Soul: A Parent's Complete Guide*, with Andrea Marks.

BARBARA KATZ ROTHMAN is a professor of sociology at the City University of New York. She has served as president of Sociologists for the Study of Social Problems and Sociologists for Women in Society. Her books include *Weaving a Family: Untangling Race and Adoption, The Book of Life, Recreating Motherhood, The Tentative Pregnancy*, and *In Labor*. She lives in Brooklyn, New York.

SHERYL BURT RUZEK is professor of health studies at Temple University. She is currently working on a second edition of her 1978 book, *The Women's Health Movement, Feminist Alternatives to Medicine Control* and is a consultant to numerous public health organizations. Her recent publications include *Women's Health: Complexities and Differences* (with Virginia

Olesen and Adele Clarke) and articles on the future of health reform.

GILLIAN SANSON is a women's health educator, researcher, and author. Her book *Mid-Life Energy and Happiness* was published in 1999, followed by *The Osteoporosis 'Epidemic': Well Women and the Marketing of Fear*. Her work has received international recognition and endorsement and was the subject of a *20/20* documentary in New Zealand in 2001. Gill lives in Auckland, New Zealand.

MEI HWEI ASTELLA SAW graduated from Northwestern University and worked as an associate editor at Seven Stories Press. A daughter of two fine doctors, she doesn't think members of the medical profession are gods.

HAGAR SCHER is a journalist and writer living in New York City. Her articles about politics, feminism, sex, women's health, fitness, sports, and first-person experiences have appeared in *Ms., Glamour, New Woman, Fitness, Ladies' Home Journal*, and *Latina* magazines. A woman of the world, Hagar was raised in Israel and Canada, and has resided in Italy and England.

LYNNE SHARON SCHWARTZ has written many books since the start of her career in the 1970s, including *Rough Strife* (nominated for a National Book Award), a collection of stories called *Referred Pain*, the novel *The Writing on the Wall*, and *The Emergence of Memory: Conversations with W.B. Sebald*, a book of interviews with the late German author. Lynne Sharon Schwartz's reviews and criticism have appeared in many leading magazines and papers. She has received grants from the Guggenheim Foundation, the National Endowment for the Arts, and the New York State Foundation for the Arts, and has taught in many writing programs here and abroad.

JULIA SCOTT is president of the National Black Woman's Health Project, and has a long history as a leader and activist in preventive health and in the struggle for the advancement of people of color. She has held a variety of other posts, including director of training for the Boston Family Planning Project, and reproductive rights field coordinator and executive director of the Foundation of Women. She has received the Gloria Steinem Women of Vision award.

SYBIL SHAINWALD'S legal career has focused almost exclusively on women's health issues. She was co-counsel in the nation's first DES daughter victory, *Bichler v. Lilly*, and she litigated thousands of cases involving drugs and devices harmful to women and their children. She co-founded Health Action International and is deeply involved with the National Women's Health Network. Shainwald was one of the first and most vocal opponents of the use of Norplant, especially its widespread use in developing nations. Her writings, lectures, and appearances before congressional subcommittees have raised the national consciousness on crucial women's health issues.

CASSANDRA SHAYLOR is an attorney and activist based in Oakland, California. She is the co-founder and co-director of Justice Now, a prison organization and training center focused on people in women's prisons in the United States. Shaylor speaks regularly to academic and activist audiences on issues of women in prison, prison abolition, and the intersections of race and sexuality in the prison-industrial complex.

SARAH J. SHEY received her MFA in nonfiction writing from Columbia University in October 1999. She has been published in such publications as the *Christian Science Monitor*, the *Philadelphia Inquirer*, and *This Old House Magazine*. She is the author of the children's books *Blue Lake Days* and *Sky All Around*.

ALIX KATES SHULMAN's twelve books include two books on the anarchist Emma Goldman, three books for children, four novels, and three memoirs (the award winning *Drinking the Rain* and *A Good Enough Daughter*). Hailed by the *New York Times* as "the voice that has for three decades provided a lyrical narrative of the changing position of women in American society," her works have been translated into eleven languages. Her most recent memoir, *To Love What Is*, was published in September 2008.

KATIE SINGER is certified to teach Fertility Awareness by the Ovulation Method Teachers' Association. She teaches at Women's Health Services in Santa Fe, New Mexico. Her first novel, *The Wholeness of a Broken Heart*, has recently been published by Riverhead Books. Her other writings include *The Garden of Fertility, Honoring Our Cycles: A Natural Family Planning Workbook*, and articles about Fertility Awareness.

Katie is currently working on a new novel and essays about fertility and ecology.

MARGOT SLADE is deputy editor, special sections, of the *New York Times* and the mother of twins, Emma and Jacob.

ELIZABETH CADY STANTON, the boldest and most brilliant of the nineteenth-century American feminists, was born in 1815 in upstate New York. For more than fifty years, there seemed to be no impediment to women's full equality that Elizabeth did not notice and attempt to route: besides suffrage, she campaigned for birth control, property rights for wives, custody rights for mothers, equal wages, cooperative nurseries, coeducation, and "deliverance from the tyranny of self-styled medical, religious, and legal authorities." Through it all Elizabeth was a doting, hands-on mother of five sons and two daughters.

EDITH STEIN was a German philosopher, a Carmelite nun, martyr, and saint of the Catholic Church who died at Auschwitz. In 1922, she converted to Christianity, was baptized into the Roman Catholic Church, and was received into the Discalced Carmelite Order in 1934. She was canonized as Saint Teresa Benedicta of the Cross (her Carmelite monastic name) by Pope John Paul II in 1998.

GLORIA STEINEM is one of the most influential writers, editors, and activists of our time. She travels worldwide as a lecturer and feminist organizer, and is a frequent media spokeswoman on issues of equality. In the words of her biographer, Carolyn Heilbrun, "She is most honored and most cherished by people throughout the country who remember her speaking, her helping to start their rape crisis center, her timely support for their various burgeoning organizations." Gloria co-founded *Ms.* in 1971 and was one of its editors for fifteen years. She continues to write and lecture on various political and feminist issues.

KOFI TAHA is a writer, activist, entrepreneur, and renowned philanthropist. His poems, essays, and articles have been published in various forms, ranging from academic journals to newspapers to hip-hop tabloids. He is the author of a book of poetry entitled *Postdiluvian America: Drought of Humility.*

LEORA TANENBAUM is the author of *Slut! Growing Up Female with a Bad Reputation.* Her writing has appeared in *Newsday, Seventeen, Ms.,* and other newspapers and magazines. She lives in New York City. Her most recent books are *Catfight: Rivalries Among Women—from Diets to Dating, from the Boardroom to the Delivery Room* and *Bad Shoes & the Women Who Love Them.*

NOY THRUPKAEW is a senior correspondent for the *American Prospect.* Previously she was the news editor of *Sojourner: The Women's Forum,* a national feminist newspaper based in Boston. She has lived in Japan and Thailand, and frequently writes on international women's human rights, welfare policy, and Southeast and East Asian literature and film.

LEONORE TIEFER is an author, educator, researcher, therapist, and activist who has specialized in many areas of sexuality. Dr. Tiefer has written widely about the medicalization of men's and women's sexuality. She has been interviewed by news media around the world and appeared on many news shows as the foremost critic of "disease-mongering" trends in the medical management of women's sexual problems. The website of her educational anti-medicalization campaign, newviewcampaign.org, is a major resource on this topic for journalists, colleagues, and the public. Dr. Tiefer has written over 150 scientific and professional publications.

ANDREA TONE is a professor of history at McGill University. She is the author of several books and edited volumes, including *Devices and Desires: A History of Contraceptives in America,* which was named one of the best books of the year by the *Washington Post* and, most recently, *Medicating Modern America: Prescription Drugs in History,* with Elizabeth Siegel Watkins. Her work has been featured on ABC News, PBS, National Public Radio, the Canadian Broadcasting Corporation (CBC), the History Channel, and in the *New York Times.*

SOJOURNER TRUTH was born into slavery in New York State. She won her freedom in 1827, when that state emancipated its slaves. Sojourner Truth consistently and actively identified herself with the cause of women's rights. She was the only black woman present at the First National Woman's Rights Convention in Worcester, Massachusetts, in 1850.

SARI TUDIVER is the resource coordinator at the Women's Health Clinic, a community health center in Winnipeg, Manitoba and an editor of *A Friend Indeed*, an international newsletter for women on menopause and midlife. An anthropologist by training, she has been involved in research, writing, education, and advocacy on many aspects of women's health, including reproductive technologies and the international pharmaceutical industry. She is a founding member of the Canadian Women's Health Network.

LILA A. WALLIS is clinical professor of medicine at Cornell University Medical College and an attending physician at the New York Hospital in New York City. Dr. Wallis is an internationally recognized expert on estrogen replacement therapy, menopause, and osteoporosis. She is also celebrated for her contributions to women's health and medical education through her organizational activities, lectures, and publications. Dr. Wallis is senior author of *The Whole Woman— Take Charge of Your Health in Every Phase of Your Life*, published in May 1999.

ELIZABETH SIEGEL WATKINS has a PhD in the history of science from Harvard University, from which her book *On the Pill* is derived. She is a historian with the Historical Society of Western Pennsylvania in Pittsburgh, and writes, teaches, and consults in Pennsylvania. Her most recent books are *The Estrogen Elixir: A History of Hormone Replacement Therapy in America* and *Medicating Modern America: Prescription Drugs in History* with Andrea Tone. Both were published in 2007.

ERICA WARREN is a freelance writer living in Brooklyn, New York.

KATHRYN WATTERSON, who teaches writing at the University of Pennsylvania, has written several prize-winning nonfiction books, including, most recently, *Not by the Sword*, which won the 1996 Christopher Award. Her first book, *Women in Prison*, is considered a classic on the subject and was the basis for the ABC documentary *Women In Prison*.

MARILYN WEBB is one of the early founders of the Second Wave of the women's movement. An organizer, speaker, and writer, she also began *Off Our Backs*, one of the first feminist newspapers, the nation's first college-based women's studies program, and

Sagaris, a feminist think-tank. Most recently she has become a leader of a new movement to improve the care of the dying. She is the author of the influential book, *The Good Death: The New American Search to Reshape the End of Life*.

ELAINE WEISS has conducted dozens of domestic violence training sessions around the country. Her writings about domestic abuse have appeared in local and national publications and are used as teaching resources in a number of battered women's shelters. Dr. Weiss is an adjunct professor at the University of Utah School of Medicine, in the Department of Family and Preventive Medicine. There, she teaches medical students and faculty how to recognize and support patients who are victims of domestic violence.

Author and neuroscientist NAOMI WEISSTEIN, known for her powerful oratory, is a Professor of Psychology at SUNY, Buffalo. A Guggenheim Fellow and a Fellow of the American Association for the Advancement of Science and the American Psychological Society, she has written over sixty articles on science, feminism, culture, and politics, including her famous "Kinder, Kirche, Kuche," credited for starting the discipline of the psychology of women.

EDITH WHITE, the author of *Breastfeeding and HIV/AIDS: The Research, the Politics, the Women's Responses*, spent more than twenty-five years teaching breast-feeding management to health professionals, and was one of the founders of the International Board of Lactation Consultants. She is now executive director of the South Shore AIDS Project, Inc. in Plymouth, Massachusetts.

FRANCES CERRA WHITTELSEY is an award-winning journalist, magazine editor, and author who teaches journalism part-time at Hofstra University.

NAOMI WOLF was born in San Francisco in 1962. Her essays have appeared in various publications including: *The New Republic, Wall Street Journal, Glamour, Ms., Esquire*, the *Washington Post*, and the *New York Times*. Her books include *The Beauty Myth, Fire With Fire: The New Female Power And How It Will Change The 21st Century, Promiscuities: The Secret Struggle for Womanhood*, and *Misconceptions*, a book on the politics of motherhood in America. Wolf's most recent book is *The End Of America: A Letter of Warning to a Young Patriot.*

ALICE WOLFSON is an attorney specializing in defending the rights of insurance policy holders for the firm Bourhis, Wolfson, and Schlichtmann in San Francisco, California. She is one of the founders of the National Women's Health Network.

SUSAN WOOD is a research professor in the Department of Environmental and Occupational Health at George Washington University. A long-time champion of women's health, Dr. Wood previously served as Director for Policy and Program Development at the US Department of Health and Human Services in the Office on Women's Health. Professor Wood has been honored with the FDA Commissioner's Special Citation (2004), the DHHS Secretary's Distinguished Service Award (2003), and the Keystone Award in Women's Health Research (2000), among other awards.

IRENE XANTHOUDAKIS works with the New York Abortion Access Fund and the Haven Coalition as well as other agencies committed to ending homelessness and providing services to formerly incarcerated individuals. Irene graduated with a Masters of Public Administration from the School of International and Public Affairs at Columbia University in February 2007.

LAURA YEAGER has published fiction in such magazines as *Paris Review, Missouri Review, North American Review, Ohio Short Fiction,* and *Kaleidoscope.* She has taught at Kent State University, Walsh University, Malone College, and Rhode Island School of Design. Laura holds a BA from Oberlin College, an MA in English from Iowa State University, and an MFA in English from the University of Iowa.

ABOUT THE EDITORS

BARBARA SEAMAN was a founding member of the women's health movement. In 1969, her landmark book on hormonal contraceptives, *The Doctors' Case Against the Pill*, sparked Congressional hearings into the safety of birth control pills and catapulted women's health issues into the national spotlight. Her work led to the creation of the world's first patient packet insert (now included in most pharmaceutical products) as well as other innovations for patient safety. In 1975 she co-founded the National Women's Health Network, an advocacy and watchdog group in Washington DC that worked to eliminate quotas for women in medical schools and give women the right to information about medical treatments and alternatives. The organization remains one of the few women's advocacy groups that refuses all money from drug and device makers. In her book, *The Greatest Experiment Ever Performed on Women*, she demonstrated the failure of the FDA and the medical establishment to demand rigorous testing of hormone therapy before mass prescribing took place and castigated the pharmaceutical industry for putting profits above women's lives. Since 2003 she has written passionately on the dangers of fertility drugs and unnecessary gynecological procedures. She is the author of seven books on women's health. She died in February 2008 at the age of seventy-two.

LAURA ELDRIDGE is Barbara Seaman's long-time collaborator and associate. She has been researching and writing about women's health topics for nearly ten years. She contributed to Seaman's *The Greatest Experiment Ever Performed on Women: Exploding the Estrogen Myth* and coauthored *The No-Nonsense Guide to Menopause*. She is the author of the book *In Our Control: The Complete Guide to Contraceptive Choices for Women*. Eldridge has degrees from Barnard College and New York University and lives and writes in Brooklyn, New York.

Index

medication withheld, 201

early clamping or milking of umbilical cord, 210

elective induction of labor, 203–4

episiotomy as routine in, 207, 209–10

father-child contact prevented, 213–14

first breastfeeding delayed, 212

food and drink withheld from normal unmedicated woman, 205

forceps routinely used in, 209

fundal pressure to facilitate, 208

hospitals required for all normal women during, 203

infant deaths with, 195–97, 200

mother separated from familial support during, 204–5

mothers moved to delivery room for, 206–7

mothers required to assume lithotomy position, 207–8, 210

mothers separated from newborn infant, 211–12

mothers uninformed about coping with, 202–3

nighttime feedings withheld from newborns, 213

normal laboring women confined to bed, 205

nursing personnel assigned to mothers or babies, 213

obstetrical intervention in placental expulsion, 211

pelvic relaxation and, 209

restricting newborns to 4-hour feeding schedule, 213

room requirements with restrictions, 214

sexual response, 209–10

shaving birth area, 205

sibling visitations restricted, 214

suctioning with nasogastric tube as routine, 211

water and formula offered to breast-fed newborn, 212–13

child-rearing, sharing of, 67–68

children. *See also* babies; motherhood

adoption and, 231, 233–34, 308–19

autism in, 286–88, 292–98

deaths among breast-fed and artificially fed, 202

molestation of, 89–90

mother blaming and, 290–92, 293

nonmothers on, 278–81

writing about mothers, 245–48

China, 177

Cisler, Lucinda, 366

Civil Rights Act, 117

class. *See* middle class; ruling class; upper class; working class

clear cell cancer, 118, 121–22, 126, 412. *See also* diethylstilbestrol; diethylstilbestrol litigation

clinical trials

DES with and without, 118–22, 127n18

drug, 62

estrogen, 129–30

in Puerto Rico, 129–30, 164, 169–70

Clinton, Bill, 53, 94, 307, 321, 341

Clinton, Hillary, 308, 420

Clomid, 268–69, 270–72

Cody, Pat, 126

Coffee, Linda, 366–70

Cohen, Mike, 302

Cohen, Rona, 301

Cohn, Victor, 49

Collier, Peter, 39

Collins, Dan, 107–8

Collins, John, 271

Collip, Bertram, 40

colonies, U.S., midwives in, 26

Comnena, Anna, 25

Comstock Laws, 27, 131

concert of action theory, 127n22

condoms, 174

Congressional Caucus for Women's Issues, 52

Connell, Elizabeth, 149, 150

consciousness raising (CR) discussions, 49

contraceptives, 27. *See also* birth control pill, for men; sterilization; *specific types of*

contraceptives

birth control and corporatization of, 130–34

birth control pills, 48, 49–50, 61, 80–83, 129–30

Catholic Church's view on, 78

commerce with doctors, 132

DES as morning-after, 50, 85, 119

health insurance with, 75

morning-after, 50, 84–86, 119

Norplant, 130, 169–74

sterilization as, 280

Cooke, Lawrence H., 122

Corfman, Eunice (wife), 160

Corfman, Minnie (grandmother), 160

Corfman, Philip, 50, 169, 323

interview, 159–63

Correll, Martha, 346

cosmetics industry, poisons in, 41–42

costs

fertility treatments, 269

gynecological surgery and annual, 351–52

of motherhood, 305

OTC drug advertisements, 303

patenting genes, 255–56

Premarin, 339–40

cough syrup, 39–40

Cowan, Belita, 50

interview, 84–87

as NWHN founder, 83, 84

Cox, Claire, 332

Cox, Nial Ruth, 140

Craft, Ian, 268

Crawford, Lester, 337

CR discussions. *See* consciousness raising discussions

crimes

female sexuality as, 9–10

healing and helping as, 11

medical and obstetrical skill as, 10

organizing, 10–11

of witches, 9–11

Cronkite, Walter, 146

Crout, Richard, 180, 334

Croxatto, Horacio, 170

culture, menopause influenced by, 347

Curry, Edward, 327

VOICES OF THE WOMEN'S HEALTH MOVEMENT

Voices of the Women's Health Movement

VOLUME TWO

Contents